DISABILITY STUDIES

PAIN MANAGEMENT YEARBOOK 2009

DISABILITY STUDIES

Joav Merrick - Series Editor
National Institute of Child Health and Human Development,
Ministry of Social Affairs, Jerusalem

Contemporary Issues in Intellectual Disabilities
V.P. Prasher (Editor)
2010. ISBN: 978-1-61668-023-7

Disability from a Humanistic Perspective: Towards a Better Quality of Life
Shunit Reiter (Editor)
2011. ISBN: 978-1-60456-412-9

Pain Management Yearbook 2009
Joav Merrick (Editor)
2011. ISBN: 978-1-61209-666-7

Pain Management Yearbook 2010
Joav Merrick (Editor)
2011. ISBN: 978-1-61209-972-9

Pain. Brain Stimulation in the Treatment of Pain
Helena Knotkova and Ricardo Cruciani Joav Merrick (Editors)
2011. ISBN: 978-1-60876-690-1

Cancer in Children and Adults with Intellectual Disabilities: Current Research Aspects
Daniel Satgé and Joav Merrick (Editors)
2011. ISBN: 978-1-61761-856-7

Neural Plasticity in Chronic Pain
Helena Knotkova, Ricardo A. Cruciani and Joav Merrick (Editors)
2011. ISBN: 978-1-61324-657-3

Rett Syndrome: Therapeutic Interventions
Meir Lotan and Joav Merrick (Editors)
2011. ISBN: 978-1-61728-080-1 (Softcover)
2011. ISBN: 978-1-61728-614-8 (Hardcover)

DISABILITY STUDIES

PAIN MANAGEMENT YEARBOOK 2009

JOAV MERRICK
EDITOR

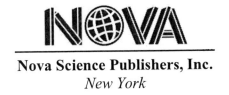

Nova Science Publishers, Inc.
New York

Copyright ©2012 by Nova Science Publishers, Inc.

All rights reserved. No part of this book may be reproduced, stored in a retrieval system or transmitted in any form or by any means: electronic, electrostatic, magnetic, tape, mechanical photocopying, recording or otherwise without the written permission of the Publisher.

For permission to use material from this book please contact us:
Telephone 631-231-7269; Fax 631-231-8175
Web Site: http://www.novapublishers.com

NOTICE TO THE READER

The Publisher has taken reasonable care in the preparation of this book, but makes no expressed or implied warranty of any kind and assumes no responsibility for any errors or omissions. No liability is assumed for incidental or consequential damages in connection with or arising out of information contained in this book. The Publisher shall not be liable for any special, consequential, or exemplary damages resulting, in whole or in part, from the readers' use of, or reliance upon, this material. Any parts of this book based on government reports are so indicated and copyright is claimed for those parts to the extent applicable to compilations of such works.

Independent verification should be sought for any data, advice or recommendations contained in this book. In addition, no responsibility is assumed by the publisher for any injury and/or damage to persons or property arising from any methods, products, instructions, ideas or otherwise contained in this publication.

This publication is designed to provide accurate and authoritative information with regard to the subject matter covered herein. It is sold with the clear understanding that the Publisher is not engaged in rendering legal or any other professional services. If legal or any other expert assistance is required, the services of a competent person should be sought. FROM A DECLARATION OF PARTICIPANTS JOINTLY ADOPTED BY A COMMITTEE OF THE AMERICAN BAR ASSOCIATION AND A COMMITTEE OF PUBLISHERS.

Additional color graphics may be available in the e-book version of this book.

Library of Congress Cataloging-in-Publication Data

ISSN: 2163-7504

ISBN 978-1-61209-666-7

Published by Nova Science Publishers, Inc. † New York

TABLE OF CONTENTS

Introduction   xi
    Joav Merrick, MD, MMedSci, DMSc

Section One - Intellectual Disability   1

Chapter 1   Pain Sensation of Individuals with Rett Syndrome: A Literature Review   3
    Meir Lotan, BPT, MScPT and Alon Kalron, BPT, MScPT

Chapter 2   Assessing Pain in Children with Intellectual Disability   13
    Lynn M Breau, PhD, RPsych

Chapter 3   Pain in Individuals with Intellectual and Developmental Disabilities   27
    Frank J Symons, PhD, Tim F Oberlander, MD
    and Lois J Kehl, DDS, PhD

Chapter 4   The Triptych of Pain in Art   37
    Gisèle Pickering, MD, PhD, DPharm

Chapter 5   Pilot Study of the Feasibility of the Non-Communicating Children's Pain Checklist Revised for Pain Assessment for Adults with Intellectual Disabilities   45
    Chantel Burkitt, Lynn M Breau, PhD., R Psych, Shoneth Salsman,
    BSc(Pharm), PhC, Tracie Sarsfield-Turner, BA, BSW, CGN, RSW
    and Robert Mullan, MD

Chapter 6   Facial Expression of Pain in Children with Intellectual Disabilities Following Surgery   61
    Lynn M Breau, PhD, R. Psych, G Allen Finley, MD, FRCPC,
    Carol S Camfield, MD, FRCPC and Patrick J McGrath, OC, PhD, FRSC

Chapter 7   Prerequisite Abilities for the Use of Hypnosis for Pain Management in Children with Cognitive Impairment   77
    Marc Zabalia, PhD and Fanny Esquerré, R Psychol

Section Two - Various Aspects of Pain   85

Chapter 8 Mechanical and holistic paradigms in sexology: Viagra® represents a mechanical worldview and may cause female sexual pain   87
Søren Ventegodt, MD, MMedSci, EU-MSc-CAM and Joav Merrick, MD, MMedSci, DMSc

Chapter 9 A Q-methodological study to explore the low back pain beliefs and attitudes of low back pain health professionals   101
Carol Campbell, BSc (Hons), MA, PhD

Chapter 10 Impact of relaxation training on the variability of psychophysics and psychometrics tests   129
Gisèle Pickering, MD, PhD, DPharm, Agathe Gelot, PhD, Sylvia Boulliau, Agathe Njomgang and Claude Dubray, MD

Chapter 11 A National Survey of the United Kingdom NHS Pain Management Services   133
Neil Collighan, MBChB, FRCA FFPMRCA and Sanjeeva Gupta, MD, DNB, FRCA, FIPP, FFPMRCA

Chapter 12 Opioid dependence among older pre-spine surgery patients. A prospective study   141
M Sami Walid, MD, PhD

Chapter 13 Combination of evidence-based medications for neuropathic pain: Proposal of a simple three-step therapeutic ladder   147
Katsuyuki Moriwaki, MD, PhD, Kazuhisa Shiroyama, MD, PhD, Mikako Sanuki, MD, Minoru Tajima, MD, Tomoaki Miki, MD, Akihiko Sakai, MD and Ken Hashimoto, MD, PhD

Chapter 14 Psychosocial predictors of health status in fibromyalgia: A comparative study with rheumatoid arthritis   155
Paula Oliveira, PhD and Maria Emília Costa, PhD

Chapter 15 Pain management in a neonatal intensive care unit   167
Edna Aparecida Bussotti, RN and Eliseth Ribeiro Leão, RN, PhD

Chapter 16 Sex differences in anxiety sensitivity among children with chronic pain and non-clinical children   173
Jennie CI Tsao, PhD, Subhadra Evans, PhD, Marcia Meldrum, PhD and Lonnie K Zeltzer, MD

Chapter 17 Nursing quality: Pain management in the emergency room   187
Rafaela Aparecida Marques Caliman, RN, Maria Fernanda Zorzi Gatti, RN, MSc and Eliseth Ribeiro Leão, RN, PhD

Chapter 18	A cognitive-behavioural group intervention for chronic pain patients: First findings *Maaike J de Boer, MSc, Gerbrig J Versteegen, PhD and Theo K Bouman, PhD*	**193**
Chapter 19	Chronic pain in injured workers *Policarpo Rebolledo, MD, Alonso Mújica, MD, Luis Guzmán, MD, Verónica Herrera, MD and Ricardo Acuña, LLB*	**207**
Chapter 20	Invasive pain management procedures: High expectations lead to perceived poor outcomes *Carol Campbell, BSc (Hons), MAEd, PhD*	**215**
Chapter 21	Children's drawings of pain faces: A comparison of two cultures *Jacqueline A Ellis RN, PhD, Eufemia Jacob, RN, PhD and Bryan Maycock, MA*	**225**
Chapter 22	Catastrophizing ways of coping and pain beliefs in relation to pain intensity and pain-related disability *Christina Knussen, PhD and Joanna L McParland, PhD*	**237**
Section Three - Brain Stimulation and Pain		**253**
Chapter 23	Brain changes related to chronic pain: Implications for stimulation treatment *Herta Flor, PhD*	**255**
Chapter 24	Introduction to electrotherapy technology *Marom Bikson, PhD, Abhishek Datta, MS, Maged Elwassif, MS, Varun Bansal and Angel V Peterchev, PhD*	**265**
Chapter 25	Principles and mechanisms of transcranial magnetic stimulation *Monica A Perez, PT, PhD and Leonardo G Cohen, MD*	**275**
Chapter 26	Principle and mechanisms of transcranial Direct Current Stimulation (tDCS) *Andrea Antal, PhD, Walter Paulus, MD and Michael A Nitsche, MD*	**287**
Chapter 27	Non-invasive brain stimulation approaches to fibromyalgia pain *Baron Short, MD, Jeffrey J Borckardt, PhD, Mark George, MD, Will Beam, BS and Scott T Reeves, MD*	**299**
Chapter 28	Non-invasive brain stimulation therapy for the management of complex regional pain syndrome (CRPS) *Ricardo A Cruciani, MD, PhD, Santiago Esteban, MD, Una Sibirceva, MD and Helena Knotkova, PhD*	**321**
Chapter 29	Safety of transcranial direct current stimulation (tDCS) in protocols involving human subjects *Arun Sundaram, Veronika Stock, MD, Ricardo A Cruciani, MD, PhD and Helena Knotkova, PhD*	**331**

Chapter 30	The potential role of brain stimulation in the management of postoperative pain *Jeffrey J Borckardt, PhD, Scott Reeves, MD and Mark S George, MD*	343
Chapter 31	Deep brain stimulation for chronic pain *Morten L Kringelbach, DPhil, Erlick AC Pereira, MBChB, Alexander L Green, FRCS (SN), Sarah LF Owen, Dphil and Tipu Z Aziz, D Med Sci*	349
Chapter 32	Invasive treatment of chronic neuropathic pain syndromes: Epidural stimulation of the motor cortex *Dirk Rasche, MD and Volker M Tronnier, MD, PhD*	367
Chapter 33	Electrical stimulation of primary motor cortex for intractable neuropathic deafferentation pain *Youichi Saitoh, MD, PhD*	383
Chapter 34	Brain stimulation for the treatment of pain: A review of costs, clinical effects, and mechanisms of treatment for three different central neuromodulatory approaches *Soroush Zaghi, BS, Nikolas Heine, BS and Felipe Fregni, MD, PhD*	397
Chapter 35	Efficacy of anodal transcranial direct current stimulation (tDCS) for the treatment of fibromyalgia: Results of a randomized, sham-controlled longitudinal clinical trial *Angela Valle, Suely Roizenblatt, Sueli Botte, Soroush Zaghi, BS, Marcelo Riberto, Sergio Tufik, Paulo S Boggio and Felipe Fregni, MD, PhD*	413
Chapter 36	Cathodal tDCS over the somatosensory cortex relieved chronic neuropathic pain in a patient with Complex Regional Pain Syndrome (CRPS/RSD) *Helena Knotkova, PhD, Peter Homel, PhD and Ricardo A Cruciani, MD, PhD*	425
Section Four - Cancer and Pain		**431**
Chapter 37	Bisphosphonates in combination with radiotherapy for the treatment of bone metastases: A literature review *Shaelyn Culleton, BSc(C), Amanda Hird, BSc(C), Janet Nguyen, BSc(C), Urban Emmenegger, MD, Sunil Verma, MD, Christine Simmons, MD, Elizabeth Barnes, MD, May Tsao, MD, Arjun Sahgal, MD, Cyril Danjoux, MD, Gunita Mitera, MRTT, MBA, Emily Sinclair, MRTT and Edward Chow, MBBS*	433

Chapter 38	Are baseline ESAS symptoms related to pain response in patients treated with palliative radiotherapy for bone metastases? *Shaelyn Culleton, BSc (C), Jocelyn Pang, BSc (C), Liying Zhang, PhD, Roseanna Presutti, BSc (C), Janet Nguyen, BSc (C), Gunita Mitera, MRT(T), Emily Sinclair, MRT(T), Elizabeth Barnes, MD, May Tsao, MD, Cyril Danjoux, MD, Arjun Sahgal, MD and Edward Chow, MBBS*	449
Chapter 39	Improvement of ESAS symptoms following palliative radiation for bone metastases *Shaelyn Culleton, BSc(C), Liying Zhang, PhD, Emily Sinclair, MRT(T), Elizabeth Barnes, MD, May Tsao, MD, Cyril Danjoux, MD, Sarah Campos, BSc(C), Philiz Goh, BSc and Edward Chow, MBBS*	457
Chapter 40	Impact of pain flare on patients treated with palliative radiotherapy for symptomatic bone metastases *Amanda Hird, BSc(C), Rebecca Wong, MD, Candi Flynn, BSc, Stephanie Hadi, BSc(C), Eric de Sa, BSc, Liying Zhang, PhD, Carlo DeAngelis, PharmD and Edward Chow, MBBS*	467
Chapter 41	Validation of meaningful change in pain scores in the treatment of bone metastases *Edward Chow, MBBS, Amanda Hird, BSc(C), Rebecca Wong, MD, Liying Zhang, PhD, Jackson Wu, MD, Lisa Barbera, MD, May Tsao, MD, Elizabeth Barnes, MD and Cyril Danjoux, MD*	475
Chapter 42	Exploring the optimal definitions of partial response and pain progression in patients receiving radiation treatment for painful bone metastases? A preliminary analysis *Roseanna Presutti, BSc(C), Liying Zhang, PhD, Amanda Hird, BSc(C), Melissa Deyell, BMSc and Edward Chow, MBBS*	483
Chapter 43	A multidisciplinary bone metastases clinic at Sunnybrook Odette cancer centre: A review of the experience from 2006-2008 *Janet Nguyen, BSc(C), Emily Sinclair, MRT (T), Albert Yee, MD, Joel Finkelstein, MD, Michael Ford, MD, Anita Chakraborty, MD, Macey Farhadian, RN, Robyn Pugash, MD, Gunita Mitera, MRT (T), Cyril Danjoux, MD, Elizabeth Barnes, MD, May Tsao, MD, Arjun Sahgal, MD and Edward Chow, MBBS*	511
Chapter 44	The test-retest reliability of the European Organization for Research and Treatment of Cancer Quality-of-Life Group Bone Metastases Module (EORTC QLQ-BM22) questionnaire *Candi J Flynn, MSc(C), Mark Clemons, MD, Liying Zhang, PhD and Edward Chow, MBBS*	523
Chapter 45	Determining reliability of patient perceptions of important bone metastases quality of life issues *Sarah Campos, BSc(C), Liying Zhang, PhD and Edward Chow, MBBS*	533

Chapter 46	Shortening the bone metastases quality of life instrument tool *Lying Zhang, PhD, Janet Nguyen, BSc (C), Amanda Hird, BSc (C) and Edward Chow, MBBS*	547
Chapter 47	Surgical stabilization of severely destructive upper cervical lytic bone metastases *Janet Nguyen, BSc(C), Matthew Chung, BSc(C), Michael Ford, MD, Philiz Goh, BSc, Joel Rubenstein, MD, Emily Sinclair, MRT(T), Gunita Mitera, MRT(T) and Edward Chow, MBBS, PhD, FRCPC*	559
Chapter 48	When all else fails: Simple bracing for the relief of intractable pain *Roseanna Presutti, BSc(C), Sarah Campos, BSc(C), Joel Finkelstein, MD, Joel Rubenstein, MD, Emily Sinclair, MRTT, Gunita Mitera, MRTT and Edward Chow, MBBS*	565
Chapter 49	Cemented hemiarthroplasty, percutaneous acetabular cementoplasty and post operative radiation for a high risk lesion of the hip *Jocelyn Pang, BSc(C), Richard Jenkinson, MD, Gunita Mitera, MRTT, Andrea Donovan, MD, Robyn Pugash, MD, Maureen Trudeau, MD, Cindy Quinton, MD, Emily Sinclair, MRTT, Janet Nguyen, BSc(C), Roseanna Presutti, BSc(C) and Edward Chow, MBBS*	573
Chapter 50	Remineralization of an impending fracture from an osteolytic metastasis in a breast cancer patient from palliative radiotherapy and bisphosphonate. A case report *Gunita Mitera, BSc, MRT(T), Joel Rubenstein, MD, Joel Finkelstein, MD, Melanie TM Davidson, PhD and Edward Chow, MBBS*	579
Chapter 51	Need for post procedure radiation therapy after kyphoplasty or vertebroplasty/cementoplasty for bony metastatic disease *Edward Chow, MBBS, May Tsao, MD, Arjun Sahgal, MD, Elizabeth Barnes, MD, Cyril Danjoux, MD, Gunita Mitera, MRT(T) and Emily Sinclair, MRT(T)*	587

Section Five – Acknowledgments	589
About the editor	591
About the National Institute of Child Health and Human development in Israel	593
Section Six - Index	593

INTRODUCTION

Joav Merrick, MD, MMedSci, DMSc[1,2,3,4,5*]

[1]National Institute of Child Health and Human Development
[2]Office of the Medical Director, Division for Mental Retardation,
Ministry of Social Affairs, Jerusalem
[3]Zusman Child Development Center, Soroka University Medical Center, Beer-Sheva, Israel
[4]Interuniversity College for Health and Development, Castle of Seggau, Graz, Austria
[5]Kentucky Children's Hospital, University of Kentucky, Lexington, United States

In the year 2008 we started the new journal "Pain management" under the auspicies of the National Institute of Child Health and Human Development in Israel in collaboration with Nova Science in New York in order to facilitate an outlet for peer-reviewed papers in the areas of pain and pain management from a holistic, practical and clinical point of view.

Pain is an alert mechanism designed to alert us when our body malfunctions, but in some populations the deciphering of the signals arising from that mechanism by an external observer might represent some difficulties. Such difficulties particularly exist in populations with communicative limitations, such as individuals with intellectual disability (ID).

Individuals with ID often present medical conditions that necessitate a variety of painful medical procedures, yet, their inability to validly report their pain experience, often leaves them improperly treated. This lack of appropriate management has been reported in cases were individuals with ID received less post-surgery analgesics as compared to people without ID, in delayed diagnosis and management of painful medical conditions, in painful situations treated as behavioral problems (1) and in setbacks in hospitalization and even death (2).

Despite the severity of the issue, pain behaviors in adults with ID have seldom been investigated due to several reasons, mainly to the difficulty of evaluating pain in this population. One shortcoming in creating an interest in researching this group lays in the fact that individuals with ID are a weak minority group, which does not suggest any high pedestals for its researchers. Therefore it leaves only the passion of the researcher to adhere to this group of participants.

---

[*] **Correspondence:** Professor Joav Merrick, MD, MMedSci, DMSc, Medical Director, Division for Mental Retardation, Ministry of Social Affairs, POBox 1260, IL-91012 Jerusalem, Israel. E-mail: jmerrick@zahav.net.il.

The fact that some professionals working with individuals with ID, express a possibility that this group of clients feels pain to a lesser degree than the general population, might have impeded proper pain management for this population. Yet recent articles have revealed that such premises holds no real ground and therefore such thoughts should be eliminated to prevent pain mismanagements from reoccurring.

Another setback preventing proper pain evaluation and management for this population is due to their unconventional pain behaviors, the lack of clear verbal communication, and the masking of pain behaviors by ambiguous sounds and behaviors. Such difficulties might necessitate the development and the use of complex multi-dimensional pain assessment tools, thereby complicating the task of the researcher as well as the health care professional caring for this population.

When examining the majority of articles evaluating pain in different populations, we found that self-report has been accepted by many researchers as the "gold standard" of pain evaluation, and we also found reservations as to the acceptance of behavioral measures as a valid report of pain. Yet, it is believed that when it comes to individuals with limitations in verbal communication, pain behaviors should be considered as a non verbal path of self report. Therefore, they should be accepted as the "gold standard" of individuals with ID.

It seems that there are a number of factors that prevents individuals with ID from receiving a "best practice" pain management as the rest of us do, and therefore it is our responsibility to become advocates for this group of clients, and to see that through proper care and proper research this situation is overturned.

In the first section of the yearbook 2009 we attempted to cover the issue of pain in individuals with ID by introducing the topic as well as suggesting a model for pain in this population. A couple of articles suggest different approaches to the complex subject of evaluation in this group of clients, and also in depth approaches to specific syndromes. It is the hope that researchers will be interested to further their efforts in understanding, researching and caring for individuals with ID, with a sincere interest to enhance the quality of life of these individuals.

In this yearbook for 2009 you will find research published from the **Journal of Pain Management** by leading researchers from all over the world and it is our hope that these researchers and practitioners will continue to produce sound and evidence based research that can help mankind to suffer less and enjoy life and a good quality of life.

References

[1] Gunsett RP, Mulick JA, Feranald WB, Martin JL. Brief report: Indication for medical screening prior to behavioral programing for severely and profounding mentally retarded clients. J Autism Dev Disord 1989;19(1):167-72.

[2] Jancar J, Speller CJ. Fatal intertinal obstruction in the mentally handicapped. J Intellect Disabil Res 1994;38:413-22.

SECTION ONE - INTELLECTUAL DISABILITY

In: Pain Management Yearbook 2009
Editor: Joav Merrick

ISBN: 978-1-61209-666-7
©2012 Nova Science Publishers, Inc.

Chapter 1

PAIN SENSATION OF INDIVIDUALS WITH RETT SYNDROME: A LITERATURE REVIEW

Meir Lotan, BPT, MScPT[*,1,2,3,4] *and Alon Kalron, BPT, MScPT*[3]

[1]Israeli Rett Center, National Evaluation Team, Chaim Sheba Medical Center, Tel HaShomer, Ramat Gan
[2]Zvi Quittman Residential Centers, Israel Elwyn, Jerusalem
[3]Department of Physical Therapy, Ariel University Center of Samaria, Ariel
[4]National Institute of Child Health and Human Development, Office of the Medical Director, Division for Mental Retardation, Ministry of Social Affairs, Jerusalem, Israel

Abstract

Rett syndrome (RS) is a developmental disorder caused by a faulty gene on the X chromosome. Since RS is characterized by an arrest of brain development individuals with RS are challenged daily by a multitude of difficulties, among them immature sensory processing. Despite the fact that this issue has been mentioned repeatedly, no actual research has investigated the sensory system of individuals with RS. Reduced pain sensation has been mentioned in the past in regard to this population, but it has remained an observed phenomenon. Due to the importance of our pain system as an alert mechanism it was the intention of this article to explore the literature in an attempt to collect data that will shed light on the phenomenon of pain sensation by individuals with RS. Each section initially presents the up-to-date knowledge regarding normative function of the pain system in the human body and than presents the corresponding findings in regards to pain system of individuals with RS. The collected evidence suggests that many sub-systems within the pain sensation/processing route are functioning abnormally for individuals with RS. It seems that the overall abnormalities of the pain system of individuals with RS suggest towards a reduce pain sensation in this population, but this assumption needs further scientific investigation before it could be considered as evidence based.

---

[*]**Correspondence:** Rehov Rothschild 67, IL-44201 Kfar-Saba, Israel. E-mail: ml_pt_rs@netvision.net.il

Keywords: Rett syndrome, intellectual disability, disability, pain, sensory processing.

Introduction

Although pain is a vital alert mechanism designed to inform us of bodily dysfunctions and damage, its presence may cause anxiety and mental distress exerting a negative influence on performance, sleep and mood and all aspects of our daily lives (1). When evaluated for their painful experiences individuals with intellectual and developmental disability (IDD) were found at risk for suffering pain. The findings showed that as many as 73%–83% of children with IDD were found to suffer constantly from episodes of pain (2,3).

People with IDD experience pain due to their underlying medical conditions and the fact that they usually have surgery, physical therapy and other diagnostic and therapeutic procedures that cause pain (4). Complicating proper treatment is the inability of individuals with IDD to accurately communicate the presence and intensity of pain, thus leaving pain untreated (4,5).

Previous studies have reported under-treatment of painful events in this population as they received less post-surgery analgesics compared to controls without IDD (6). This increased their suffering and harmed their quality of life. At worst, underestimating pain has delayed diagnosis and management of painful medical conditions causing setbacks in hospitalization and even death (7). Over the years scientifically unsupported remarks have been made relating to abnormal pain sensation of individuals with IDD (8,9), some suggesting elevated pain threshold as the cause (10). Yet, an in-depth evaluations of pain responses of this population indicated that pain threshold was actually reduced in this population compared with controls without IDD (11), and that atypical pain expression was probably due to delayed brain pain processing (12). An example of the obscurity of the pain experience of individuals with IDD could be presented, when examining the pain processing in a subgroup of this population; individuals with Rett syndrome (RS).

RS is a neurological disorder expressed mainly in females (13), it is characterized by loss of fine and gross motor skills and communicative abilities, deceleration of head growth, and the development of stereotypic hand movements, occurring after a period of normal development. It is considered to be the second most common cause (after Down syndrome) of multi-disabling genetic disorder in females (14). The development of the disorder is characterized by normal birth and apparently normal psychomotor development during the first 6-18 months of life (15). The child then enters a short period of developmental stagnation followed by rapid regression in language and motor skills. The trademark of the disease is the repetitive stereotypical hand movements appearing, when the child enters stage II of RS. Additional characteristics at the breakthrough of the disorder includes autistic like behavior, panic-like attacks, bruxism, breathing irregularities, episodic of apnea and/or hyperpnea, gait ataxia and tremors, apraxia, and acquired microcephaly (15). After this period of rapid deterioration, despite the relatively stable manner of the disease, the person with RS is likely to develop dystopia and if not ambulant, might also develop foot and hand deformities (16) as they grow up. Seizures occur in up to 85% (15) of individuals with RS. Females with Rett syndrome typically survive into adulthood and their estimated life expectancy is about 50 49 years (17).

The Sensory System of Individual with RS

The sensory system of RS population was investigated in the past, and assumptions regarding the state of the sensory system in RS have also been hypothesized from individual behaviors. Some observations have been made by Lindberg (18) from her personal experience as a special education teacher working with this population, as well as reports from parents. Through her observations Lindberg suggested that individuals with RS present difficulties in all areas of the sensory system: receiving, deciphering and processing of information through cerebral centers.

Lindberg reported (18) that persons with RS reject superficial touch in facial areas (especially around the mouth) implying hypersensitivity of the tactile system of individuals with RS in this area. From our own clinical experience (ML) some individuals with RS show a dislike to being held by their forearms, probably due to similar tactile over-sensitivity in this area.

Some reports linked with sensorial abnormalities of the taste and olfactory systems (19). The findings by Ronnett and her associates (20), suggested that compared with age-matched controls, there were far fewer mature olfactory receptor neurons and significantly greater numbers of immature neuron-specific tubulin-positive present in the nasal epithelium of persons with RS. Moreover, abnormal sensors structure was found in biopsies(19).

The visual sensory system is considered to work within the norm (19,21). In fact, eye sight of extremely physically disabled individuals with RS was found to function within the norm even in late adulthood (15), except for some cases showing short or near sightedness (19). Moreover it was found that visual evoked potentials were normal in all patients with RS (22).

The evidence from the auditory system is controversial, since some authors (23) reported pathological findings suggesting multilevel impairment of the auditory nervous system, while others reported that the auditory sensory system appears to be working within the norm (23).

Nevertheless the fact that individuals with RS are extremely keen on music and use their eyes to communicate and convey different communicational acts enhance the notion that the auditory and the visual elements of the sensory system should be considered as the points of strength of individuals with RS.

The primary dysfunction of the sensory system may be attributed to findings by Guerrini et al (24), regarding incoming sensory information of individuals with RS. They reported slow neural conduction through ascending dorsal routes, as well as the dorsal lamniscal and thalmo-cortical tracts. This reduction in conduction, 3-4 times slower than the norm, causes a delay in transfer of sensory information to the pre-central cortical areas correlated with the sensitized body organ.

General Reports and Assumptions Regarding Pain Reaction of Individuals with RS

To the best of our knowledge, there has not been studies conducted or published evaluating pain experience of individuals with RS, but comparing existing knowledge on pain conduction, pain processing and pain sensation in populations without RS will gives us some comparison into the pain experience of individuals with RS.

The aberrant observed pain reaction of individuals with RS include cases in which a child with RS has fallen backwards experiencing a severe blow to the head with no apparent reaction, or existing reports regarding bone fractures that were only discovered days after the traumatic incident due to reduced pain reaction of the child (19). The scarce, yet existing literature related to pain behaviors of individuals with RS give some possible explanations regarding pain experience of this population. Coleman et al (25) mentioned that 88% of individuals with RS were suspected by parents of having a reduced pain sensation, but Hagberg (15) suspected that the observed reduced pain reaction of individuals with RS should be attributed not to lack of sensitivity to pain, but rather to a very late reaction to a painful stimulus caused by disorganization of the reception and processing parts of the related neural systems.

Kerr and Witt-Engerstrom (21) also believed that pain processing was the cause for the observed late pain reaction reported by parents rather than the inability of individuals with RS to feel pain. This assumption is also supported by Hunter (19), who suggests that the pain sensation of individuals with RS is unaffected, but rather claims the abnormal freezing and withdrawal behavior common to individuals with RS, gives the observer the feeling of hyposensitivity to pain. It should be mentioned however that a similar freezing/withdrawal behavior have been found common in individuals with IDD, when exposed to a painful stimulus (26). The extreme reaction of individuals with RS to internal/visceral pain and in contrast a slight, sometimes undetected reaction to external pain stimulus (such as injections) is another phenomenon that has been reported (18,19).

The Evaluation of Pain Sensation in Individuals with RS

In verbally non-communicative populations such as: neonates, demented elderly and children with IDD (27), the evaluation of pain experience is usually performed through observation of behaviors. In individuals with RS aberrant emotional and behavioral conduct has been observed, as for example Mount et al (28), who reported that 29%-71% showed an indifferent facial appearance apparently masking pain expression. Many other behaviors presented by this population might interfere with the external deciphering of pain reaction in RS. Such behaviors were: facial grimaces (up to 76%), expressions of anxiety, fear and general distress such as self mutilation (49%) and screaming (33%). Due to these aberrational behaviors, pain evaluation of individual with RS by an external assessor could not be considered extremely reliable and a search for other, more evidence based, sources of information regarding the pain experience of this population should be conducted.

Scientific Findings Reports Regarding Different Aspects of the Pain Systems in Rett Syndrome

A. The Peripheral System

Nerve Growth Factor (NGF) plays an important factor in modulating the sensitivity of the sensory nervous system to noxious stimuli. The evidence that NGF levels increase during inflammation makes a strong case for NGF being a critical mediator of inflammatory pain. NGF clearly has a powerful neuroprotective effect on small-diameter sensory neurons, and NGF levels have been shown to change in a number of models of nerve injury (29).

Lack of NGF in the early development of a child might cause potential pain sensors type A to transform into mechano-receptors instead of becoming pain receptors (30). Since reduced levels of NGF have been found in individuals with RS, due to impaired critical developmental signals required for early NGF production, the clinical significance of these findings might be that the individuals with RS do not hold the full capacity of peripheral pain sensors (31) in comparison with the general population.

Substance-P is a significant chemical involved in the transfer of pain sensation. It is regarded as a pain modulator chemical usually involved in the enhancement of pain sensation in the spinal area (32). In RS a significant decrease of the level of this protein throughout the peripheral and central nervous system, especially at the posterior ganglions, was found in some studies (33,34). In all investigated sites the protein levels did not exceed values corresponding to those of with a two month old infant. Due to the importance of substance-P in the enhancement of pain input, these reduced levels might suggest a diminishing effect on the transference of external pain stimuli into the central nervous system.

Another factor influencing sensory input is nerve conduction. It has been found that adolescents (ages: 9-19) with RS present secondary damage to peripheral nerve system (35). This secondary damage is expressed by elongation of peripheral nerve conduction, due to reduction in the number of posterior ganglions of the spine (36). Such a reduction is estimated to suppress different sensory input in to the central nervous system, including pain related signals.

Different studies regarding nerve conduction in this population have reported contradicting findings. At a young age (6-9 years) giant conduction potentials have been associated with hyperactivity of the cerebrum (37). On the other hand at older ages (above 9 years of age) Verma et al (38) reported a slight reduction in neural conductivity, while Kalmanchey (22) found a significant slowing of nerve conduction by individuals with RS. These findings further support the accumulating reports suggesting a reduced pain sensation by individuals with RS mostly individuals at age older than 9 years of age.

B. The Spinal Level

The dorsal horn of the spinal cord is the major receiving zone for primary axons that transmit information from sensory receptors in the skin, viscera, joints and muscles of the trunk and limbs to the central nervous system. Nociceptive primary axons terminate almost exclusively in the dorsal horn, and it is therefore the site of the first synapse in ascending pathways that convey to the brain sensory information that underlies triggers conscious perception of pain. The synaptic contacts made between afferent terminals and dorsal horn neurons are highly organized, both topographically (to reflect their location) and by sensory fiber type. This important synapse, avergingaveraging incoming information with excitatory and inhibitory transmission, provides accurate transfer regarding the onset, duration, location and quality of peripheral nociceptive pain (39). The dorsal ganglions have been found to be reduced in number in individuals with RS as compared to controls without RS (36). These findings suggest that the flow of incoming nociceptive information from the periphery to the central nervous system might be reduced in individuals with RS.

The importance of NGF in the development and maintenance of sensorial neurons in the posterior ganglion have been documented (30). On the other hand, investigations into the levels of NGF in the cerebrospinal fluid of children with RS (40) have repeatedly demonstrated reduced level of this substance. These finding may support the reduction or ill development of sensorial neurons in the dorsal horns of the spinal ganglions, reducing incoming sensory information in ascending nociception tracts.

Biochemical studies of the cerebro-spinal fluid (CSF) of 34 participants with RS aged 2.5-15 years showed high levels of beta-endorphins (41), and this finding was corroborated by others (24,42). Since the endogenous opioid system is one of the most studied innate pain-relieving systems producing analgesia (43), these findings suggests an increase in central opiate activity in girls with Rett syndrome (24). On top of that, Bader et al (44,45) reported that the ascending neural pathways through the upper spinal cord were delayed, suggesting a general impairment of central conduction time.

C. The Cerebrum

There are a number of pathways that transmit nociceptive information from the spinal cord to the forebrain. Consequently, multiple regions of the forebrain are activated due to the complexity of the pain experience. Cortical regions activated by during a painful incoming massages include: limbic, paralimbic and sensory areas, notably anterior cingulated cortex, insular cortex, prefrontal cortex, and primary and secondary somatosensory cortices.

Although general analgesic effects of opiates on the peripheral and spinal areas are considered an important factor, receptors in the cingulated cortex may be particularly important for opiate-related changes in the emotional aspects of pain. According to Numora and Segawa (46) the basic dysfunction in RS cerebrum is the lack of development of the monoaminergic system.

According to these researchers (46) the dysfunctional monoaminergic system, which influences the development of higher systems in the brain, causes a cascade of events leading to abnormalities of intra-cortical transmission caused by failure in dendrite branching of the cortical neurons, as shown in neuro-pathological observations. The same monoaminergic dysfunction also causes the hypo-activation of the noradrenergic and serotonergic systems thus leading to slowing down of background and disorganization of electrical activities of the brain in awake subjects with RS (47,48) indicating an abnormal neuronal activity occurring at all cortical areas of individuals with RS (49).

On top of that, secondary damage is expressed by elongation of nerve conduction, in the phonetic pathways in the brainstem as well as the lamniscal areas and up to the cortex level (36). The low dendrite branching typical of all persons with RS (50) is bound to cause impaired synaptic transmission (49) affecting different central brain processing, mainly complex systems such as the pain system.

Conclusion

This article has examined existing evidence that might propose an insight into the pain behavior and experiences of individuals with Rett syndrome (RS). According to existing evidence post-natally processes of neural development in each young baby and child are accompanied by structural and functional reorganization of sensory connections. Due to the fact that such changes are dependent upon normal neural activity and the maturation of normal neural structures (51), one might speculate that the abnormal neural formation and activity related to RS in early life may therefore cause long term changes in pain processing for this population.

Despite of the fact that we did not find articles specifically addressing the issue of pain sensation and observation of pain behaviors of individuals with RS, the accumulating evidence of neuro-anatomical and chemical findings relating to sensory/pain conduction, and processing represent the following picture:

- The development of cutaneous pain sensors is probably deficient in RS (31).
- The peripheral nerve conduction of individuals with RS has been found to reduce with age and with the progression of the disorder (22).
- The dorsal ganglions, a major station in peripheral pain pathways, have been found to show reduced number of neurons compared to controls without RS (36).
- The CSF of individuals with RS has been found with high levels of Beta-endorphins, which have been connected to reduction in peripheral pain (41).
- Substance-P, a protein involved in pain transmission throughout the nervous system has been found in significantly reduced quantities in persons with RS in comparison to individuals without RS(33).
- The arrest in brain development typical of RS (52) causes reduction in dentritic branching across all brain regions (50), which probably reduces brain affectivity in processing incoming stimulus of all kinds mainly affecting the more complex multi centered systems (i.e. pain sensation).
- The decreased levels of many neurotransmitters, suggests a defective brain maturation mechanism which might cause overall reduction of brain activity (53).
- EEG findings of individuals with RS actually suggestsEEG findings of individuals with RS actually suggest a general slowing down of cerebral neural activity (54).

All the above findings contribute to reduction in the intake, transmission and processing of painful stimuli by individuals with RS. Our knowledge that abnormal activity related to pain in early life has the potential to cause long term changes in pain processing (51) supports the notion that this system is not functioning properly from an early age in this population.

On the other hand, one of the theories explaining major defects in the central neural system of individuals with RS is the pathology of the monoaminergic system (46). Such pathology creates a chain reaction diminishing neurotransmitter activity in the seotonregic and neuroadrenergic systems. These neurotransmitters are also used in the neural system as pain reduction agents. Therefore the lack of these elements will actually elevate pain threshold for the population of RS. Moreover it seems that the lack of neuro-chemical activity causes synapse hyper-sensitivity which therefore also acts as a pain enhancer.

We conclude this inquiry by stating that the accumulating evidence clearly imply that pain reception, conduction and processing is abnormal for the individual with RS, in regards to individuals without this condition. Since most abnormalities within the neural system react as pain reducers, it stands to reason to assume that pain sensation by individuals with RS is reduced in comparison to individuals without RS, supporting observations by parents (19) and professionals (18). We believe strongly suggest that further research should be conducted in this population in order to scientifically investigate the pain system of individuals with RS.

Clinical Application

To be on the safe side we should therefore accept that the person with RS has a reduced pain perception and clinicians working with this population must take extra care, when applying different manual techniques such as manipulations. Moreover, due to the difficulties of the person with RS to verbally express herself, it is recommended that any change in behavior should alarm the caretaker to physically examine the person with RS in order to detect or rule out a possible trauma as the cause for the observed change in behavior.

References

[1] Blomqvist K, Hallberg IR. Recognizing pain in older adults living in sheltered accommodation: The view of nurses and older adults. Int J Nurs Stud 2001;38:305-18.
[2] Stallard P, Wiilaims L, Lenton S, Velleman R. Pain in cognitively impaired, non-communicating children. Arch Dis Child 2001; 85:460-2.
[3] McGrath PJ, Breau LM, Camfield C, Finley GA. Caregivers management of pain in cognitively impaired children with severe speech impairments. 5th Int Symp Pediatr Pain, London, 18-21 Jun 2000.
[4] Nalviya S, Voepel-Lowins T, Tait AR, Merkel S, Lauer A, Munro H, Farley F. Pain management in children with and without cognitive impairment following spine fusion surgery. Paediatric Anaesth 2001;11:453-58.
[5] Krauss MW, Gulley S, Sciegaj M, Wells N. Access to specialty medical care for children with mental retardation, autism, and other special health care needs. Ment Retard 2003;41(5):329-39.
[6] Gauthier JC, Finley GA, McGrath PJ. Children's self-report of postoperative pain intensity and treatment threshold: determining the adequacy of medication. Clin J Pain 1998;14(2):116-20.
[7] Carter G, Jancar J. Sudden death in the mentally handicapped. Psychol Med 1984;14:691-5.
[8] Ellenor GL, Zimmerman S, Kriz J. An interdisciplinary approach to dental care of the mentally disabled. J Am Dent Assoc 1978;97:491-5.
[9] Kauanaugh JH. Caveati hip fractures in the mentally deficient. Ortho Clin North Am 1981;12(1):165-74.
[10] Biersdorff KK. Incidence of significantly altered pain experience among individuals with developmental disabilities. Am J Ment Retard 1994; 98(5):619-31.
[11] Defrin R, Pick CG, Peretz C, Carmeli E. A quantitative somatosensory testing of pain threshold in individuals with mental retardation. Pain 2004;108:58–66.
[12] Hennequin M, Morin C, Feine JS. Pain expression and stimulus localization in individuals with Down's syndrome. Lancet 2000;356:1882-7.
[13] Amir RE, Van den Veyver IB, Wan M, Tran CQ, Francke U, Zoghbi HY. Rett syndrome is caused by mutations in X-linked MECP2, encoding methyl-CpG-binding protein 2. Nat Genet 1999;23(2):185-8.

[14] Ellaway C, Christodoulou J. Rett syndrome: Clinical characteristics and recent genetic advances. Disabil Rehabil 2001;23:98-106.
[15] Hagberg B. Rett Syndrome clinical and biological aspects. Cambridge: Cambridge Univ Press, 1993.
[16] Sponseller P. Orthopedic update in Rett syndrome. Rett Gazette 2001;1:4-5.
[17] Percy AK. International research review. IRSA 12th Ann Conf, Boston, MA, 24-27 May 1996.
[18] Lindberg B. Understanding Rett Syndrome, 3rd ed. Toronto: Hogrefe Huber, 2006.
[19] Hunter K. The Rett syndrome handbook. Washington DC: IRSA, 1999.
[20] Ronnett GV, Leopold D, Cai X, Hoffbuhr KC, Moses L, Hoffman EP, Naidu S. Olfactory biopsies demonstrate a defect in neuronal development in Rett's syndrome. Ann Neurol 2003;54(2):206-18.
[21] Kerr AM, Witt-Engerstrom I. The clinical background to the Rett disorder. In: Kerr AM, Witt-Engerstrom I, eds. Rett disorder and the developing brain. Oxford: Oxford Univ Press, 2001:1-26.
[22] Kalmanchey R. Evoked potentials in the Rett syndrome. Brain Dev 1990;12(1):73-6.
[23] Pillion JP, Rawool VW, Naidu S. Auditory brainstem responses in Rett syndrome: effects of hyperventilation, seizures, and tympanometric variables. Audiology 2000;39:80–7.
[24] Genazzani AR, Zappella M, Nalin A, Hayek Y, Facchinetti F. Reduced cerebrospinal fluid B-endorphin levels in Rett syndrome. Child Nerv Syst 1989;5(2):111-3.
[25] Coleman M, Brubaker J, Hunter K, Smith G. Rett Syndrome: A survey of North American patients. J Ment Def Res 1988;32:117-24.
[26] Defrin R, Lotan M, Pick CG. Evaluation of acute pain in individuals with cognitive impairment: A differential effect of the level of impairment. Pain 2006;124(3):312-20.
[27] Breau LM, Camfield C, McGrath PJ, Rosmus C, Finley GA. Measuring pain accurately in children with cognitive impairments: refinement of a caregiver scale. J Pediatr 2001;138:721–7.
[28] Mount RN, Hastings RP, Reilly S, Cass H, Charman T. Behavioral and emotional Features in Rett Syndrome. Disabil Rehabil 2001;23(3/4):129-38.
[29] McMahon SB, Bennett DLH, Priestly JV, Shelton DL. The biological effects of endogenous NGF in adult sensory neurons revealed by a trkA-IgG fusion molecule. Nature Med 1995;1(8):774-80.
[30] Meyer RA, Campbell JN, Raja SN. Peripheral neural mechanisms of nociception. In: Wall PD, Melzack R, eds. Text book of pain. New York: Churchill Livingstone, 1994:13-44.
[31] Lipani JD, Bhattacharjee MB, Corey DM, Lee DA. Reduced nerve growth factor in Rett syndrome postmortem brain tissue. J Neuropathol Exp Neurol 2000;59(10):889-95.
[32] Snijdelaar DG, Dirkwen R, Slappedel R, Crul, BJP. Substance P. Eur J Pain 2000;4:121-35.
[33] Armstrong DD, Kinney H. The neuropathology of the Rett disorder. In: Kerr AM, Witt-Engerstrom I, eds. Rett disorder and the developing brain. Oxford: Oxford Univ Press, 2001:57-84.
[34] Matsuishi T, Nagamitsu S, Yamashita Y, Murakami Y, Kimura A, Sakai T, Shoji H, Kato H, Percy AK. Decreased cerebrospinal fluid levels of substance P in patients with Rett syndrome. Ann Neurol 1997;42:978–81.
[35] Jellinger K, Grisold W, Armstrong D, Rett A. Peripheral nerve involvment in the Rett syndrome. Brain Dev 1990;12(1):109-14.
[36] Witt-Engerstrom I, Hagberg B. The Rett Syndrome: Gross motor disability and neural impairment in adults. Brain Dev 1990;12(1):23-6.
[37] Yoshikawa H, Kaga M, Suzuki H, Sakuragawa N, Arima M. Giants somatosensory evoked potentials in the Rett syndrome. Brain Dev 1990;12(1):36-9.
[38] Verma P, Nigro MA, Hart CH, Rett A. Rett syndrome a gray matter disease. Electroencephalogr Clin Neurophysiol 1987;67:327-9.
[39] Willis WD, Coggeshall RE. Sensory mechanisms of the spinal cord. New York: Kluwer, 2004.
[40] Lappalainen R, Lindholm D, Riikonen R. Low levels of nerve growth factor in cerebrospinal fluid of children with Rett syndrome. J Child Neurol 1996;11(4):296-300.

[41] Budden SS, Myer ED, Butler IJ. Cerebrospinal fluid studies in Rett syndrome: Biogenic amines and B-Endorphins. Brain Dev 1990;12;(1):81-4.
[42] Myer EC, Tripathi HL, Dewey WL. Hyperendorphinism in Rett syndrome: cause or result? Ann Neurol 1988;24:340–1.
[43] Holden JE, Jeong Y, Forrest JM.The endogenous opioid system and clinical pain management. AACN Clin Issues 2005;16(3):291-301.
[44] Bader G, Witt-Engerstrom I, Hagberg B. Neurophysiological findings in Rett syndrome. II. Visual and auditory brainstem, middle and late evoked responses. Brain Dev 1989;(11):110-4.
[45] Bader G, Witt-Engerstrom I, Hagberg,B. Brain stem and spinal cord impairment in Rett syndrome: somatosensory and auditory evoked responses investigations. Brain Dev 1987;(9):517-22.
[46] Nomura Y, Segawa M. The monoamine hypothesis in Rett syndrome. In: Kerr AM, Witt-Engerstrom I, eds. Rett disorder and the developing brain. Oxford: Oxford Univ Press, 2001:1-26.
[47] Verma NP, Chheda RL, Nigro MA, Hart ZH. Electroencephalographic findings in Rett syndrome. Electroencephalogr Clin Neurophysiol 1986;64:394–401.
[48] Ishizaki A, Inoue Y, Sasaki H, Fukuyama Y. Longitudinal observation of electroencephalograms in the Rett syndrome. Brain Dev 1989;11:407–12.
[49] Nomura Y. Neurophysiology of Rett syndrome. Brain Dev 2001;23(Suppl 1):S50-7.
[50] Nihei K, Naitoh H. Cranial computed tomographic and magnetic resonance imaging studies on the Rett syndrome. Brain Dev 1990;12(1):101-4.
[51] Fitzgerald M, Walker S. The role of activity in developing pain pathways. Progress in pain research and management. Seattle, WA: IASP Press, 2003.
[52] Armstrong DD. The neuropathology of Rett Syndrome overview 1994. Neuropediatrics 1995;26:100-4.
[53] Armstrong DD. Rett syndrome neuropathology review 2000. Brain Dev 2001;23(Suppl 1):S72-6.
[54] Guerrini R, Bonanni P, Parmeggiani L, Santucci M, Parmeggiani A. Sartucci F. Cortical reflex myodomus in Rett syndrome. Ann Neurol 1998;43(4):472-9.

Chapter 2

ASSESSING PAIN IN CHILDREN WITH INTELLECTUAL DISABILITY

Lynn M Breau, PhD, RPsych*

School of Nursing, Department of Pediatrics, Department of Psychology, Dalhousie University
and Complex Pain Team, IWK Health Centre, Halifax,
Nova Scotia, Canada

Abstract

Children with intellectual and developmental disabilities may be more susceptible to pain than typically developing children due to their medical conditions, treatment for those conditions that may cause pain, and greater risk for injury. Despite this, research to develop better pain management for them has lagged behind that for the general child population. In the past 15 years, research regarding pain assessment for this group has emerged. This is important because pain assessment is the foundation of good pain management. Research at this time suggests that only a minority of children with an intellectual disability are capable of providing self-report using scales developed for typical children and that the abilities they do exhibit may be compromised during pain due to the nature of the experience. Because of this, observational measures of pain are recommended for most children in this population. Of those currently available, the Non-communicating Children's Pain Checklist appears to have the most sound psychometric properties for acute or chronic pain. It has also shown preliminary validity with adults, which can assist with ongoing assessment as children reach adulthood. Tools such as this only provide estimates of pain intensity, one dimension of pain. Thus, a comprehensive approach is recommended for ongoing pain, including assessment of pain intensity, location, temporal patterns. Changes in function and maladaptive behaviour should also be considered as they may reflect pain. A bio-ecological approach is encouraged, encompassing child, family and the social and cultural context of the child's pain.

Keywords: Assessment, pediatric pain, behavioural scales, assessment tools, intellectual disability.

---

* **Correspondence:** Lynn M Breau, Dalhousie University, 5869 University Avenue, Halifax, Nova Scotia, B3H 3J5, Canada. E-mail: lbreau@dal.ca

Introduction

Pain can be an adaptive part of everyday life. Its role is to warn us of injury or illness, so that action can be taken or help sought. Without pain, we risk repeated injuries and illness that can go unchecked. However, pain can also become maladaptive; as is the case when chronic pain persists long after tissue has healed. Pain's adaptive function is also curtailed when a person is unable to take action and has less ability to seek help, as is the case for infants and young children, the elderly with dementia, and those with intellectual or developmental disabilities.

In contrast to the main body of pain research, the bulk of research aimed at understanding the pain of children with intellectual or developmental disabilities has only emerged in the past decade, following about 10 years behind research of pain in typically developing children and infants. Because these children may have limited verbal abilities, they have been excluded from most studies of pain in which children are asked about their pain. Unlike research in the general population, however, pain research aimed at those with intellectual disabilities (ID) has emerged first for children, with studies of adult pain only recently being added. This may stem from the fact that methods used to assess pain in those with ID, and the issues involved in assessment, are more similar to those of typical children than typical adults.

Many children with ID suffer pain related to co-morbid physical disabilities and/or medical problems or to treatments for those problems (1). Poor detection of more common health problems may also lead to untreated pain (2), and injuries are also more common in this group (3), especially those who are mobile (4). Research also suggests that pain has substantial impacts on children's daily function (5) and may lead to unwanted behavior such as self-injury (6). This mounting body of evidence, therefore, makes it clear that pain presents a serious problem for children with ID.

`Families and caregivers of these children are also affected by a child's pain. Parents report that they struggle with healthcare professionals when seeking care for pain. They believe professionals have difficulty assessing and treating their child's pain and that their child's pain is treated differently than that of typical children (7). Some parents report a feeling of isolation and inordinate responsibility because professionals, who have difficulty with treating their child, refer decisions back to the parent (2). Parents also report anger that their child must suffer pain in addition to their other problems, but also a sense of helplessness and emotional turmoil (8). These accounts highlight the fact that the children's suffering due to pain also impacts their family.

Pain Assessment as a Foundation for Pain Management

Pain assessment is the foundation of good pain management, so it is the key to improving care for children with ID. In many cases, treatments for the pain these children experience do exist, but are not used because pain remains undetected. The effectiveness of treatments may also be questioned because pain is not monitored, sometimes leading to the abandonment of attempts to manage the child's pain. Good pain assessment is, therefore, crucial at all stages of pain management; from detection, to monitoring treatment, to prevention in situations where pain may occur, such as during medical procedures.

Self-report is considered the "gold standard" for pain assessment. For self-report to be appropriate, however, the individual with pain must be capable of appraising their pain and of communicating that internal experience to others. For many people with ID this isn't possible. In the absence of self-report, observational tools can be used to measure an individual's pain based on overt behavior. This approximation is usually an underestimate, since not all aspects of the pain experience are expressed in overt behavior. However, correspondence between observational estimates and self-report can be good under the correct circumstances.

Accounting for Biased Observers

One requirement for good assessment is that biases or preconceived beliefs of those observing pain behavior not cloud objective evaluation of the evidence they may see or hear from someone with pain. This can be problematic for children with ID because some reports have suggested that people with ID are insensitive or indifferent to pain (9) and this belief could lead to underestimates of pain or discounting of potential pain. However, these suggestions have been based primarily on anecdotal reports or un-validated pain assessment methods. In contrast, research suggests that some adults believe that children with ID may over-react to pain (10), which could also lead to less than adequate management if parents feel the reaction does not reflect the true severity of the child's pain. The use of a sound assessment tool can reduce the likelihood that evaluation is tainted with preconceived beliefs, but cannot eliminate the potential for minimizing the importance of pain for children with ID, regardless of whether the observer believes these children over- or under-react to pain. For example, in a study by Fanurik et al., 29% of parents reported that they believe their child's pain is treated differently solely because of their ID (7). For the professional, awareness of their personal beliefs regarding pain in this group may be the best guard against unintentional influence on clinical care.

Evaluating Psychometrics of Assessment Tools

A second requirement for good pain assessment is that the observational pain tool being used has proven psychometric properties. This may be more important with this population because of biases and that professionals may have relatively less experience with the way these children show pain. Pain intensity is the focus of most pain tools, and reflects only one component of the pain experience. Nonetheless, it is a useful parameter clinically and appears to be the most easily quantified quality of the multidimensional pain experience. An understanding of the key psychometric aspects of a pain tool is especially important when looking at those for use with children with ID. Many of the tools that exist are still under study, meaning that ongoing research can show limitations or extensions of their use. Thus, professionals should keep basic psychometric concepts in mind when deciding which tool to use.

A sound pain assessment tool must be both valid and reliable. A valid tool specifically measures the desired construct and nothing else. In the case of pain, that means ensuring that the tool measures pain specifically, not anxiety or distress or illness. Validity is tested by comparing the scores from a tool to other measures of pain taken at the same time, either by other observers or from the individual who has pain in the form of self-report. It can also be determined by comparing scores during pain to those when pain is absent or after pain has been treated. A reliable tool provides the same score each time it is used or when used by different people. Pain assessment tools should provide consistently low scores when people do not have pain and consistently higher scores when they do have pain. If the tool is designed for use by multiple observers, then scores from these should not differ substantially. Validity and reliability are context-dependent; they may vary due to the setting (e.g. hospital or home), the person completing the tool (caregiver or family member), the type of pain and context of pain (e.g. chronic pain versus acute procedural pain) and the person who has pain (adult versus child, intellectual disability alone versus intellectual and physical disabilities). This means research must be conducted to evaluate the validity and reliability of a tool in numerous contexts before it can be considered valid and reliable for general use. Until that time, it should only be considered sound in those circumstances in which it was tested or in very similar ones.

Pain Assessment Methods

Early Research Regarding Pain in People with ID

Although the bulk of recent research regarding pain in children with ID has focused on assessment, early research in this area focused primarily on individual cases or on the apparent differences in response to pain by people with ID (11,12). The first study to show pain leads to consistent behaviors appeared in 1965 (13). Reynell provided evidence that children with ID experience pain under circumstances most children would be expected to have pain, following surgery, that their pain behavior was observable, and that it did not vary due to level of impairment. Cases studies predominated the literature for 30 years after Reynell's first report (14-16). Then, in 1995, Giusiano et al (17) recorded pain behavior observed during a physical exam by 100 individuals aged 2 to 33 years in a long-term care facility. This seminal study provided the first indication that a set of common pain behaviors could be observed and aggregated into a basic assessment tool for people with ID. Since then, two main approaches have been undertaken in efforts to improve assessment for this group. On the one hand, studies have explored whether tools designed for typical children are valid when used with children who have ID. On the other, studies have been conducted to develop new instruments, most often based on empirical evidence for observable pain responses by the children.

Pain Assessment Tools Designed for Typical Children

Facial Expression. Studies with children with ID have reported differing results when trying to use facial expression to detect pain. In the first study published, Oberlander et al (18) found no significant change in facial reaction to pain during a mock and real immunization for eight adolescents with spastic quadriplegia (18). Similarly, Hadden et al (19) observed no change in facial expression during home physiotherapy exercises in 19 children with cerebral palsy, although pain ratings using the Non-communicating Children's Pain Checklist did increase during stretches. In contrast, Nader et al (20) did report increased facial activity in 21 children with autism when they were observed during intravenous needles, as well as greater facial activity relative to controls. These three studies used the Child Facial Coding System (21), which has shown some validity with typical children (22,23). However, the differences in results here raise questions as to whether this research tool has potential for children with ID. Mercer and Glenn (24) found facial response in 8 infants with developmental delay who were receiving immunizations did change with needle insertion. Facial expression was also not diminished, but was more diffuse than in a comparison group of 30 infants without ID, when they used the Maximally Discriminative Facial Movement Coding System.

Thus, the tool used may underlie differences in results among these studies. However, there is clearly a great deal of work to be done in this area before clinical use of any facial expression tool is feasible. Not only must more support for their validity be found. But also, most current systems are time-consuming and coded from videotape, making bedside application impractical.

Multidimensional Tools

Although the development of observational tools to assess pain in people with ID has proceeded quickly since the 1990s, some research of tools designed for typical children has also occurred in parallel. One group examined the validity of the FLACC scale (Faces, Legs, Activity, Cry, Consol ability) for measuring pain in children with ID after surgery (25). Revisions improved the reliability (26), but cut-offs developed with the original scale may no longer be appropriate for the revised scale because mean scores differed after the changes. The revised scale also allows for personalization of items by a caregiver or parent. However, it is not clear how this would affect cut-off values. More research is needed before the FLACC is used clinically for people with ID.

Soetenga et al (27) used the University of Wisconsin Children's Hospital Pain Scale with 74 children admitted to hospital, 15 of whom were over age 3 years, but nonverbal. This scale contains four subscales: Vocal, Facial, Behavior and Body Movement. Scores were significantly lower after analgesic administration and inter-rater reliability was excellent. However, subgroup analyses for the nonverbal children in the sample are not provided, so it is difficult to conclude whether the psychometrics presented would be similar had the scores for the subgroup been examined separately.

Most recently, Solodiuk and Curley (28) suggested the use of an individualized visual analogue scale (VAS) for children with severe cognitive impairments. A caregiver is asked to provide descriptors for the 0 and 10 anchors and points between. They report this has worked well clinically, but have not yet reported data on the validity or reliability of this measure.

Overall, there is not convincing evidence that the tools above are satisfactory for children with ID. Although further research may provide additional evidence to support their use clinically, they should not be used clinically at this time.

Self-Report Pain Tools

Since self-report is the "gold standard" of pain assessment, it is important to consider it as a possibility when assessing pain in individuals with ID. Fanurik et al (29) were the first to explore the self-report abilities of children with borderline to profound ID. They found only half of children with borderline ID and less than 30% of the group with mild ID could pass tests indicating they understood order and magnitude, two concepts encompassed in commonly used scales of pain intensity. Benini et al (30) found the number of children in their study who chose a rating indicating pain after venepuncture varied depending on whether a standard or modified scale was used. The scales they included were the Eland Color Scale (31) and an adaptation of that scale, and the Facial Affective Scale (32), along with a modified version. This is contrasted by several studies that have asked children or adults with ID to rate hypothetical pain situations using various types of pain scales (33-35). They have found higher rates of successful use of self-report pain rating scales that the studies conducted by Benini or Fanurik's groups. This discrepancy suggests that people with ID may appear more capable when rating hypothetical pain than they are in real-life pain situations. Research with the general population indicates cognitive abilities are usually reduced during pain, and those with ID are not likely exempt from this effect. In fact, Benini et al. reports fear reduced success in their study (30). This is relevant to clinical situations, where professionals often ask children to "practice" using a scale by rating hypothetical events, such as scraping a knee. The child's ability in using the tool for these trials may not reflect her ability during actual pain.

Observational Tools Designed for Children with ID

Echelle Douleur Enfant San Salvador (DESS). Since their first study published in 1995 (36), Collignon and Giusiano and their group (36) have continued their development of the DESS. In a second study, they reduced the original 22 behaviors to 10 items and report that a score of 2 indicates "pain is possible", while a score of 6 indicates "definite pain needing treatment" (36). A strength of this scale is that it was based on research with children and adults, making it useful across age groups. However, several weaknesses undermine the scale's psychometrics. Overlap among items means that crying behaviors carry an inordinate weight in scoring and some items incorporate the subjective opinion of caregivers. Unfortunately, the DESS is also designed so that items are rated in relation to the individual's typical behavior. This may be possible, or even preferred in some situations, but makes the tool less valid when observers do not know the person's typical behavior. Using change from typical behavior also means that scores cannot be used across situations (e.g. home versus school/hospital) as children often exhibit pain differently in hospital where they feel more inhibited in front of staff. Finally, validation of the DESS was conducted in French. Caution should be taken in using those cut-off values if using an English version of the scale until systematic translation and validation in English is completed. Cultural and language differences can impact both pain behavior displayed and our perception of pain behavior.

The Pediatric Pain Profile (PPP)

This scale was developed through interviews with 121 caregivers of children with ID (37). From an original pool of 56 items, a set of 20 was selected. Inter-rater reliability between parents and a caregiver was reported to be good. Scores also decreased significantly after analgesics were given. Although a cut-off score is provided, it only identifies moderate pain. In a second study of a subgroup of the original sample, scores in a home setting were compared during videotaped daily activities thought to be painful for children with chronic pain conditions but not those without chronic pain (38). However, the cut-off varied slightly from the first study and a different method of computing scores was used. One positive attribute of the scale is that the developers have created a package that caregivers can complete to document their child's baseline behavior when he is pain free and behavior during common pains. This might be particularly helpful in cases where children have multiple conditions that cause chronic or recurrent pain, as it might help to untangle the temporal patterns of specific pains. However, with only two studies to date, some change in the cut-off values, data from only one population and no data in a hospital setting, the Pediatric Pain Profile needs more research support before it is used widely for on the spot pain assessment.

The Non-communicating Children's Pain Checklists (NCCPC's)

In the mid-1990's, a series of studies began that reported the development, testing and revision of the Non-communicating Children's Pain Checklist. The original scale included yes/no responses to 30 items in seven categories: Vocal, Eating/Sleeping, Social/Personality, Facial Expression, Activity, Body and Limbs, and Physiological (39). In the original study, which included children and adults, no differences in scores were found due to age (3 to 44 years) of the person with ID. A further study of the NCCPC–Postoperative Version (NCCPC-PV) investigated its use for postoperative pain (40). Items from the Eating/Sleeping subscale were excluded and more detailed responses from observers were added, such that they now provided ratings to indicate whether each item was observed "not at all", just a little", "fairly often" or "very often" during 10 minute pre- and postoperative observations of 24 children. A cut-off score for moderate to severe pain (equivalent to 3+ out of 10 on a 10 cm visual analogue scale) was set at 11 and detected 88% of cases. Later, a score of 6 to 10 was developed to detect mild pain (< 3 /10 on a 10 cm visual analogue scale of pain), with 75% accuracy. Caregivers' (parents and primary caregivers) and researcher' total scores increased after surgery, as would be expected. Total scores between the two observers were also significantly correlated, indicating good inter-rater reliability. This is especially important , because it indicates scores from an observer who is unfamiliar with the child (researcher) are valid.

The original NCCPC was also revised for the home setting, and renamed the NCCPC-Revised (NCCPC-R). The 30 items were retained, but the frequency scoring used for the NCCPC-PV was adopted. It was re-examined in a home setting with a larger sample than the first study (39), and based on two-hour observations of children. Scores for children who had pain during the observations were compared to scores for children who did not have pain. A total score of 7 detected pain in 84% of cases. The results also indicated total NCCPC-R scores were consistent across the two episodes of pain, as were the number of items children displayed. This is important because it has been suggested that children with ID show pain inconsistently. This result negates that; revealing that their pain response is consistent between two episodes of pain due to two different causes.

The NCCPC's were specifically designed for children who had very limited verbal abilities due to their ID. However, Hadden and von Baeyer have also used the NCCPC-R with children with cerebral palsy with varying levels of verbal abilities. Parents identified items from the checklist that occurred when their child had pain. The reported presence of 24 items from the NCCPC-R did not vary due to the children's communication ability (41). In a subsequent study by the same authors, 129 children with cerebral palsy who had a wide range of verbal abilities, were observed during home physiotherapy exercises that were expected to cause pain (19). Although children's facial expression did not change significantly during active stretching, scores on the NCCPC-PV were significantly higher. Thus, there is some evidence that the NCCPC's may be valid for higher functioning children with physical impairments. Breau et al. also examined whether the NCCPC-R is valid for children who display self-injurious behavior (6). This is a concern because, despite evidence to the contrary, some believe that these children may be insensitive to pain. There were no significant differences in NCCPC-R total scores for observed episodes of pain in children with (n = 44) and without (n = 57) a history of ongoing self-injury. The results also suggested that children who had chronic pain might show a different pattern of self-injury, suggesting self-injurious behavior might be a reaction to pain in some children.

The NCCPC's have also been translated into several languages. Although a recent study of 24 children in a rehabilitation hospital indicated good reliability and validity when used by parents or caregivers, it also suggested a cut-off score of 5 was more appropriate for the Swiss-German version (42). This highlights the need for validating translated scales, because interpretations of items may differ due to language constraints or cultural factors. Children may also display behavior differently depending on cultural norms regarding appropriate pain expression. A French translation of the NCCPC- PV, developed in Canada and France, is currently being validated in hospitals in Canada and France. This study also incorporated a change in the observation time needed, in an attempt to improve feasibility of the NCCPC-PV in a clinical setting. Observations were reduced from the 10 minutes of previous research, to 5 minutes. Preliminary data for the «Grille d'Évaluation de la douleur - déficience intellectuelle» with 77 participants aged 3 to 57 suggest scores increase after surgery and may be similar to those found with the English version (43). Mean pre-operative scores were below 7.0, while mean post-operative scores were over 14.0. Further detailed analyses will reveal whether the scores differ due to age (child/adult) or culture.

Very recently, the NCCPC–R has also been used with 159 adults with ID who received vaccinations (44). Although scores differed prior to the immunization due to level of ID, they increased significantly after vaccination regardless of level of ID. New data, using the NCCPC-R for chronic pain in 17 adults with an average age of 42 years, reveals mean total NCCPC-R scores of 4.8 (SD = 5.2) when pain is absent and 32.3 (SD = 13.8) when pain is present (Burkitt and Breau, manuscript submitted for publication). This study also incorporated a reduced observation time of 5 minutes. Although further research is needed to provide more psychometric evidence for use of the NCCPC's with adults, these early studies suggest that the NCCPC's have the potential to be used throughout the lifespan, which can ease transition to adult care.

Summary

There are more similarities than differences among scales created for children and adults with ID. This supports the argument that pain behavior is consistent in this population and that a standardized scale can be developed for children with ID. The basis on which to choose a scale then becomes a matter of the amount of research supporting the tool's psychometric properties. To date, the NCCPC's have the most evidence to support their use clinically for children with ID and there is some data to suggest that they may continue to be used as youth transition to adulthood, which may be helpful in documenting long-term or recurrent pain problems that can span years. The NCCPC's have been used across a number of studies by different research groups. These have included children and adults and have taken place in home, hospital and residential facilities, suggesting the NCCPC- R and NCCPC- PV can be used widely within the population of children and adults with ID. For current clinical use, the NCCPC-PV is recommended because its shorter observation period (currently 10 minutes) makes it more feasible. Cut-offs are available for mild pain (Total score = 6-10) and moderate to severe pain (Total score = 11+).

Putting Research into Practice

Parents have identified pain as an area of concern for their children who cannot communicate verbally (45). They also express concern that some professionals may discount their reports that their child has pain (2) and that their child's pain is treated differently than that of typical children (7). In interview studies, parents also report that familiarity with their child is required to assess their child's pain (2,8). No professional would argue the fact that each child is unique, whether or not she has ID. However, parents' beliefs about the inability of professionals to manage their child's pain may reflect assumptions based on past experience in which professionals failed in attempts to discern pain due to lack of training, little literature to provide guidance, and the unavailability of structured tools to help them to assess pain. The landscape has changed dramatically in the past 10 years, with increased research and awareness of issues regarding pain assessment for this particular group.

Among the important advancements that have been made is the understanding that variation in children's pain behavior does not preclude the use of validated measures that have been empirically and scientifically evaluated with this population. When provided with information in a structured way, or using a validated tool, observers who are unfamiliar with children with ID may provide very reliable judgments. For example, the good inter-rater reliability between parents and a researcher reported by Breau et al. (40) suggests use of a structured tool may facilitate agreement and reduce the impact of preconceived beliefs during pain assessment. Professionals may also be very adept at putting aside preconceived beliefs regarding a group, when dealing with one child in a clinical situation using a tool that helps them to structure their evaluation.

Thus, pain assessment for children with ID should follow the same principles as that for other groups. Self-report is always the preferred method of obtaining information about pain intensity. However, it is advisable to test the child's abilities to understand the underlying concepts when possible. Training a child in how to use a scale, by having him rate hypothetical situations (46) may improve his skills if he understands the concepts necessary for using a self-report scale. However, the possibility that the child's abilities may be reduced during actual pain should be kept in mind. The NCCPC-PV should be used when self-report is not possible, whether for chronic or acute pain. It has fewer items that the NCCPC-R and a shorter (10 minute versus 2 hour) observation time, and new data is suggesting that information regarding eating and sleeping patterns (included in the NCCPC-R) may not be necessary for accurate pain assessment. These aspects of behaviour are more difficult to assess because they cannot be judged over a short time frame, and they may be more difficult for observers who are unfamiliar with a child to evaluate, since they require some knowledge of the child's typical eating and sleeping patterns. When chronic or recurrent pain is suspected, multiple applications of the NCCPC-PV can provide information regarding the temporal pattern of pain and can help to disentangle behaviour changes due to pain from those due to factors such as illness or sleep problems. Records of a child's pain history, using a format such as that provided with the Paediatric Pain Profile (37) can also be useful for helping to untangle multiple sources of pain and for developing a dossier that can be used to help with diagnosis of pain problems.

Although ratings of pain intensity may be sufficient to inform management of acute pain due to procedures or injury, additional information may be helpful for cases of chronic pain. Any information regarding pain quality and location that can be collected will assist with diagnosis. Some research suggests that self-injury may also be a cue, not only of pain presence, but also of pain location and temporal pattern (6). Changes in a person's functioning may also help assess pain presence, as well as alert caregivers to potential skill losses that may occur due to pain and reduce daily functioning and independence (5).

Pain is multidimensional, affecting multiple areas of a person's life and having sensory, cognitive and emotional components. Bronfenbrenner's Bio-ecological Model (47) has been proposed as a model for comprehensive pain management for typical children with chronic pain (48). This model may serve children with ID just as well, since it is based on the premise that children are evolving beings, each with their own growth trajectory. Thus, it allows for the fact that children with ID may differ in their developmental path from typical peers. The model also incorporates the idea that each child's unique set of environments impact the pain experience, which is very important to consider for this particular group of children who may be exposed to situations and experiences not common for most children, such as residential care or repeated medical procedures or hospitalizations. The model also accounts for the fact that pain itself becomes part of the child's environment, interacting with the child, family and society and changing their dynamic relations. Finally, the model emphasizes the importance of the child's internal characteristics, among which is her ability to comprehend pain and its causes and treatments. Children with ID may have limited abilities to understand abstract aspects of pain or to follow the logic of treatments, which may affect their willingness to report pain or to cooperate with treatment. At the same time, they may have extensive experience with pain and many memories of painful experiences, which can add to emotional reactions to pain. This complex internal environment is not inconsequential and should be taken into account with each child. Discussion with a child regarding his experience should be frequent, so that his perceptions can be taken into account when making treatment decisions. Information should not be kept from him. This could lead to a lack of trust and an attempt by him to hide pain. Finally, all information and assessment methods should be appropriate to the child's cognitive or mental age and not based on standards for the general child population, chronological age, or assumptions that a long history of pain has increased the child's comprehension of pain.

All pain assessment activities should be coordinated within a comprehensive pain management plan that should be from a multi-disciplinary approach whenever possible. Untreated pain can lead to mood and anxiety problems, maladaptive behaviour and functional impairments for people with ID, a group who can sorely afford any additional burdens to reaching their fullest potential. Research regarding pain in children has advanced a great deal in the past 15 years, but much is still unknown, particularly about the long-term consequences for these children who already have burdens that can hinder development. Pain is an unnecessary burden in most cases, because actions could be taken to prevent or treat it. Because of its pivotal role in pain management, good pain assessment is vital to any attempt to improve care for this vulnerable group of children.

Acknowledgments

The author is supported by a New Investigator Salary Award from the Canadian Institutes of Health Research.

References

[1] Breau LM, Camfield CS, McGrath PJ, Finley GA. The incidence of pain in children with severe cognitive impairments. Arch Pediatr Adolesc Med 2003;157(12):1219-26.

[2] Hunt A, Mastroyannopoulou K, Goldman A, Seers K. Not knowing--the problem of pain in children with severe neurological impairment. Int J Nurs Stud 2003; 40(2):171-83.

[3] Braden K, Swanson S, Di Scala C. Injuries to children who had preinjury cognitive impairment: a 10-year retrospective review. Arch Pediatr Adolesc Med 2003; 157(4):336-40.

[4] Breau LM, Camfield CS, McGrath PJ, Finley GA. Risk factors for pain in children with severe cognitive impairments. Dev Med Child Neurol 2004; 46(6):364-71.

[5] Breau LM, Camfield CS, McGrath PJ, Finley GA. Pain's impact on adaptive functioning. J Intellect Disabil Res 2007; 51(Pt 2):125-34.

[6] Breau LM, Camfield CS, Symons FJ, Bodfish JW, Mackay A, Finley GA et al. Relation between pain and self-injurious behavior in nonverbal children with severe cognitive impairments. J Pediatr 2003; 142(5):498-503.

[7] Fanurik D, Koh JL, Schmitz ML, Harrison RD, Conrad TM. Children with cognitive impairment: Parent report of pain and coping. J Dev Behav Pediatr 1999;20(4):228-34.

[8] Carter B, McArthur E, Cunliffe M. Dealing with uncertainty: parental assessment of pain in their children with profound special needs. J Adv Nurs 2002;38(5):449-57.

[9] Biersdorff KK. Pain insensitivity and indifference: alternative explanations for some medical catastrophes. Ment Retard 1991; 29(6):359-62.

[10] Breau LM, MacLaren J, McGrath PJ, Camfield CS, Finley GA. Caregivers' beliefs regarding pain in children with cognitive impairment: relation between pain sensation and reaction increases with severity of impairment. Clin J Pain 2003;19(6):335-44.

[11] Couston TA. Indifference to pain in low-grade mental defectives. Br Med J 1954;1(4871):1128-9.

[12] Stengel E, Oldham AJ, Ehrenberg AS. Reactions of low-grade mental defectives to pain. J Ment Sci 1958;104(435):434-8.

[13] Reynell JK. Post-operative disturbances observed in children with cerebral palsy. Dev Med Child Neurol 1965;7(4):360-76.

[14] Mette F, Abittan J. Essais d'évaluation de la douleur chez le polyhandicapé. Annales Kinésithérapie 1988;15:101-4.

[15] L'automutilation: expression de la douleur chez le sujet deficient mental profond. La Douleur de l'Enfant Quelles Resposes?; 92 A.D. Dec 15; Paris: UNESCO, 1992. [French]

[16] Collignon P, Giusiano B, Porsmoguer E, Jimeno ME, Combe JC. Difficultes du diagnostic de la douleur chez l'enfant polyhandicape. Ann Pediatr 1995;42(2):123-6. [French]

[17] Giusiano B, Jimeno MT, Collignon P, Chau Y. Utilization of a neural network in the elaboration of an evaluation scale for pain in cerebral palsy. Methods Inf Med 1995;34:498-502.

[18] Oberlander TF, Gilbert CA, Chambers CT, O'Donnell ME, Craig KD. Biobehavioral responses to acute pain in adolescents with a significant neurologic impairment. Clin J Pain 1999;15:201-9.

[19] Hadden KL, von Baeyer CL. Global and Specific Behavioral Measures of Pain in Children With Cerebral Palsy. Clin J Pain 2005; 21(2):140-6.

[20] Nader R, Oberlander TF, Chambers CT, Craig KD. Expression of pain in children with autism. Clin J Pain 2004;20(2):88-97.

[21] Chambers CT, Cassidy KL, McGrath PJ, Gilbert CA, Craig KD. Child facial coding system: A manual. Nova Scotia: Dalhousie Univ, Univ British Columbia, 1996.

[22] Breau LM, McGrath PJ, Craig KD, Santor D, Cassidy KL, Reid GJ. Facial expression of children receiving immunizations: A principal components analysis of the Child Facial Coding System. Clin J Pain 2001;17(2):178-86.

[23] Gilbert CA, Lilley CM, Craig KD, McGrath PJ, Court C, Bennett SM et al. Postoperative pain expression in preschool children: Validation of the child facial coding system. Clin J Pain 1999; 15(3):192-200.

[24] Mercer K, Glenn S. The expression of pain in infants with developmental delays. Child Care Health Dev 2004;30(4):353-60.

[25] Voepel-Lewis T, Merkel S, Tait AR, Trzcinka A, Malviya S. The reliability and validity of the Face, Legs, Activity, CRY, Consolability observational tool as a measure of pain in children with cognitive impairment. Anesth Analg 2002;95:1224-9.

[26] Malviya S, Voepel-Lewis T, Burke C, Merkel S, Tait AR. The revised FLACC observational pain tool: improved reliability and validity for pain assessment in children with cognitive impairment. Pediatr Anesth 2006;16(3):258-65.

[27] Soetenga D, Pellino TA, Frank J. Assessment of the validity and reliability of the University of Wisconsin Children's Hospital pain scale for preverbal and nonverbal children. Pediatr Nurs 1999; 25(6):670-6.

[28] Solodiuk J, Curley MA. Pain assessment in nonverbal children with severe cognitive impairments: the Individualized Numeric Rating Scale (INRS). J Pediatr Nurs 2003;18(4):295-9.

[29] Fanurik D, Koh JL, Harrison RD, Conrad TM, Tomerlin C. Pain assessment in children with cognitive impairment: An exploration of self-report skills. Clin Nurs Res 1998;7(2):103-24.

[30] Benini F, Trapanotto M, Gobber D, Agosto C, Carli G, Drigo P et al. Evaluating pain induced by venipuncture in pediatric patients with developmental delay. Clin J Pain 2004;20(3):156-63.

[31] Eland JM. The child who is hurting. Semin Oncol Nurs 1985; 1(2):116-22.

[32] McGrath PA, deVeber LL, Hearn MJ. Multidimensional pain assessment in children. In: Fields HR, Dubner R, Cevero F, eds. Advances in pain research and therapy, Vol 9. New York: Raven Press, 1985.
[33] Zabalia M, Jacquet D, Breau LM. Rôle du niveau verbal sur l'expression et l'évaluation de la douleur chez des sujets déficients intellectuals. Doul et Analg 2005;2:65-70. [French]
[34] Boldingh EJ, Jacobs-van der Bruggen MA, Lankhorst GJ, Bouter LM. Assessing pain in patients with severe cerebral palsy: development, reliability, and validity of a pain assessment instrument for cerebral palsy. Arch Phys Med Rehabil 2004; 85(5):758-66.
[35] Bromley J, Emerson E, Caine A. The development of a self-report measure to assess the location and intensity of pain in people with intellectual disabilities. J Intellect Disabil Res 1998;42:72-80.
[36] Collignon P, Giusiano B. Validation of a pain evaluation scale for patients with severe cerebral palsy. Eur J Pain 2001;5(4):433-42.
[37] Hunt A, Goldman A, Seers K, Crichton N, Mastroyannopoulou K, Moffat V et al. Clinical validation of the paediatric pain profile. Dev Med Child Neurol 2004;46(1):9-18.
[38] Hunt A, Wisbeach A, Seers K, Goldman A, Crichton N, Perry L et al. Development of the paediatric pain profile: role of video analysis and saliva cortisol in validating a tool to assess pain in children with severe neurological disability. J Pain Symptom Manage 2007; 33(3):276-89.
[39] Breau LM, McGrath PJ, Camfield C, Rosmus C, Finley GA. Preliminary validation of an observational pain checklist for persons with cognitive impairments and inability to communicate verbally. Dev Med Child Neurol 2000;42(9):609-16.
[40] Breau LM, Finley GA, McGrath PJ, Camfield CS. Validation of the Non-Communicating Children's Pain Checklist - Postoperative version. Anesthesiology 2002;96(3):528-35.
[41] Hadden KL, von Baeyer CL. Pain in children with cerebral palsy: common triggers and expressive behaviors Pain 2002;99(1-2):281-8.
[42] Kleinknecht M. [Reliability and validity of the german language version of the "NCCPC-R"]. Pflege 2007;20(2):93-102. [German]
[43] Breau LM, Gregoire M, Lévêque C, Hennequin M, Bureau N, Wood C. Validation en français de la Grille d'Évaluation de la Douleur-Déficience Intellectuelle. Société Française d'Etude et de Traitement de la Douleur. In press. [French]
[44] Defrin R, Lotan M, Pick CG. The evaluation of acute pain in individuals with cognitive impairment: a differential effect of the level of impairment. Pain 2006;124(3):312-20.
[45] Stephenson JR, Dowrick M. Parent priorities in communication intervention for young students with severe disabilities. Educ Training Ment Retard Dev Disabil 2000;35(1):25-35.
[46] Cassidy KL, Reid GJ, McGrath PJ, Smith DJ, Brown TL, Finley GA. A randomized double-blind, placebo-controlled trial of the EMLA patch for the reduction of pain associated with intramuscular injection in four to six-year-old children. Acta Paediatr 2001; 90(11):1329-36.
[47] Bronfenbrenner U. The ecology of human development: Experiments by nature and design. Cambridge, MA: Harvard Univ Press, 1979.
[48] Breau LM. A bio-ecological approach to pediatric pain assessment. J Pain Managet. In press.

In: Pain Management Yearbook 2009
Editor: Joav Merrick

ISBN: 978-1-61209-666-7
©2012 Nova Science Publishers, Inc.

Chapter 3

PAIN IN INDIVIDUALS WITH INTELLECTUAL AND DEVELOPMENTAL DISABILITIES

Frank J Symons, PhD[*1], *Tim F Oberlander, MD*[2] *and Lois J Kehl, DDS, PhD*[3]

[1]Department of Educational Psychology, University of Minnesota, Minniapolis, United States of America
[2]Department of Pediatrics, Center for Community Child Health Research, University of British Columbia, Vancouver, Canada
[3]Department of Anesthesiology, University of Minnesota, MinniapolisMinneapolis, United States of America

Abstract

Historically, pain among individuals with intellectual and developmental disabilities (IDD) has received very little scientific attention and as study participants individuals with IDD have been systematically excluded from pain research. Clinically, the expression of pain by individuals with IDD is frequently ambiguous and its recognition by caregivers and health care providers can be highly subjective. For these reasons we know less scientifically than we should about the nature of pain among individuals with IDD. The purpose of this introductory article is to highlight a number of the issues and challenges associated with the problem of pain in IDD. Many fundamental questions remain unanswered, however, regarding how the pain system functions when its underlying neural substrate is altered. In turn, these barriers limit our understanding of how best to assess and manage pain in individuals with developmental disabilities. We assert, however, that directly addressing the problem of pain among individuals with IDD provides a tremendous opportunity to reexamine at many levels our understanding of what constitutes this universal but highly subjective personal human experience.

Keywords: Pain, intellectual disability.

---

[*] **Correspondence:** Frank Symons, PhD, Department of Educational Psychology, Education Sciences Building 56 River Road, University of Minnesota, MN 55455, United States. E-mail: symon007@umn.edu

Introduction

Pain is a universal human experience that is an essential component necessary for health by alerting us to danger but is also associated with tremendous suffering that compromises our quality of life when under recognized or poorly treated. Until recently pain in people with intellectual and developmental disabilities (IDD) received very little scientific attention and as study participants individuals with IDD have been systematically excluded from pain and related research (1). Expression of pain by individuals with IDD is frequently ambiguous and its recognition by caregivers and health care providers can be highly subjective. This presents a tremendous challenge for clinicians, researchers, individuals with disabilities and their families. Even when pain-specific behaviors are present, such behaviors may be regarded as altered, blunted or confused with other sources of generalized stress, arousal, or, in the extreme, misinterpreted as a reflection of a behavior disorder of psychiatric origin. However, there is no reason to believe that pain is any less frequent in the lives of someone with an intellectual or related developmental disability that alters the way they communicate, or that such an individual would be insensitive or indifferent to pain.

From a developmental perspective, the ability to communicate pain and distress is an integral part of human existence and a necessary component of the assessment and management of pain (2). Gaffney and others (3-5) have described the age-related developmental course children follow in their understanding of pain and in the use of language to communicate pain/distress during childhood. Typically a child's understanding of pain progresses from vague, nonspecific terms in the preschool period to abstract concepts of pain causality in adolescence. Similarly, words used to describe pain become increasingly specific, differentiated and informative with increasing age. This work highlights the importance of accounting for developmental level when attempting to understand pain. The principle, although often overlooked, may be no less applicable to children and adolescents with IDD. Recent work specific to IDD from Defrin, Lotan and Pick (6) highlights this issue, in part, with their findings showing that level of cognitive impairment was related to different patterns of pain expression during a noxious experience depending on the type of nonverbal behavioral measurement tool being used. In other words, whether a pain response was observed depended not only of the type of measure selected but also on the degree of developmental disability.

Regardless of the degree of disability and the underlying neurological condition, functional limitations frequently confound the presentation of pain in individuals with intellectual and developmental disabilities (7). How can pain be assessed and managed when typical means of verbal or nonverbal communication or cognition are altered or absent? In the absence of easily recognized verbal or motor-dependent forms of communication, it remains uncertain if the pain experience itself is different or whether only the expressive manifestations are altered. Indeed, without easily recognizable means of communication or functional motor skills, pain may remain under recognized and under treated. In spite of the potential for altered nociception and pain expression, there is no evidence that cognitively or motor impaired individuals are spared any of the miseries of a noxious experience (8).

Over the past decade there has been a growing recognition of the need to study pain in individuals with developmental disabilities (9). The purpose of this introductory article is to highlight a number of the issues and challenges associated with the problem of pain in IDD.

We assert that directly addressing the problem of pain among individuals with IDD provides a tremendous opportunity to reexamine at many levels our understanding of what constitutes this universal but highly subjective personal human experience. Many fundamental questions remain unanswered, however, regarding how the pain system functions when its underlying neural substrate is altered. In turn, these barriers limit our understanding of how best to assess and manage pain in individuals with developmental disabilities. These challenges include the following issues.

What are the translational issues facing the study of pain in developmental disabilities? In other words, what barriers may interfere with moving knowledge from research to practice? The complex and challenging nature of pain in individuals with IDD and the inherently interdisciplinary nature of this field make it likely that collaborative opportunities may be overlooked. Addressing an issue like pain in individuals with IDD requires an interdisciplinary approach based on multiple converging but often divergent assumptions, perspectives, and research traditions (10). An interdisciplinary approach is filled with the promise of generating novel solutions for long-standing problems. Although within-discipline inquiry in pharmacology, physiology, molecular biology, genetics, and psychology has led to remarkable advances in understanding pain, it is likely that the next advances will come from the intersections of these fields (11). In addressing pain in individuals with IDD, the field requires us to build interdisciplinary networks investigating multiple interrelated components of the brain, behavior, and clinical sciences that ultimately lead to transforming new knowledge into novel therapeutic approaches. Beyond the obvious need for new basic knowledge, there are professional contextual barriers that need to be crossed. These range from fundamental technical, jargon-specific to a given discipline to broad cultural differences among scientists and clinicians, within their specific disciplinary backgrounds and professional ladders for career advancement. Recognition of such barriers is important and should be acknowledged to help facilitate initial discussions and foster the growth of interdisciplinary working groups focused on pain in IDD.

Conceptual, Definitional, and Ethical Issues Related to the Study and Management of Pain in Individuals with IDD

The core of our understanding requires addressing conceptual, definitional, and ethical issues inherent in any discussion of pain in individuals with IDD. Such a foundational discussion needs to include understanding of historical and contemporary conceptual and definitional issues of the pain experience, as discussed by Craig (12). There are also ethical issues raised by the problems created by conventional definitions of pain with direct health care implications regarding the necessity of analgesia and broader social issues concerning quality of life (8).

The experience of pain includes sensory perception of painful stimuli, such as tissue inflammation or nerve injury, by pain-sensing nerve fibers in conjunction with an individual's affective or emotional response to these stimuli. Typically the 'afferent component' of pain is perceived or experienced before any behavioral response such as self-report or behavioral changes occur. Feeling and reporting pain are often parallel and related phenomena, but self-report, nonverbal expression and evidence of tissue damage can be highly discordant, particularly among individuals with disabilities. Many developmental disabilities are associated with painful conditions that require recurrent noxious and invasive procedures, resulting in increased pain during daily life. This is compounded by difficulties in communicating distress and motor impairments needed to solicit help, which in turn may lead to an increased incidence, severity and duration of pain. Thus, current knowledge about what we know about measurement of pain in developmental disability including a critical examination of state of the art assessment technologies remains an urgent need. Finally, there is evidence that individuals may be denied appropriate and timely pain management because caregivers may not accept that the pain is "real" when the ability to communicate their experiences with discrete words and motor movements is limited.

In all areas of science, advances in methodology and measurement go hand in hand with advances in substantive knowledge. New technologies for studying the human brain make it possible to engage in systematic study of the neural circuitry and mechanisms underlying the complexities of the human pain experience. Despite substantial advances in our understanding of the neurobiological basis of pain, we still have much work to do to readily translate this knowledge into reliable and valid interventions with measurable real-world effects. As mentioned previously, there can be numerous barriers to interdisciplinary research. In addition to substantive issues specific to disciplinary inquiry, there are at least two 'meta-level' challenges that can limit the realization of a translational research agenda predicated on interdisciplinary research (13). The first may be referred to as a 'linkage' problem: How do we build sustainable and productive links among disciplines? The second may be referred to as a 'levels of analysis' problem: How do we integrate findings based on different scales (metrics), time frames (slow vs. fast reactivity), account for reactivity system discordances (i.e., biological and behavioral discordances or typical developmental processes that are inherently discordant), and cross different categories of measurement specific to any given discipline? The linkage problem requires a sound understanding of the social and empirical context of research and being informed of the opportunities for sustainable collaboration that cross disciplinary lines. The level of analysis problem involves moving back and forth between the basic neurobiological substrates of pain and pain behavior in social contexts.

As Salzinger (14) observed, writing from a different position on translational research issues, there can be serious interpretive problems when we seek to correlate the blood levels of metabolites of some single neurotransmitter, measured correctly to the nearest nanogram, with behavioral ratings measured correctly to the nearest rater. In short, the precision of measurement has to be balanced against the ambiguity of interpretation when all relevant pieces of the phenomenon under investigation remain unknown. Quite often, interpretive ambiguity is the context in which we find ourselves when trying to fit the pieces of the pain puzzle together in IDD.

Scope of Pain among Individuals with IDD

A further barrier is the overall scope of the problem itself. Beyond our knowledge that pain is common and poorly treated among adults and children with disabilities, our understanding of the scope and impact of pain across the spectrum of disabilities continues to limit research and clinical care. There is good reason to believe that pain is much more a part of the daily lives of most of these children than is the case for those without disabilities (15).

At present, there are no satisfactory population level epidemiological data regarding the incidence or prevalence of chronic or acute pain in populations of children with disabilities. While the etiology of the underlying conditions vary, making this a heterogeneous population, the additive effects of pain in the presence of a disability are common to many of the conditions associated with IDD. Therefore, even by crude indirect methods it might be reasonable to estimate that pain is more common among children and adults with IDD than among children and adults in general, highlighting this as an area for urgent discussion and future study.

Similarly, efforts to understand pain require an evaluation of the functional impact of the pain, its role in the quality of life and its compounding interaction with the disability itself (16). Studies of pain typically focus on describing symptoms, duration and intensity of pain without accounting for the functional consequences of the symptom even though this is likely to have a major impact on the individual. The measurement of functional disability related to adult pain outcomes has received considerable attention because of issues related to work and cost-related effects. However, analogous work in pediatric and adolescent populations with IDD is limited, further highlighting the urgent need for a critical evaluation of what we know and what we need to know. Recent work by Breau and colleagues (17) has begun to address this issue in relation to the effects of recurrent pain on the development of adaptive behavior.

Pain and an Altered Neurobiological Substrate

There is an urgent need to undertake a detailed examination of the basic and clinical phenomenology of pain in relation to the underlying neural impairment. Current advances in the two primary spheres of research in pain—brain and behavior—provides an opportunity to make new connections between basic preclinical data and clinical observations that can inform assessment, treatment and practice (18). The relations among these expressions of pain need to be organized in a comprehensive conceptual framework that includes psychological, developmental and biological processes that influence the pain experience.

For example, the neurobiological mechanisms that explain why some individuals with IDD experience analgesic failure after exposure to optimal pain treatment remain unclear. Predicting who will and who will not respond to a given analgesic regimen currently relies on clinical trial and error. Complicating this clinical reality are findings from ongoing genetic and metabolic research (19) showing that genetic polymorphisms may account for significant variability in enzymatic activity underlying the metabolism of different compounds. A key system – the cytochrome P450 family of enzymes – is the main enzymatic system responsible for drug metabolism (20). Underlying genetic variability in the P450 system means that metabolic capacity may be enhanced or diminished for different individuals. Thus, observed variability in analgesic response may be a function of whether the individual is an efficient or inefficient drug 'metabolizer' (21). Sacchetti et al (22), for example, reported on the reduced clearance of lorazepam in individuals with Gilbert syndrome.

Although there is only limited empirical work to date including individuals with IDDs, in studies examining hepatic P450 isoenzyme variability (both genetic and pharmacological related enzymatic induction or inhibition), it would seem prudent to consider metabolic differences as a potential cause for analgesic failure or associated adverse effects. This clinical problem is compounded further by the fact that individuals with IDD frequently have altered cognitive and communicative capacities making it difficult to distinguish pain from other stress/arousal behaviors and to determine the specific need for analgesia. This problem is significant as individuals with IDD experience markedly higher rates of pain (30-50%) than their typically developing peers (15) with enormous associated costs (extended hospital stays, emotional cost of suffering, reduced adaptive function).

Impact of Developmental Disabilities on the Pain Experience

Current diagnostic and therapeutic approaches to pain management with IDD are further limited by our narrow understanding of whether altered sensory regulatory mechanisms may differentially contribute to pain in the various etiologic conditions associated with IDD (i.e., congenital abnormalities, spasticity, neural tube defects, muscle strain, metabolic disorders, etc.). Although imaging methods (i.e. MRI, CT Scan) may offer 'windows' to help define the nature of pain in the presence of an altered neurological substrate and may assist diagnosis in some cases, imaging findings by themselves frequently have a low correlation to pain and disability levels found upon physical evaluation. This may be because biochemical or metabolic alterations, which are frequently undetectable by current imaging, are contributing to a chronic pain state. Whether, because of the elusive nature of pain in IDD -due to problems related to self-report and cognitive, motor, and sensory impairments, or lack of a basic understanding of pain in this setting, therapeutic decisions are frequently based on trial and error, a situation frustrating to both physician and patient (and their families). To improve therapeutic outcomes and quality of life for sufferers of chronic pain associated with developmental disorders, there is an urgent clinical need to develop advanced diagnostic tools based on an expanded understanding of the mechanisms underlying chronic pain. Identification of biochemicals uniquely associated with pain in distinct IDD diagnostic subgroups is one approach that may yield objective measures (i.e. biomarkers) to distinguish etiologic mechanisms or predict therapeutic outcome in these patients.

Future Steps

This special issue reviews current knowledge and raises new topics to stimulate further discussion about, recognition of, and research into the problem of pain in individuals with IDD. Individuals with neurodevelopmental disorders do not come to us with neatly compartmentalized difficulties, but rather their problems are inextricably intertwined across traditionally distinct academic divisions. Although investigation within the disciplines of pharmacology, physiology, molecular biology, genetics, and psychology has led to remarkable advances in understanding pain, it is likely the next advances will come from the intersections of these fields. Absent from much of the dialogue is a discussion specific to what a translational research agenda might look like successfully linking the disciplines (13). In all areas of science, advances in methodology and measurement go hand in hand with advances in substantive knowledge. New technologies in studying the human brain make it possible to engage in systematic study of the neural circuitry and mechanisms underlying the complexities of the human pain experience. Despite the contributions of neuroscience to fundamental advances in research on pain, we still have little understanding of the process by which basic findings can be translated reliably and validly into interventions with measurable real world effects.

We hope that this special issue provides a platform from which to launch a critical discussion of pain in the context of IDD. Central to this process will be the task of defining the most effective use of interdisciplinary and translational research to address the problem of pain in developmental disability. Such a framework could include: a) further refining the definition of what constitutes the behavioral phenomenology of pain in the absence of verbal self-report; b) more detailed and larger scale epidemiology studies (including incidence and prevalence); c) approaches that incorporate what is currently known about pain mechanisms (at the neural level) to address the issue of whether the underlying circuitry mediating the pain signal associated with an IDD is altered; d) continued development of interventions and tests of their relative efficacy and effectiveness for a given pain problem among individuals with IDD (e.g., what evidence-based approaches should be used in a randomized trial for the treatment of chronic pain associated with spasticity among individuals with communicative impairments?) and e) given the challenges of understanding biological and behavioral signals associated with pain associated with verbal, cognitive and motor impairments, we need to explore and develop novel approaches to identifying pain-related biomarkers.

There are a number of related clinical reasons for the development and application of bio-behavioral assessment technologies built around a biomarker approach to assess pain in individuals with cognitive and communicative impairments. Such an approach would

1. Better inform a primary health care provider's diagnosis;
2. Provide guidance toward rational treatment strategies;
3. Provide a benchmark from which to evaluate treatments; and
4. Assist the identification of pain correlates thereby providing more information about the occurrence of pain and the setting in which it occurs.

A search for biomarkers of the pain experience among individuals with IDD should be guided by an understanding that pain reactivity lies on a spectrum shared by a variety of responses to all external and internal challenges to our psychological and physiological homeostasis. In this sense a search for biomarkers related to pain will require evaluation of biomarkers shared by a variety of responses to stress in general. In addition, the multitude of possible biological causes of pain makes it unlikely that a single marker for the experience of pain will be identified. In the absence of a single biomarker, there are likely to be multiple factors identified that are predictive of pain severity and type. It is known that neuropathic, inflammatory, and cancer-related pain is associated with different changes in protein expression and are differentially responsive to therapeutic agents (23). The ability to distinguish between these and other potential causes of pain in an individual with significant neurological impairment could significantly improve therapeutic outcomes.

Although interest in pain has been longstanding and the advances brought by scientific inquiry in the past 100 years have been remarkable, there has been comparatively little attention to the unique problems posed by intellectual and developmental disabilities. Contemporary research programs in pain represent a stunning example of our progress in understanding the structure of the nervous system and its function in relation to a universal human condition. In turn, a forum to discuss unmet clinical and research needs on pain in

IDD should provide a venue to organize a discussion of what we know and do not know about an under acknowledged topic in the pain field and map future policy and practice strategies that lead to improved outcomes.

Acknowledgments

This work was supported, in part, by a University of Minnesota Futures Grant from the Office of the Vice President for Research and NIH Grant No. 47201.

References

[1] Oberlander TF, Craig KD. Pain and Children with developmental disabilities. In: Schechter NM, Berde CB, Yaster M, eds. Pain in infants, children and adolescents, 2nd ed. Baltimore: Lippincott Williams Wilkins, 2003:599-619.
[2] Craig KD. Social modeling influences: pain in context. In: Sternbach RA, ed. The psychology of pain, 2nd ed. New York: Ravens Press, 1986.
[3] Gaffney A. How children describe pain: A study of words and analogies used by 5-14 year-olds. In: Dubner R, Gebhart GF, Bond MR, eds. Proceedings of the Vth World Congress on Pain. Amsterdam: Elsevier, 1988:341-7.
[4] Gaffney A, Dunne EA. Developmental aspects of children's definitions of pain. Pain 1986;26(1):105-17.
[5] Tesler M, Savendra M, Ward JA, Holzemer WL, Wilkie D. Children's language of pain. In: Dubner R, Gebhart GF, Bond MR, editors. Proceedings of the Vth World Congess on Pain. Amsterdam: Elsevier, 1988:348-52.
[6] Defrin R, Lotan M, Pick CG. The evaluation of acute pain in individuals with cognitive impairment: a differential effect of the level of impairment. Pain 2006;124(3):312-20.
[7] Abu-Saad HH. Challenge of pain in the cognitively impaired. Lancet 2000;356(9245):1867-8.
[8] Sobsey D. Pain and disability in an ethical and social context. In: Oberlander TF, Symons FJ, eds. Pain in children and adults with developmental disabilities. Baltimore, MD: Paul H Brookes, 2006: 19-39.
[9] Oberlander TF, Symons FJ, ed. Pain in children and adults with developmental disabilities. Baltimore, MD: Paul H Brookes, 2006.
[10] Ness T, Wesselmann U, Stone L, Mantyh P, Neubert J. The American Pain Society and Translational Pain Research: A Postion Statement from the American Pain Society, 2007.
[11] Mao J. Translational pain research: bridging the gap between basic and clinical research. Pain 2002;97(3):183-7.
[12] Craig KD. The construct and definition of pain in developmental disability. In: Oberlander TF, Symons FJ, eds. Pain in children and adults with developmental disabilities. Baltimore, MD: Paul H Brookes, 2006:7-18.
[13] Symons FJ, Oberlander TF. Translational research perspectives and priorities. In: Oberlander TF, Symons FJ, eds. Pain in children and adults with developmental disabilities. Baltimore, MD: Paul H Brookes, 2006:227-34.
[14] Salzinger K. Connections: a search for bridges between behavior and the nervous system. Ann N Y Acad Sci 1992;658:276-86.

[15] Bottos S, Chambers CT. The epidemiology of pain in developmental disabilities. In: Oberlander TF, Symons FJ, ed. Pain in children and adults with developmental disabilities. Baltimore, MD: Paul H Brookes, 2006.

[16] Rivard P. Acute postoperative pain control for children with chronic disabilities. Orthop Nurs 2001;20(1):17-21.

[17] Breau LM, Camfield CS, McGrath PJ, Finley GA. Pain's impact on adaptive functioning. J Intellect Disabil Res 2007;51(Pt 2):125-34.

[18] Kehl LJ, Goldetsky G. Overview of pain mechanisms: Neuroanatomical and neurophysiological processes. In: Oberlander TF, Symons FJ, ed. Pain in children and adults with developmental disabilities. Baltimore, MD: Paul H Brookes, 2006.

[19] Goldstein DB, Need AC, Singh R, Sisodiya SM. Potential genetic causes of heterogeneity of treatment effects. Am J Med 2007;120(4 Suppl 1):S21-S25.

[20] Bernard SA, Bruera E. Drug interactions in palliative care. J Clin Oncol 2000;18(8):1780-99.

[21] Taddio A, Oberlander TF. Pharmacological management of pain in children and youth with significant neurological impairments. In: Oberlander TF, Symons FJ, ed. Pain in children and adults with developmental disabilities. Baltimore, MD: Paul H Brookes, 2006:193-211.

[22] Sacchetti A, Turco T, Carraccio C, Hasher W, Cho D, Gerardi M. Procedural sedation for children with special health care needs. Pediatr Emerg Care 2003;19(4):231-9.

[23] Woolf CJ. Pain: moving from symptom control toward mechanism-specific pharmacologic management. Ann Intern Med 2004;140(6):441-51.

In: Pain Management Yearbook 2009
Editor: Joav Merrick

ISBN: 978-1-61209-666-7
©2012 Nova Science Publishers, Inc.

Chapter 4

THE TRIPTYCH OF PAIN IN ART

Gisèle Pickering[*], MD, PhD, DPharm
Clinical Pharmacology Department, Faculty of Medicine/University Hospital, Clermont-Ferrand, France

Abstract

Pain is a subjective and multidimensional phenomenon with a combination of sensory, emotional/affective and cognitive facets. This emotional component is precisely the communication link between the painter and the observer as to elicit and suggest feelings in the latter. Different techniques are developed by painters to deliver an appropriate emotion to the observer.

Introduction

The expression of human pain and suffering is a theme that is present throughout the history of painting. With a descriptive, suggestive or psychoanalytical approach, this recurrent subject of interest sheds light on man's experience of, and reaction to painful situations, both his own and those of others. Over the centuries, the expression of pain and suffering in painting has reflected the political, religious or cultural influences of the time. Pain is a subjective and multidimensional phenomenon with a combination of sensory/perceptual/discriminative, emotional/affective and cognitive domains (1). This emotional component is precisely the communication link between the painter and the observer as to elicit and suggest feelings in the latter. Observers however may experiment different chronological feelings when looking at a painting with a "pain" component. Artists have used several approaches to pass the message to the observer and these interactions in emotions may be classified in three sections.

---

[*] **Correspondence:** Gisèle Pickering, MD, PhD, DPharm, Clinical Pharmacology Department, INSERM U766, Medical Faculty, University of Auvergne, Medical Consultant, INSERM 501, University Hospital, Clermont-Ferrand, France. Tel: 33 4 73 17 84 16; E-mail: gisele.pickering@u-clermont1.fr

First, physical pain and its expression of intense human suffering may be obvious as in many paintings dealing with the crucifixion of Christ. The presence of pain is rapidly identified, easily understood with a predominant accent on the facial expression of pain: it is mainly the sensory aspect of pain that is presented.

Secondly, the painful situation may be expressed by the general atmosphere of the painting, without any obvious sign of physical pain in the painting or in the main character : this is where emotion and empathy play a part, and the skill of the artist is precisely to make us understand, guess and feel the tension and to interpret the thoughts and feelings of those portrayed. The suggestion of an emotional atmosphere in the painting will engender corresponding feelings in the observer. A number of mystical paintings follow this approach, such as in the deposition of Christ from the Cross. This is the affective/emotional aspect of pain that is suggested.

Thirdly, there may be no obvious facial and/or body expression of pain in the person depicted who however is clearly in a difficult situation of physical and psychological suffering as in Frida Kahlo's self-portrait. The cognitive capacity of the observer is then solicited and modulates the genesis of his emotion.

Along the course of these three approaches, moving from the depiction of raw physical pain to a painful, emotionally rich environment and then to a "cold" but suggestive and cognitively demanding painful situation, the implication of the observer becomes more and more dynamic and powerful and the three dimensions of pain are represented.

Raw Physical Pain

Physical pain and suffering are evident in many paintings, especially associated with mystical and religious paintings and particularly with the figure of Christ. The expression of physical pain and human suffering fill the central panel of the German artist Matthias Grünewald's multi-paneled Isenheim Altarpiece, Crucifixion (1510-1515) (see figure 1). This artist of the Gothic era has excelled in exposing the horror of suffering and visualized anatomically the agony of the dying Christ, especially in this painting that had been commissioned for the monastic hospital of Isenheim to bring support to patients suffering from skin diseases which were common at the time. His representation of Christ is far from the beautiful athletic representation of Christ found in the Renaissance time. The details of "the swollen and torn skin following flagellation, the contorted hands, the contracted feet and torn right ankle, the elongated arms dragging the crossbar of the crucifix that bends under the weight of the victim are a powerful scream of suffering". The tension involves all muscles and the top of the body is crouched on the legs as a sign of impending death.

Some artists have the skill of offering paintings full of expression of pain with the face displaying a plethora of emotions. Martyrdom, torture and mythological paintings have also been extraordinary records of disfiguring and intense human suffering. Mimetic and facial muscles are unique and the face is the predominant actor of the scene. The flaying of Marsyas (Jusepe de Ribera, 17th century) is the sinister description of Apollo's punishment because Marsyas the flautist had challenged him and lost. With his head upside down, Marsyas shows a pain expression which is obvious in what appears as a cry of terror and pain with a skinned right leg and an impassive Apollo. Likewise, but much more static, Gerard David in "le juge venal écorché vif (1498/99)", where the judge Sisamne was skinned alive on the order of the king Cambyse, the tension of the face of the martyr, his clenched hand on the ropes that attach him to the leg of the anatomy table show the crude pain of an individual surrounded by indifferent people. Closer to our time, in Pablo Picasso, Weeping woman (1937), the tears of Dora Maar, Picasso's mistress, her contorted mouth, the greyish handkerchief, the power of bright, bitter and primary colours all accentuate the sorrow and pain. Representation of emotions is quite a challenge for the artist to achieve an impact on the observer. Researchers have been and are interested in the management of this emotional load. Duchenne de Boulogne, a French clinician of the 19th century often noted by Darwin in "The expression of emotions in man and in animals" explored deeply the human face with localised electric current. Specific muscles have the possibility to express a specific emotion such as the eyebrow for pain, and his research helped artists with the expression of emotions.

The face has been the centre of attention for researchers who have focused on the association of actions and pain (2). They have shown that four actions showed evidence of a consistent association with pain: brow lowering, tightening and closing of the eyelids and nose wrinkling/upper lip raising. The " Laokoon's brow" named after the sculpture "the Laokoon's Group" discovered in Rome in 1506 is characterised by a brow line that is exaggerated in painful or tragic situations and is well illustrated in figures of Memling (15th century) in "the Last Judgement".

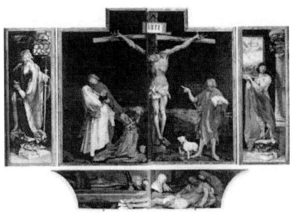

Figure 1. Isenheim Altarpiece by Matthias Grünwald.

The American Geriatrics Society Guidelines for Persistent Pain in Older persons have also identified facial expressions (grimacing, frowning, tightened eyes) as indicators of pain and these are used routinely in pain evaluation of individuals with cognition disorders.

Experimental pain provoked in the laboratory by cold pressure exposure (3) showed that these facial reactions were most salient at onset of pain, indicating blends of startled adaptive reaction, emotional expression, and pain, but they declined in intensity over time, although self-report of pain continued to mount. The relation between subjective distress and facial expression was greatest at the beginning of noxious stimulation, as a sign of acute rather than chronic, long-standing pain. It is precisely the instantaneous acute pain report of these paintings that makes them so powerful.

Over the last ten years, imaging has suggested how emotion and pain share common anatomical networks and has underlined the emotional component in pain. Recent neuroimaging and neuropsychological work has begun to shed light on how the brain responds to the viewing of facial expressions of emotion (4). Facial expressions of pain were found to engage cortical areas also engaged by one's own experience of pain, including anterior cingulate cortex and insula. A number of studies lend support to the idea that common neural substrates are involved in representing one's own and others' affective states. Therefore, considering the representation of the sensory/perceptual/discriminative of raw pain triggers these pathways in the observer for the genesis of a feeling.

Emotion and Empathy

In many paintings, the harrowing intensity of pain is brought about not only by the central figure of the painting but by the empathy and the grief of the traumatized relatives, friends or witnesses that are present. Among great episodes of the story of Christ, the Crucifixion and Deposition of Christ have inspired many artists, and empathy to pain gives power to the painting. Painters have worked on physical and facial expressions to emphasize the horror and tension of the situation.

In Grünewald's Small Crucifixion (1511/20), the figure of Christ takes most of the space, with Mary standing upright; in the later version of this painting, Crucifixion, more space has been allocated to other people, especially Mary. She is dramatically pale in her white gown, as white as a sheet, collapses into herself, eyes closed, back arched, hands joined and clutched together, her whole body swirled by intense suffering and giving up in face of the traumatic vision of her dying son. In Rogier van der Weyden's (1435), "Christ and her Mother echo the same position : He falls from the cross physically dead; she falls to the ground emotionally dead".

It is the same in the Deposition Borghese of Raphael (1507-1509) with Mater Dolorosa and the saintly women surrounding her. In the hands of this great Italian artist, the removal of Christ's body from the Cross is a moment of intense drama and pain. Painters have explored the degrees of suffering, grief and emotion to express pain. St John in despair and flinging back his arms in Giotto's (1304-1313) is stoic and grave in Crucifixion and in Roger van der Weyden's Deposition. In this painting as in Master of the Avignon's Pieta (1470) (see figure 2), a painting of an unknown painter of the south of France there is a poignant distress in the faces and attitudes. This intense relationship between on the one hand the friends/family and the sufferer or on the other hand between the spectators, ourselves, and the personages of the painting can be ascribed to empathy.

Various definitions of empathy have been given ranging from not only an affective response to another person but also the cognitive capacity to take the perspective of the other person while keeping one's self and the other' differentiated (5).

It is obvious in the paintings that emotional arousal comes from this connection between self and other. A number of studies have shown the occurrence in newborn babies of imitations of body attitudes and also of emotional expressions (6). Abundant literature in the domain of perception and action has supported the notion of automatic mapping between self and other, with an automatic activation of one's own representations of a given behaviour (7). It has also been shown that mirror neurons in monkeys in the ventral premotor and posterior parietal cortices fire both during action and observation of action in others (8).

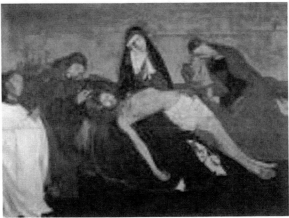
Figure 2. Master of Avignon's Pieta.

Decoding the Presence of Pain

The communication of pain requires a sufferer to encode and transmit the experience and an observer to decode and interpret it (9). In some paintings however pain expression and facial clues of any suffering are totally absent while the body wears the stigmata of dramatic physical or mental trauma. This discrepancy between the lack of pain expression on the painting and the feelings this very painting will generate in the observer involves a very dynamic interpretative effort on the part of the spectator. Factual trauma, potential pain, absent emotions : the observer may decipher (or not) the presence, the intensity of pain and the feelings of the impassive sufferer.

One of the best examples of this situation is represented by Frida Kahlo and her broken column in her painting called "The broken column", 1944 (see figure 3). No expression of pain, a placid face but a torn body. The observer will have his own interpretation in the light of his past experience and of his cultural background.

A number of studies have focused on pain judgment and showed how observers with a positive family history of chronic pain attributed greater pain to the patients than those with a negative family history of chronic pain. They also demonstrated how professionals' pain judgements are lower than those of subjects in the control group (10). Memory of our own pain is not very reliable despite the fact that we might have been fully immersed in it (11) and Singer et al (12) suggested it does not involve the entire "pain matrix", only the affective and not the sensory components of pain. Jackson et al (13) opened a window into the neural processes involved in empathy and showed that there is a partial cerebral commonality between perceiving pain in another individual and experiencing it oneself. They showed subjects a series of still photographs of hands and feet in situations that are likely to cause pain, and a matched set of control photographs without any painful events.

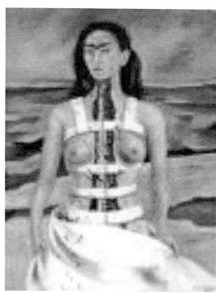

Figure 3. Frida Kahlo «The broken column».

The results of the tests demonstrated that perceiving and assessing painful situations in others was associated with significant bilateral changes in activity in several brain regions (the anterior cingulate, the anterior insula, the cerebellum, and to a lesser extent the thalamus), regions known to play a significant role in pain processing. Finally, the activity in the anterior cingulate cortex was strongly correlated with the participants' ratings of the others' pain, suggesting that the activity of this brain region is modulated according to subjects' reactivity to the pain of others. Interestingly, cognition has been shown to have a major role in the control of emotions (14) and it is possible to cognitively change the meaning of emotionally evoked stimuli. These observations may explain our large inter-individual variability when considering "painful" artistic productions.

Conclusion

In the context of the observation of a painting that depicts an obvious or hidden painful situation, the observer displays multiple reactions, from pure indifference to intense emotion ; the artist uses different techniques to let the message get through, from shocking representation to subtly suggested pain. Many parameters hence are at work to elicit the budding of an emotion in the observer, but, when progressing in the three domains of pain, sensory/discriminative, emotional/affective and cognitive, we note that a larger dynamic involvement of the observer becomes required, with an enhanced cognition for his understanding of the art piece. Thence, our first appreciation of a "painful" painting may be quite different from the secondary or further feeling we experiment because of the ping-pong game of emotion, empathy, cognition and new emotions that are solicited and that contribute to build up our judgement.

References

[1] Melzack R. From the gate to the neuromatrix. Pain 1999;Suppl 6:S121-6.
[2] Prkachin KM. The consistency of facial expressions of pain: a comparison across modalities. Pain 1992;51(3):297-306.
[3] Craig KD, Patrick CJ. Facial expression during induced pain. J Pers Soc Psychol 1985;48(4):1080-91.
[4] Botvinick M, Jha AP, Bylsma LM, Fabian SA, Solomon PE, Prkachin KM. Viewing facial expressions of pain engages cortical areas involved in the direct experience of pain. Neuroimage 2005;25(1):312-9.
[5] Batson CD, Batson JG, Slingsby JK, Harrell KL, Peekna HM, Todd RM. Empathic joy and the empathy-altruism hypothesis. J Pers Soc Psychol 1991;61(3):413-26.
[6] Meltzoff AN, Decety J. What imitation tells us about social cognition: a rapprochement between developmental psychology and cognitive neuroscience. Philos Trans R Soc Lond B Biol Sci 2003;358(1431):491-500.
[7] Preston SD, de Waal FB. Empathy: Its ultimate and proximate bases. Behav Brain Sci 2002;25(1):1-71.
[8] Rizzolatti G, Fogassi L, Gallese V. Mirrors of the mind. Sci Am 2006;295(5):54-61.
[9] Prkachin KM, Berzins S, Mercer SR. Encoding and decoding of pain expressions: A judgement study. Pain 1994;58(2):253-9.
[10] Prkachin KM, Solomon P, Hwang T, Mercer SR. Does experience influence judgments of pain behaviour? Evidence from relatives of pain patients and therapists. Pain Res Manag 2001;6(2):105-12.
[11] Rainville P, Doucet JC, Fortin MC, Duncan GH. Rapid deterioration of pain sensory-discriminative information in short-term memory. Pain 2004;110(3):605-1.
[12] Singer T, Seymour B, O'Doherty J, Kaube H, Dolan RJ, Frith CD. Empathy for pain involves the affective but not sensory components of pain. Science 2004;303 (5661):1157-62.
[13] Jackson PL, Meltzoff AN, Decety J. How do we perceive the pain of others? A window into the neural processes involved in empathy. Neuroimage 2005;24 (3):771-9.
[14] Ochsner KN and Gross JJ. The cognitive control of emotion. Tr Cogn Sc 2006; :242-9.

Chapter 5

PILOT STUDY OF THE FEASIBILITY OF THE NON-COMMUNICATING CHILDREN'S PAIN CHECKLIST REVISED FOR PAIN ASSESSMENT FOR ADULTS WITH INTELLECTUAL DISABILITIES

Chantel Burkitt[1], Lynn M Breau[*2], PhD., R Psych,
Shoneth Salsman[3], BSc(Pharm), PhC,
Tracie Sarsfield- Turner[4], BA, BSW, CGN, RSW
and Robert Mullan[5], MD*

[1]Department of Psychology, Saint Mary's University
[2]School of Nursing, Dalhousie University, Halifax, Nova, Scotia, Canada
[3]Pharmacist, Kings Regional Rehabilitation Centre
[4]Social Worker, Kings Regional Rehabilitation Centre
[5]Medical Director, Kings Regional Rehabilitation Centre, Waterville, Nova Scotia, Canada

Abstract

It is suspected that those with intellectual disabilities (ID) experience more pain, more frequently then the general population, yet there are currently no well-validated measures for pain assessment in adults with ID. This research aimed to respond to this need by validating the Non-Communicating Children's Pain Checklist - Revised (NCCPC-R) for use with adults with ID during chronic or recurrent pain. Staff at a regional residential facility observed participants ($N = 16$) during two conditions (pain; no-pain) for 5-minute periods. The two staff independently completed both the NCCPC-R and a 10 cm visual analogue scale (VAS) of pain. Analyses indicated 6 of the 30 items should be removed from the NCCPC-R. Internal consistency (Cronbach's alpha = .86), inter-rater reliability (ICC = .83) and

---

* **Correspondence:** Lynn Breau, Dalhousie University School of Nursing, 5869 University Ave, Halifax, Nova Scotia, B3H 3J5 Canada. E-mail: lbreau@dal.ca

construct validity ($t(15) = 7.03$ $p < .001$) of a new 24-item scale indicate good psychometric properties. A cut-off score of 10 provided 94% sensitivity and 87% specificity for pain. Our results indicated revisions should be made to the NCCPC-R to improve psychometric properties when used for chronic or recurrent pain in adults with ID. Our new scale, which we have called the Chronic Pain Scale for Nonverbal Adults with Intellectual Disabilities (CPS-NAID), displays good psychometric properties in this pilot study. Future studies should include both the NCCPC-R and the CPS-NAID to confirm the results we found here.

Keywords: chronic pain, pain assessment, intellectual disability, mental retardation.

Introduction

Accurate assessment is the first and most vital step towards effective pain management. This is an ongoing challenge for those with intellectual disabilities (ID), where pain is more difficult to assess because of limited communication. Assessment challenges also arise due to behaviour problems and inconsistencies often associated with the intellectual disability. This may be further complicated when adults with ID demonstrate behaviours thought to reflect pain (e.g. agitation or facial changes) when no pain is occurring. Thus, self-report assessment tools used with typical adults may not be feasible for use by those with these limitations and caregiver estimates may also be inaccurate due to behavioural idiosyncrasies.

Pain in Adults with Intellectual Disabilities

The lack of validated tools for assessing pain in people with ID is particularly troublesome because this group appears to experience a great deal of pain. Research indicates people with ID are more likely to have medical problems than the general population of adults and that many of these conditions are associated with pain. In an early study, Minihan (1) found that 99% of residents in a New York State facility had at least one chronic medical condition that required continued monitoring. More recently, a population study by a group in Australia revealed that people with mental retardation had an average of 5.4 medical conditions each (2). For many people with ID, their medical conditions result in pain. For example, Cooper et al. report that 5.5% of residents of institutions in the UK they studied who were under age 65 had arthritis, 9.6% had an orthopedic problem, 2.7% ulcers, and 16.4% a gastrointestinal disorder (3).

Specific medical problems that can cause pain have also been studied. It has been reported that 75% of women with Down Syndrome have menstrual pain, compared to 50% in the general population (4). Cerebral palsy is a common diagnosis for those with ID, and as many as 67% of those with cerebral palsy report chronic pain (5). High rates of fractures (6) and injuries (7) are also reported, as are greater rates of dental problems (8) and respiratory infections (9). Thus, evidence increasingly suggests that this population has a higher incidence of both medical conditions in general and painful medical conditions specifically.

Pain Assessment for Adults with Intellectual Disabilities

There is currently no well-validated observational assessment tool specifically designed to measure pain in adults with ID. Data to support the psychometrics of the Pain and Discomfort Scale (PADS) are presented in a study of pain during a dental scaling procedure (10). The PADS was developed from the Non-communicating Children's Pain Checklist – Revised (NCCPC-R; (11) for use during a physical examination. Thirteen items from the NCCPC-R were removed and one item added. The results of the dental study indicated good inter-rater reliability and sensitivity, but the design did not allow for examination of specificity, item analysis or development of cut-off scores. Given that dental scaling reflects only mild procedural pain, these results are insufficient to support use of the PADS for general use with adults with ID at this time.

The NCCPC-R has previously been used to assess pain during vaccination in adults (12). These researchers found that NCCPC-R scores did increase significantly during injection. However this study did not include item analyses. More recently, Lotan and colleagues conducted a large-scale study of the NCCPC-R for vaccination pain in 228 adults with ID (Lotan, Ljunggren, Johnsen, Defrin, Pick and Strand, submitted). They concluded that removal of nine items was necessary, based on item analyses, for this type of acute pain situation. Although these results do provide preliminary evidence of good psychometrics of the NCCPC-R, vaccination pain differs from chronic pain in frequency, intensity and duration. The pain of vaccination is generally rated as very mild by those experiencing it. Further, it may last only seconds which may not be sufficient for an individual to display some of the behaviours described in the NCCPC-R or for observers to detect fleeting displays of these behaviours. The NCCPC-R has not been used to evaluate injection pain in children and it is very possible that major changes to the scale, such as those recommended by Lotan et al., are needed to make it valid and reliable for this particular type of pain in adults with ID.

The purpose of this pilot study was to provide preliminary support for a program of research aimed at improving chronic pain assessment for this population. The hope is that improved assessment will lead to better pain management in this vulnerable group who are often not able to reliably communicate to caregivers that they have pain. The first step towards this development is determining whether an observational pain tool that was designed for children with ID, the Non-Communicating Children's Pain Checklist - Revised (NCCPC-R; (13)) can be used for adults with intellectual disabilities in a residential care centre. The pain behaviour of typical children and adults may differ for many reasons (14), suggesting these differences may also exist between children and adults with ID. Thus, several aspects of the NCCPC-R, when used to assess chronic or recurrent pain in adults, were evaluated.

A sound pain assessment tool must be both valid and reliable. A valid tool specifically measures the desired construct and nothing else. In the case of pain, that means ensuring that the tool measures pain, not anxiety or distress or illness. Validity is tested by comparing the scores from a tool to other measures of pain taken at the same time, either by other observers or from the individual who has pain in the form of self-report. It can also be determined by comparing scores during pain to those when pain is absent. A reliable tool provides the same score each time it is used or when used by different people. Pain assessment tools should provide consistently low scores when people do not have pain and consistently higher scores when they do have pain. If the tool is designed for use by multiple observers, then scores from these should not differ substantially. Validity and reliability are context-dependent; they may vary due to the setting (e.g. hospital or home), the person completing the tool (caregiver or family member), the type of pain and context of pain (e.g. chronic pain versus acute procedural pain) and the person who has pain (adult versus child, intellectual disability alone versus intellectual and physical disabilities). This means research must be conducted to evaluate a tool's validity and reliability in numerous contexts before it can be considered valid and reliable for general use. Until that time, it should only be considered sound in those circumstances in which it was tested, or very similar ones.

This study examined these important psychometric constructs by evaluating NCCPC-R scores derived from 5-minute observations of two staff members who watched an individual with ID residing in a residential centre when he/she did and did not have pain. In addition, analyses were conducted to examine whether removal of items from the NCCPC-R would improve validity or reliability. For example, items from the Eating/Sleeping Subscale of the tool can be more difficult to evaluate in a short time period. Thus, analyses were conducted to learn whether this subscale could be omitted without negatively affecting the psychometrics of the scale. Finally, analyses were conducted to determine cut-off scores for pain. This pilot study is a necessary step towards building an evidence base for use of this tool for adults. The NCCPC-R is commonly used clinically for children with ID who are 18 years or under. However, at this time, it is not known whether it has sufficient psychometric qualities to recommend it for use with adults.

Methods

Participants

Residents of the Kings Regional Rehabilitation Centre (KRRC) in Waterville, Nova Scotia, Canada were invited to take part in this pilot study. The KRRC provides services to 197 residents in the Centre itself, in small-options homes, supervised apartments and other community programs. Approximately 50% of the residents are considered nonverbal meaning that they typically produce utterances of two-words or less.

This study was approved by the Dalhousie University Research Ethics Board and the KRRC Ethics Board. Few residents of KRRC are capable of providing informed consent or assent. Thus, consent was obtained from the 17 participants' next of kin. Potential participants were selected based on a review of their health records and discussion with staff to ascertain which residents met the criteria for participation. Participants were selected if they resided at KRRC or in one of the community homes associated with the Centre, were suspected of having chronic or recurrent pain, and their ability to communicate verbally did not exceed two-word utterances.

Measures

Information from the participants' health records was collected. This included the participants' age, gender, etiology of intellectual disability and known medical conditions that could cause pain (e.g. arthritis, constipation). One staff person, who was familiar with each resident, completed the Vineland-II Adaptive Behaviour Scales (15) to provide an indication of that resident's functional level. The Vineland II provides age equivalents for functioning in the following areas: communication, daily living skills, socialization, and motor skills.

The NCCPC-R was scored for 5-minute observations. Items received a rating of 'not at all' (0), 'just a little' (1), 'fairly often' (2), or 'very often' (3). Items which were scored as 'not applicable' by an observer were given a value of '0'. This procedure is standard practice when using the NCCPC-R with children (11). This scoring allowed participants to receive a score ranging from 0-90 for the 5-minute observation. The subscale scores were totaled for each of the seven subscales (Vocal, Social, Facial, Activity, Body/Limb, Physiological Signs, and Eating/Sleeping). A total score was also computed. Previous research has employed a 2-hour observation for the NCCPC-R, a 10-minute observation period has proven sufficient to produce good psychometrics in the version of the scale designed for postoperative use (NCCPC-PV; (16). However, a decision was made to use a 5-minute observation here because it would enhance feasibility of the scale. This was based on new evidence that a 5-minute observation may be sufficient for children (17).

A visual analogue scale (VAS) of pain was completed for each 5-minute observation by both observers independently. This scale consisted of a 10-cm line with the left end anchored by "no pain at all" and the right end anchored by "worst pain ever". When scoring this scale the number of millimeters from the left was recorded providing a possible score from 0-100.

Procedure

Two KRRC staff who were involved in each participant's care watched the individual simultaneously. Observation periods were selected based on the staffs' judgment that the resident did or did not have pain based on their previous experience caring for that individual. The two staff members chose a 5-minute period during which they determined the resident was not experiencing pain (no-pain condition). They watched the participant for this 5-minute period without interacting with each other or the participant. The two staff then completed the NCCPC-R and independently rated the participant's pain on the 10-cm VAS of pain. This procedure, using both the NCCPC-R and the visual analogue scale, was repeated during another 5-minute period during which the staff members believed the resident was experiencing pain (pain condition). Due to the logistics of completing the observations in a residential centre with 24 hour care, the observers for the pain condition and the no-pain condition were generally not the same for each participant.

Statistical Analysis

Data was collected for 17 participants. However, one participant's scores were removed from analysis due to having more than 10% of scores for the NCCPC-R missing. Examining the data once the one participant was excluded revealed that the remainder of the data ($N=16$) included only .002% uncompleted scores. For those scores which were left blank (.002 % in the pain condition and .002% in the no-pain condition) the mean of the scores for that item for the respective condition (pain or no-pain) was used to replace the missing score.

Data analysis was conducted using SPSS for Windows version 15.0.1(18). Power analyses were conducted for the Repeated Measures Analysis of Variance (RM ANOVA) using tables prepared by Stevens (19). Alpha level was set at .05 with Bonferroni corrections applied to maintain alpha for sets of analyses at .05. Scores for the NCCPC-R were computed using the original scale (30 items/7 subscales) then recalculated when items were removed. For each observation one rater of the two was randomly chosen as the primary rater. All analyses are conducted on scores from this primary rater with the exception of inter-rater reliability analyses which required use of scores from the two raters. In one case the secondary rater's data was used because the primary rater failed to record the time and date of the observation.

Analyses were conducted to determine whether subscales and or items should be removed to improve psychometrics. A repeated measures analyses of variance (RM ANOVA) was conducted on the original NCCPC-R (30 items) to explore the sensitivity of the overall scale to pain and to determine if differences in scores between pain and no-pain conditions varied due to subscale. This was followed by post hoc paired samples t-tests to examine the difference between pain and no-pain scores for individual subscales. After removal of 6 items, a paired samples t-test was used to determine if total scores remained sensitive to pain.

Cronbach's alpha was used to assess the internal consistency of the scale; calculations first used all 30 items (7 subscales). Corrected item-total correlations were examined to determine whether items should be removed from the scale. Cronbach's alpha was recalculated after items were deleted.

After selection of items for the final scale was complete, additional analyses were conducted to further examine the psychometric properties of the scale. Construct validity was measured by computing a paired samples t-test comparing the scores for the pain condition to those for the no-pain condition. Concurrent validity was tested by generating a Pearson correlation between the total revised pain scale score and the VAS pain total score during the pain condition. Inter-rater reliability was determined by conducting an Intraclass Correlation Coefficient (ICC). Because rater pairs varied by participant, a one way random model was chosen. A Receiver Operating Characteristic (ROC) curve was then generated to determine potential cut off scores for pain with the final version of the scale. Sensitivity and specificity were also determined.

Results

Demographic Information

The mean chronological age of participants at the time of data collection was 43 years and 6.6 months ($SD = 12.3$ months). Participants included 9 males and 7 females, all of whom have significant functional limitations as displayed by the age equivalents generated for them with the Vineland-II Adaptive Behaviour Scales. Participant's mean age equivalent for 'communication' was 3 years, 7.4 months ($SD = 27.5$ months), 'daily living skills' was 3 years, 1 month ($SD = 49.2$ months), 'socialization' was 1 year, 5.3 months ($SD = 20.8$ months), and 'motor skills' was 1 year, 4.7 months ($SD = 18.7$ months). The etiologies of the intellectual disability as well as the known painful medical conditions abstracted from health records of each participant are displayed in Table 1.

Table 1. Etiology of intellectual disability and known painful medical conditions ($N = 16$)

Participant	Etiology of Intellectual Disability	Chronic Painful Medical Conditions
1	Down's Syndrome	Scoliosis, dysmenorrhea, constipation
2	Perinatal Complications	Constipation, seizures, paraplegia
3	Unknown	Congenital hip displacement, osteoporosis, self-injury, constipation
4	Unknown	Constipation, seizures, cerebral palsy, spastic quadriplegia, scoliosis
5	Unknown	Spastic quadriplegia, dysmenorrhea, constipation
6	Unknown	Cerebral palsy, self-injury, constipation, gastroesophegeal reflux
7	Unknown	Scoliosis, seizures, dysmenorrhea
8	Unknown	Leg contractions, hips dislocated, scoliosis
9	Unknown	Constipation, poor circulation lower extremities, spasticity
10	Unknown	Self injury, deformed feet
11	Down's Syndrome	None listed
12	Chromosomal Abnormality	Constipation, dysmenorrhea
13	Traumatic Brain Injury	Osteoporosis – previous fracture, contractures, spasticity, dysmenorrhea
14	Down's Syndrome	Deformed feet, arthritis, constipation
15	Autism	Constipation, headaches, upset stomach
16	Extreme Prematurity	Scoliosis, cerebral palsy, gastroesphegeal reflux, contractures

Descriptive Statistics

Mean item scores and the proportion of participants displaying each item during pain and no-pain conditions are depicted in Table 2. Mean subscale scores and total scores for the NCCPC-R for both pain and no-pain conditions are depicted in Table 3. Mean VAS pain scores for the pain condition ($M = 54.81$, $SD = 21.64$) were significantly higher than those for the no-pain condition ($M = 3.31$, $SD = 4.87$; $t(15) = 9.58$, $p < .001$).

Psychometric properties of the original NCCPC-R

Construct Validity

A paired samples t-test revealed total scores differed between the pain and no-pain conditions ($t(15) = 7.76$, $p < .001$). A RM ANOVA of the seven subscales also resulted in significant effects for Time ($F(1, 15) = 60.26$, $p < .001$), Subscale ($F(3.65, 54.75) = 19.06$, $p < .001$), and the Time by Subscale interaction ($F(3.65, 54.74) = 6.74$, $p < .001$). This indicates that overall, NCCPC-R scores differed between pain and no-pain conditions. However, the interaction indicates that the differences between pain and no-pain varied by subscale. A RM ANOVA using 6 subscales (excluding the Eating/Sleeping subscale) resulted in significant effects for Time ($F(1, 15) = 58.01$, $p < .001$), Subscale ($F(3.67, 55.07) = 16.35$, $p < .001$) and the Time by Subscale interaction ($F(3.50, 52.52) = 4.76$, $p = .003$). Paired samples t-tests of the subscales indicated that, after Bonferroni corrections, the difference between pain and no-pain scores were significant for all subscales except the Eating/Sleeping Subscale ($p = .03$). Thus, the Eating/Sleeping subscale was not sensitive to pain. A second paired samples t-test of total scores for these 27 items (6 subscales, excluding the Eating/Sleeping subscale) revealed total scores continued to differ significantly between pain ($M = 31.13$, $SD = 13.54$) and no-pain conditions ($M = 4.69$, SD 5.17; $t(15) = 7.62$, $p < .001$).

Internal Consistency

Cronbach's alpha revealed that the internal consistency of the scale when all 7 subscales were included ($\alpha = .81$) was increased by removal of the Eating/Sleeping subscale ($\alpha = .82$). Item-total correlations were also examined to evaluate the relation of items to total scores (Table 2). These ranged from -.39 to .61 for the 7 subscale version. However, this was improved when only items from 6 subscales (excluding the Eating/Sleeping subscale) were included, ranging from -.34 to .67.

The lowest item-total correlations for this latter version were -.34 for "jumping around", -.06 for "screaming" and .04 for the "floppy".

Due to their negative item-total correlations suggesting they were negatively related to pain, "screaming" and "jumping around" were removed. The item "floppy" ($r = .04$) was only slightly positively correlated and the frequency of individuals displaying the item during the pain condition was identical to that of individuals showing it during the no-pain condition. Thus, this item was also removed. With these items removed it was decided that the division of items into subscales would no longer be useful because they are not used clinically. Therefore no further analyses of subscale scores were computed.

Because the tests of sensitivity and internal consistency indicated removal of 6 items from the original scale, we repeated the analysis of construct validity with the remaining 24 items. Further analyses of the concurrent validity and inter-rater reliability of scale totals were then computed using the 24-item version. Mean total scores for this version are displayed in Table 3.

Table 2. Statistics for NCCPC-R Items during Pain and No-pain Conditions (*N*=16)

NCCPC-R Item	Mean (SD) Pain Condition	Mean (SD) No-pain Condition	% Displaying Pain Condition	% Displaying No-pain Condition	Item Total Correlation during Pain 30 Items	27 Items	24 Items
Vocal Subscale							
Moaning, whining, whimpering (fairly soft)	1.31 (1.14)	.50 (.89)	63	31	.51	.48	.52
Crying (moderately loud)	1.50 (1.32)	.06 (.25)	63	6	.43	.44	.50
Screaming/yelling (very loud)	0.81 (1.05)	.13 (.50)	50	6	-.10	-.06	-
A specific sound or word for pain (e.g. a word, cry or type of laugh)	1.25 (1.39)	.00 (.00)	50	0	.44	.36	.40
Social Subscale							
Not cooperating, cranky, irritable, unhappy	1.69 (1.40)	.44 (.89)	69	25	.58	.64	.64
Less interaction with others, withdrawn	0.94 (1.12)	.00 (.00)	50	0	.57	.60	.56
Seeking comfort or physical closeness	1.00 (1.21)	.00 (.00)	50	0	.58	.61	.65
Being difficult to distract, not able to satisfy or pacify	1.50 (1.37)	.19 (.54)	63	13	.61	.67	.66
Facial Subscale							
A furrowed brow	2.19 (1.11)	.38 (.81)	88	25	.61	.59	.55
A change in eyes, including: squinching of eyes, eyes opened wide, eyes frowning	2.56 (.73)	.38 (.81)	100	25	.52	.54	.50
Turning down of mouth, not smiling	2.19 (1.11)	.81 (.83)	88	63	.46	.53	.46
Lips puckering up, tight, pouting, or quivering	1.13 (1.26)	.38 (.89)	50	19	.54	.55	.61
Clenching or grinding of teeth, chewing or thrusting tongue out	1.38 (1.46)	.31 (.79)	50	19	.29	.28	.22
Activity Subscale							
Not moving, less active, quiet	0.56 (1.09)	.00 (.00)	25	0	.21	.11	.18
Jumping around, agitated, fidgety	1.13 (1.26)	.19 (.40)	50	19	-.39	-.34	-

Table 2. (Continued)

NCCPC-R Item	Mean (SD) Pain Condition	Mean (SD) No-pain Condition	% of Participants Displaying Item Pain Condition	% of Participants Displaying Item No-pain Condition	Item Total Correlation during Pain 30 Items	Item Total Correlation during Pain 27 Items	Item Total Correlation during Pain 24 Items
Body/Limb Subscale							
Floppy	0.44 (0.96)	.31 (.70)	19	19	.03	.04	-
Stiff, spastic, tense, rigid	1.44 (1.26)	.38 (.50)	69	38	.33	.36	.36
Gesturing to or touching part of the body that hurts	0.44 (1.03)	.00 (.00)	19	0	.39	.40	.40
Protecting, favoring or guarding part of the body that hurts	0.31 (0.87)	.00 (.00)	13	0	.10	.08	.08
Flinching or moving the body part away, being sensitive to touch	0.75 (1.13)	.00 (.00)	38	0	.26	.23	.26
Moving the body in a specific way to show pain (e.g. head back, arms down, curls up etc)	1.38 (1.41)	.00 (.00)	57	0	.25	.21	.27
Physiological Subscale							
Shivering	0.38 (0.72)	.00 (.00)	25	0	.31	.28	.31
Change in colour, pallor	1.25 (1.34)	.00 (.00)	57	0	.56	.55	.55
Sweating, perspiring	0.63 (1.09)	.13 (.34)	31	13	.26	.21	.22
Tears	0.88 (1.26)	.00 (.00)	38	0	.38	.42	.45
Sharp intake of breath, gasping	1.25 (1.24)	.06 (.25)	56	6	.25	.23	.25
Breath holding	0.31 (0.87)	.06 (.25)	13	6	.28	.29	.32
Eating/Sleeping Subscale							
Eating less, not interested in food	0.50 (0.89)	.06 (.25)	31	6	-.01	-	-
Increase in sleep	0.31 (0.79)	.06 (.25)	19	6	.05	-	-
Decrease in sleep	0.38 (0.72)	.00 (.00)	25	0	.25	-	-

Table 3. NCCPC-R Total and Subscale Scores (*N* = 16)

NCCPC-R Score	Mean (*SD*) Pain	Mean (*SD*) No-pain	Paired Samples t-test * *t*=	*p* value
Original NCCPC-R (30 items):				
Vocal Subscale	5.00 (2.90)	0.69 (1.08)	5.43	<.001
Social Subscale	5.13 (4.41)	0.63 (1.20)	3.80	<.001
Facial Subscale	9.44 (3.61)	2.25 (3.68)	6.02	<.001
Activity Subscale	1.69 (1.20)	0.19 (.40)	5.48	<.001
Body/Limb Subscale	5.19 (3.80)	0.69 (0.70)	4.60	<.001
Physiological Signs Subscale	4.69 (3.65)	0.25 (0.45)	4.62	<.001
Eating/Sleeping Subscale	1.19 (1.80)	0.13 (0.50)	2.35	.03**
Total	32.31 (13.78)	4.81 (5.18)	7.76	<.001
27 Item Version Total	31.13 (13.54)	4.69 (5.17)	7.62	<.001
24 Item Version Total (Chronic Pain Scale for Nonverbal Adults with Intellectual Disabilities; CPS-NAID)	28.19 (13.63)	4.06 (4.45)	7.03	<.001

Note: * *df* for all t-tests = 15. ** NS.

Psychometrics of Revised Scale

Construct Validity
A paired samples t-test of the 24-item NCCPC-R revealed total scores differed between the pain and no-pain conditions (*t* (15) = 7.03, *p* < .001; Table 3).

Internal consistency
Cronbach's alpha of the new 24-item scale was α = .86. Item-total correlations (Table 2) ranged from .08 ("protects part of body") to .66 ("difficult to distract").

Concurrent validity
A significant Pearson correlation was found between total scores for the 24-item NCCPC-R and the VAS pain rating (*r* = .66, *p* = .005) during the pain condition.

Inter-Rater Reliability
An Intraclass Correlation Coefficient between the two observers of the pain condition for the 24-item NCCPC-R scores indicated a high level of agreement (*ICC* = .83).

Cut-off Scores

A Receiver Operating Characteristic (ROC) curve was generated to determine potential cut off scores for pain with the new 24-item scale. The cut off score was determined to be 10. This provided 94 % sensitivity and 87 % specificity for the presence of pain.

Discussion

These results provide preliminary evidence that revision is required to the NCCPC-R to obtain validity and reliability for assessing chronic or recurrent pain in adults with ID. Our analyses indicate that the Eating/Sleeping subscale is not sensitive to chronic pain in this group of adults. Of note, Defrin et. al. (12) also reported improved reliability of the NCCPC-R during vaccination when items of this subscale were removed. In their study observers found it difficult to judge these items during a short observation. This may be the reason for the poor performance in this current study and removal of the items may make it easier for the scale to be used by those who are unfamiliar with an individual or in situations where an observer does not have information regarding the individual's eating and sleeping over the past day or several hours. In addition, 3 items "screaming", "jumping around" and "floppy" were removed because of poor item total correlations or no variation between pain and no-pain conditions. After removal of the 6 items, this pilot suggests the new scale shows good construct and concurrent validity as well as good inter-rater reliability and internal consistency. Because items were removed from several subscales, subscales were not evaluated for the final version here because subscale scores are not used clinically but were only used to categorize items and were not based on factor analysis or other empirical evidence of co-occurrence of items.

The observation time for the pain and no-pain conditions was only five minutes in this study, decreased from previous studies which used the NCCPC-R (11) for two hours or the NCCPC-PV (13) for ten minutes. The significant results here for analyses of several aspects of the scale's psychometric properties provide evidence that the checklist can be used for this decreased time. This is especially clinically relevant as it promotes the increased usability and efficiency of the scale.

Strengths and Limitations

There are some limitations of this study that must be considered. The main limitation is the small sample size of 16 participants. However, significant results were found and the psychometric properties of the scale were good despite a heterogeneous sample with varied etiologies for their ID and diverse diagnoses of painful medical conditions. This adds to the generalizability of the results.

A major strength of this study is found in the real-life context of this project. The study was conducted in a non-experimental natural environment. Staff members familiar with the participants scored the questionnaires during conditions normally seen at the facility. The real-life quality of this study strengthens the results found.

Implications

These results indicate that the original NCCPC-R should not be used with adults with ID to assess chronic pain. Instead, this revised scale (Appendix), which we are calling the *Chronic Pain Scale for Nonverbal Adults with Intellectual Disabilities (CPS-NAID)*, appears to have more sound psychometric properties when tested with this sample. Further research should be conducted to replicate these results with larger samples and to establish the psychometric properties of the CPS-NAID in other settings and for other types of pain.

Chronic Pain Scale for Nonverbal Adults with Intellectual Disabilities (CPS-NAID)

Please indicate how often this person has shown the signs referred to in *items 1-24* in the *last 5 minutes*.
Please circle a number for each item. If an item does not apply to this person (for example, this person cannot reach with his/her hands), then indicate "not applicable" for that item

0 = Not present at all during the observation period. (Note if the item is not present because the person is not capable of performing that act, it should be scored as "NA").
1 = Seen or heard rarely (hardly at all), but is present.
2 = Seen or heard a number of times, but not continuous (not all the time).
3 = Seen or heard often, almost continuous (almost all the time); anyone would easily notice this if they saw
the person for a few moments during the observation time.
NA = Not applicable. This person is not capable of performing this action.

0= NOT AT ALL	1= JUST A LITTLE	2=FAIRLY OFTEN	3= VERY OFTEN
	NA=NOT APPLICABLE		

1. Moaning, whining, whimpering (fairly soft)	0	1	2	3	NA
2. Crying (moderately loud)	0	1	2	3	NA
3. A specific sound or word for pain (e.g., a word, cry or type of laugh)	0	1	2	3	NA
4. Not cooperating, cranky, irritable, unhappy	0	1	2	3	NA
5. Less interaction with others, withdrawn	0	1	2	3	NA
6. Seeking comfort or physical closeness	0	1	2	3	NA
7. Being difficult to distract, not able to satisfy or pacify	0	1	2	3	NA
8. A furrowed brow	0	1	2	3	NA
9. A change in eyes, including: squinching of eyes, eyes opened wide, eyes frowning	0	1	2	3	NA
10. Turning down of mouth, not smiling	0	1	2	3	NA
11. Lips puckering up, tight, pouting, or quivering	0	1	2	3	NA
12. Clenching or grinding teeth, chewing or thrusting tongue out	0	1	2	3	NA
13. Not moving, less active, quiet	0	1	2	3	NA
14. Stiff, spastic, tense, rigid	0	1	2	3	NA
15. Gesturing to or touching part of the body that hurts	0	1	2	3	NA
16. Protecting, favoring or guarding part of the body that hurts	0	1	2	3	NA
17. Flinching or moving the body part away, being sensitive to touch	0	1	2	3	NA
18. Moving the body in a specific way to show pain (e.g. head back, arms down, curls up, etc.)	0	1	2	3	NA
19. Shivering	0	1	2	3	NA
20. Change in color, pallor	0	1	2	3	NA
21. Sweating, perspiring	0	1	2	3	NA
22. Tears	0	1	2	3	NA
23. Sharp intake of breath, gasping	0	1	2	3	NA
24. Breath holding	0	1	2	3	NA

TOTAL SCORE : _____

SCORING:

1. Add up the scores for each item to compute the Total Score. Items marked "NA" are scored as "0" (zero).
2. Check whether the score is greater than the cut-off score.
    A score of 10 or greater means that there is a 94% chance that the person has pain.
    A score of 9 or lower means that there is an 87% chance that the person does not have pain.

Version 01.2008 © 2008 Breauurkitt, Burkittreau, Salsman, Sarsfield-Turner, Mullaen

Conclusion

Adults with ID experience pain more frequently than typical adults. However, their pain is frequently left untreated due to assessment difficulties, particularly in cases where the individual may have very severe communication limitations. We evaluated the psychometric properties of the NCCPC-R, a tool that has shown validity and reliability with children who have ID, with a sample of adults. Our results indicated that major revisions were required to improve the tool's psychometrics. To this end, we propose a new scale, called the CPS-NAID, based on the NCCPC-R which is more suitable for adults. Evidence of a tool's psychometric properties is cumulative, suggesting that further research is needed to verify the superior psychometrics of this new scale. Thus, future studies should be conducted that include both the NCCPC-R and the CPS-NAID to confirm the results we found here.

Acknowledgments

The authors wish to acknowledge the assistance of the staff at the Kings Regional Rehabilitation Centre, including Betty Mattson, Chief Executive Officer, and Darren Shupe for assistance with organizing this project. This project was the result of a Nova Scotia Health Research Foundation Research Capacity Award to Dr. Lynn Breau. Chantel Burkitt was supported by a Summer Studentship from the Nova Scotia Cooperative Employment Program. Lynn Breau is supported by a New Investigator Award from the Canadian Institutes of Health Research.

References

[1] Minihan PM. Planning for community physician services prior to deinstitutionalization of mentally retarded persons. Am J Public Health 1986;76(10):1202-6.
[2] Beange H, McElduff A, Baker W. Medical disorders of adults with mental retardation: a population study. Am J Ment Retard 1995;99(6):595-604.
[3] Cooper SA. Clinical study of the effects of age on the physical health of adults with mental retardation. Am J Ment Retard 1998;102(6):582-9.

[4] Kyrkou M. Health issues and quality of life in women with intellectual disability. J Intellect Disabil Res 2005;49(Pt 10):770-2.
[5] Schwartz L, Engel JM, Jensen MP. Pain in persons with cerebral palsy. Arch Phys Med Rehabil 1999;80(10):1243-6.
[6] Glick NR, Fischer MH, Heisey DM, Leverson GE, Mann DC. Epidemiology of fractures in people with severe and profound developmental disabilities. Osteoporos Int 2005;16(4):389-96.
[7] Loebl D, Willems B, Nordin M. Database analysis of injury patterns in an institution for developmental disabilities. J Occup Rehabil 1995;5(3):169-84.
[8] Cumella S, Ransford N, Lyons J, Burnham H. Needs for oral care among people with intellectual disability not in contact with Community Dental Services. J Intellect Disabil Res 2000;44(1):45-52.
[9] Chaney RH, Eyman RK. Patterns in mortality over 60 years among persons with mental retardation in a residential facility. Ment Retard 2000; 38(3):289-93.
[10] Phan A, Edwards CL, Robinson EL. The assessment of pain and discomfort in individuals with mental retardation. Res Dev Disabil 2005;26(5):433-9..
[11] Breau LM, McGrath PJ, Camfield CS, Finley GA. Psychometric properties of the non-communicating children's pain checklist-revised. Pain 2002; 99(1-2):349-57.
[12] Defrin R, Lotan M, Pick CG. The evaluation of acute pain in individuals with cognitive impairment: A differential effect of the level of impairment. Pain 2006;124:312-20.
[13] Breau LM, Finley GA, McGrath PJ, Camfield CS. Validation of the non-communicating children's pain checklist postoperative version. Anesthesiology 2002;96(3):528-35.
[14] McGrath PA. Pain in children: Nature, assessment and treatment. New York: Guilford, 1990.
[15] Sparrow SS, Cicchetti DV, Balla DA. Vineland-II Adaptive Behavior Scales. Circle Pines, MN: American Guidance Service, 2005.
[16] Breau LM, Finley GA, McGrath PJ, Camfield CS. Validation of the Non-communicating Children's Pain Checklist-Postoperative Version. Anesthesiology 2002;96(3):528-35.
[17] Breau G, Grégoire MC, Breau LM, Wood C, Zabalia M, Lévêque C. Validation in French of "La Grille de la Douleur Des Personnes Avec Des Déficience Intellectuelles". Pain Res Manage 2005;10(2):106.
[18] SPSS. Chicago: SPSS Inc., 2006.
[19] Stevens J. Applied multivariate statistics for the social sciences, 3rd ed. Mahwah, NJ: Lawrence Erlbaum, 1996.

Chapter 6

FACIAL EXPRESSION OF PAIN IN CHILDREN WITH INTELLECTUAL DISABILITIES FOLLOWING SURGERY

Lynn M Breau, PhD, R. Psych[*1], *G Allen Finley, MD, FRCPC*[2], *Carol S Camfield, MD, FRCPC*[3] *and Patrick J McGrath, OC, PhD, FRSC*[4]

[1]School of Nursing, and Departments of Pediatrics and Psychology, Dalhousie University and Complex Pain Team and Division of Child Neurology, IWK Health Centre
[2]Departments of Anaesthesia and Psychology, Dalhousie University and Pediatric Pain Service and Department of Paediatric Anaesthesia, IWK Health Centre
[3]Department of Pediatrics and Psychology, Dalhousie University and Division of Child Neurology, IWK Health Centre
[4]VP Research, IWK Health Centre and Departments of Psychology, Pediatrics and Psychiatry, Dalhousie University; Halifax, Nova Scotia, Canada

Abstract

Many children with intellectual disabilities cannot provide reports of their pain postoperatively and behavioural measures that have been developed to date may not be appropriate for all of these children. This study examines the Child Facial Coding System (CFCS), a detailed measure of facial reaction to pain to determine whether it has potential to measure postoperative pain in children with intellectual disabilities. 26 children were filmed for up to 60 minutes while in the post-anesthesia care unit (PACU) following surgery. Videotape was divided into five 10-sec segments and coded with the CFCS by a research assistant. Visual analogue scale ratings of pain and sedation were also collected from videotape. Children's facial reaction to pain did not vary over 50 minutes in the PACU. PCA analyses indicated a "pain face" was present similar to that reported for typically developing children. This set of facial actions was related to pain ratings and analgesic administration, but not to ratings of sedation. The frequency of facial actions appeared greater than that reported for typically developing children.

---

* **Correspondence:** Lynn Breau, Dalhousie University School of Nursing, 5869 University Ave, Halifax, Nova Scotia, B3H 3J5 Canada. E-mail: lbreau@dal.ca

This study indicates a subset of facial actions from the CFCS appears to reflect postoperative pain in children with intellectual disabilities. Development of a bedside version of the CFCS is warranted as this may provide an alternative to more gross behavioural measures of postoperative pain in these children.

Keywords: postoperative pain, intellectual disabilities, pain assessment, pediatric pain.

Introduction

Many children with intellectual disabilities (ID) cannot provide accurate or reliable pain reports postoperatively. This may be one reason they receive fewer postoperative analgesics than children without ID (1). For example, Fanurik et al (2) reported that only 10 of 120 children scheduled for surgery displayed the abilities needed to use a 0 to 5 pain scale. Observational pain assessment tools such as the Non-communicating Children's Pain Checklist – Postoperative Version (3) and the Paediatric Pain Profile (4) have shown potential. However, they have not been evaluated in the immediate postoperative period, when children may show reduced responses due to the continued presence of perioperative analgesics or sedatives.

The Child Facial Coding System (CFCS)(5) may be a viable alternative for children with severe ID in this situation. Facial expression has been recognized as a method for measuring pain for some time. This began with studies of adults (6) using Ekman and Friesen's Facial Action Coding System (FACS)(7). The Neonatal Facial Coding System (NFCS) (8) was developed from a subset of facial actions that reflect pain in adults. The CFCS was then derived from both the FACS and the NFCS to detect pain in toddlers and school age children and has shown sensitivity to procedural (9;10) and postoperative pain (11) in typically developing children.

Several studies indicated facial action, measured using the FACS (7), does change with pain in individuals with ID. Two studies examined facial action in institutionalized adults with ID during injections. In one, pain-related facial activity did not vary due to ability to self-report pain and was significantly higher during insertion of the needle (12). In the other, facial response to pain did increase during insertion of the needle, but varied due to level of impairment (13). FACS scores of those with mild to moderate impairments increased with insertion, but not those for participants with severe or profound impairments. In another study of 8 adolescents with severe cognitive impairments, neither FACS nor CFCS scores increased during vaccination (14). However, the injection observed was judged by observers as only mildly painful. In a larger study of 21 younger children with autism, the same group found that children displayed a more substantial reaction to pain due to venepuncture, based on the CFCS, than a comparison group of typically developing children (15).

Although no study has examined postoperative facial reaction to pain in individuals with ID, these studies of procedural pain do suggest that facial reaction may be a viable alternative for postoperative pain assessment for children with ID. The present study is a preliminary exploration of whether the Child Facial Coding System (CFCS) could detect pain in children with ID in the immediate postoperative period.

Methods

Participants

Twenty-six children with severe intellectual disabilities and their caregivers participated. They were recruited from a cohort taking part in longitudinal research regarding pain in children with severe ID. The IWK Health Centre's Research Ethics Board approved this study and all caregivers provided informed consent.

Measures

The Child Facial Coding System (5) was used to code the discrete facial movements of the children from videotape. This system includes 13 facial actions (FAs). Ten FAs are coded for intensity (0-2; absent, slightly present, distinctly/maximally present). Three FAs (blink, flared nostril, open lips) are coded as present or absent (0-2). The 0-2 coding for binary FAs was necessary to equate their weighting with that of facial actions receiving an intensity score (0, 1 or 2) for use in multivariate procedures.

A Visual Analogue Scale (VAS) was used to rate the intensity of children's pain from videotape. The 100-millimetre line was anchored at the left by the phrase "no pain at all" and at the right by "worst pain ever". Similar scales have shown sensitivity to acute pain in children (14) and adults (12) with ID and has been used to assess postoperative pain in children with ID (16).

A Visual Analogue Scale (VAS) was also used to rate the amount of children's sedation from videotape. The 100-millimetre line was anchored at the left by the phrase "fully awake" and at the right by "fully sedated".

The Vineland Adaptive Behavior Scales (17), a standardized measure of functional adaptation, were administered as a structured interview to caregivers of the children. Children receive an age-equivalent in four domains: Communication, Daily Living Skills, Socialization, and Motor Skills. These were included as an indicator of children's functional level because Vineland scores are generally associated with intelligence test scores in this population (18).

Procedure

The Vineland Adaptive Behavior Scales (17) were administered to caregivers at the time children joined the cohort. This was up to 19.3 months before the day of surgery ($M = 7.2$ months, $SD = 5.9$ months). Demographic information was also collected at that time. One caregiver completed the interview 2 months after their child had surgery. Caregivers were asked to contact a research assistant if their child was scheduled for surgery.

On the day of surgery, a research assistant filmed the child in the postanesthesia care unit for up to 60 minutes from the time they were deemed "reactive" by the attending nurse. This entailed the child having achieved a combined score of 10 across five areas of functioning including respiration, energy, alertness, circulation and temperature. This occurred 15 minutes to 4 hours 5 minutes after surgery was completed ($M = 1$ hour, 12 minutes, $SD = 47$ minutes). One child was sent immediately from the operating room to the intensive care unit because of pre-existing medical conditions. Filming for that child was conducted in that setting.

Filming continued for 60 minutes or until the child left the recovery room. Children spent from 50 minutes to 5 hours, 25 minutes in the recovery room ($M = 2$ hours, 4 minutes, $SD = 1$ hour, 9 minutes). Information regarding the length of surgery, administration of analgesics in the operating room and recovery room and length of stay in the recovery room was abstracted from children's medical records.

Coding of Videotapes

Videotapes were divided into 10-minute segments. For each segment, the first 10-second interval in which the child's face was clearly visible was selected for coding. A trained research assistant coded each segment for the 13 facial actions of the CFCS. A second trained research assistant coded 7 (27%) of the tapes to assess reliability. Each segment was then independently rated for pain intensity using the 100-mm VAS by a third research assistant and a nurse who had not coded the videotapes using CFCS and had not been involved in filming the children. Several months later, the same nurse, and the second research assistant independently coded each segment for sedation using the 100-mm VAS.

Reliability for CFCS ratings were computed with the formula recommended by Ekman and Freisen (7). This provides a conservative index of agreement because it does not take into account agreement on the absence of FAs and regards disagreements in intensity values as errors. Reliability for the 13 FAs ranged from to .65 to .97 ($M = .80$, $SD = 8.8$). Reliability between VAS pain ratings and VAS sedation ratings was computed using Pearson correlation coefficients and ranged from .72 to .89 for pain and .44 to .84 for sedation.

Statistical Analysis

Data was analysed using SPSS 10.0.7 (19). Alpha was set at .05 for all tests. When multiple tests were conducted, Bonferroni corrections were used to maintain alpha at .05 for the set. Power calculations were computed using SamplePower (20) or based on tables prepared by Stevens (21).

Missing Data

Twenty-two children had film for 50 minutes, but only 15 for the full 60 minutes. Thus, analyses were conducted on the first 50 minutes of film for each child. View of two children was obscured during the second 10-minute interval, one during the third interval and one during the fourth, primarily due to staff monitoring the child's condition or caregivers comforting the child. All missing data were replaced with the median value for each FA for the remaining children during that second and that segment. This amounted to replacement of 8% of data for segments two and four, 4% for segment three and 15% for segment 5.

Descriptive Statistics

The total number of seconds and percentage of seconds that each FA was present during each segment was computed. The mean intensity for each of the 10 FAs coded for intensity was also computed for each of the five segments. To compute FA summary scores, the mean intensity of each FA across all 50 seconds was computed and this was multiplied by the number of seconds in which that action was present. Summary scores for the binary FAs were computed using the mean of the value for absent (0) and present (2).

Change in Facial Action over Time

To examine the pattern of facial action over the 5 segments coded, a 5 (segment) x 13 (mean facial action intensity) and a 5 (segment) x 10 (total facial action frequency) repeated measures analysis of covariance (ANCOVA) were conducted. The first examined the mean intensity of the 10 actions coded for intensity. The second examined the total frequency of all 13 FAs across the five segments. To include VAS pain ratings as a between-subjects factor, children were grouped as "high" or "low" pain through splitting mean VAS pain scores at the median. This resulted in 13 children in the "high" pain group with a mean VAS score of 34.3 from the researcher ($SD = 17.7$) and 10.5 ($SD = 4.1$) from the nurse. The "low" pain group had a mean VAS score of 13.0 from the researcher ($SD = 12.9$) and 2.7 ($SD = 2.4$) from the nurse. Children's mean sedation VAS score was included as a covariate. Power computations indicated 27 children were needed to achieve .80 to detect a medium one-way effect per pain group (high/low) and 13 children to detect a large effect, not accounting for the covariate, whose entry would increase power.

Structure of Facial Action

To investigate the structure of the facial action, and its meaning and relation to child characteristics, categorical principal components analyses, using optimal scaling techniques, which are appropriate for small groups, were used (22,23). The facial action summary scores for each segment were first standardized. This allowed use of the individual scores for each child's five segments because it accounts for repeated observations over time (24). Variable principal normalization was used for both analyses. For the first categorical PCA, standardized FA summary scores were entered. In addition, demographic variables were entered as supplementary variables to explore the relation between these and the FA components. Thus, they were not active in the derivation of components, but their loading with the FA components were computed to allow a determination of their relationship to the components already extracted. In order to validate the meaning of the FA components, a second categorical PCA was conducted following a procedure recommended by Kline (25) and used in previous analyses of CFCS data (10). This entailed entering the extracted components plus "marker" variables that were believed to reflect the meaning of the components. The component scores for each child for the FA components extracted in the first PCA were entered. Mean VAS pain and sedation ratings for the 5 segments were also standardized and entered, as were surgery factors.

Results

Characteristics of the Children

At the time of surgery, the children ranged in age from 3.7 to 19.6 years ($M = 11.6$, $SD = 4.3$) and 31% were girls. The children's adaptive age equivalents, based on the Vineland Adaptive Behavior Scales (17), were 12.6 months ($SD = 6.9$) for Communication, 11.9 months ($SD = 14.5$) for Daily Living Skills, 15.8 months ($SD = 19.6$) for Socialization and 6.9 months ($SD = 10.6$) for Motor Skills. The children had neurological impairments of prenatal (65%), perinatal (19%) and postnatal onset (15%). Ten children suffered neurological impairments due to dysmorphic or chromosomal syndromes, three due to traumatic brain injury, six due to asphyxia at birth. Of the remaining children, two were extremely premature and two had a neurodegenerative syndrome. One child had an intrauterine acquired condition. The cause of impairment was unknown for one child, and information was unavailable for another. Further characteristics of the children are displayed in table 1.

Characteristics of the Surgeries

The procedures the children underwent included: dental extractions (6), G-button insertions and removals (6), heelcord/tendon lengthening (3), other orthopedic surgery (2), endoscopies and biopsies (2), fundoplication (2), subcutaneous venous access device insertion (1), bilateral myringotomy tube insertion (1), strabismus repair (1) skin graft (1), and mole removal (1). Seven of the children had two procedures, with dental extractions being the most frequent procedure conducted in combination with others. Surgeries lasted from 8 minutes to 3 hours 45 minutes ($M = 74$ minutes, $SD = 64$) and length of stay in the recovery room ranged from none to 5 hours 25 minutes ($M = 1$ hour 45 minutes, $SD = 67$ minutes). Nine children received opioids intraoperatively, three children were given non-opioid analgesics in the recovery room and six were given a combination of opioids and non-opioids in the recovery room. Twelve children (46%) were given no analgesic introperatively or in the recovery room. Thirteen were admitted to hospital.

Descriptive Statistics

The total frequency of the 13 FAs and the mean intensity of the 10 facial actions that are not binary across the five segments coded are shown in table 2. The most frequent facial actions were those involving the mouth, such as open lips, and upper lip raise. Upper lip raise, vertical mouth stretch and horizontal mouth stretch were also the most intense, but were followed by eye squeeze and nasolabial furrow.

Table 1. Characteristics of the children

Characteristic		% Children
Level of Diagnosed Mental Retardation*:	Moderate	4%
	Severe	58%
	Profound	27%
Upper Limb Use:	Full	38%
	Some	41%
	None	21%
Lower Limb Use:	Full	17%
	Some	33%
	None	50%
Cerebral Palsy:		67%
Seizures:		65%
Tube Fed:		46%
Requires Medical Monitoring:	None	13%
	Monthly	54%
	Weekly	8%
	Daily	25%
Lives with Family:		89%
Medications on Regular Basis:	None	15%
	One to Three	38%
	More than Three	47%

Table 3 lists the total frequency of all FAs per segment and the mean intensity of all FAs per segment. There was little variation across segments. The correlations between FA frequency and intensity for each segment and the VAS ratings of pain and sedation are also listed in table 3. Almost all correlations between FAs and VAS pain ratings were significant after corrections for multiple tests. The exception was the correlation between FA frequency and VAS pain ratings in the first segment, and the correlations between FA frequency and intensity in the final segment. All correlations between FA frequency or intensity and VAS sedation ratings were nonsignificant.

Table 2. Total facial action frequency and mean facial action intensity across five 10-second segments

Facial Action	Total Frequency Mean	SD	Percentage of Seconds Present Mean	SD	Mean Intensity Mean	SD
Brow Lower	12.0	12.4	27	26	.39	.45
Squint	13.7	13.1	18	19	.28	.32
Eye Squeeze	9.0	9.7	38	29	.44	.38
Nose Wrinkle	18.6	14.6	14	21	.22	.36
Nasolabial Furrow	7.0	10.5	26	24	.42	.44
Cheek Raiser	12.8	12.2	24	25	.35	.41
Upper Lip Raise	34.0	18.6	68	37	1.04	.64
Lip Corner Pull	2.3	4.3	01	01	.06	.11
Vertical Mouth Stretch	29.2	17.7	58	35	.80	.59
Horizontal Mouth Stretch	24.0	16.8	48	34	.67	.54
Blink**	2.4	3.5	01	01	-	-
Flared Nostril**	7.7	11.1	15	22	-	-
Open Lips**	40.8	15.4	82	31	-	-

** Not coded for intensity.

Table 3. Total facial action frequency and mean facial action intensity per segment and partial correlations between facial action frequency and intensity and visual analogue scale ratings of pain and sedation

Segment	Total Frequency[a] Mean	SD	Mean Intensity[b] Mean	SD	Partial Correlation with VAS Rating[c] Total Frequency Pain	Sedation	Mean Intensity Pain	Sedation
1	44.6	26.9	.48	.40	.55*	.14	.60**	.14
2	40.2	22.6	.44	.37	.71**	.06	.81**	.16
3	43.0	30.1	.48	.45	.78**	-.33	.82**	-.12
4	42.7	29.5	.46	.45	.81**	-.28	.89**	-.30
5	43.4	27.2	.48	.43	.47*	.00	.51*	-.03

* $p < .05$. **Significant after corrections for multiple tests, $p < .003$. [a] Total for 13 facial actions. [b] Mean of 10 facial actions coded for intensity. [c] Nurse's 100-mm visual analogue scale ratings; correlations with pain controlled for the effects of sedation and correlations with sedation controlled for the effects of pain.

Table 4 lists the VAS pain and sedation ratings provided by the nurse and the two researchers. Overall the nurse provided lower pain ratings, but not lower sedation ratings, than the researchers. The correlations among the nurse and researcher's VAS pain ratings were all significant after corrections for multiple tests.

Table 4. Visual analogue scale ratings of nurse and researchers

Segment	VAS[a] Pain Ratings Nurse Mean (SD)	Researcher Mean (SD)	r	VAS Sedation Ratings Nurse Mean (SD)	Researcher Mean (SD)	r	Pain and Sedation VAS Ratings[b] r
1	7.9 (11.0)	20.2 (15.1)	.73*	37.3 (22.8)	40.0 (24.3)	.44	-.21
2	6.5 (11.9)	18.1 (20.5)	.89*	42.1 (21.5)	42.6 (23.0)	.74*	-.05
3	7.9 (12.0)	24.0 (24.6)	.83*	33.9 (23.6)	35.3 (23.8)	.81*	-.14
4	6.9 (12.3)	23.2 (27.9)	.85*	32.2 (23.8)	35.6 (24.6)	.75*	-.17
5	8.5 (14.7)	23.1 (25.1)	.72*	30.1 (22.6)	31.9 (23.9)	.84*	.03

* $p < .005$. [a]Visual Analogue Scale. [b]Based on Nurse's Ratings.

All but the correlation between VAS sedation ratings for the first segment were also significant.

Change in Facial Action over Time

A repeated measures analysis of covariance conducted on total frequency scores for the five segments revealed a nonsignificant main effect for segment ($F(4,92) = 1.5, p = .21$), the covariate sedation ($F(1,23) = 1.7, p = .21$), and the interaction between the two ($F(4,92) = 2.0, p = .11$). However, the main effect of pain (high/low) was significant ($F(1,23) = 8.6, p = .007$) and it did not interact with segment ($F(4,92) = 1.7, p = .16$). Children in the high VAS pain rating group displayed significantly more frequent facial action across segments ($M = 52.9, SD = 22.8$) than children in the low pain group ($M = 33.7, SD = 14.3$). Facial action did not vary across the segments, nor was it affected by sedation.

A second analysis on mean intensity scores for the 10 facial actions coded for intensity across the five segments revealed a nonsignificant main effect for segment ($F(4,92) = 0.3, p = .86$), the covariate sedation ($F(1,23) = 0.4, p = .54$), and the interaction between the two ($F(4,92) = 0.4, p = .76$). However, the main effect of pain (high/low) was again significant ($F(1,23) = 10.5, p = .004$) and it did not interact with segment ($F(4,92) = 0.9, p = .45$). Thus a similar pattern was found as for frequency. Facial action intensity was greater for children in the high pain group ($M = 0.64, SD = 0.37$) than children in the low pain group ($M = 0.29, SD = 0.15$), but it did not vary by segment or due to sedation.

Structure of Facial Action

The first categorical PCA examined the structure of the facial action summary scores. The best solution consisted of three independent components, accounting for 67% of the variance. The eigenvalues of the three components, variance accounted for, and loadings by the 13 facial actions are shown in table 5. The FA Component 1 appeared to reflect pain. FAs that loaded onto it most were those previously associated with a "pain face" in adults (6) and children (10), such as brow lower, nose wrinkle, nasolabial furrow, cheek raiser, horizontal mouth stretch and flared nostril. Eye squeeze and vertical mouth stretch, previously associated with an expectation of pain by children (10), also loaded onto this component. FA Component 2 was loaded onto most highly by open lips, followed by vertical mouth stretch and upper lip raise. This component appeared to reflect an open mouth and it was hypothesized it might pertain to children who had had dental procedures. FA Component 3 was loaded onto most highly by squint and blink and appeared to reflect eye movements only. It was hypothesized that this component might reflect awakening.

The Relation between Demographic Characteristics and Facial Action Components

Children's demographic characteristics were also entered into this analysis as supplementary variables, to explore the relation between their characteristics and the FA components. The loadings of these variables with the three components are shown in table 6. As can be seen there, few child characteristics were strongly related to the FA components. Children's age, adaptive skills age equivalents and gender were not related to the FA components. There was a tendency for FA Component 1, reflecting the "pain face" to be associated with greater upper limb impairment, suggesting children with more severe physical impairments displayed a stronger facial reaction to pain. However, it is not clear whether this is because these children display more facial reaction, or because they may have had surgeries that were more painful.

Validation of the Facial Action Components

To determine the meaning of the FA Components, a second categorical PCA was conducted on children's scores for the three FA Components and the characteristics of their surgeries. The three FA Components were entered as variables into this analysis. To ascertain whether FA Component 1 reflected pain, children's VAS pain ratings by the nurse were entered, as were the analgesics they were given intraoperatively or in the recovery room. To determine if FA Component 2 reflected having had dental procedures conducted, a variable was entered to indicate whether the child had had any dental procedures performed. To determine if FA Component 3 reflected awakening, VAS sedation ratings by the nurse were entered. In addition, length of time in surgery and length of time in the recovery room were entered.

The purpose of this study was to determine if the CFCS (5) could detect pain in children with severe ID. The results indicate the overall frequency of facial action and intensity of facial action was significantly greater in children rated as having higher pain by observers. However, facial action did not change over the course of the 50 minutes of time in the recovery room. This is similar to Gilbert et al (11), who also found no change over time in the facial action of typical children after surgery.

Table 5. Categorical principal components analysis of facial action scores across five segments

Variables Entered	Facial Action Component Loadings		
	1	2	3
Brow Lower	.83		
Squint		.36	.72
Eye Squeeze	.48	-.32	-.48
Nose Wrinkle	.86	-.31	
Nasolabial Furrow	.88		
Cheek Raiser	.83		
Upper Lip Raise	.60	.54	
Lip Corner Pull		.37	
Vertical Mouth Stretch	.55	.55	
Horizontal Mouth Stretch	.82		
Blink*			.75
Flared Nostril*	.87	-.31	
Open Lips*	.36	.68	
Eigenvalue	5.4	1.8	1.5
Percentage of Total Variance Accounted For	41.7	13.9	11.7

Note. Facial actions with loadings ≥ .30 shown.

The best solution involved three components accounting for 59.8% of the variance. The eigenvalues and loadings of the FA components and surgical variables onto these Validation Components are shown in table 7. As these loadings indicate, Validation Component 1 is loaded onto most highly by the presence of dental surgery and long length of surgery. The FA Component that loads highest onto this Validation Component is FA Component 2, consisting of FAs representing an opening of the mouth. FA Component 3, hypothesized to reflect awakening, also loads fairly highly onto this Validation Component, but in the negative direction. Thus, this set of FAs appears to represent the open mouth of children who had had dental procedures performed and to reflect to some extent their grogginess after lengthy surgeries.

Validation Component 2 was loaded onto very highly by FA Component 1 and the VAS pain ratings, supporting the hypothesis that these FAs reflect a "pain face". Analgesic administration in the recovery room also loaded with this Validation Component. This suggests the physicians who were caring for children displaying this set of FAs felt pain treatment was warranted, suggesting they believed the children had clinically significant pain. The VAS sedation ratings also loaded negatively onto this Validation Component, suggesting these FAs were most prevalent in children who were not experiencing continued sedation due to anaesthetics.

Table 6. Loadings of supplemental child characteristic variables onto facial action components

Supplemental Variables Entered	Supplemental Variable Loadings		
Facial Action Component	*1: Pain Face*	*2: Dental Surgery*	*3: Awakening*
Age (months)	-.08	.04	.08
Gender	.17	-.19	-.05
Level of Diagnosed Mental Retardation	.24	.12	-.02
Communication Age Equivalent (months)	-.17	.03	.20
Daily Living Skills Age Equivalent (months)	-.11	.00	.00
Socialization Age Equivalent (months)	-.08	.06	.00
Motor Skills Age Equivalent (months)	-.16	-.07	.08
Cerebral Palsy	-.03	.18	-.15
Seizures	.00	.14	-.26
Upper Limb Impairment	.37	.26	-.04
Lower Limb Impairment	.14	.04	.01
Tube Feeding	.27	.07	.06
Frequency of Medical Monitoring	.18	-.02	-.12

Table 7. Validation categorical principal components analysis of the facial action components and surgical factors

Variables Entered	Validation Components Extracted		
	1	2	3
Facial Action Component 1	.19	.84	.24
Facial Action Component 2	.43	.08	-.59
Facial Action Component 3	-.47	.25	-.32
VAS Pain Rating	.17	.86	.30
VAS Sedation Rating	.33	-.37	.66
Intravenous Opioids Intraoperatively	-.44		.61
Analgesic in Recovery Room (none, non-opioid, opioid)	-.07	.52	-.26
Length of Surgery (minutes)	.81	.00	.11
Length of Time in Recovery Room (minutes)	.28	-.12	.15
Any Dental Surgery	.90	.04	-.11
Eigenvalue	2.3	1.9	1.5
Percentage of Total Variance Accounted For	23.1	19.5	15.2

Validation Component 3 was loaded onto most highly be the VAS sedation ratings, followed by intravenous opioids provided intraoperatively. Two FA Components loaded negatively onto this validation component, FA Component 2, reflecting the open mouth, and FA Component 3, reflecting blinking and squinting. It is likely that these loadings represent the fact that children who were groggier produced less facial action than their counterparts who were not still experiencing the residual effects of anaesthesia.

In summary, this analysis suggests that the facial actions contained in FA Component 1 do reflect a "pain face". The FAs contained in FA Component 2, on the other hand, seem to relate to having experienced oral surgery. Finally, the FAs contained in FA Component 3, which loaded in the opposite direction as sedation on all three validation components appears to reflect the absence of sedation or awakening.

Discussion

The analyses also indicate only a subset of the CFCS FAs reflect pain in this situation. Of the three components extracted from the CFCS summary scores, only one was strongly related to the nurse's VAS pain ratings and administration of analgesics. The FAs that loaded most highly onto FA Component 1 are similar to the "pain face" reported in children during immunization (10), such as brow lower, nose wrinkle, nasolabial furrow, cheek raiser, horizontal mouth stretch and flared nostril. To a lesser extent, FAs associated with an expectation of pain by children (10), such as eye squeeze and vertical mouth stretch, also loaded onto this component. The similarity in the structure of the components found in this study and those observed during immunization suggest that a core set of FAs may be shown by children during various types of pain, a finding reported for adults (26), and that the set of FAs shown by children with ID may not differ substantially from those shown by children without impairments. However, direct comparison of children with and without impairments undergoing the same type of pain would be needed to confirm this.

The results also indicate, however, that some FAs contained in the CFCS reflected aspects of the children's surgical experience rather than pain. FA Component 2 appears most closely related to whether children underwent dental procedures. This set of FAs appeared to represent a wide open mouth. Having had a lengthy surgery and sedation were also associated with this set of FAs, suggesting that this set of facial actions may reflects factors related to oral pain or ongoing sedation. Additional studies could clarify this.

The final component, FA Component 3, was most related to blinking and squinting. It was hypothesized this component reflected awakening. Upon awakening in the recovery room, children are met by bright lights and an array of sounds, scenes and people. This was supported by the fact that the VAS sedation ratings provided by the nurse loaded negatively with this set of FAs.

These results differ somewhat from those reported by Gilbert et al. (11) who studied typically developing children's facial action after surgery. Whereas they report one component, three were found in our study. There are several possible reasons for this difference. First, in conducting their PCA, they do not report rotating their solution, which could lead to extraction of a single component reflecting within-subject similarity (25).

Secondly, it is also possible the differences are due to the nature of the surgeries the children underwent in the two studies. The children who were observed for the Gilbert et al (11) study appear to have had their pain well managed. This is suggested by the authors as one reason they did not find any relation between facial action and pain medication administered. They do not report the VAS ratings of pain conducted from videotape, so this cannot be confirmed. However, it is also notable that only 17% of the children in that study received no analgesic either intraoperatively or in the recovery room. In sharp contrast, 46% of the children in our study received no analgesic intraoperatively or in the recovery room. A study of postoperative care for children with and without impairments following spine fusion also found that children with impairments received fewer analgesics (1) relative to their unimpaired peers. It was suggested that the difference may have been related to a lack of valid, reliable pain assessment methods for the children with impairments, who were less able to provide self-report. That may also be a reason for the low rate of analgesic administration here and highlights the need for valid observational methods of judging pain in the postoperative period for children with ID.

These results, when compared to those of Gilbert et al (11), also suggest that children with ID may display more facial reaction to pain than their typically developing peers. Only four FAs were present more than 10% of the time in their sample, and the highest frequency for a facial action they report related to pain was less than 14%. In contrast, only two facial actions in this study, blink and lip corner puller, were present less than 10% of the time. The remaining facial actions were coded as present 14% to 82% of the time, with the six loading .80 or greater onto the "pain face" component present 14% to 68% of the time. This would coincide with the findings Nader et al (15), who found children with autism displayed more facial reaction to venepuncture than a control group of children without impairments. Porter and her colleagues (27), also found that elderly individuals with dementia displayed greater facial reaction to a venepuncture than elders without dementia. Thus, it is possible that individuals with intellectual or cognitive impairments exhibit a more pronounced pain expression. Whether this is aimed at compensating for their reduced ability to communicate verbally or the result of reduced social inhibition could be examined in further studies.

In summary, it is likely that the differences found between the results reported by Gilbert et al (11) and those found here reflect both statistical factors and the fact that the children in this study may have had more intense pain during the observation, leading to higher pain ratings and more facial actions. However, it is also possible that the children in this study displayed more facial activity in response to pain because of their intellectual disabilities.

Conclusion

Overall, the results suggest that facial action may be a viable method of assessing the pain of children with ID after surgery. A subset of FAs was found that is similar to those seen in children without impairments during immunization and after surgery, including changes in the eye and mouth area that resemble a Tightening or pulling back of the face. The facial action of the children in this study also did not vary due to their physical limitations. However, the Child Facial Coding System (5) is a research tool at this point, and clinical use is not feasible. Coding must be conducted from videotape and coding of one minute of videotape can take up to one hour. However, our results suggest that research aimed at refining the CFCS into a clinically feasible measure for use bedside is warranted. Further work could result in developing it into a clinically feasible tool to help healthcare professionals managing the pain of these children in the postoperative period.

Acknowledgments

This research was funded by the Hospital for Sick Children Foundation (Toronto, Canada). Support was also provided by the Canadian Institutes for Health Research through a Doctoral Fellowship to Lynn Breau and a Distinguished Scientist Award and Canada Research Chair to Patrick McGrath, and Postdoctoral Fellowships to Lynn Breau by AstraZeneca Canada Inc. and the Child Health Clinician Scientist Program of the Canadian Institutes for Health Research.

References

[1] Malviya S, Voepel-Lewis T, Tait AR, Merkel S, Lauer A, Munro H, et al. Pain management in children with and without cognitive impairment following spine fusion surgery. Paediatr Anaesth 2001;11(4):453-8.
[2] Fanurik D, Koh JL, Harrison RD, Conrad TM, Tomerlin C. Pain assessment in children with cognitive impairment: An exploration of self-report skills. Clin Nurs Res 1998;7(2):103-24.
[3] Breau LM, Finley GA, McGrath PJ, Camfield CS. Validation of the Non-Communicating Children's Pain Checklist. Postoperative version. Anesthesiology 2002; 96(3):528-35.
[4] Hunt A, Goldman A, Seers K, Crichton N, Mastroyannopoulou K, Moffat V, et al. Clinical validation of the paediatric pain profile. Dev Med Child Neurol 2004;46(1):9-18.
[5] Chambers CT, Cassidy KL, McGrath PJ, Gilbert CA, Craig KD. Child Facial Coding System: A manual. Halifax, Nova Scotia: Dalhousie Univ, Univ British Columbia, 1996.
[6] LeResche L. Facial expression in pain: A study of candid photographs. J Nonverbal Behav 1982;7(1):46-55.
[7] Ekman P, Friesen WV. Investigator's Guide to the Facial Action Coding System. Palo Alto, CA: Consult Psychol Press, 1978.
[8] Grunau RVE, Craig KD. Pain expression in neonates: facial action and cry. Pain 1987;28:395-410.
[9] Cassidy KL, Reid GJ, McGrath PJ, Finley GA, Smith DJ, Morley C, et al. Watch needle, watch TV: Audiovisual distraction in preschool immunization. Pain Med 2002;3(2):108-18.
[10] Breau LM, McGrath PJ, Craig KD, Santor D, Cassidy KL, Reid GJ. Facial expression of children receiving immunizations: a principal components analysis of the child facial coding system. Clin J Pain 2001;17(2):178-86.
[11] Gilbert CA, Lilley CM, Craig KD, McGrath PJ, Court C, Bennett SM, et al. Postoperative pain expression in preschool children: Validation of the child facial coding system. Clin J Pain 1999;15(3):192-200.
[12] LaChapelle DL, Hadjistavropoulos T, Craig KD. Pain measurement in persons with intellectual disabilities. Clin J Pain 1999;15:13-23.
[13] Defrin R, Lotan M, Pick CG. The evaluation of acute pain in individuals with cognitive impairment: a differential effect of the level of impairment. Pain 2006;124(3):312-20.

[14] Oberlander TF, Gilbert CA, Chambers CT, O'Donnell ME, Craig KD. Biobehavioral responses to acute pain in adolescents with a significant neurologic impairment. Clin J Pain 1999;15:201-9.

[15] Nader R, Oberlander TF, Chambers CT, Craig KD. Expression of pain in `children with autism. Clin J Pain 2004;20(2):88-97.

[16] Terstegen C, Koot HM, de Boer JB, Tibboel D. Measuring pain in children with cognitive impairment: pain response to surgical procedures. Pain 2003; 103(1-2):187-98.

[17] Sparrow SS, Balla DA, Cicchetti DV. Vineland Adaptive Behavior Scales: Interview Edition Survey Form Manual. Circle Pines, MN: Am Guidance Serv, 1984.

[18] Atkinson L, Bevc I, Dickens S, Blackwell J. Concurrent validities of the Stanford-Binet, 4th ed, Leiter, and Vineland with developmentally delayed children. J School Psychol 1992;30(2):165-73.

[19] SPSS 10.0.7. Chicago IL: SPSS Inc, 2000.

[20] SamplePower 1.2. Chicago, IL: SPSS Inc, 1997.

[21] Stevens J. Applied multivariate statistics for the social sciences, 3rd ed. Mahwah, NJ: Lawrence Erlbaum, 1996.

[22] Van de Geer JP. Multivariate analysis of categorical data: Theory. London: Sage, 1993.

[23] Van de Geer JP. Multivariate analysis of categorical data: Applications. London: Sage, 1993.

[24] Bijleveld C, van der Kamp L, Mooijaart A, van der Kloot W, van der Leeden R, van der Burg E. Longitudinal data analysis: Designs, models and methods. London: Sage, 1998.

[25] Kline P. An easy guide to factor analysis. New York: Routledge, 1994.

[26] Prkachin KM. The consistency of facial expressions of pain: a comparison across modalities. Pain 1992;51(3):297-306.

[27] Porter FL, Malhotra KM, Wolf CM, Morris JC, Miller JP, Smith MC. Dementia and response to pain in the elderly. Pain 1996;68(2-3):413-21.

In: Pain Management Yearbook 2009
Editor: Joav Merrick

ISBN: 978-1-61209-666-7
©2012 Nova Science Publishers, Inc.

Chapter 7

PREREQUISITE ABILITIES FOR THE USE OF HYPNOSIS FOR PAIN MANAGEMENT IN CHILDREN WITH COGNITIVE IMPAIRMENT

Marc Zabalia[*], *PhD and Fanny Esquerré, R Psychol*

Laboratoire de Psychologie des Actions Langagières et Motrices (PALM JE 2528) et pôle Modélisation en Sciences Cognitives (ModeSCo), Université de Caen Basse-Normandie, Caen, France

Abstract

Children with mild to moderate intellectual disabilities may be able to use some self-report tools to provide a rating of the intensity of their pain. They can also describe pain quality with appropriate words and use adaptative strategies to cope with their painful experiences. Objective: To test the efficiency of mental imagery and autobiographical memory as they could be involved in hypnosis techniques for pain management. Study groups: 21 adolescents with intellectual disabilities, (M= 17 years-old, ages from 13 to 20 years-old), mental age (M= 6.8 years-old, ages from 3.6 to 9.6 years-old) and 10 typical children as a baseline to the autobiographical memory test (M= 6 years-old, ages from 5 to 9 years-old). Method: To test the ability to mentally represent events, children were asked to choose a picture to complete a story they had listened to. A semi-directive interview was conducted to assess autobiographical memory for comparison to typical children. Results: Children with intellectual disabilities were able to generate a mental image while listening to a story. They were able to recall autobiographical memories of events that were personal and specific. Conclusion: Children with intellectual disabilities appear able to take advantage of hypnosis for pain management. Further research should examine their ability to use these techniques in a clinical setting.

---

[*] **Correspondence:** Marc Zabalia, Université de Caen Basse-Normandie, MRSH, 14032 Caen cedex 5, France. Tel: (33) 02 31 56 62 19; Fax : (33) 02 31 56 62 60; E-mail: marc.zabalia@unicaen.fr

Keywords: Children, intellectual disabilities, mental imagery, autobiographical memory, hypnosis .

Introduction

For a long time, the assessment and management of pain in people with intellectual disabilities was neglected. The first studies (1) to investigate the self-report skills of children with cognitive impairments assessed children's ability to use numerical rating scales of pain and to match cards depicting faces at different levels of pain. In a more recent study (2), children completed original and adapted versions of a 100 mm Visual Analogue Scale of pain, the Eland Color Scale (3), and the Faces Scale (4) after training for pain due to venipuncture. This indicated that children with mild impairments may be able to use some self-report tools to provide a first-hand rating of the intensity of their pain. Only one other study (5) investigated the ability of children with mild to moderate cognitive impairments to use a 100 mm Visual Analogue Scale of pain and a the Faces Pain Scale-Revised (6) to rate the pain of individuals depicted in vignettes. Children rated the pain they believed they would experience were they to experience the event in the vignettes. After ratings were provided, the children were also asked to describe the quality of the pain of each event. The children's pain ratings for both the vignettes and the pain they would feel in that situation did vary due to the cause of pain, suggesting they did distinguish between the pain events. They also provided up to nine words to describe the quality of the pain for the events, a number that is similar to that reported by typical children of a similar mental age, and the words were appropriate for the pain depicted (burning, pinching). Although the children did not rate their own pain for an actual experienced event, the results did indicate the children had some skill in rating pain, and most importantly, that they could describe pain quality.

In the area of pain coping skills in the population with intellectual disabilities, one study (7) has used the Pediatric Pain and Coping Inventory (PPCI) developed by Varni et al (8). Results show that children with intellectual disabilities more frequently sought social support as a method of coping with their painful experiences as compared to literature studying typical children. Seeking social support when experiencing pain is not considered to be an optimal coping strategy under typical conditions. We proposed that this might be the most effective mechanism for those with intellectual disabilities, because they do not have the ability to respond effectively without assistance.

The evidence of abilities to assess and to cope with pain in children with cognitive impairment has opened questions regarding the efficiency of functions involved in hypnosis for pain management. It is now well known that hypnosis can decrease pain and stress during painful events (9,10). It is much easier for a child to enter in an hypnotic state than an adult, because of his high abilities to use imagination as an escape (11), and the hypnotic trance state is more reachable from 7 to 14 years of age. Several hypnotic techniques have been used, depending on age and developmental level of the child (12). Distraction (13) or listening to music (14) are good supports for hypnotic techniques. However, most of the techniques employed between 6 and 12 years of age (e.g. thinking of a favorite place, or favorite hobby, listening to a story) involve mental imagery and autobiographical memory.

Research regarding mental imagery in people with cognitive impairments has yielded no evidence of a deficit, although their abilities appear to be more heterogeneous (15-17). For example, imagery processing is more efficient for visual object properties than for spatial properties. Furthermore, the use of mental imagery appears to be an efficient strategy for improving recall in people with Down Syndrome (18). Autobiographical memory is the memory of personal events we have lived and it takes supports a feeling of selfness and the feeling of continuity. Near the end of the second year of life, autobiographical memory begins to store events as "events I lived" (19). This type of memory never appears to have been studied in people with intellectual disabilities.

The aim of this study was to investigate mental imagery and autobiographical memory, as they could be involved in hypnosis techniques for pain management in children with mild to moderate intellectual disabilities.

Methods

Participants were 21 adolescents with intellectual disabilities, 14 girls and 7 boys (M= 17 years-old, ages from 13 to 20 years-old), mental age (M= 6.8 years-old, ages from 3.6 to 9.6 years-old) recruited in the place, where they attended school.

A control group of typical children was recruited to provide a baseline for the autobiographical memory test. 10 children, 5 girls and 5 boys (M= 6 years-old, ages from 5 to 9 years-old) were interviewed at a leisure centre. Authorization was obtained from the management of the institutions, from the parents and from children themselves.

Procedure

The first task was to assess the ability to mentally represent and to understand two short stories. After listening to the stories, participants were asked to choose from three pictures the one which depicted the end of the story (20). For example, for Story A (a bear having a magic dream the night before a vaccination), one of the non-target pictures was ambiguous because it showed the bear in his bed, as described at the beginning of the story. In contrast, the non-ambiguous picture depicted the bear flying on his pillow at night (target picture). For Story B (the bear's friend is ill and he must call a doctor) the target picture is not ambiguous, it shows the doctor administering an injection to the bear's friend. Children performed the task individually, and it took no more than 5 minutes.

The second task was to assess children's autobiographical memory during a semi-directed interview. Fourteen questions assessed memory for specific events (Have you been to the zoo?), four questions assessed memory for personal events (Can you remember something unpleasant that happened?) and four questions assessed flashbulb memories, memories of major events shared by a social group. Because of the cognitive impairment of participants, we focused on a current and media event.

The interview followed a guide (see table 1), however, the focus was on allowing the participant to freely express him/herself without structuring his/her responses. Before the interview, the interviewer ensured the child understood the purpose of the study, and that the questions were clear so that the child knew how to best respond with relevant information. Indices of prolixity were also calculated (the number of words divided by the number of questions). Children were individually interviewed. Interview lasted no more than 10 minutes.

Data Analysis

Data were analyzed using Statistical software. Alpha was set at p = .05 for determining significant differences.

Table 1. Percentages of children with intellectual disabilities and children in the control group who gave responses to autobiographical memory questions

Questions	% of children with intellectual disabilities	% of the control group	X^2 alpha
1. Have you ever seen the sea?	100	100	ns
2. Where was it?	76	90	ns
3. With whom were you?	43.6	100	.01
4. What did you do?	43.6	100	.01
5. Did you go into the sea? What did you feel?	43.5	90	.01
6. Have you ever gone to the zoo?	72	90	ns
Give at least one animal's name	88	89	ns
Give at least three animal's name	52	44	ns
7. How old are you?	100	100	ns
8. What did you do last Christmas?	66	90	ns
9. Where were you?	85	30	.001
10. What did you received as gifts?	86	90	ns
11. Have you ever taken a trip?	76	90	ns
12. Where did you go?	69	67	ns
13. Can you tell me something that happened during the trip?	76	80	ns
14. Tell me what you did during the last holiday.	90	60	ns
15. Can you remember an unpleasant thing that happened?	57	80	ns
16 Can you remember a pleasant thing that happened?	38	90	.01

Questions	% of children		X² alpha
	with intellectual disabilities	of the control group	
17. Do you know the name of the French President?	52	80	ns
18. Have you ever seen him?	47	60	ns
19. Can you remember where it was?	23	30	ns
20. When did he win the election?	14	20	ns

Data Analysis

Data were analyzed using Statistic software. Alpha was set at p = .05 for determining significant differences.

Results

Mental Imagery Task

Children with intellectual disabilities performed better for Story B than Story A ($X^2[2]$= 35,48 p<.001). For story A, 52% were able to select the correct picture to complete the story ($X^2[2]$= 16,89 p<.001), while 38% chose the ambiguous picture. For Story B, 90 % of the children chose the correct picture ($X^2[2]$= 67,67 p<.001).

Autobiographical Memory Task

To compare the group of children with intellectual disabilities with the control group in the autobiographical memory interview, indices of prolixity were calculated. Over questions 1 to 16, there was a significant difference between the groups (t(29)= 1,82 p<.05). All children were able to give responses to the questions about personal events. Children in the control group displayed a mean index of prolixity of 13 words per question? (max: 19; min: 4). The mean indices of prolixity for children with intellectual disabilities was 9 words per question (max: 23; min: 1). There was notable dispersion in both groups (see figure 1). However, if we look at the ability to give a response to questions about specific events, the groups only differ in the evocation of a pleasant memory.

There was no significant difference between the groups in the ability to give responses regarding flashbulb memory questions, but they shown different indices of prolixity (t(29)= 2,06 p<.05). Nevertheless, 52% of the children with intellectual disabilities are able to give the name of the French President, while 80% of children in the control group could do so.

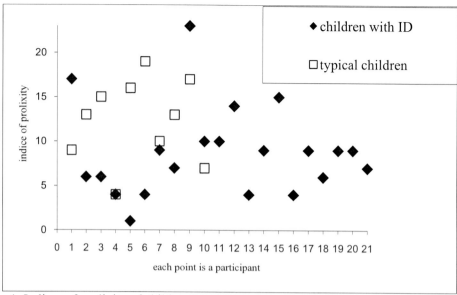

Figure 1. Indices of prolixity of children by group.

Discussion

These results show that children with intellectual disabilities were able to generate mental images regarding what was happening in a story read to them. The image seems to have been sufficiently vivid to help them to choose a picture depicting the end of the story. However, as suggested by their great difficulty with Story A, stories may have to be simple with no ambiguous nor unreal events. This appears more suited to their cognitive level.

The assessment of autobiographical memory here shows that this kind of memory may be elicited in children with intellectual disabilities. Compared to the typical children in our control group, they were able to recall personal and specific events. According to recent data (5), cognitive impairments seem to limit the prolixity of recall statements rather than the probability that an individual will recall an event. Although there was variability in the ability to respond in both groups of children, our results suggest that we can elicit recall of memories in people with intellectual disabilities if we pay attention to the verbal level of the questions. Cognitive impairment appears to be more of an issue when precise elements of the memories are sought; with these, a difference emerges between children with and without intellectual disabilities.

There is now building evidence that children with mild to moderate intellectual disabilities are capable of reporting aspects of their pain experience and of taking some steps to cope with their pain (2,5,7). The results of this study support the idea that hypnosis has potential for pain management is a relevant technique in this population as well as it is for young typical children. It is now necessary to test the use of hypnosis in clinical pain situations. This would provide evidence as to whether the stress caused by the pain experience attenuates the cognitive abilities and coping skills of these children, making hypnosis less effective for them as a pain management strategy.

Conclusion

We know that people with intellectual disabilities experience more pain than the general population. In spite of the growing number of studies about pain management in this population, there are yet no specific methods currently in clinical use for helping them to cope with their pain. This work suggests that mental imagery and autobiographical memories are functional, an important finding because they are involved in hypnosis for pain management. We have now good reason to develop clinical studies to investigate hypnosis as a potential pain management strategy for children with mild to moderate intellectual disabilities. This would provide caregivers and health professionals with non-pharmacological strategies that could minimize children's pain in a group where polypharmacy is frequently a concern when it comes to administering pain medications.

References

[1] Fanurik D, Koh JL, Harrison RD, Conrad TM, Tomerlin C. Pain assessment in children with cognitive impairment: An exploration of self-report skills. Clin Nurs Res 1998;7:103-24.

[2] Benini F, Trapanotto M, Gobber D, Agosto C, Carli G, Drigo P et al. Evaluating pain induced by venipuncture in pediatric patients with developmental delay. Clin.J Pain 2004;20:156-63.

[3] Eland JM. The child who is hurting. Semin Oncol Nurs. 1985;1:116-122.

[4] Wong DL. Baker CM. Pain in children: comparison of assessment scales. Ped Nurs 1988;14:9-17.

[5] Zabalia M, Jacquet D, Breau LM. Rôle du niveau verbal sur l'expression et l'évaluation de la douleur chez des sujets déficients intellectuels. Doul. et Analg 2005;2:65-70.

[6] Hicks CL, von Baeyer CL, Spafford PA, Van KI, Goodenough B. The Faces Pain Scale - Revised: toward a common metric in pediatric pain measurement. Pain 2001;93:173-83.

[7] Zabalia M, Duchaux C. Stratégies de faire-face à la douleur chez des enfants porteurs de déficience intellectuelle. Revue Francophone de la Déficience Intellectuelle 2006 ;17 :53-64.

[8] Varni JW, Waldron SA, Cragg RA, Rapoff MA, Bernstein BH, Lindsley CB, Newcomb MD. Development of the Waldron/Varni pediatric pain coping inventory. Pain 1996;67:141-50.

[9] Wild MR, Epsie CA. The efficacy of hypnosis in the reduction of procedural pain and stress in pediatric oncology: a systematic review. Dev Behav Pediatrics 2004;25:207-13.

[10] Butler LD, Symons BK, Henderson SL, Shortliffe LD, Spiegel D. Hypnosis reduces distress and duration invasive medical procedure for children. Pediatrics 2005;115:77-85.

[11] Morgan A, Hilgard E. Ages differences in susceptibility to hypnosis. Int J Clin Exp Hypn 1973;21:78-85.

[12] Olness K, Cohen DP. Hypnosis and hypnotherapy in children. New York: Grunne Stratton,1996.

[13] Gupta D, Argawal A, Dhiraaj S, Tandon M, Kumar M, Singh RS, Songh PK, Sing U. An evaluation of efficacy of balloon inflation on venous cannulation pain in children: a prospective, randomized, controlled study. Anesth Analg 2006;02(5):1372-5.

[14] Hatem TP, Lira PI, Mattos SS. (). The therapeutic effects of music in children following cardiac surgery. J Pedia (Rio J) 2006;82(3):166-8.

[15] Courbois Y. Evidence for visual imagery deficits in persons with mental retardation. Am J Ment Retard 1996;101:130-48.

[16] Courbois Y, Lejeune L. Étude expérimentale de la génération d'images mentales chez des adolescents retardés mentaux. Revue Francophone de la Déficience Intellectuelle 2000;11(l):73-84.

[17] Courbois Y. Proposition d'un cadre théorique pour l'étude de la cognition visuelle des personnes retardées mentales. Revue Francophone de la Déficience Intellectuelle 2002;13(2):101-13.

[18] Gibson L, Glynn SM, Takahashi T, Britton BK, Imagery and the prose recall of mildly retarded children. Contemp Educ Psychol 1995;20(4):476-82.

[19] Howe ML, Toth S, Cicchetti D. Memory and developmental psychopathology. In: Cicchetti D, Cohen D, eds. Developmental psychopathology, 2nd ed. Volume 2: Developmental neuroscience New York: Wiley;2006;2:629-55.

[20] de la Iglesia C, Buceta J, Campos A. Prose learning in children and adults with Down syndrome: The use of visual and mental image strategies to improve recall. J Intellect Dev Disabil 2005;30(4):199-206.

SECTION TWO - VARIOUS ASPECTS OF PAIN

Chapter 8

MECHANICAL AND HOLISTIC PARADIGMS IN SEXOLOGY: VIAGRA® REPRESENTS A MECHANICAL WORLDVIEW AND MAY CAUSE FEMALE SEXUAL PAIN

Søren Ventegodt, MD, MMedSci, EU-MSc-CAM[*,1,2,3,4,5] *and Joav Merrick, MD, MMedSci, DMSc*[5,6,7,8]

[1]Quality of Life Research Center, Copenhagen, Denmark; [2]Research Clinic for Holistic Medicine and [3]Nordic School of Holistic Medicine, Copenhagen, Denmark; [4]Scandinavian Foundation for Holistic Medicine, Sandvika, Norway; [5]Interuniversity College, Graz, Austria; [6]National Institute of Child Health and Human Development, [7]Office of the Medical Director, Division for Mental Retardation, Ministry of Social Affairs, Jerusalem, Israel and [8]Kentucky Children's Hospital, University of Kentucky, Lexington, United States

Abstract

Males tend to go for genital potency, while women tend to go for deeper emotional and spiritual experiences in sexuality. Men often live in practical, simplistic, mechanical paradigms, while women live in complex, social, emotional, and spiritual paradigms. Male sexual dysfunction indicates fundamental problems in the couple's sexual interaction; the solution to male sexual erectile dysfunction is therefore not a drug increasing genital hardness, but rather sexological couple therapy, developing the couple's sexual consciousness and the understanding of the genders different characters. The conflict between mechanical and holistic worldviews is classical in sexology. Kegel found that sexual dysfunctions including dyspareunia, lack of desire and orgasm was caused by weakness in the

---

[*] **Correspondence:** Søren Ventegodt, MD, MMedSci, EU-MSc-CAM, Director, Quality of Life Research Center, Classensgade 11C, 1 sal, DK-2100 Copenhagen O, Denmark. Tel: +45-33-141113; Fax: +45-33-141123; E-mail: ventegodt@livskvalitet.org

pubococcygeus muscle, while Reich believed that low orgasmic potency was caused by a blockage in the life-energies that should flow through the whole body and be fully integrated in the human character. Freud believed sexual dysfunctions to be caused by the repression of sexuality into the unconscious. Jung believed that orgasmic potency came from our ability to accept and meet out inner anima/animus – the opposite gender in our sexual shadow. In the tradition of erotic tantra the sexual energies are cultivated and circulated through body, mind, spirit, and heart. The optimal sexological treatment is multi-paradigmatic and allows the couple to analyze their sexual paradigms to come to an understanding of self and the partners physical, emotional, and spiritual needs in sexuality. Viagra® does not always solve the psychosexual problems related to erectile dysfunction and likely to increase female dyspareunia.

Keywords: Integrative medicine, holistic health, behavioral science, sexology, sex counseling, human development, mental health.

Introduction

Sexuality was an object for intensive research in the first half of the 20th century, with great discoveries that lead to establishment of the medical science of sexology around 1960. Since then thousands of sexologist, some of them physicians and other therapists, have helped millions of patients with sexual dysfunctions. Recently the pharmaceutical industry has contributed to sexology with the development of sildenafil citrate (Viagra ®) for male erectile dysfunction. In spite of the understandable popularity of this drug among impotent men, the effect on their female partner has not really been discussed. Tiefer (1) has reflected on the fact that the pharmaceutical industry has systematically withheld the data from the partner-survey from publication. This is likely to indicate lack of a positive effect on the female partner's sexual satisfaction, or even worse that the female partner is experiencing more problems and sexual pain because of the drug.

In our sexological clinical practice we often heard female partners express their disappointment with Viagra®, as it has not improved her sex-life. The real need of a female, she will say, is not "hard sex" but a relationship that is playful, experimental, deeply emotionally involving, and even spiritually enlightening. These concepts are often fundamentally lacking in the male universe, making the women feel his male energy somewhat hard, mechanical, simplistic and alien – sometimes even described as an emotionally and spiritually wasteland. Insensitive penetration causes often pain, which is the most common female complain in the sexological clinic, and it is insensitive penetration that makes her reject him sexually giving him problems with his sexual self-confidence and these emotional problems rare the true cause of his erective dysfunction. The couple's sexual problems are thus going deeper that just being an evil circle that can be broken with Viagra®.

To rehabilitate female orgasmic potency, with all its elements of desire, excitement, enjoyment and lack of pain – it is often necessary not only to work mechanically on strengthening her pelvic floor musculature, but also to help her develop self-confidence, acceptance and even to heal emotional wound from her youth- and childhood sexual traumas. It often takes a great existential awakening to help a woman back to full orgasmic potency (2,3).

Men's sexual problems are normally connected with lack of erectile potency and premature ejaculation; both these are well known from sexological research (2) to be strongly connected with psychological factors. It is worth remembering the fact that Masters and

Johnson were able to cure almost all impotent men in just 14 days using a competent female substitute partner, documenting the psychological dimensions in erectile dysfunction. Confidence, self-insight, acceptance of own body and sexuality, and a deep understanding of the differences in men's and women's sexuality seems to be what is needed to be a sexually able man. This is also what a woman needs to open op emotionally and spiritually for the man, not just a hard member, as many men seemingly still believe.

Sexological paradigms

The word *paradigm* refers to Kuhn's famous work on scientific paradigms (4). In sexology the sexological inadequacies have been understood in very different ways.

The mechanical paradigm

Kegel (4,5) saw most sexual problems coming from the simple mechanical weakness of the pelvic floor muscles, primarily the pubococcygeus muscle around the vagina. In 1948 Kegel found that the ability to tighten the vagina around the male penis, an ability that he documented varies much from women to woman, is essential for good sexual functioning; he therefore developed the famous "Kegel exercises" to strengthen the pelvic floor musculature (4). In the second paper in 1952 Kegel wrote (6): "Summary. Findings in the present series indicate that sphincteric and sensory sexual function of the vagina is practically always potentially present, and can be developed through muscle education and resistance exercise. Every woman with sexual complaints should be investigated for possible dysfunction of the pubococcygeus muscle. In a large percentage of cases it will be found that "lack for vaginal feeling" and so-called frigidity can be traced to faulty development of function of the pubococcygeus muscle (6). Graber and Kline-Graber continued this research (7).

Hartman and Fithian wrote in 1972 (8): "It is important to determine whether there is any sensation or awareness in the vagina. Some women are unaware if the examining finger or if the speculum is in or out. What we attempt to do is to get her to focus on the feeling in the vagina, with an examining finger in the vagina. We found that often nothing has ever been in the vagina long enough for her to have developed any perception, and because of this, she may describe any movement as pain. This is easily determined if the pain is inconsistent in location." (8, page 81). "About one out of ten women that we see are not able to move their vaginal muscles at all. In these women the vagina is often gapping and open, and they usually have some problem with stress-incontinence. In such cases we have difficulty in getting them to move the muscle enough to identify it so that they can learn to do the vaginal exercises. However, if they can learn to do the exercises and will do them, remarkable changes can take place in the physiology of the vaginal barrel, even where here has been extensive trauma in childbirth" (8, page 82). "The woman has the organ of accommodation and can develop a tight vaginal vault where she can receive much more friction and feeling trough vaginal exercises. This is not only positive for her in the vagina, but also a tight vagina will cause more movement of the foreskin over the clitoral shaft which will increase her satisfaction and pleasure. We feel that it is to the advantage of both the female and male …" (8, page 89-90).

"If there is a tear or lesion in the wall of the vagina and we insert a finger in that area or we flick the band where there is any fibrosity, this can often be painful and the woman frequently responds by saying, "What is that? That is exactly what happens in intercourse, but I have never been able to find out what it is." We can assure the woman that it is simply a fibrous band or a separation on the vaginal wall and can easily be filled in or corrected by her doing the suggested vaginal exercises (Kegel pelvic contractions)" (8, page 86).

"A well-conditioned vagina is long and narrow. It should be remembered that a vagina is not an actual space, but a potential. It is by inserting a finger and moving is against the wall we ascertain the contour, since the fleshy part of the vagina meets the resistance of the vaginal muscles when palpated with a finger. If you notice again our illustration, you will see that the bottom left-hand boxes, which are divided into thirds, identify the vaginal barrel right and left by lower, middle and upper third, which have different markings on them. The top third of than indicate no observable muscle. It is in poor condition with a lot of fibrosity indicated by the x. The lower third has a circle with an X, which indicates there is some muscle response there, but here is fibrosity or sessions in the muscle. The lower part indicates the muscle is in better shape having less fibrosity in the right side still not too good. If you look at the last set of boxes, you see that in a year's time the mobility has markedly changed" (8, page 92).

The mechanical logic is clear, and the text leaves no doubt that a woman, who is able to catch her partners member in a strong, dynamic grip will have her vagina and clitoris well stimulated this way, offering also the man the physical stimulation needed, thus bringing them both to full orgasm. You could say that this is the first, basic level of genital sexuality: When there is a functioning intercourse the rest is just details so as a sexologist you would be wise to focus here. And if you believe that a harder member can compensate for a weaker vagina, Viagra® is a good solution to the problem of male erectile dysfunction. Clearly a man with an artificial erection can have intercourse, but this is not automatically giving the woman sexual pleasure; only the most chauvinistic of men believe today that a hard member is enough to satisfy a woman. The emotional contact is the most important thing for a woman and as the couple's emotional problems are also in most cases the true cause of the erectile dysfunction; therefore the emotional problems must be solved to increase sexual satisfaction for both the male and the female.

Holistic paradigms

The word "holistic" means "with regard to the wholeness". The first part of the 20th century gave birth to several holistic sexological paradigms.

Sigmund Freud (1856-1939). The most influential has without doubt been the understanding of human sexual development by Sigmund Freud, from the oral to the anal and finally the genital sexuality (9). In spite of the simplicity of this idea is has lead to highly complex intervention restoring the patients sexual ability though regression all the way into early infancy, to rehabilitate sexuality at its very roots. Freud's early idea was that sexuality was repressed through childhood traumas, but later he believed that it was human nature to repress sexuality as we, the Ego, were destined to inner conflicts between out animalistic side, the Id, and our social consciousness, the Super-Ego. The conflict theory put sexual transference and counter-transference in the center of psychodynamic psychotherapy.

Wilhelm Reich (1897-1957). The person who in reality created the science of sexology was Wilhelm Reich. Reich succeeded in mapping the sexual cycle in the curve of orgasm, which is the basis of all sexological understanding today. He understood the orgasm as the release of sexual energy, which had build op between the genitals and the rest of the body. The higher developed sexually a person was, the more sexual energy could be charged on this inner battery. Therefore the whole body was involved in sexuality, not only the genitals. The whole character of the person should integrate the genitals and the sexual energy and become what Reich called a *genital character* (3,10). Reich found that sexual bodywork combined with psychodynamic psychotherapy helped the patient to heal not only sexual dysfunctions, but also somatic and mental health, including in some cases schizophrenia and cancer. In the last half of the 20th century researchers like Searles (11) and Levenson (12) took these ideas to the next level and developed cures for schizophrenia respective cancer that are still under scientific investigation with regard to their efficacy.

Carl Gustav Jung (1875-1961) was strongly inspired by the Eastern concept of sexuality, where sexual energy is seen to circulate through the whole human being and thus energizing and integrating body, mind and spirit into the abstract human "heart" (13). Jung saw sexual tension as a building up between the persons own gender, which is expressed outwardly, and an inner core of opposite sexuality, which Jung called the anima/animus. The Eastern idea that we are total, all-inclusive beings found its expression in human sexuality. According to this model all sex is masturbatory; when we engage in sexuality we only project our inner male or female part into our partner. The more sexually healthy we are, the more can we accept our anima/animus, and the more sexual energy can we accumulate in our system, and the stronger can we project sexual attractiveness into our sexual partner. The whole tradition of erotic tantra is close to this understanding (14).

Sexological treatments according to paradigms

The treatment of sexual dysfunction is strongly depending on how the patient and the sexologist understand sexuality. In a mechanical paradigm the goal will basically be to get the intercourse going. The man can be helped with Viagra, and the women with pelvic floor exercises ("Kegel's").

The sexological examination

A more integrative approach has been the sexological examination developed by several clinicians (8,15-20). The sexological examination is actually a series of interventions that are both explorative and therapeutic-educational at the same time (a medical concept often called "clinical medicine"); the four steps are described by Hoch in 1986 (16, p. 768):

- *Gynecological examination:* The gyneco-sexologist first proceeds with the gynecological examination. Inspection and palpation of the external genitalia may reveal involuntary contractions of the pubococcygeal muscle, in which case it is advisable to ask the patient to contract and relax the anal sphincter, thus teaching her how to control the perivaginal musculature. In order to familiarize the patient with her own body, she is instructed to introduce first her own fingers and then the examiners fingers into the vagina.

- *Vaginal acupressure:* The examiners fingers are moved to and fro, starting on the posterior vaginal wall and then slowly proceeding toward the lateral and anterior aspects of the vaginal canal. Touching and light pressure are alternatively used on every part. Proper lubrication of the fingers is necessary during this part of the examination. The patient is asked to concentrate and to indicate her sensory feelings during stimulation of the different vaginal regions. Her reactions are recorded.
- *Vaginal sexological examination:* If she indicates discomfort, pain, or no special sensation, the fingers are slowly moved on, until an erotically reactive area is identified. Stimulation is then continued on the area for a while, but never longer that required for reaching the excitement phase of beginning plateau phase of her sexual cycle. When stimulating the anterior vaginal wall, pressure applied to the second hand on the suprapubic region proved to be very helpful in enhancing the patient's sensation. This bimanual stimulation is performed in a steady circular fashion, almost bringing the two examining hands together. The external hand of the examiner is then replaced by the patients hand, teaching her how to locate, through her abdominal wall, the intravaginal examining fingers.
- *Partner exercise:* The last step is giving the couple sexological exercises for home practice.

There are today several types of sexological examinations, the "Hoch" type is very medical and oriented towards pathology and dysfunctions, although it clearly includes the emotional aspect of sexology, while the "Pomeroy-Brown" type is much more holistic. Pomeroy and Brown rebelled against Hoch (15) in 1982: "This difference between a sexological exam, as advocated by Hoch and our own system emphasizes the fundamental difference between a medical (i.e. a pathological) approach and a pleasure approach to sexuality. The former focuses on illness, deviance, and pathology and is the most common approach used in Europe and elsewhere outside the US. Fortunately, in the US we have finally realized that the medical model is inappropriate and are now concerned with health, pleasure, communication, sensitivity, and awareness which allows for change and growth far beyond that conceptually possible, employing the medicinal model" (17, page 73). "For a non-medically oriented type of sexological examination, since the focus is on gathering and imparting information on anatomy, physiology, arousal patterns, response cycles, and pleasure zones, any knowledgeable and sensitive sex therapist should be able to conduct the procedure skillfully. Medical training is not necessary for this nor is it necessary in order to know how to insert a speculum. This skill can be gained rapidly – evidence by the many women's self-help groups that have sprung up throughout the country. The women in these groups learn to insert specula both in themselves and other women and learn to examine the cervices, vaginal walls, etc. Furthermore, Hoch's manner of examining the female appears to be too medically focused and lacking in relaxation, since the woman is on an examining table with her feet in stirrups, as in a regular gynecological exam. In our sexological exams, we try to have the woman reclining on large, overstuffed pillows in order to eliminate the elements of fear and tension that are often present in a medical atmosphere" (17, page 74).

Hoch is also insisting on not involving the patients whole body, while Pomeroy and Brown insist that: "A sexological examination that does not include at least total body mapping, i.e. rating on a scale of –3 to +3 where and how a person enjoys being touched, is not a true indicator of a person's sexual responses" (17, page 75). This must be understood as a clear indication of Pomeroy and Brown "going holistic".

Vaginal acupressure/ vaginal massage/ Hippocratic pelvic massage

The vaginal acupressure part of the sexological examination have always been an integral part of bodywork, physical therapy and physiotherapy and was practiced by the European doctors all the way back to Hippocrates and his students, where it is described in the Corpus Hippocraticum (21). Many medieval sources describe interventions almost identical to the sexological examination, including the provocative element of direct sexual stimulation (22-28). Vaginal acupressure/pelvic massage have in a number of studies been found highly efficient for sexual dysfunctions including pelvic pain (29-37). In spite of the common use of this kind of therapy, it must be realized that "there are no standard treatment protocols guiding the manual therapy" (37, page 518). There seems to be a general agreement among researchers that every therapist most find his own way here and include the elements that he or she finds most usable.

The technique of pelvic and genital bodywork has therefore also been described and practiced in many different ways. We saw Hoch's description of vaginal massage in step two above; a more contemporary description of pelvic physical therapy was given by Rosenbaum in 2005, who concluded that: "Physicians recognizing and treating women presenting with vaginismus and dyspareunia should consider physiotherapists as vital members of the interdisciplinary team" (39, page 337). "The physiotherapist's assessment of the vulva differs from the gynecological examination. Both the external and internal exam focus on the mobility and integrity of the muscular, fascial and connective tissue components. The vulvar and pelvic floor exam consists of the following: a) Observation of the vulva, perineum, and anus to note areas of redness, raised areas, scar tissue or edema; b) palpation to note tenderness to touch; c) internal exam to assess pelvic floor muscle tension and tightness to touch; c) internal exam to assess pelvic floor muscle tension and tightness, tone, range of motion, and hymeneal presence and thickness; d) assessment of internal muscle trigger points; e) determination of the integrity of the pelvis organs and possible presence of prolapse of the bladder, uterus, or rectocele and f) anorectal internal exam" (39, page 335). "Conclusion: Physical therapy treatment of pelvic pain is an integral component of the multidisciplinary approach to CCP (chronic pelvic pain) and associated sexual dysfunctions. (38, page 513). "Manual techniques including massage, stretching, and soft tissue and bony mobilizations, are important components of treatment..." (38, page 517). "In assessing the pelvic floor muscle tone, important markets include muscle length, muscle tension, muscle stiffness, presence of trigger point, and pelvic floor synergy or presence of dysenergia" (38, page 517).

Weiss described in 2001 pelvic physiotherapy this way: "In contrast to external muscle group that physiotherapists treat manually with 1 or 2 hands, internal muscle groups limit the practitioners to 1-finger treatment via the rectum or vagina. Tenderness, tightness or taut bands are located. They are then treated with compression, stretching, strumming at right angles to the affected muscle bundles or allowing the finger to glide between fibres to seek toe direction of least resistances, termed following the well" (33, page 2227). "Any tender points are then eradicated by compression and stretching" (33, page 2228). "Treatment should continue until tenderness and tightness have dissipated, which requires 1 to 2 visits weekly for 8 to 12 weeks depending on the duration and severity of symptoms. (33, page 2228).

Bergeron et al (31) treated 35 women with vulvar vestibulitis: "Physical therapy yielded a complete or great improvement for 51.4% of the participants, a moderate improvement for 20.0% of participants, and little to no improvement for the other 28.6%. Treatment resulted in a significant decrease in pain experienced both during intercourse and gynecological examinations; it also resulted in a significant increase in intercourse frequency and levels of sexual desire and arousal. ... Finds demonstrate that physical therapy is a promising treatment modality for dyspareunia associated with vulvar vestibulitis" (31, page 183-184). They concluded: "Physical therapy is one of the few treatment for vulvar vestibulitis that is non-invasive and has no known negative side effects. (31, page 184-185). They described their method as "physical therapy sessions": "Manual techniques used for proprioception, normalization of muscle tone, pain modification, and mobilization were applied on the surface of the perineum and internally by vaginal and sometimes anal palpation. These techniques included, among others, myofascial release, trigger-point pressure, and massage" (31, page 185).

Vaginal acupressure is different from the sexological examination. Hoch wrote (15): "Stimulation then proceeds [in the sexological examination] to the external genitalia involving the vestibule, urethral region, labia minora, and clitoris. There are no standard techniques for successful clitoral stimulation. Different patients react differently to various sites, pressures, pace, and form of clitoral stimulation, but it will generally be successful if one common condition is met: The moment we have located what is best for our patient, stimulation should be continuous and uninterrupted until a beginning plateau level is reached. Here again it is the patient's responsibility to provide the examiner with exact instructions for the achievement of successful stimulation" (15, page 61).

To us vaginal acupressure is a most simple procedure that is already an integral part of the standard pelvic examination: "It is important to understand that the procedure of acupressure through the vagina, is the same exploration part of the standard pelvic examination by a gynecologist, but in this case done so slowly that the woman can feel the emotions held by the different tissues contacted by the finger of the physician. It can be used in combination with the pelvic examination and as the woman always will contact some feelings while examined in her vagina, the situation is really that every pelvic examination contains an element of acupressure through the vagina. Often the awakening of unpleasant feelings is very emotionally painful for the woman and if not taken care of by the physician/gynecologist it will make the standard pelvic examination difficult for the woman, as many women actually experience. Just ignoring the fact that the woman is a living human being reacting emotionally to the pelvic examination is not going to help the woman not to feel" (40).

All the researchers seems to agree that there are no side effects of the manual sexological treatments, but there is some warning that most of patients with pelvic and genital pain has psychiatric co-morbidity (41). This does not at all mean that one should not help sexually dysfunctional mentally ill patients, but that the therapist needs to work with special attention to the patient's emotional problems as well as their mental, spiritual, and existential problems.

Even in the most mechanical and physical therapy, only rational approach when is comes to the sexological patient is holistic. Just taking care of the body is not an option. Most interestingly it has so often been found that therapeutic work in the pelvic and sexological area can cure not only pain and sexual dysfunction, but also cure the patient's seemingly unrelated mental and somatic illness (42). This strongly indicates that unsolved psychosexual developmental problems are causing severe and chronic somatic and psychological imbalance, distress, illness and disease.

Ethical considerations

Hoch (15) wrote: "The sexological examination of the female patient, as performed in our Center, has proved to be an essential and almost indispensable diagnostic and therapeutic tool for the treatment of female sexual dysfunction" (15, page 58). Hoch did not, in the light of the patient's obvious need of cure find any ethical problems in the procedure, but admitted that there was a problems in taking a female patient all the way to orgasm during the sexological examination: "Special care is taken to avoid high preorgasmic levels of sexual response, or orgasmic release, which might often evoke in the partner unnecessary fears of having "to compete" with the more knowledgeable (and often male) physician (15, page 62).

Alzate and Londoño (43) described the ethical problems in a research project with sexological examination, where the patients were taken all the way to orgasm: "Some comments on the ethical implications of this research are in order here, since in absence of any practical alternative the subjects reached climax with the help of the male examiner. Although there seems to be a consensus among sexologists on the rules that should govern sex therapist/patient (client) interactions, and on the limitations of the sexological examination conducted in a therapeutic setting (but not on the professionals qualified to perform it), apart from the minimal requirements of professionalism, confidentiality, and consent, the ethics of sex research should be flexible enough not to hinder the advancement of knowledge, once the human subject's protection has reasonable been taken into account. Therefore, we believe that our examination procedure, which might be improper in a therapeutic setting, is ethically acceptable as long as the examiner keeps from being erotically involved with the subject, which was the case in this study (43).

The researchers seem all to agree about the Hippocratic ethical rule of not having sex with the patients, but it is highly doubtful that sexological work can be done without some sexual excitement of the therapist as both Freud and Searles have admitted (44,45). Yalom (46) also argued that this is absolutely normal and should not be considered a problem: "I have been sexually aroused by patients and so have every therapist I know". The therapist's sexual arousal, which is often higher in the beginning of his sexological carrier when everything is still new, is not a problem if the therapist knows how to control his behavior. In our experience the experienced sexologist easily controls the level of sexual arousal, sexual mentation and sexual behavior.

As manual sexological therapy has no side effects all researchers seems to agree that there is not ethical problems with manual sexological treatment, e.g. the sexological examination, if only the therapist respect the Hippocratic ethics. Recently the Hippocratic ethical rules has been re-formulated in a practical formulation useful for sexologist by the International Society of Holistic Health (47).

Discussion

Men and women are psychosexually very different in accordance with their historical sex-roles. In the modern uni-sex culture, where both genders are taking all kinds of jobs and social functions we forget that sex is about biology and biology does not change as fast as culture. We therefore need to acknowledge nature and respect the differences of male and female. One of the most important differences seems to be the female's need for respect, safety, security and care, to open up emotionally and sexually. Sexuality is often quite mechanical for a man; a tight vagina is to some extend what he always dreams about. The woman's sexual dreams are much more romantic, and sexuality is really rewarding without a deep feeling of love and devotion. The sexologist must understand these differences, and train the two genders to understand and respect each other. Interestingly most male sexual dysfunctions, erectile impotency, and premature ejaculation, come directly from emotional problems in the relationship, the man feeling insecure and uneasy in the sexual situation. In the same way most female sexual dysfunction come from her partner not holding her emotionally and spiritually also; even the hardest and most persistent penetration is rarely enough to bring her to high levels of pleasure and orgasm; often insensitive penetration is actually the direct course of sexual pain, making about half of the world's women complain about dyspareunia. Therefore correction of penile hardness with a drug like Viagra ® is not the whole story.

Viagra® has become a money machine, because millions of impotent men desperately want to become sexually potent today. But keeping up appearances is not solving the sexual problems, which are not really inside the man, but lies in the interaction between the partners. The physician having the patient's confidence for a moment before prescribing Viagra can therefore help the male, who is in deep trouble by pinpointing the real problems. We all know that it takes one minute to prescribe a drug, but many hours to help a man solve his real problems. So the next time you think of prescribing Viagra® to a patient please consider the true needs of this man and his female partner.

When it comes to sexual dysfunctions talking is not enough, reviews have shown that bodywork is actually needed (48). Meston and Bradford (49) concluded recently that "medical treatments for women's sexual dysfunctions have largely failed to outperform placebo treatments but may be useful in specific clinical subgroups" and "despite widespread clinical acceptance in many cases, few psychosocial treatments for women's sexual dysfunction are empirically supported. Little is known about which treatment components are most effective" (49). Marinoff and Turner (50) concluded already in 1991 that "too often patients with vulvar symptoms are shunted from one gynaecologist to another and finally told they should seek psychiatric help." Another thing that clearly does not help much in dyspareunia is antibiotic drugs, which are also often prescribed; the reason for this is simple: "Although some authors have proposed that the vulvar vestibulitis syndrome may reflect an infection agent such as Candida albicans, our results showed little evidence of an infections etiology, even after multiple samplings at various sites ... We found that dyspareunia was present at first intercourse in 44% of the patients, suggesting a primary form of this syndrome in a relatively large proportion of affected woman (51).

The more "sterile" and orderly, mechanical type sexological treatment is also inefficient: "Approximately 15% of woman have chronic dyspareunia that is poorly understood, infrequently cured, often highly problematic and distressing. Chronic dyspareunia is an urgent health issue…the traditional treatment of vaginismus with vaginal "dilatation" plus psycho education, desensitisation, and so forth is not evidence-based… Pelvic floor therapies for dyspareunia may be effective" (52). Schultz's group (52) were very positive to the "educational gynecological sexological examination": "When conducted correctly, it can be highly therapeutic." "Through this examination, the foundation is laid for a meaningful discussion afterwards, in which all the findings are explained and at which time further sexual complaints may come to light…" (52). Schultz et al (52) concluded: "Ideally a multidimensional, multidisciplinary approach for sexual pain is recommended, with attention to the following areas: the experience of pain, the emotional/psychological profile, any context of past mutilations or sexual abuse; the genital mucose membrane; the pelvic floor; and sex and partner therapy…Psychological issues (as well as interpersonal issues) should be addressed early on with psychotherapy" (52).

Rosenbaum and Owens (38) concluded: "Physical therapy treatment of pelvic pain is an integral component of the multidisciplinary approach to chronic pelvic pain and associated sexual dysfunctions (38). There thus seem to be an agreement among the researchers that manual sexological treatment is needed for curing sexual dysfunctions. Conversation therapy cannot do this alone. Pharmacological treatment is also not always helpful and neither is psychiatric treatment. And very few believe surgery to be the answer to genital pain.

Conclusions

Researchers seem to agree that manual sexological procedures combined with conversation therapy is the cure of choice in most sexual dysfunctions. Couple therapy is often recommended. Erective dysfunction can be symptomatically treated with Viagra®, but we do not believe this to be a good solution for the female partner, and therefore not for the couple. We do not believe it to be helpful at all in the long run. The reason is erectile impotency mostly is caused by emotional problems and lack of emotional contact with the female partner and that mechanical penetration without emotional contact is the primary cause of female dyspareunia. Sexual intercourse is a mutual thing; only when the sexual interaction is emotionally and spiritually deep and energetically dynamic can both participants reach optimal sexual pleasure and full orgasm.

The sexologist must have more than a mechanical approach to sexology; it takes a fully developed holistic approach to give the necessary attention to all relevant aspects of the human being - body, mind and spirit - to help a couple reach the highest levels of sexual pleasure. Very often both somatic and psychiatric problems are solved in this process of sexual healing. The patient's psychosexual development and the whole field of sexology therefore seem to be of utmost importance in medicine.

Sexual problems are almost always caused by emotional problems, which cannot be solved with a drug. Sexology must focus not only on the genitals, but also on the whole person. Developing on the patient's understanding of the different natures of male and female and involving the partner in the solution of sexual problems are indispensable steps in the healing of sexual dysfunctions.

Acknowledgments

The Danish Quality of Life Survey, Quality of Life Research Center and The Research Clinic for Holistic Medicine, Copenhagen, was from 1987 till today supported by grants from the 1991 Pharmacy Foundation, the Goodwill-fonden, the JL-Foundation, E. Danielsen and Wife's Foundation, Emmerick Meyer's Trust, the Frimodt-Heineken Foundation, the Hede Nielsen Family Foundation, Petrus Andersens Fond, Wholesaler C.P. Frederiksens Study Trust, Else and Mogens Wedell-Wedellsborg's Foundation and IMK Almene Fond. The research in quality of life and scientific complementary and holistic medicine was approved by the Copenhagen Scientific Ethical Committee under the numbers (KF)V. 100.1762-90, (KF)V. 100.2123/91, (KF)V. 01-502/93, (KF)V. 01-026/97, (KF)V. 01-162/97, (KF)V. 01-198/97, and further correspondence. We declare no conflicts of interest.

References

[1] Tiefer, L. Sexology and the pharmaceutical industry: the threat of co-optation. J Sex Research 2000;37:273-83.
[2] Masters WH, Johnson VE. Human sexual inadequacy. Philadelphia, PA: Lippincott Williams Wilkins, 1966.
[3] Reich W. [Die Function des Orgasmus]. Köln: Kiepenheuer Witsch, Köln, 1969. [German]
[4] Kuhn TS. The structure of scientific revolutions. Chicago: Univ Chicago Press, 1962.
[5] Kegel AH. Progressive resistance exercise in the functional restoration of the perineal muscles. Am J Obstet Gynecol 1948;56(2):238-48.
[6] Kegel AH. Sexual function of the pubococcygeus muscle. Western J Surg Obstet Gynaecol 1952;60(10):521-4.
[7] Graber B, Kline-Graber G. Female orgasm: Role of pubococcygeus muscle. J Clin Psychiatry 1979;40(8):348-51.
[8] Hartman WE, Fithian MA. Treatment of sexual dysfunction. Long Beach, CA: Center Marital Sex Stud, 1972.
[9] Jones E. The life and works of Sigmund Freud. New York: Basic Books, 1961.
[10] Reich W. Character analysis. New York: Farrar Straus Giroux, 1990.
[11] Knight RP. Preface. In: Searles HF. Collected papers on schizophrenia. Madison, CT: Int Univ Press, 1965:15-8.
[12] Levenson F B. The causes and prevention of cancer. London: Sidgwick Jackson, 1985.
[13] Jung CG. Man and his symbols. New York: Anchor Press, 1964.
[14] Anand M. The art of sexual ecstasy. The path of sacred sexuality for Western lovers. New York: Tarcher/Perigree (Putnam), 1989.
[15] Hoch Z. A commentary on the role of the female sexological examination and the personnel who should perform it. J Sex Res 1982;18(1):58-63.
[16] Hoch Z. Vaginal erotic sensitivity by sexological examination. Acta Obstet Gynecol Scand 1986;65(7):767-73.

[17] Pomeroy WB, Brown M. A reaction to Hoch's commentary on the female sexological examination. J Sex Res 1982;18(1):72-6.
[18] Hartman WE, Fithian MA. In Magnus Hirschfeld archive for sexuality. Accessed 2008 Dec 01. http://www2.hu-berlin.de/sexology/ECE5/sexological_examination.html
[19] Grafenberg E. The role of urethra in female orgasm. Int J Sexol 1950;3(3):145-8.
[20] Goldberg DC, Whipple B, Fishkin RE, Waxman H, Fink PJ, Weisberg M. The Grafenberg spot and female ejaculation: A review of initial hypothesis. J Sex Marital Ther 1983;9;1:27-37.
[21] Jones WHS. Hippocrates. Vol. I–IV. London: William Heinemann, 1923-1931.
[22] Spencer WG. Aulus Cornelius Celsus: On medicine. Cambridge, MA: Harvard Univ Press, 1935.
[23] Temkin O. Soranus of Ephesus: Gynecology. Baltimore, MD: Johns Hopkins Press, 1956:140-70.
[24] Adams F. Aretaeus Cappadox: The extant works of Aretaeus the Cappadocian. London: Sydenham Society, 1856.
[25] Siegel R. Galen of Pergamon: De Locis Affectis. New York: Karger, 1976.
[26] Ricci JV. The gynaecology and obstetrics of the sixth century AD. Philadelphia: Blakiston, 1950
[27] Radicchio R. Mustio [Moschion]. La Gyneacia di Muscione. Pisa: Giardini, 1970:122.
[28] Maines R. The technology of orgasm. Baltimore, MD: Johns Hopkins Univ Press, 1999.
[29] Lukban J, Whitmore K, Kellogg-Spadt S, Bologna R, Lesher A, Fletcher E. The effect of manual physical therapy in patients diagnosed with interstitial cystitis, high-tone pelvic floor dysfunction, and sacroiliac dysfunction. Urology 2001;57(6 Suppl 1):121-2.
[30] Markwell SJ. Physical therapy management of pelvi/perineal and perianal pain syndromes. World J Urol 2001;19(3):194-9.
[31] Bergeron S, Brown C, Lord MJ, Oala M, Binik YM, Khalifé S. Physical therapy for vulvar vestibulitis syndrome: a retrospective study. J Sex Marital Ther 2002;28(3):183-92.
[32] Schultz WCMW, Gianotten WL, van der Meijden WI, van de Wiel HBM, Blindeman L, et al. Behavioral approach with or without surgical intervention to the vulvar vestibulitis syndrome: a prospective randomized and non-randomized study. J Psychosom Obstet Gynecol 1996;17:143-8.
[33] Weiss JM. Pelvic floor myofascial trigger points: Manual therapy for interstitial cystitis and the urgency-frequency syndrome. J Urol 2001;166(6):2226-31.
[34] Wurn BF, Wurn LJ, King CR, Heuer MA, Roscow AS, Hornberger K, Scharf ES. Treating fallopian tube occlusion with a manual pelvic physical therapy. Altern Ther Health Med 2008;14(1):18-23.
[35] Wurn LJ, Wurn BF, King CR, Roscow AS, Scharf ES, Shuster JJ. Increasing orgasm and decreasing dyspareunia by a manual physical therapy technique. Med Gen Med 2004;6(4):47-53.
[36] Ventegodt S, Clausen B, Merrick J. Clinical holistic medicine: Pilot study on the effect of vaginal acupressure (Hippocratic pelvic massage). ScientificWorldJournal 2006;6:2100-16.
[37] Polden M, Mantle J. Physiotherapy in obstetrics and gynecology. Stoneham, MA: Butterworth Heinemann, 1990.
[38] Rosenbaum TY, Owens A. The role of pelvic floor physical therapy in the treatment of pelvic and genital pain-related sexual dysfunction (CME). J Sex Med 2008;5(3):513-23.
[39] Rosenbaum TY. Physiotherapy treatment of sexual pain disorders. J Sex Marital Ther 2005;31(4):329-40.
[40] Ventegodt S, Clausen B, Omar HA, Merrick J. Clinical holistic medicine: Holistic sexology and acupressure through the vagina (Hippocratic pelvic massage). ScientificWorldJournal 2006;6:2066-79.
[41] Wylie KR, Hallam-Jones R, Coan A, Harrington C. A review of the psychophenomenological aspects of vulval pain. Sex Marital Ther 1999;14(2):151-64.
[42] Ventegodt S, Thegler S, Andreasen T, Struve F, Enevoldsen L, et al. Clinical holistic medicine (mindful, short-term psychodynamic psychotherapy complemented with bodywork) in the treatment of experienced impaired sexual functioning. ScientificWorldJournal 2007;7:324-9.

[43] Alzate H, Londoño ML. Vaginal erotic sensitivity. J Sex Marital Ther 1984;10(1):49-56.
[44] Freud S. Further recommendations in the technique of psychoanalysis: Observations on transference love. In: Rieff P, ed. Therapy and techniquere. New York: Collier Books, 1915:168.
[45] Searles HF. (1965) Oedipal love in the countertransference In: Searles HF. Collected papers on schizophrenia. Madison, CT: Int Univ Pres, 1965:284-303.
[46] Ventegodt S, Kandel I, Merrick J. Clinical holistic medicine: avoiding the Freudian trap of sexual transference and countertransference in psychodynamic therapy. ScientificWorldJournal 2008;8:371-83.
[47] de Vibe M, Bell E, Merrick J, Omar HA, Ventegodt S. Ethics and holistic healthcare practice. Int J Child Health Human Dev 2008;1(1):23-8.
[48] O'Donohue W, Dopke CA, Swingen DN. Psychotherapy for female sexual dysfunction: A review. Clin Psychol Rev 1997;17(5):537-66.
[49] Meston CM, Bradford A. Sexual dysfunctions in women. Annu Rev Clin Psychol 2007;3:233-56.
[50] Marinoff SC, Turner ML. Vulvar vestibulitis syndrome: an overview. Am J Obstet Gynecol 1991;165(4 Pt 2):1228-33.
[51] Bazin S, Bouchard C, Brisson J, Morin C, Meisels A, Fortier M. Vulvar vestibulitis syndrome: an exploratory case-control study. Obstet Gynecol 1994;83(1):47-50.
[52] Schultz, W.W., Basson, R., Binik, Y., Eschenbach, D. Wesselmann, U. van Lankveld, J. Women's sexual pain and its management. J Med Sex 2005;2:301-16.

In: Pain Management Yearbook 2009
Editor: Joav Merrick

ISBN: 978-1-61209-666-7
©2012 Nova Science Publishers, Inc.

Chapter 9

A Q-METHODOLOGICAL STUDY TO EXPLORE THE LOW BACK PAIN BELIEFS AND ATTITUDES OF LOW BACK PAIN HEALTH PROFESSIONALS

Carol Campbell*, BSc (Hons), MA, PhD
School of Social Sciences and Law, University of Teesside,
Middlesbrough, United Kingdom

Abstract

Low back pain continues to be a common and costly problem both to sufferers, their families and health services. Despite its prevalence, proven efficacious treatments remain elusive. Little attention has been given to the attitudes and beliefs that health professionals who work with low back pain sufferers hold. This is an important omission as low back pain sufferers will encounter many different health care personnel in their care trajectory. Objective: To explore beliefs relating to low back pain held by health care professionals working in secondary or tertiary low back pain management facilities. Study group: Thirty-four health care professionals working in the North East of England. Methods: Employing Q-methodology, the Q-sorts of thirty-four health care professionals (comprising orthopaedic surgeons, anaesthetists, nurses, physiotherapists, occupational therapists, pharmacists and psychologists in specialised low back pain units) were factor analysed. Results: Six factors were generated to identify accounts of these professional views of low back pain. The six accounts highlighted the different views that the different health professional groups held with regards to low back pain. Conclusions: The differences between these professional groups play an important part in how individual professionals' beliefs regarding low back pain are communicated to patients and consequently how these may be perceived and interpreted by sufferers. The findings have important ramifications for the delivery of multidisciplinary low back pain management and the implications of this are discussed.

Keywords: Low back pain, Q-methodology, health care professionals

---

* **Correspondence:** Carol Campbell, School of Social Sciences and Law, University of Teesside, Borough Road, Middlesbrough, TS1 3BA United Kingdom. Tel: 01642 342385; Fax: 01642 342399; Email: carol.campbell@tees.ac.uk

Introduction

Low back pain (LBP) has a long and detailed history, yet remains one of the most commonly experienced forms of disabling pain in western societies (1). The increasing prevalence of low back pain since 1945 has seen a paralleled augmentation of confusion within the medical profession over how to treat and manage it. This confusion has been attributed to the lack of an intelligible relationship between expressed patient symptoms and pathological signs that can be observed in sufferers' musculo-skeletal systems and as such it continues to be a pervasive health care problem (2). It is estimated that 60% to 90% of the western population will have at least one experience of LBP during their lifetime and approximately 10 to 15% of sufferers will progress to develop chronic LBP and related disability (3). As such, there are considerable individual and societal costs associated with its development (4), intransigence and treatment.

The presence of LBP leads sufferers to seek relief and consulting a health care professional 'is a primary treatment strategy for those who have chronic or persistent pain' (5). However, of those who consult primary care physicians only one quarter are likely to be fully recovered after a period of one year (6). Consequently, referral to secondary and/or tertiary care providers is actively sought by both primary care physician and sufferer. Furthermore, LBP sufferers differ from other patient groups by seeking the care of a variety of health care professionals. However, it has been highlighted that there is no standard or agreed definition of chronic LBP (7) and there remains continuing uncertainty and disagreement within the medical and health professions related to its cause, nature and treatment. This is problematic not least because a failure to reach consensus regarding the cause and nature of LBP can lead to 'inconsistencies in the advice and subsequent treatment that is given to individuals suffering with low back pain' (8), but also because inconsistent and conflicting advice may contribute to the chronification process (3).

Consideration of the beliefs and attitudes relating to LBP held by health professionals is a relatively recent addition to the research literature with the majority of studies instead having focused on the interaction between patient and health care provider and the resulting satisfaction with and expectations of treatment (9). Despite this paucity of literature the few studies that have examined the beliefs and perceptions of health care professionals are worthy of review because it not only frames current thinking about the management of LBP but also reveals the limitations in the research methods used.

In an early study, general practitioners' (GP) perceptions of LBP patients were investigated using semi-structured interviews (10). The ten GPs who were interviewed provided six principal differentiations of the LBP patients they encountered during the treatment and management of their pain. The six differentiations highlighted patients who presented with a predominantly psychological overlay to their pain; those who presented with acute versus chronic LBP; those who lacked motivation to comply with treatment; those who appeared genuine in their pain complaint; the social background of the patient; and finally the sex and occupation of the person in pain. These six principal forms of patient differentiation highlighted how the GPs segmented their LBP patient population into ideal types based on stereotypical characteristics and in so doing influenced their decisions in relation to treatment choice and pain management options. However, only ten GPs from a very small geographical region in the United Kingdom participated in this study and so caution must be applied in drawing too great an inference from the extracted themes. Nevertheless, the findings are important because they highlight the cognitive biases that GPs may invoke in the presence of particular LBP sufferers and in so doing provide insight into the reasons why some LBP patients express dissatisfaction with their care and engage in active treatment seeking from other GPs and related health professionals.

The measurement of attitudes and beliefs within and between health care professional groups, as stated above, has only recently attracted research attention. It has been shown that beliefs and attitudes influence health care professionals' LBP management practices (11). However, the mechanisms by which this occurs and how these beliefs and attitudes influence practice behaviour are not fully understood (12). The main method employed to elicit attitudes and beliefs about LBP from health care professionals has been conducted via surveys or questionnaires. Werner et al (13) sent questionnaires asking about LBP beliefs to LBP physicians, physiotherapists and chiropractors. They found significant differences between the three professional groups in answers to two out of five statements relating to LBP treatment and management (regarding spontaneous recovery and surgery for disc herniation). The greatest discordance in their answers were between the physicians and the chiropractors, with the physiotherapists answering somewhere in between. Whilst this brief survey was able to identify clear differences in attitudes toward LBP management between the three professional groups it is limited in that only a few statements were asked. Nevertheless the highlighted disparities may provide some evidence to account for the often expressed dissatisfaction by LBP patients as to the different experiences they perceive when being treated by different professional groups. However the narrow scope of the questionnaire items means that caution must be given to these findings.

Specific attitude questionnaires have also been devised to elicit attitudes, beliefs and practice behaviour of different groups of health care practitioners. Despite the proliferation of clinical guidelines that collectively advise maintaining normal activities, avoiding bed rest and passive treatments and returning to or staying in work (14) adherence to the guidelines is poor (15).

Bishop, Thomas and Foster (16) in their critical review of the literature found five tools that have been used with different health care professional groups to determine attitude strength, LBP beliefs and impact on LBP management practice behaviour. The five tools (Attitudes to Back Pain Scale for musculoskeletal practitioners; Fear avoidance beliefs tool; Fear Avoidance Beliefs Questionnaire; Health Care Providers' Pain and Impairment Relationship Scale; and Pain Attitudes and Beliefs Scale for Physiotherapists) however are lacking in empirical testing particularly in relation to their reliability. Furthermore little use has been made of these scales within a UK setting. One exception to this being Pincus et al (17) who used the Attitudes to Back Pain Scale for musculoskeletal practitioners with groups of chiropractors, osteopaths and physiotherapists. Findings revealed that all three professional groups endorsed a psychosocial approach to LBP treatment and management but significant differences were found between the groups for some of the dimensions on the questionnaire. Most notably, physiotherapists reported that they limited the number of treatment sessions more than the chiropractors and osteopaths, and osteopaths reported limiting sessions more than chiropractors. Additionally, both physiotherapists and chiropractors reported more willingness to engage in psychological issues with LBP patients than osteopaths. Furthermore, physiotherapists were less concerned about the quality of the treatment that they delivered to their patients than either of the other two groups. Whilst this study does highlight the attitudinal similarities and differences between these three health practitioner groups in relation to their practice, there are methodological limitations that need to be considered. The health practitioners recruited to explore attitudes in this study were also the same practitioners involved in the initial development of the scale. Therefore, the participants may have been primed in their responses due to their earlier involvement with the project. Additionally, there were more physiotherapists than chiropractors in the sample which may account for the differences in attitudes observed between these groups. Finally, whilst the authors suggest that they are measuring attitudes toward back pain within their questionnaire, scrutiny of the factors that comprise the scale indicate that what is actually being measured by the nineteen items is more an examination of the practitioners personal viewpoint in relation to treatment. The scale considers Personal Interaction and Treatment Orientation but fails to explore attitudinal positions regarding LBP development and presentation in any depth.

Most recently findings have been reported from a postal survey that employed the Pain Attitudes and Beliefs Scale and a clinical vignette of a person with LBP with general practitioners (GPs) and physiotherapists in the United Kingdom (UK) (18). A diverse response set between the physiotherapists and GPs was found but most importantly over a quarter of the entire sample indicated that they would recommend, contrary to current guidelines, that the individual within the vignette be advised to stay off work. Reported attitudes and beliefs were significantly related to a biomedical orientation in those professionals recommending staying away from work. The authors concluded that a 'considerable proportion of health care practitioners in the UK ...continue to practice predominantly within a biomedical model' (p.192). Whilst the response rate was disappointing in this study; these findings are of particular interest as they highlight the continuing dominance of the biomedical model in contemporary health care practice in the UK and a decrease in biopsychosocial attitude suggesting that further scrutiny of attitudes and beliefs of those individuals involved in LBP management are warranted not least because it has been suggested that patients' beliefs relating to their LBP may result from the projected beliefs of their own health care provider (19).

With all of these studies there is a need to think critically about the methods used and how these may impact on the findings derived. A major criticism of these self-report measures is that bias may be introduced with social desirability answering being especially pertinent (16). Furthermore, the different attitudes that are being considered within these studies are explicit. Little research is available that has compared explicit and implicit attitudes however, the work that is available suggests that the relationship between them is at best weak but that both are related to treatment recommendations (20). There is a clear need to understand further the beliefs and attitudes of practitioners not least because their personal orientation to treatment will undoubtedly influence their initial decisions during patient care encounters. Depending on their educational and professional training backgrounds (and hence attitudinal position) could mean that the endorsement of either a biomedical or biopsychosocial approach would empahsise either predominantly physical factors or multidimensional perceptions in their management of LBP.

The attitudes held by different health practitioner groups also have important implications not least for the adherence to clinical guidelines. Across the many professional groups that are involved in the management of LBP there is a broad consensus as to what constitutes best care. However, despite agreement on what this comprises, adherence to these guidelines is poor with some practitioners reluctant to change their clinical practice in line with best practice recommendations. This may be because health professionals 'advise and treat individual patients but the evidence on which they base many of their decisions is drawn from research populations' (p.1084) (21). Moreover, the tension between treating individual patients and the nature of evidence upon which best practice guidelines are based is problematic with many health care professionals perceiving difficulty in applying such guidelines to individual patients (22). It is clear therefore, that the study of beliefs and attitudes towards LBP and its treatment is complex and multifaceted and worthy of further study. What is of particular interest however is that despite the paucity of research in this area, studies that have considered beliefs and attitudes have excluded hospital based doctors, psychologists and nurses as well as other health care professionals that are involved in the management of LBP focusing instead (almost exclusively) on physiotherapists, chiropractors and osteopaths.

One study that has focused on the various medical personnel that are often involved in pain management employed a social constructionist analysis of how sense was made of the causes of chronic pain (23). By examining patients' and professionals' understandings of the causes of chronic pain using Q-methodology the authors revealed four accounts representing the participant sample and identified the themes of responsibility, blame and the need to protect identity as common to each of the accounts. They concluded that a shift in perception by the practitioner regarding the patient is needed, in order to appreciate individual constructs of identity. Whilst this study focused on chronic pain in general rather than chronic LBP in particular it is nevertheless one of the few studies to consider the breadth of personnel that are involved in pain treatment and management. Emphasising the importance of the beliefs of the many different health care professionals with whom LBP patients may come into contact, is then an important, if albeit neglected area of research. Indeed, it is suggested that 'we need to know more about the origins of beliefs and attitudes of health-care practitioners about back pain' (p.173) (17) and this would appear to be even more pertinent when consideration is given to the many different health care professionals involved in multidisciplinary pain management teams and the fact that their beliefs may be related to actual behaviour (24).

In order to examine this issue further a preliminary study to explore the beliefs and understandings about LBP from a range of health professionals who were involved in the secondary or tertiary treatment and management of LBP in the North East of England was undertaken. Q-methodology was employed to address the following question: What are your beliefs relating to chronic low back pain and its management?

Methods

Brief overview of Q methodology

Q-methodology was devised by Stephenson (25) and elaborated and developed by Brown (26) as a simple alternative methodology to those used in traditional psychometric assessment. Q-methodology is based on the twofold premise that subjective points of view are communicable and always advanced from a position of self reference (27). Q-methodology offers a research tool (the Q-sample) to explore and describe the diverse population of meanings and understandings that a given group of participants has about a specified phenomenon – in this case health professionals and LBP. The Q-sample is presented usually in the form of statements that represent the broadest variety of attitudes and perspectives on a given topic. Each participant is required to rank order each item within the Q-sample from 'most agree' (+6) to 'most disagree' (-6) sorting all of the items within the Q-sample into a quasi-normal distribution placing each statement in a grid that is provided. Each completed grid represents an ipsative construction of the Q-sample (28), whereby all statements have been sorted in relation to each other. The completed sorts are factor-analysed by person rather than by variables or statements and the resulting factors reflect clusters of individuals who sorted the statements in the most similar way as well as also indicating dimensions of the underlying phenomenon. Each factor is then interpreted and explained in terms of commonly shared perspectives.

Producing the Q-set (the item sample)

In order to ground the item sample in concrete existence (29) and to generate the broadest concourse of potential item statements as possible a range of sources were used in order to construct the sample of items. A focus group, unstructured interviews and informal conversations as well as a review of the academic literature that had reported qualitative findings of LBP research were undertaken. The focus group consisted of seven health care professionals who had experience of treating and managing the LBP of sufferers over a number of years. The professionals represented different practitioner groups and comprised: an orthopaedic surgeon; an anaesthetist; a physiotherapist; a clinical psychologist; a nurse; an occupational therapist; and an osteopath. The group were asked to discuss freely their experiences in treating and managing LBP and to explore what their understanding of LBP was. From this 223 statements were derived.

Unstructured interviews were undertaken with five other practitioners, who were unable to join the focus group. The interviews followed a similar format to the focus group whereby the professionals were asked to discuss their experiences relating to LBP management as well as exploration of their understanding of LBP. They comprised: a GP with a particular interest in LBP management; a chiropractor; an acupuncturist; a pharmacist; and a medical sociologist. From these interviews 167 statements were derived. Combined with the data derived from informal conversations and from a search of the academic literature the large statement set was systematically checked and an initial set of seventy-eight statements was produced. A sample of statements that is representative is one that samples the diversity of the subject domain adequately without favouring some beliefs and perceptions to the exclusion of others and without omitting sections of known constructions of belief (30). Through this preliminary stage and reflecting the broad professional base consulted four constructions emerged, namely: biomedical; psychological; social; and cultural.

A pilot sample of four participants critically examined and sorted the initial statements prior to the main study. The purpose of this pilot stage was to ensure that the statements were unambiguous in their terminology, germane to the research question and able to discriminate between participants. From this scrutiny, twenty-two items were removed leaving a total of fifty-six to be used in the main study, which is more than an adequate item sample size (31).

The final list of statements is shown in Table 1. Each of the individual fifty-six statements was then printed onto a card and a number from one to fifty-six written on the reverse.

Table 1. Q-set (item sample)

1.	Aggression and power are linked to low back pain onset
2.	Our culture encourages people to talk about their low back pain
3.	The culture in which we are brought up plays an essential role in how we feel and respond to low back pain
4.	Low back pain differs from person to person, culture to culture
5.	Within different cultures the presence of low back pain is seen as an honour
6.	Low back pain is just a feeling
7.	Low back pain is just an emotion
8.	Low back pain is just a physical state
9.	Low back pain is just a mental state
10.	Low back pain develops because the person has done something wrong
11.	All low back pain is real regardless of its cause
12.	Chronic low back pain isolates people because it demands all of their attention and energy
13.	People with chronic low back pain are preoccupied with pain and ill health
14.	Chronic low back pain is not a sign of injury
15.	Low back pain means many things to many people
16.	The presence of low back pain can be seen as a punishment
17.	Chronic low back pain has no useful function
18.	The meaning people give to their low back pain influences the way they feel their pain
19.	Chronic low back pain is an obstacle and a threat to the sufferer
20.	Low back pain is so common that it could be said to be part of normal everyday life
21.	Exercise is an important part in the management of chronic low back pain
22.	People suffering with low back pain may see many different health professionals and end up with little or no help
23.	People suffering with chronic low back pain may see many medical specialists several times without experiencing any significant pain relief
24.	Some health professionals expect people from different social, cultural or religious backgrounds to respond to low back pain in different ways
25.	Drugs have a valuable role in the management of chronic low back pain
26.	The effect of many treatments for chronic low back pain is short-lived
27.	Psychological help can be useful for people who suffer with chronic low back pain
28.	Many health professionals don't believe that patients have chronic low back pain
29.	A psychologist can often help people to reach a better understanding of the nature of chronic low back pain
30.	The prescribed treatments for chronic low back pain are a complete waste of time
31.	In this day and age you would think that there was something that could be given or that could be done to cure chronic low back pain
	Health professionals do not always have a good reputation among patients because they cannot always relieve their low back pain
33.	People who have low back pain are vulnerable to the things that health professionals

	say to them
34.	People who have chronic low back pain and take morphine will become addicted

Table 1. (Continued)

35.	Past experiences of low back pain lead sufferers to develop tactics for tolerating and reducing their pain
36.	Elderly people cope better than anyone else with chronic low back pain
37.	People who suffer from chronic low back pain wish to be cured
38.	People with chronic low back pain can see no connection between emotion and pain
39.	Individuals suffering from chronic low back pain have lost the ability to cope well with their disability and distress
40.	People who have chronic low back pain cannot see the negative effects of seeking a cure for their pain
41.	People who have chronic low back pain are frequently told to take things easy
42.	Sufferers are unwilling to learn ways that could help them manage their low back pain
43.	People who have chronic low back pain will try anything to get to the bottom of what is causing the pain
44.	People expect a miracle cure for their low back pain
45.	People with chronic low back pain would allow themselves to be experimented on to get rid of their pain
46.	People don't want to learn to manage their low back pain, they want rid of it
47.	People use their chronic low back pain to obtain welfare benefits
48.	People fake low back pain to get sympathy and draw attention to themselves
49.	Chronic low back pain usually means that the person has to stop working and rely on benefits
50.	The family and friends of a person with low back pain should do as much as they can to stop the pain getting worse
51.	There are social costs and benefits of revealing chronic low back pain
52.	People with chronic low back pain are malingerers
53.	Because chronic low back pain is invisible, sufferers put on a performance for those around them
54.	Chronic low back pain leads to invalidity
55.	People with chronic low back pain reduce their working and social life because the pain they feel indicates that further damage is being done
56.	People who have chronic low back pain exaggerate their symptoms to gain sympathy

Participants

Sampling within Q-methodology is different to that employed in conventional methodology. Here participants are represented as variables rather than sample elements. The sample therefore is each participants completed sorting of the Q-set and each distribution of the Q-set becomes the data that are analysed. Research participants should be individuals who have pertinent viewpoints on the topic domain, with the breadth and diversity of the sample more appropriate than proportionality (29). Following university and host hospital research ethical approval, participants were recruited from several specialist National Health Service (NHS) LBP and pain management units in the North East of England. The final sample comprised thirty-four LBP health practitioners representing several different professional groups. These were: eight pain nurse specialists; three orthopaedic surgeons; four anaesthetists specialising in pain management; seven physiotherapists; five occupational therapists; four psychologists; and three pharmacists. Each participant was involved in most, if not all, of their working time in the treatment and management of LBP.

Procedure

Participants completed the sorting individually and were instructed to first read through all fifty-six of the statements in order to familiarise themselves with the Q-set. After the initial reading they were instructed to initially sort the statements into three piles: either agree, disagree or neutral/unsure. They were then asked to select the one statement that they most agreed with from the agree pile and place this in the most extreme right hand box on the blank grid that was provided to them (see figure 1). They were then asked to select the statement that they most disagreed with from the disagree pile and place this in the most extreme left hand box on the grid. They were asked to continue this process until all of the cards from the Q-set had been placed on the grid. Once all of the items had been sorted each participant was asked to re-examine the positioning of each item and if necessary rearrange any items until they were happy with the final array. The number and position of each card was noted on a smaller grid and these data were entered into a spreadsheet using SPSS (version 13.0).

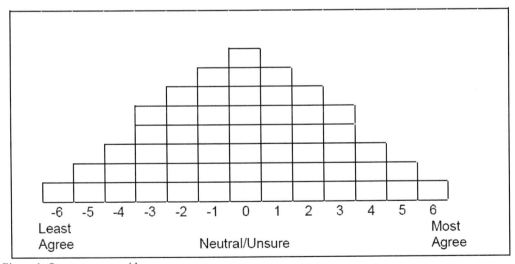

Figure 1. Q-set response grid.

Results

The thirty-four completed sorts were analysed using factor analysis. The extraction of the factors was achieved using principal components analysis, and varimax rotation with kaiser normalisation. Using an eigenvalue greater than unity (> 1.00), the original 34 sorts reduced to 6 independent orderings at the 0.05 level that explain 53% of sample variance. Factor loadings for each (pseudonymised) participant are shown in table 2. Of the thirty-four participants, twenty-one loaded significantly and exclusively on one of the six factors. Significance was taken at =0 .50. The remaining thirteen sorts which did not achieve the level of significance were not used to define any of the resulting six factors.

Table 2. Rotated factor matrix

Sorter	Factor 1	Factor 2	Factor 3	Factor 4	Factor 5	Factor 6
Molly	76	30	06	08	01	12
Lottie	77	06	11	06	02	09
Chris	60	38	19	07	01	-27
Sarah	69	-10	11	39	00	-08
Keith	64	20	25	16	21	27
Ray	68	20	09	15	27	01
Jen	23	62	29	15	16	14
Alan	12	65	-01	08	-06	27
Karen	29	71	09	-13	28	04
Tracy	13	-07	73	14	-02	00
Jack	11	22	73	20	18	09
John	47	24	65	-11	02	20
Mark	33	22	36	56	28	-25
May	36	02	-17	56	-17	-13
Jane	32	-03	19	72	32	03
Phil	-04	00	21	74	22	38
Jim	02	18	-18	15	57	-05
Vic	11	06	09	21	70	25
Julie	05	39	27	11	63	14
Adam	33	37	14	18	18	57
Briony	07	12	07	00	21	77
Les	29	43	25	47	-15	03
Eddie	19	45	36	15	15	-30
Fran	33	19	-11	46	04	05
Paul	-15	16	06	07	43	32
Joe	00	43	10	05	05	16
Jill	49	26	48	-03	06	02
Lisa	39	-23	33	00	47	08
Jan	00	00	-05	-03	07	41
Julie	13	45	49	11	13	01
Wes	-04	-10	46	13	02	15
Dean	48	26	22	41	-02	-09
Kate	19	45	22	-09	26	-21
Sam	06	-05	24	-01	04	06

Note. Factor exemplars by factor are shown in shaded areas. Decimal points omitted from loadings.

Once the defining Q-sorts had been identified for each factor further calculations were undertaken in order to determine the magnitude of the extent to which each individual sort contributed to the aggregated factor. Each defining sort was proportionately weighted and this weighting applied to each Q-item. The scores for each item were then summed and then rank ordered into the original Q-sort. Subsequently idealised Q-sorts for each of the six factors was produced and constitutes the factor arrays. Factor arrays for the six factors are shown in table 3. Scrutiny of the factor arrays enables the researcher to identify how the Q-items are distinguished across each of the factors and in so doing facilitates the interpretation of each of the factors.

Table 3. Factor arrays: scores against each item by factor

Q item		F1	F2	F3	F4	F5	F6
1.	Aggression and power are linked to low back pain onset	-3	-5	-1	+2	-2	-4
2.	Our culture encourages people to talk about their low back pain	-4	-3	-3	-2	-2	0
3.	The culture in which we are brought up plays an essential role in how we feel and respond to low back pain	+3	+1	+1	+2	-1	-1
4.	Low back pain differs from person to person, culture to culture	+4	0	-2	+2	0	0
5.	Within different cultures the presence of low back pain is seen as an honour	+1	-1	-1	-2	0	-5
6.	Low back pain is just a feeling	-6	-2	-4	-4	-5	-4
7.	Low back pain is just an emotion	-5	-3	-4	-6	-4	-3
8.	Low back pain is just a physical state	-4	-3	-5	-4	-4	-6
9.	Low back pain is just a mental state	-5	-4	-5	-4	-3	-3
10.	Low back pain develops because the person has done something wrong	+2	-3	+1	0	-4	-4
11.	All low back pain is real regardless of its cause	+6	+3	+4	+3	-1	+2
12.	Chronic low back pain isolates people because it demands all of their attention and energy	+5	0	-2	+2	-3	-3
13.	People with chronic low back pain are preoccupied with pain and ill health	+2	+4	+1	-2	-1	0
14.	Chronic low back pain is not a sign of injury	-2	-1	-3	+2	0	-2
15.	Low back pain means many things to many people	-1	-1	+5	+1	-2	+1
16.	The presence of low back pain can be seen as a punishment	-3	-6	-1	-1	-2	-3
17.	Chronic low back pain has no useful function	-2	-2	0	-3	+4	-1
18.	The meaning people give to their low back pain influences the way they feel their pain	0	+1	+3	+1	-1	-5
19.	Chronic low back pain is an obstacle and a threat to the sufferer	-1	-2	-1	+3	+2	-2
20.	Low back pain is so common that it could be said to be part of normal everyday life	-1	+2	+1	-5	+1	+5
21.	Exercise is an important part in the management of chronic low back pain	+3	+5	+2	+3	+2	+2
22.	People suffering with low back pain may see many different health professionals and end up with little	+3	+1	0	-2	-1	+1

	or no help						

Table 3. (Continued)

Q item		F1	F2	F3	F4	F5	F6
23.	People suffering with chronic low back pain may see many medical specialists several times without experiencing any significant pain relief	+5	+1	+1	+3	+3	+3
24.	Some health professionals expect people from different social, cultural or religious backgrounds to respond to low back pain in different ways	0	+1	0	0	-3	-1
25.	Drugs have a valuable role in the management of chronic low back pain	+1	0	+4	+5	+5	+3
26.	The effect of many treatments for chronic low back pain is short-lived	-1	0	+2	+4	-1	0
27.	Psychological help can be useful for people who suffer with chronic low back pain	+4	+3	+2	0	+2	-1
28.	Many health professionals don't believe that patients have chronic low back pain	+1	-2	-2	-1	+1	+3
29.	A psychologist can often help people to reach a better understanding of the nature of chronic low back pain	+2	+3	+5	0	+2	-1
30.	The prescribed treatments for chronic low back pain are a complete waste of time	0	-1	-2	-1	-6	+4
31.	In this day and age you would think that there was something that could be given or that could be done to cure chronic low back pain	+1	-4	+4	+2	0	+1
32.	Health professionals do not always have a good reputation among patients because they cannot always relieve their low back pain	+1	-1	+2	0	-2	0
33.	People who have low back pain are vulnerable to the things that health professionals say to them	+2	0	+3	+1	+1	-2
34.	People who have chronic low back pain and take morphine will become addicted	-2	-3	0	+5	+3	0
35.	Past experiences of low back pain lead sufferers to develop tactics for tolerating and reducing their pain	-1	+2	+1	-3	0	-1
36.	Elderly people cope better than anyone else with chronic low back pain	0	-2	-3	-3	-5	+3
37.	People who suffer from chronic low back pain wish to be cured	+3	+6	+2	+6	+4	+2
38.	People with chronic low back pain can see no connection between emotion and pain	+2	+2	-3	-1	0	-2
39.	Individuals suffering from chronic low back pain have lost the ability to cope well with their disability and distress	+2	0	+3	+1	+1	0

40.	People who have chronic low back pain cannot see the negative effects of seeking a cure for their pain	+4	0	-1	0	+1	+1

Q item		F1	F2	F3	F4	F5	F6
41.	People who have chronic low back pain are frequently told to take things easy	+1	+5	+3	+1	-2	+3
42.	Sufferers are unwilling to learn ways that could help them manage their low back pain	-2	-1	-3	0	0	-3
43.	People who have chronic low back pain will try anything to get to the bottom of what is causing the pain	+1	+4	-1	+4	+6	+4
44.	People expect a miracle cure for their low back pain	0	+3	+6	+1	+3	+2
45.	People with chronic low back pain would allow themselves to be experimented on to get rid of their pain	0	+2	+2	+3	+5	+5
46.	People don't want to learn to manage their low back pain, they want rid of it	+3	-2	-2	+4	+1	+6
47.	People use their chronic low back pain to obtain welfare benefits	-1	+4	+1	-1	+3	+1
48.	People fake low back pain to get sympathy and draw attention to themselves	-3	+1	0	-2	+2	+4
49.	Chronic low back pain usually means that the person has to stop working and rely on benefits	-3	0	-6	-5	+1	+2
50.	The family and friends of a person with low back pain should do as much as they can to stop the pain getting worse	-4	-5	+2	-3	-3	0
51.	There are social costs and benefits of revealing chronic low back pain	0	+1	0	-3	0	-2
52.	People with chronic low back pain are malingerers	-2	+2	0	-1	-1	+2
53.	Because chronic low back pain is invisible, sufferers put on a performance for those around them	-1	+2	-1	+1	-3	-2
54.	Chronic low back pain leads to invalidity	-3	-4	-4	0	+2	-1
55.	People with chronic low back pain reduce their working and social life because the pain they feel indicates that further damage is being done	0	+3	+3	-1	+3	+1
56.	People who have chronic low back pain exaggerate their symptoms to gain sympathy	-2	-1	0	-2	+4	+1

The qualitative interpretation of the emergent factors is the final stage in Q-methodology. This is advanced in terms of consensual and divergent subjectivity, with attention given to the relevance of such patterns to existing or emerging theories, propositions, and the like [27]. Detailed exposition of the six factors, which together explain 53% of the variance, is presented below. The factor score for each statement is given in parentheses after each item.

Interpretation of factors

FACTOR ONE - 'The sufferers perspective'

Participants who loaded exclusively onto this factor demonstrated an understanding of chronic LBP that is centred on the lived experience of pain and to a certain extent reflects the LBP sufferers' perspective. Within this factor a strong biopsychosocial understanding of LBP is acknowledged with respondents supportive of psychological help as well as recognising the potentially isolating force of living with LBP.

Six participants (Molly, Lottie, Chris, Sarah, Keith and Ray), all nurse specialists, defined this factor. This factor accounted for 28.69% of the total variance and this was the only factor that strongly endorsed the following items:

11. All low back pain is real regardless of its cause (+6)
12. Chronic low back pain isolates people because it demands all of their attention and energy (+5)
23. People suffering with chronic low back pain may see many medical specialists several times without experiencing any significant relief (+5)
27. Psychological help can be useful for people who suffer with chronic low back pain (+4)
40. Most people who have chronic pain cannot see the negative effects of seeking a cure for their pain (+4)
4. Low back pain differs differ from person to person, culture to culture (+4)

This view of LBP also acknowledges the physical and psychological demands that LBP sufferers endure as they continually strive to negotiate the health care system in order to receive relief from their pain, whilst conceding that this search for a cure can be counterproductive. Respondents to this factor also strongly disagreed with the following items:

6. Low back pain is just a feeling (-6)
9. Low back pain is just a mental state (-5)

Whilst this factor most strongly rejected these items, scrutiny across all of the factor arrays sees that each of the six factors also did not agree with these statements, suggesting that where pain is proposed as unidimensional, strong responses across the participant sample have been elicited and may reflect professional (as proposed to lay) knowledge that pain is multidimensional.

The participants who loaded onto this factor also disagreed with the following items:

2. Our culture encourages people to talk about their low back pain (-4)
48. People fake low back pain to get sympathy and draw attention to themselves (-3)

Rejection of these items may be due to the fact that these pain nurse specialists tend to spend more time with LBP sufferers either via out-patient clinics, or LBP management programmes and therefore become more familiar (over time) with the individual circumstances that LBP sufferers face. This factor therefore, identifies with the position that psychological evaluation is an important part of pain management and that cultural background must also be considered for effective understanding of LBP manifestation. It demonstrates the importance of believing patients, even without physical evidence of the nature of the pain, but also points to the damaging effects that can occur when patients continue in their search for a cure. Respondents to this factor demonstrate a belief in the impact that chronic low back pain has on the individuals who experience and live with it and suggests a rejection of the medical model in favour of a more person-centred, biopsychosocial approach to LBP management.

FACTOR TWO - 'The active/passive perspective'

Participants who loaded exclusively onto this factor demonstrated an understanding of chronic low back pain that is somewhat ambivalent insofar as LBP is perceived as all-encompassing and leading to preoccupation by the sufferer and that mixed messages in relation to LBP management perpetuate this passivity. This factor also exclusively acknowledged the role of exercise as important to LBP management.

Three participants (Jen, Alan and Karen) all physiotherapists, defined this factor. This factor accounted for 8.26% of the total variance. This was the only factor that strongly endorsed the following items:

21. Exercise is an important part in the management of chronic low back pain (+5)
41. People who have chronic low back pain are frequently told to take things easy (+5)
13. People with chronic low back pain are preoccupied with pain and ill health (+4)

Item 37 was the most strongly endorsed by respondents loading onto this factor but this was not exclusive to this factor, with factor 4 also strongly agreeing with the statement

37. People who suffer from chronic low back pain wish to be cured (+6)

As well as being the only factor that strongly endorsed the item relating to exercise, respondents to this factor also most strongly endorsed the item related to LBP being used for personal gain, as in item 47:

47. People use their chronic low back pain to obtain welfare benefits (+4)

The perspective endorsed by factor 2 is one where individual responsibility for LBP management is given primacy. This perspective rejects the view that people within the social world of the sufferer should facilitate pain management; likewise a considered view relating to pharmacological management is evident here:

50. The family and friends of a person with low back pain should do as much as they can to stop the pain getting worse (-5)

25. Drugs have a valuable role in the management of chronic low back pain (0)
34. People who have chronic low back pain and take morphine will become addicted (-3)

Maintaining beliefs related to individual responsibility, rather than a cultural view of LBP causation and management this was the only factor that strongly rejected the following items:

1. Aggression and power are linked to low back pain onset (-5)
16. The presence of low back pain can be seen as a punishment (-6)

Collectively, the respondents endorsing factor 2 demonstrate beliefs relating to LBP that is focused on the patient as an active individual insofar as pain is perceived by the individual almost to the exclusion of other influences and thus LBP management will be achieved by the efforts of the individual sufferer. Somewhat cynically this factor views LBP sufferers as preoccupied with their pain, searching for a cure, yet using their LBP to take advantage of secondary and tertiary gains. The three respondents who loaded exclusively onto this factor were all physiotherapists and may account for the emphasis on physical exercise as an effective way to manage LBP; the fact that LBP sufferers are frequently told to take things easy and a rejection of the help from family and friends that defines this factor also supports a 'patient as active' orientation. This 'active/passive' perspective resonates with the biomedical model with little emphasis given to psychological aspects and an ambivalent stance towards social or cultural elements in chronic LBP development.

FACTOR THREE - 'The psychological perspective'

Participants who loaded exclusively onto this factor demonstrated an understanding of chronic LBP that is patient focused but also where chronic LBP is viewed as a concept unique to each individual. Additionally, this factor views LBP as being constructed by each individual sufferer yet promotes a hopeful outlook for LBP management.

Three participants (Tracy, Jack and John) all psychologists defined this factor. This factor accounted for 7.34% of the total variance and this was the only factor that strongly endorsed the following items:

44. People expect a miracle cure for their low back pain (+6)
15. Low back pain means many things to many people (+5)
29. A psychologist can often help people to reach a better understanding of the nature of chronic low back pain (+5)
11. All low back pain is real regardless of its cause (+4)
31. In this day and age you would think that there was something that could be given or that could be done to cure chronic low back pain (+4)

The beliefs highlighted in this factor acknowledge the unique subjective phenomenon of LBP whilst also conceding that those who suffer with LBP would rather be without it! It demonstrates an understanding of LBP that is rooted within the sufferers' perspective but more so in the psychological domain than that which is shown in factor 1. There is also acknowledgement of the role of wider social influences on LBP sufferers and their management of their pain with the inclusion of item 50:

50. The family and friends of a person with low back pain should do as much as they can to stop the pain getting worse (+2)

Respondents to factor 3 were alone in their endorsement of item 50 and may suggest that where family and friends are unsupportive towards the LBP sufferer this may compound the suffering. Likewise, positive endorsement of items 18 and 33 were the most strongly rated by this factor:

18. The meaning people give to their low back pain influences the way they feel about their pain (+3)
33. People who have low back pain are vulnerable to the things that health professionals say to them (+3)

Support for these two items emphasises the affective and emotional elements inherent in pain perception and serves to further define this factor as more psychologically focused.

Respondents who loaded onto this factor also most disagreed with the following items:

49. Chronic low back pain usually means that the person has to stop working and rely on benefits (-6)
9. Low back pain is just a mental state (-5) (with factor 1)
38. People with low back pain can see no connection between emotion and pain (-3)

Disagreement with these items maintains the beliefs that LBP is multifaceted yet also sees the LBP sufferer as agentic insofar as they are active in their own understanding of the complexities inherent in LBP development and management and that this should not preclude sufferers from maintaining an active role in their work by remaining in employment. This factor demonstrates the importance of understanding the many different levels of the person that pain can act upon and reflects a strong psychological understanding of LBP to the (almost) exclusion of biomedical principles.

FACTOR FOUR - 'The solution focused perspective'

Participants who loaded exclusively onto this factor demonstrated beliefs that centred on the resolution to LBP whilst cognisant of pain existing at this present point in time. Within this factor there is a sense that solutions for LBP management are transient as well as a rejection of items that suggest LBP interferes with the social lives of sufferers.

Here the emphasis is evenly distributed between the desire to have the pain cured and the interventions that are prescribed in an attempt to achieve this.

Four participants (Mark, May, Jane and Phil), two occupational therapists, one physiotherapist and one pharmacist defined this factor. This factor accounted for 5.25% of the total variance and was the only factor that strongly endorsed the following items:

26. The effect of many treatments for chronic low back pain is short-lived (+4)
34. People who have chronic low back pain and take morphine will become addicted (+5)

The most strongly endorsed item (number 37) was also endorsed by respondents to factor 2:

37. People who suffer from chronic low back pain wish to be cured (+6)

Interestingly within this factor, respondents endorsed items that were in opposition to the pattern seen across the other factors with such items as:

1. Aggression and power are linked to low back pain onset (+2)

and item 14 being positively endorsed by respondents to this factor

14. Chronic low back pain is not a sign of injury (+2)

Endorsement of these items suggests an understanding of LBP whereby causes other than physical factors may be involved in the onset and development of LBP. Respondents to this factor also disagreed with the following items:

7. Low back pain is just an emotion (-6)
20. Low back pain is so common it could be said to be part of normal everyday life (-5)
35. Past experiences of low back pain lead sufferers to develop tactics for tolerating and reducing their pain (-3)
51. There are social costs and benefits of revealing chronic low back pain (-3)
55. People with chronic low back pain reduce their working and social life because the pain they feel indicates that further damage is being done (-1) (the only negative endorsement across all factors of this item)

Respondents were neutral in relation to the following items:

27. Psychological help can be useful for people who suffer with LBP (0)
29. A psychologist can often help people to reach a better understanding of the nature of their chronic low back pain (0)

The beliefs relating to chronic LBP and its treatment evident within this factor are resonant of the stereotypical LBP sufferer that is most readily identified within LBP clinical practice. LBP patients who present to secondary or tertiary health care facilities often have undiagnosed chronic non-specific LBP, they long to have the pain cured, undergo (repeated) treatments despite their known limited efficacy, and believe that stronger pain relief will remedy their pain yet are wary of either the side effects or dependence due to prolonged use. They also do not perceive any benefit in being seen by a psychologist. Respondents to this factor believe in the elimination of LBP whilst acknowledging that the pain is unlikely to be cured because the treatments are either ineffective or have undesirable risks associated with them. The respondents also repudiate any social costs to living with LBP and demonstrate ambivalence to the benefits to be gained from psychological help thereby suggesting a preference for a biomedical approach to LBP management whilst acknowledging the failings with this model.

FACTOR FIVE - 'The biomedical perspective'

Participants who loaded exclusively onto this factor demonstrated beliefs that reflected a predominantly biomedical perspective and viewed LBP as a bodily state amenable to physical intervention and pharmacotherapy. This perspective also believes that the patients use their LBP for secondary gains and may become disabled as a consequence of its presence.

Three participants (Jim, Vic and Julie), all anaesthetists specialising in pain management defined this factor. This factor accounted for 5.09% of the total variance and strongly endorsed the following items:

43. People who have chronic low back pain will try anything to get to the bottom of what is causing their pain (+6)
17. Chronic low back pain has no useful function (+4)

Respondents to this factor also positively endorsed item 25, a ranking also shared by factor 4:

25. Drugs have a valuable role in the management of low back pain (+5)

This view of LBP places treatment seeking by patients as a primary factor and endorses the use of medication as a key LBP management tool. The positive endorsement of item 17 also acknowledges that LBP serves no bodily purpose to the sufferer yet the endorsement of the following two items suggests that the sufferer may find a purpose for their pain.

56. People who have chronic low back pain exaggerate their symptoms to gain sympathy (+4)
54. Chronic low back pain leads to invalidity (+2)

This factor recognises the predominantly biomedical facets of the chronic LBP experience, but is on the whole a generally negative view of chronic LBP and the individuals who live with it. The participants who loaded onto this factor most disagreed with the following items:

30. The prescribed treatments for chronic low back pain are a complete waste of time (-6)
36. Elderly people cope better than anyone else with chronic low back pain (-5)

They also disagreed with the following two statements that specifically address issues related with health professionals:

24. Some health professionals expect people from different social, cultural or religious backgrounds to respond to low back pain in different ways (-3)
32. Health professionals do not always have a good reputation among patients because they cannot always relieve their low back pain (-2)

Factor five, defined by three anaesthetists that specialise in pain management, can be seen therefore, to reflect beliefs of LBP that are embedded within a biomedical domain with endorsement of items that support treatment, medicine, and the health care professionals that prescribe them.

FACTOR SIX - 'The pessimistic perspective'

Participants who loaded exclusively onto this factor demonstrated beliefs that viewed LBP as a negative but unavoidable experience and one where the only goal is to eliminate it. This factor, similar to factor 5, is embedded within a biomedical domain but with a stronger tendency towards viewing LBP sufferers as only intent on removing the pain rather than finding ways to manage it.

Two participants (Adam and Briony), both orthopaedic surgeons, defined this factor. This factor accounted for 4.54% of the total variance. The items that were strongly endorsed by the two participants were:

46. People don't want to learn to manage their low back pain, they want rid of it (+6)
20. Back pain is so common that it could be said to be part of normal everyday life (+5)

They also endorsed item 45 that was equally endorsed by respondents in factor 5:

45. Some people with chronic pain would allow themselves to be experimented on to get rid of their pain (+5)

These first three items reflect a view of LBP as a pervasive problem that is so undesirable that sufferers cannot live with it. They also agreed with the following items:

30. The prescribed treatments for chronic low back pain are a complete waste of time (+4)
48. People fake low back pain to get sympathy or draw attention to themselves (+4)
36. Elderly people cope better than anyone else with chronic low back pain (+3)

The two respondents defining this factor exclusively agreed with items 30 and 36. They also strongly disagreed with the following items:

8. Low back pain is just a physical state (-6)
18. The meaning people give to their low back pain influences the way they feel their pain (-5)

Furthermore, they were the only respondents to disagree with item 27, albeit with a weak negative response:

27. Psychological help can be useful for people who suffer with chronic low back pain (-1)

Both participants who loaded onto this factor were orthopaedic surgeons and their responses to these salient items reflect rather pessimistic and negative beliefs of LBP experience and its management presenting a view whereby prescribed LBP treatment techniques are perceived as futile. They disagree that psychological input can help sufferers and do not strongly endorse any items that are outside the biomedical domain.

Discussion

This study explored the beliefs of chronic low back pain that were held by a range of health care professionals working in specialised low back pain units in the North East of England. Using Q-methodology, six distinct factors were identified and interpreted. The six factors accounted for 53% of the total variance. These factors were labelled "the sufferers' perspective", "the active/passive perspective", "the psychological perspective", "the solution focused perspective", "the biomedical perspective" and "the pessimistic perspective". All six factors represent different clusters of beliefs related to chronic LBP and its management. Whilst these factors accounted for just over half of the variance within the sample, it is evident that amongst these different practitioner groups there are clear differences in their beliefs related to LBP.

What is particularly striking from the resulting six factors is that the respective professionals have tended to sort in similar ways with only one mixed factor emerging (factor 4). Nurse specialists loaded exclusively onto factor 1 and can be seen to hold beliefs that are aligned with a viewpoint that places the sufferers at the centre of their understanding of LBP and endorses a patient-focused and biopsychosocial model of LBP management. Physiotherapists loaded onto factor 2 reflecting beliefs that activity is important to the management of LBP but where messages received by sufferers often run contrary to this. Factor 2 supports a biomedical orientation with little recognition given to wider social or psychological factors in the progression or management of LBP. Psychologists loaded exclusively onto factor 3 and demonstrated beliefs in the unique subjectivity of the lived LBP experience and whilst this factor emphasised psychological and social influences it also weakly endorsed biomedical intervention thus indicative of a biopsychosocial orientation.

Factor 4 was solution focused and the only factor which participants from different professional backgrounds loaded onto (two occupational therapists, one physiotherapist and one pharmacist). Here there is a sense of pain being viewed in the here and now and where the stereotypical LBP patient (undertaking several treatments, requiring medication etc.) is at the fore. This factor was distinct from others in that there was ambivalence demonstrated toward psychological support for LBP management and a belief that elimination of pain is what is desired by sufferers. Factor 4 endorses a biomedical approach to LBP management whilst acknowledging its limitations. Anaesthetists specialising in pain management loaded exclusively onto factor 5 and reflected beliefs that were entrenched within the biomedical domain. Physical interventions and pharmacological solutions were favoured, with few items that related to psychological or social factors in the pain experience being strongly endorsed. The final factor, factor 6 was exclusively endorsed by two orthopaedic surgeons and reflects rather negative beliefs relating to LBP. Similar to factor 5, factor 6 endorsed items reflecting a biomedical orientation with elimination of LBP (being seen as ubiquitous) the only desired outcome but with agreement that prescribed treatments for LBP may not be effective. This may suggest an underlying belief that surgery is perceived as the only effective way of removing the pain.

Such demarcation between the different professional groups was unexpected but does follow a similar sorting pattern to other research [23]. Furthermore, as in the studies discussed above (13,17,18) showed comparable differences between practitioner groups although the number of different professional groups involved in those studies was not as extensive as was included here. The differences in practitioner beliefs found in this study are important because they suggest that educational background may be a more powerful determinant in forming the schema of professional practice of each of these individuals and thus may represent the guiding principles that underpin such practice than previously thought. If, as is believed, that both implicit and explicit attitudes are related to treatment recommendations (20) and the giving of information and advice (7) then the disparate beliefs revealed within this study (if they are translated into practice) may account for the expressed dissatisfaction by patients of their encounters with health care providers and the resulting outcomes of such encounters (9). This would seem to be of even greater relevance when consideration is given to the aims of pain management programmes.

Pain management programmes are designed to bring together health specialists from different professional disciplines (e.g. medicine, nursing, physiotherapy, occupational therapy, psychology and pharmacy) in order to meet the complex needs of patients who have chronic pain, or specific pain problems such as LBP. Within such programmes each specialist takes responsibility for interventions guided by their respective disciplines, and so, to a certain extent, the loading by respondents from similar backgrounds onto factors that defined and reflected their professional training would suggest a desired commonality for the purposes of pain management programmes. Indeed, the clinical effectiveness of these programmes has been clearly demonstrated (32). However, the rationale of multidisciplinary pain management programmes is to adopt a biopsychosocial treatment philosophy targeting the many facets of a patient's life that may prevent them from successfully managing their pain. The findings revealed in the six factors in this study however, would suggest that far from a widespread adoption of the biopsychosocial approach, the respondents remained fixed within the boundaries defined by their professional disciplines and, whilst collectively they may achieve the desired outcomes of the programmes, individually (perhaps with the exception of the nurses and psychologists) they appear to be falling somewhat short of this ideal. The roles of the different health specialists may overlap and so it is important that there is an integration of, and consistency in the messages that are delivered to the LBP sufferers. This has particular relevance as it has been shown that 'a lack of integration can ... (result) in increased patient dissatisfaction, provider frustration and less than satisfactory treatment outcomes' (p.588) (33). Competing agendas advanced by different professional groups can therefore, interfere with successful patient outcomes and may in fact undermine the principles upon which the programmes are designed.

The continuing dominance of the biomedical model evidenced across the emergent factors in this study is also of particular interest because it reinforces and perpetuates the view of the patient as passive. This disease-based model of health has established what Foucault (34) has called the gaze, the way in which disease, illness and health care are thought about and viewed. Within the clinical gaze, Foucault argues that the bodies of patients become docile and yield to the power and authority of the scientific/medical discourse. This medical discourse has the power to diagnose or label individuals as healthy/unhealthy or able bodied/disabled and as a result ultimately determine the positioning of individuals within a society. Those who do not meet the (labelled) criteria for normality can be considered deviant or abnormal, creating the category of 'other' which can then be legitimately studied by members of the dominant group. The act of naming or labelling is an act of power of one group over another, and once labelled, groups can be studied, dissected, and theorised about by experts from the dominant group. This process of 'othering', is conceptualised as a discourse for dominating, restructuring, and having authority over the other (35). Competing discourses must struggle for recognition and legitimacy, or remain marginalised and it would appear from the findings presented here that the hegemony afforded to the biomedical model serves to limit the impact of psychosocial influences across these professional groups.

Whilst two of the factors did demonstrate beliefs that placed LBP management within a biopsychosocial domain, this model too is not without its criticisms. Stam (36) has argued that what is problematic in the biopsychosocial model is its claim to comprehend all aspects of existence and to provide professional management for disease and health. Biopsychosocial medicine still favours the technological management of existence evidenced by the way it biases intervention toward technical and professionalised treatment and in so doing continues many of the traditions of the medical model. As a result the biopsychosocial model can be seen as a powerful deceptive metaphor that converts non-scientific, non-technological treatments of disease, and particularly LBP, into techniques that can be owned by modern professions. Crossley (37) also argues that the biopsychosocial model represents no more than a multiple explanatory framework in which various physical, emotional and behavioural factors are thrown together in a seemingly fragmented way with little theoretical understanding of how they actually connect together. As a result medically prescribed pain treatments and practices remain the most socially desired and respected despite their limited efficacy and applicability when viewed within a wider social framework. So the dominance by the medical professions persists perpetuated by the educational remit of the respective health care professionals and the patients who covet their services.

The findings also raise interesting practice based issues, not least for those LBP practitioners who endorse a biomedical orientation. In describing what is a 'good back consultation' it has been suggested that in addition to maintaining open communication relating to the LBP problem, greater focus should be given to psychosocial issues with particular attention given to how LBP impacts on the various roles of everyday living (38). What is not considered however is that even where questions may be posed with the aim of eliciting this information, what is of greater relevance is how the practitioner uses this information to determine an appropriate course of treatment. Many pain practitioners profess to work within a biopsychosocial perspective yet this is often not reflected in their practice whereby physical/bodily symptoms and programmes of physical rehabilitation are given clinical primacy over psychosocial (and possibly less tangible) issues.

It must also be remembered that there is a substantial proportion of LBP sufferers who do not appear to benefit from any of the treatment modalities that are currently available. The majority of research that has been undertaken to consider treatment efficacy, pain management programme outcomes and treatment compliance has done so with the LBP patient groups as the main grouping variable. It is proposed that one way to address this problem is to improve the match between the treatment and the relevant characteristics of the patient (39). However, what may be more propitious is the match between the characteristics of the patient and those of the health care provider. Rather than assume that the treatments are inefficacious, it may be that the beliefs that are held by that practitioner are at odds with those of the LBP patient and that it is perhaps, at this psychosocial level, that good LBP management is effected.

The rich data that has been derived from this study is by virtue of the methodology chosen. This perspective is invaluable for insights into service provision and utilisation. Questionnaires provide too rigid a framework, and interviews expose themselves to social desirability answering. It is doubtful whether such perspectives would have emerged in face to face interviews. Whilst it must not be forgotten that these six factors have only accounted for just over half of the variance within the sample, and that the sample was generated from only the North East of England, it does nevertheless, reveal a range of beliefs derived from a large number of LBP practitioners. Q-methodology, therefore, has allowed for the study of participant subjectivity in a way that enables the individual to communicate his or her point of view. Consequently, each individual participant has 'modelled' their beliefs of LBP and its management on a matter of subjective importance. The only potential constraint being the domain of subjectivity that is imposed by the researcher however considerable effort was taken when producing the Q-set to ensure that the broadest collection of viewpoints relating to LBP were included.

This study serves as a starting point from which further investigation into the beliefs of health professionals specialising in LBP within secondary and tertiary care facilities can begin. Future research should concentrate on the disparities between what these services perceive to be providing and what the LBP patient is expecting. There is also great scope to explore the different paradigms within which the different professional groups are practising, and to examine further whether particular patients benefit more from being referred to specific specialists within these services based on their beliefs related to LBP. So too would a deeper understanding of how the collective efforts of the pain management specialists, regardless of their practice orientation, achieve successful outcomes from pain management programmes and whether the LBP patients who derive greatest benefit from these programmes equally endorse the biopsychosocial orientation of it.

Conclusion

This is a tentative first study that has examined the attitudes and beliefs of a group of health professionals working within the domain of low back pain management within secondary or tertiary health care settings and builds on the emerging body of literature that has begun to explore the attitudes and beliefs of LBP practitioners. The findings have identified a range of perspectives that appear to be embedded within the professional background of each of the practitioner groups and suggest that the biomedical model of LBP management remains dominant despite research evidence that propounds the application of a biopsychosocial approach. Interdisciplinary differences in held beliefs and attitudes relating to LBP manifestation and management can, and do, lead to patient confusion, frustration and despair and probably account for the oft cited admonishment that patients receive many different messages from as many different pain practitioners that they see. Health professionals need to recognise that their perspectives may not be shared by their patients, and that they should avoid inflicting their own culturally specific values onto patients [40, 41, 42]. Furthermore, there is a continuing assumption that patients are passive and at the behest of the treatments prescribed and the practitioners that prescribe them. Little consideration is given to the dynamism between the practitioner, the patient and the treatment and this is an area that warrants further examination. Effective pain management requires coherency amongst the different practitioner groups. Acknowledgement of the different attitudes and beliefs of these different practitioners may be one way to achieve this.

Acknowledgments

I would like to thank all of the health professionals who participated at each stage of this research study.

References

[1] Clinical Standards Advisory Group. Report of a CSAG Committee on back pain. London: HMSO, 1994.
[2] Waddell G. A new clinical model for the treatment of low back pain. Spine 1987;12:632-43.
[3] Waddell G. The back pain revolution. Edinburgh: Churchill Livingston, 1998.
[4] Maniadakis N, Gray A. The economic burden of back pain in the UK. Pain 2000;84:95-103.
[5] Shi Q, Langer G, Cohen J, Cleeland CS. People in pain: How do they seek relief? J Pain 2007;8:624-36.
[6] Croft PR, Macfarlane GJ, Papageorgiou AC, Thomas E, Silman AJ. Outcome of low back pain in general practice: a prospective study. BMJ 1998;316:1356-9.
[7] Evans G, Richards S. Low back pain: An evaluation of therapeutic interventions. Bristol: Health Care Evaluation Unit, Univ Bristol, Univ Bristol Print, 1996.
[8] Campbell C, Muncer SJ. The causes of low back pain: A network analysis. Soc Sci Med 2005;60:409-19.
[9] Verbeek J, Sengers M-J, Riemans L, Haafkans J. Patient expectations of treatment for back pain. Spine 2004;29:2309-18.
[10] Skelton AM, Murphy EA, Murphy RJL, O'Dowd TC. General practitioner perceptions of low back pain patients. Fam Pract 1995;12:44-8.
[11] Daykin AR, Richardson B. Physiotherapists' pain beliefs and their influence on the management of patients with chronic low back pain. Spine 2004;29:783-95.
[12] Bonnetti D, Pitts NB, Eccles M, Grimshaw J, Johnston M, Steen N, et al. Applying psychological theory to evidence-based clinical practice: identifying factors predictive of taking intra-oral radiographs. Soc Sci Med 2006;63:1889-99.
[13] Werner EL, Ihlebaek C, Sture Skouen J, Laerum E. Beliefs about low back pain in the Norwegian general population: Are they related to pain experiences and health professionals? Spine 2005;30:1770-6.
[14] van Tulder M, Becker A, Bekkering T, Breen A, del Real MT, Hutchinson A, et al. European guidelines for the management of acute non-specific low back pain in primary care. Eur Spine J 2006;15(Suppl 2):S169-91.
[15] Rainville J, Carlson N, Polatin P, Gatchel RJ, Indahl A. Exploration of physicians' recommendations for activities in chronic low back pain. Spine 2000;25:2210-20.

[16] Bishop A, Thomas E, Foster NE. Health care practitioners' attitudes and beliefs about low back pain: A systematic search and critical review of available measurement tools. Pain 2007;132:91-101.
[17] Pincus T, Foster NE, Vogel S, Santos R, Breen A, Underwood M. Attitudes to back pain amongst musculoskeletal practitioners: A comparison of professional groups and practice settings using the ABS-mp. Manual Ther 2007;12:167-75.
[18] Bishop A, Foster NE, Thomas E, Hay EM. How does the self-reported clinical management of patients with low back pain relate to the attitudes and beliefs of health care practitioners? A survey of UK general practitioners and physiotherapists. Pain 2008;135:187-95.
[19] Rainville J, Bagnall D, Phalen L. Health care providers' attitudes and beliefs about functional impairments and chronicl back pain. Clin J Pain 1975;11:287-95.
[20] Houben RM, Vlaeyen JW, Peters M, Ostelo RW, Wolters PM, van den Berg SG. Health care providers attitudes and beliefs towards common low back pain: factor structure and psychometric properties of the HC-PAIRS. Clin J Pain 2004;20:37-44.
[21] Griffiths F, Green E, Bendelow G. Health professionals, their medical interventions and uncertainty: A study focusing on women at midlife. Soc Sci Med 2006;62:1078-90.
[22] Summerskill Williams SM, Pope C. I saw the panic rise in her eyes and evidence-based medicine went out of the door. An exploratory qualitative study of the barriers to secondary prevention in the management of coronary heart disease. Fam Pract 2002;19:605-8.
[23] Eccleston C, Williams A, Stainton Rogers W. Patients' and professionals' understandings of the causes of chronic pain: Blame, responsibility and identity protection. Soc Sci Med 1997;45:699-709.
[24] Linton SJ, Vlaeyen J, Ostelo R. The back pain beliefs of health care providers: Are we fear-avoidant? J Occupat Rehabil 2002;12:223-32.
[25] Stephenson W. Techniques of factor analysis. Nature 1935;136:297.
[26] Brown SR. Political subjectivity: Applications of Q methodology in
[27] political science. New Haven, MA: Yale Univ Press, 1980.
[28] McKeown B, Thomas D. Q methodology. Newbury Park, CA: Sage, 1988.
[29] Jones S, Guy A, Ormrod JA. A Q-methodological study of hearing voices: A preliminary exploration of voice hearers' understanding of their experiences. Psychol Psychother 2003;76:189-209.
[30] Brown SR. Q Methodology and qualitative research. Qual Health Res 1996;6:561-7.
[31] Stephenson W. The study of behaviour: Q-technique and its methodology. Chicago, IL: Univ Chicago Press, 1953.
[32] Dennis KE. Q-methodology: Relevance and application to nursing research. Adv Nurs Sci 1986;8:6-17.

[33] Morley S, Eccleston C, Williams AC. Systematic review and meta-analysis of randomized controlled trials of cognitive behaviour therapy and behaviour therapy for chronic pain in adults, excluding headache. Pain 1999;80:1-13.
[34] Brown KS, Folen RA. Psychologists as leaders of multidisciplinary chronic pain management teams: A model for health care delivery. Prof Psychol Res Pr 2005;36:587-94.
[35] Foucault M. The birth of the clinic. New York: Vintage Books, 1975.
[36] Said EW. Orientalism. New York: Vintage Books, 1979.
[37] Stam HJ. The body and psychology. London: Sage, 1998.
[38] Crossley ML. Rethinking health psychology. Buckingham: Open Univ Press, 2000.
[39] Laerum E, Indahl A, Skouen JS. What is 'the good back-consultation'? A combined qualitative and quantitative study of chronic low back pain patients' interaction with and perceptions of consultations with specialists. J Rehabil Med 2006;38:255-62.
[40] Vlaeyen JWS, Crombez G, Goubert L. The psychology of chronic pain and its management. Phys Ther Rev 2007;12:179-88.

[41] Helman CG. Culture, health and illness, 3rd ed. Oxford: Butterworth Heinemann, 1994.
[42] Kotarba J. Chronic pain: Its social dimensions. Beverley Hills, CA: Sage, 1983.
[43] Parsons EP. Cultural aspects of pain. Surg Nurs 1992;5:14-6.

In: Pain Management Yearbook 2009
Editor: Joav Merrick

ISBN: 978-1-61209-666-7
©2012 Nova Science Publishers, Inc.

Chapter 10

IMPACT OF RELAXATION TRAINING ON THE VARIABILITY OF PSYCHOPHYSICS AND PSYCHOMETRICS TESTS

Gisèle Pickering, MD, PhD, DPharm[*,1,2], *Agathe Gelot, PhD*[2], *Sylvia Boulliau*[1], *Agathe Njomgang*[1] *and Claude Dubray, MD*[1,2]

[1]CHU Clermont-Ferrand, INSERM CIC501, France, and [2] Université d'Auvergne, INSERMU766, Clermont-Ferrand, France

Abstract

Clinical trials with analgesics in healthy volunteers often show a large variability. This randomized controlled study (n=40) evaluates if relaxation improves the reproducibility of psychophysics and psychometrics tests. Method: Two sequences are separated, in the relaxation group, by training to relaxation and in the control group, by no relaxation. During one sequence, each volunteer completes two pain tests and a psychometric test (CRT). Result: Relaxation does not modify the results of pain or psychometrics tests, but diminishes the variability of CRT ($p<0.05$). Conclusion: This suggests the limited benefit of adding relaxation to the preparation of analgesics clinical trials.

Keywords: Trial, pain, vigilance

Introduction

A frequent difficulty encountered in clinical trials dealing with analgesics is the variability of the responses to psychophysics and psychometrics tests: one of the main reasons is that pain has a large subjective component. Indeed, the two domains explored with analgesics are, on

---

* **Correspondence:** Gisèle Pickering, MD, PhD, DPharm, Clinical Pharmacology Centre, Bâtiment 3C, CHU, Hopital G Montpied, 63001 Clermont-Ferrand cedex, France. Tel : 33(0)4 73 17 84 16; Fax 33(0)4 73 17 84 12; E-mail :gisele.pickering@u-clermont1.fr

the one hand, the potency and analgesic property of the drug, analysed with specific psychophysical pain tests, and, on the other hand, the central nervous system side-effects using psychometrics tests to explore attention, concentration or vigilance. Optimization of these tests is very important in phase I clinical trials with healthy volunteers and will determine the future development of the drug. For more than 30 years has been described a physiological "relaxation response" opposed to the response to stress. While the response to stress is innate in human beings, the response to relaxation requires to learn a technique. Relaxation is reported to improve the well-being of individuals and has been integrated in many studies on pain, migraine, depression or sleep difficulties (1). The aim of the present trial is to study if relaxation could improve the reproducibility of psychophysics and psychometrics tests used in clinical trials with healthy volunteers.

Methods

This study with two parallel groups is randomized and controlled. 40 healthy volunteers (24 +/-2 years old; 20 male, 20 female) were selected in this study after approval by the Regional Ethics Committee. Exclusion criteria included a known inefficacy of relaxation, lack of concentration and unsatisfactory results to the psychophysics training tests during two training sessions. The study has two sequences, S1 and S2, separated 1- in the relaxation group (R), by a training period to the relaxation technique during five weeks, 45 minutes twice a week; 2 – in the control group (C), by visits to the investigation centre to avoid any placebo effect of the visit, without any cognitivo-behavioural technique. During S1 and S2, the volunteer repeats three times each of the tests: pain tests with an electrical stimulus (Pain matcher®), with a thermal stimulus (thermotest), and a psychometrics test: the Choice reaction time (CRT). Just before the tests, the subjects are asked to remind themselves of the relaxation technique they have acquired.

The Pain Matcher (Cefar, France) is a pain autoevaluation tool based on the electrical stimulation of the median nerve. The volunteer is instructed to place the electrode box, between the first and second finger of the dominant hand, taking a firm grip. This device gives constant current stimulation with a frequency of 10 Hz and an amplitude of 10 mA. The subjects determine the pain detection threshold when they begin to feel pain in response to increasing intensity of the stimulus and release the fingers from the device. The value reached (0-90 units) is directly related to the pulse displayed on a liquid crystal display screen, saved in the memory, and considered as the pain detection threshold.

The thermotest (Somedic AB, Stockholm, Sweden) consists of a 2.5 x 5cm thermode with series-coupled Peltier elements. Heat pain thresholds are determined on the thenar aspect of the dominant hand with a baseline temperature of 37°C, a 1°C / sec rate change and a cut-off limit of 52°C. The subject indicates the threshold by pressing a button connected to the thermotest. Each threshold is calculated as the average of five tests performed with intervals of about 15 sec between stimulations.

Visual choice reaction time evaluates the psychomotor performance and is determined with the Psychomotor tester (Leeds Psychomotor test, Guilford, England. The subject faces a tray equipped with a central button sensitive to touch and six diodes displayed in a fan-formation around the central point. The subject must as fast as possible move his index finger from the central button towards the activated bulb. The mean of fifty consecutive presentations is recorded in milliseconds as choice reaction time (CRT). Any vigilance impairment will manifest itself in a longer CRT.

The relaxation technique is the commonly used Schultz method (2), a system of very specific auto suggestive formulas that have the purpose to relieve tensions, and is used for stress and psychosomatic disturbances management. Training is acquired in the investigation centre in 8 sessions of 45 min.

Statistics

All results are expressed as means ± SD. For each of the three tests, the variability (coefficient of variation (CV) SD/mean), is calculated in sequence S1 and sequence S2. For each test, variability differences between R and C are compared by ANOVA and Student t-tests with a significance at $p < 0.05$.

Results

Control and relaxation groups are not significantly different at baseline as regards any of the tests (p=NS). Concerning pain tests, electrical pain thresholds (in units) as well as thermal pain thresholds (in °C) are not significantly modified by relaxation training (electrical thresholds for R : 9.6 ± 1.4 (S1); 10.8 ± 1.1 (S2); for C: 9.2 ± 1.2 (S1); 10.2 ± 1.0 (S2); thermal thresholds for R : 44.1 ± 1.3 (S1); 45.3 ± 1.0 (S2); for C: 44.4 ± 1.2 (S1); 45.3 ± 1.1 (S2), all p=NS. The variability of electrical (CV 15% (S1) vs 11% (S2) and thermal thresholds (CV: 3% (S1) vs 2.2% (S2) with relaxation are not significantly modified either.

Concerning psychometrics tests, Choice reaction time (in msec) is not significantly diminished by relaxation: for R: 755±44: (S1); 722±31:(S2) (p=0.09); for C: 750±40 :(S1); 742±42 :(S2) (p=NS). There is however a significant diminution of the variability of CRT in R between S1 and S2: 3%(S1) vs 2 %(S2)(p=0.03) while the variability in the control group C is maintained.

Discussion

The aim of this study was to find out if the practice of relaxation by healthy volunteers before clinical trials could improve the variability of the tests used when studying analgesics in clinical pharmacology. The main finding is a slight but significant diminution of the variability of the choice reaction time in the group of patients who had the relaxation sessions. This is particularly important especially when testing drugs with an action on the central nervous system, and the practice of relaxation could allow to obtain more homogeneous results during successive psychometrics trials. CRT values themselves have not however been significantly modified by relaxation, underlining that the relaxation technique used in this study has therefore little effect on vigilance or concentration performances when the patient is confronted to a visual stimulus.

Concerning pain tests, the variability and the values of the pain thresholds are not modified by relaxation. In this study, as in any study performed in our laboratory, prior to the protocol, the subjects are trained to the tests in order to get accustomed and to have acquired sufficient mastery of the tests before the beginning of the trial. No change in the performance indicates that the subjects were already at the best of their performance and did not need any additional training to obtain consistent responses. Several authors have reported that the relaxation response may alter pain perception as a protective mechanism against excessive pain, antagonizing the potentially harmful effects of pain and its associated stress. This effect has been shown to be critically mediated by catecholamines, NO, serotonin or dopamine, and cerebral structures involved in emotions like the limbic system are particularly at play. Most studies however concern patients with chronic pain and not volunteers with experimental pain, like in this study. The overall very low benefit we gain in this study with relaxation is probably linked to the fact that applied pain is acute and experimental rather than chronic, disturbing and part of the everyday life of suffering patients.

Considering the results of this randomized controlled study in healthy volunteers and the small benefit gained from relaxation, we do not recommend to add relaxation to improve the reproducibility of psychophysics and psychometrics tests. Introduction of relaxation in a study is time and staff-consuming and does not add much to the quality of the tests, as long obviously, as the subjects have been trained adequately to the different tests of the protocol.

References

[1] Salamon E, Esch T, Stefano GB. Pain and relaxation. Int J Mol Med 2006;18(3):465-70.
[2] Durand de Bousingen R. Schultz' autogenic training. A relaxation method using concentrated auto-decontraction. Soins Psychiatr 1985;(61):9-12.

Chapter 11

A NATIONAL SURVEY OF THE UNITED KINGDOM NHS PAIN MANAGEMENT SERVICES

Neil Collighan[*], MBChB, FRCA FFPMRCA and Sanjeeva Gupta, MD, DNB, FRCA, FIPP, FFPMRCA

Department of Anaesthesia, Pain Management and Intensive Care, Bradford Teaching Hospitals NHS Foundation Trust, Bradford, England

Abstract

With the support of the British Pain Society Interventional Pain Medicine Special Interest Group we completed a postal survey of all consultant members, who had expressed an interest in receiving postal material. We asked a series of questions based around four sections: Acute pain, staffing and time management, equipment and out-patient clinics. This article is the outcome of those respondent's answers. We compared our outcomes with previously produced benchmarking surveys with the aim to set out the current status of pain management in the United Kingdom and allow practitioners to compare their situation with others. Responses appear to indicate an improvement in pain service provision as identified by these data sets and the Royal College of Anaesthetists guidance 'Pain management services. Good practice' (2003). However it is possible that only those pursuing best practice responded, in which case the percentages presented in the current survey may be inflated.

Keywords: Pain, pain management, pain service, survey.

Introduction

The facilities, practices and staffing available can vary between pain management centres. We found few surveys had ever occurred with this in mind. In 1999 the Clinical Standards

---

[*]**Correspondence:** Neil Collighan, MBChB, FRCA, Specialist Registrar, Department of Anaesthesia, Pain Management and Intensive Care, Bradford Teaching Hospitals NHS Foundation Trust, Bradford, BD9 6RJ England. Tel: 01274 364065; Fax: 01274 366548; E-mail: neil@collighan.co.uk

Advisory Group (CSAG) produced a report 'Services for Patients with Pain' which aimed to show the way in which specialist pain services were being delivered in the United Kingdom (1). In 2003 Dr. Foster produced a survey looking more at the delivery of pain management in the Primary care sector in the UK (2). This was followed in 2003 by a report to the Pain Society by Lee, Baranowski and Hester with the intention of benchmarking the state of pain management and to assess Consultant views about current resources and working practices (3).

We have done a postal survey which has allowed us to assess current pain practices in the UK and compare them with the previous studies. The postal survey was performed under the auspices of the British Pain Society Interventional Pain Medicine Special Interest Group.

Methods

A questionnaire, with tick boxes for ease of completion, was developed within the Bradford Pain management team and posted to the 290 Consultant members of the British Pain Society who had agreed to receive postal mail. The questionnaire asked about both acute and chronic pain provision by the Consultant members. It contained four sections and these were Acute Pain, Staffing and Time management, Equipment and Out-Patient Clinics. Within each section it was aimed to assess time involved in pain management and more specifically equipment used in interventional practice.

Results

Of the 136 (47%) respondents, 46 (34%) were involved in acute pain management and 120 (88%) were involved in chronic pain management. 30 (22%) provided both acute and chronic pain sessions. Of those who ticked the boxes 18 (15.3%) provide a full-time commitment to chronic pain management whilst 100 (84.7%) provide a part-time commitment to pain.

Section one – acute pain

Clinicians were asked with regards the number of acute pain sessions (each session is about 4 hours) they attended. 13 (28%) did less than 2 sessions per month, 19 (41%) did 2-4 sessions per month, 9 (19%) 4-6 sessions, 2 (4%) 6-8 sessions, 2 (4%) 8-10 sessions and 2 (4%) >10 sessions per month (Figure 1). Within these sessions the number of patients involved was queried. 11(24%) saw less than 5 patients per session, 13(28%) saw between 5 and 10 patients, 9 (20%) saw 10-15 patients, 3 (7%) saw 15-20 patients and 5 (11%) saw more than 20 patients per acute pain session. 39 Consultants are accompanied by pain nurses during their acute pain sessions of which 28 are specifically acute pain nurses but replies also indicated that 21 nurses had chronic pain responsibilities.

Section two – staffing and time management

18 (15%) Consultants who answered were full time chronic pain specialists and 100 (85%) were part-time chronic pain specialists.

With regards treatments (interventional procedures), 12 (10%) doctors did less than 2 chronic pain treatment sessions per month, 28 (24%) did between 2 and 4 treatment sessions per month, 37 (31%) 4-6 sessions, 9 (8%) 6-8 sessions, 16 (13%) 8-10 sessions and 17 (14%) did more than 10 chronic pain treatment sessions per month (see figure 1). Within each treatment session we questioned the number of patients involved and the results are shown in table 1.

The number of chronic pain nurses in the pain management departments is shown in figure 2 and their attendance at treatment sessions and clinics is shown in table 2.

Table 1. Percent of patients involved within each interventional procedure (treatment) session

No. of patients per session	An average treatment session	Your last treatment session
<4	7%	13%
4-6	33%	34%
6-8	29%	24%
8-10	25%	18%
>10	7%	11%

Table 2. Are chronic pain nurses in attendance at your interventional procedure (treatment) sessions and out-patient clinics?

	Never	Sometimes	Always
Treatment Sessions	32%	47%	20%
Out-patient clinics	26%	28%	46%

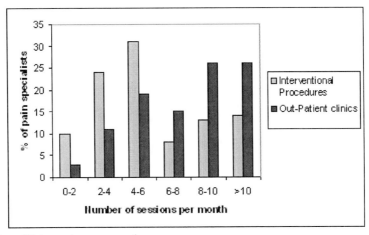

Figure 1. Number of Pain sessions per month.

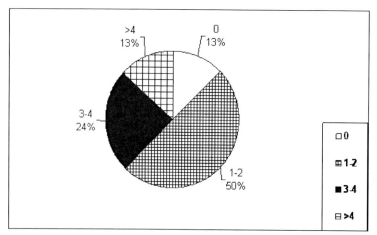

Figure 2. Number of chronic pain nurses in each department.

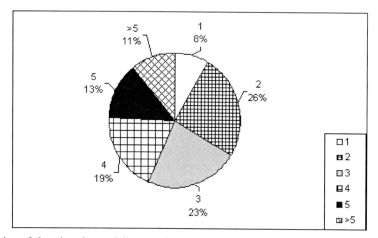

Figure 3. Number of chronic pain specialists per department.

Finally we queried the number of chronic pain specialists within each respondent's hospital and this is shown in figure 3.

Section three – equipment

113 (97.4%) of respondents had access to a fluoroscopy machine whilst 3 (2.6%) did not. Of these 110 (97%) had C-arm fluoroscopy machines available, 3 (3%) had fixed fluoroscopy machines for interventional techniques whilst 12 (10.6%) had both types of fluoroscopy machines available.

74 (72.5%) use a Quincke type of needle, 25 (24.5%) use a Pencil-point type of needle and other preferences noted were 'both', 'BD spinal' and 'Yale'.

93 (80%) respondents had access to a lesion generator for Radiofrequency lesioning and Pulsed Radiofrequency, 23 (20%) did not. For needles used during interventions see table 3.

Table 3. Needles used for pain procedures. [a] 1 (1.6%) Practitioner used both types of non-insulated tip; [b] 1 (3%) Practitioner used both types of non-insulated tip

	18G	20G	22G	24G	25G	Active tip 5mm	Active tip 10mm
General Non-RF inter-ventional procedures	-	20 (18.6%)	82 (76.8%)	1 (0.9%)	4 (3.7%)	-	-
RF Facet joint denervation	3 (3.8%)	23 (29.5%)	52 (66.6%)	-	-	58[a] (79.4%)	14[a] (19%)
RF Lumbar Sympathectomy	2 (4%)	19 (38%)	29 (58%)	-	-	20[b] (44%)	24[b] (53%)

Section four – out-patient clinics

The number of clinics done per month by each clinician was requested. 4 (3.4%) did 0-2 clinics per month, 13 (11%) did 2-4 per month, 22 (18.6%) did 4-6 per month, 18 (15.3%) did 6-8 per month, 30 (25.4%) did 8-10 per month and 31 (26.3%) did greater than 10 clinics per month.

Within each clinic 3 (2.6%) saw less than 4 patients in an average clinic, 13 (11%) saw 4-6 patients, 26 (22%) saw 6-8 patients, 43 (36.4%) saw 8-10 patients and 33 (28%) saw more than 10 patients in an average clinic (see figure 4).

In each clinic 14 (12%) saw 1-2 new patients, 64 (54.7%) saw 3-4 new patients (58%) and 39 (33.3%) saw more than 4 new patients in an average clinic (30%). No clinicians held an average clinic where they saw no new patients.

The time allocated to see a new patient and a follow-up patient is shown in figure 5 and figure 6 respectively. We have incorporated full and part-time sessional involvement into the accompanying figures.

For overall clinic time, 1 (0.8%) clinician's clinic lasted, on average, less than 2.5 hours, 4 (3.4%) lasted between 2.5 and 3 hours, 36 (31%) lasted between 3 and 3.5 hours, 59 (50.4%) lasted between 3.5 and 4 hours and 17 (14.5%) clinicians said their average clinic lasted longer than 4 hours.

48 (40.7%) of respondents stated that they held multi-disciplinary out-patient clinics (when using the criteria of the presence of 3 or more disciplines in the clinic).

Of these, 47 (81%) involved a physiotherapist, 11 (19%) involved a pharmacist and 49 (84%) involved a psychologist. Other specialties noted to be involved in the multidisciplinary clinics included hypnotherapist, massage, neurologist, neurosurgeon (4), occupational therapist (6), palliative care physician, psychiatrist, rheumatologist (2), 'spinal surgeons', TENS nurse, nurse (12), nurse consultant (2), nurse psychologist, nurse psychiatrist, 'pain nurse specialist', CBT therapist, 'ENT/Max-Fax surgeon', general practitioner, gynaecologist, paediatrician (2) and rehabilitation consultant.

Discussion

The results are a snapshot of the current practices occurring in the United Kingdom's different pain management practices. The aim of the survey was to set a starting point upon which to build and then to monitor henceforth. This initial data will allow individual clinicians to compare and contrast their own service with their fellow pain clinicians and hopefully provoke further debate.

When these results are compared with previous outcomes there appears to be an improvement in the provision of pain services in the UK. The Clinical Standards Advisory Group (1) remarked that over a third of consultants were working alone whilst in our study only 8% of Consultants replied that they were single handed. Only half of the pain services in the UK had a specialist pain nurse whilst our study shows only 13% that did not have a specialist pain nurse. The lack of availability of multidisciplinary teams in pain management was also raised as problematic but our study shows that approximately 40% of practices now run multidisciplinary clinics involving a pharmacist, a psychologist and/or a physiotherapist. As a long list shows many specialities are involved indirectly.

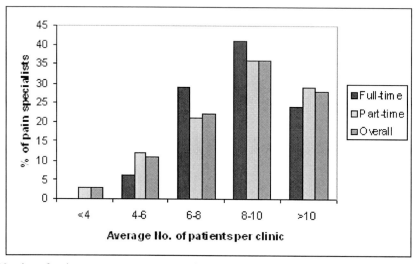

Figure 4. Number of patients on average per out-patient clinic for full-time and part-time pain specialists.

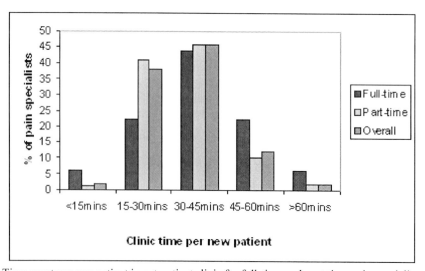

Figure 5. Time spent per new patient in out-patient clinic for full-time and part-time pain specialists.

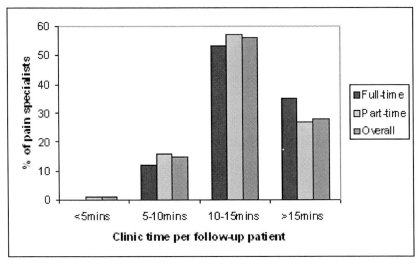

Figure 6. Time spent per follow-up patient in out-patient clinic for full-time and part-time pain specialists.

Lee, Baranowski and Hester (3) showed a balance of Consultant pain session commitments where 83% did this in combination with anaesthesia and 14% worked exclusively in chronic pain (2% were involved in palliative care). We have shown similar outcomes with 85% and 15% respectively. They presented the average time allocated with a new patient as 39 minutes (mean minimum time 20 minutes, mean maximum time 65 minutes) and the average time allocated for a follow up patient as 16 minutes (mean minimum time 8 minutes, mean maximum time 37 minutes). Whilst the allocation of time for a new patient is similar to our findings the time for our follow-up patients seems slightly shorter with the majority of patients having between 10 and 15 minutes for their consultation. Lee, Baranowski and Hester also noted that their timings were longer for doctors working exclusively in pain management (new patient 46 minutes, follow up patient 19 minutes) and our results seem to correlate with full-time pain specialists appearing to see more new patients per clinic, spend more time with new patients and spend more time in clinic than part-time pain specialists.

Dreyfuss (4) and Bogduk (5) suggested that better results can be obtained for facet joint radiofrequency denervation procedures by using larger gauge needles. Our survey suggested that most of the clinicians are using 22G needles which may not be ideal for optimal outcome.

In 2003 The Royal College of Anaesthetists, London, in conjunction with The Pain Society produced guidance 'Pain Management services; Good Practice' with regards provision of pain services (6). As suggested by our survey a multi-disciplinary approach to pain management is occurring but further advances need to be made. Close links with other medical specialties appears to be in existence. There now appears to have been a movement in response to the 2003 CSAG report where the Royal College of Anaesthetists report raised concerns that none had been made. The number of nurse specialists/consultants is on the increase and this is for the better and finally, whilst not everybody had the equipment required for providing all the services available to the specialty of Pain management these numbers are increasing. However it should also be noted that the current survey reflects the practice of only 47% of those surveyed (the response rate). It is possible that only those pursuing best practice responded, in which case the percentages presented in the current survey are inflated.

It is our intention to repeat this study in the future but focussing upon different points of interest as dictated by our pain colleagues.

Acknowledgments

Thank you to the British Pain Society for their support with this survey.

References

[1] Clinical Standards Advisory Group. Services for Patients with Pain. 1 84182 157 8. CSAG, PO Box 777, London SE1 6HX. 1999.
[2] Dr Foster in conjunction with the Pain Society. Adult Chronic Pain Management Services in the UK. Dr Foster Ltd., Sir John Lyon House, 5 High Timber Street, London EC4V 3NX. 2003.
[3] Lee J, Baranowski A, Hester J. Pain Management benchmarking questionnaire for medical consultants. London: Pain Soc, 2004.
[4] Dreyfuss P, Halbrook B, Pauza K, Joshi A, McLarty J, Bogduk N. Efficacy and validity of radiofrequency neurotomy for chronic lumbar zygapophyseal joint pain. Spine 2000;25:1270-7.
[5] International Spine Intervention Society. Percutaneous radiofrequency lumbar medial branch neurotomy. In: Bogduk N, Ed. Practice guidelines. Spinal diagnostic and treatment procedures. San Francisco: Int Spine Intervent Soc, 2004:188-218.
[6] The Royal College of Anaesthetists and the Pain Society. Pain Management services. Good practice. London: Royal Coll Anesth Pain Soc, 2003.

In: Pain Management Yearbook 2009
Editor: Joav Merrick

ISBN: 978-1-61209-666-7
©2012 Nova Science Publishers, Inc.

Chapter 12

OPIOID DEPENDENCE AMONG OLDER PRE-SPINE SURGERY PATIENTS. A PROSPECTIVE STUDY

M Sami Walid[*], *MD, PhD*

Medical Center of Central Georgia, Macon, Georgia, United States of America

Abstract

Back pain patients are highly exposed to prescription painkiller abuse and opioid-dependence (OD). This study was conducted in order to investigate the relationship between age and OD in patients admitted for spine surgery. This study is a prospective study in a community hospital with a convenience sample of 186 preoperative pre-spine-surgery patients using opioids for pain relief. The prevalence of OD was calculated by means of a questionnaire based on the WHO and DSMIV guidelines for the diagnosis of OD defining "dependence" as the presence of at least three of the following six criteria—strong desire, binge use, withdrawal, tolerance, neglect and use despite harm. We evaluated the relationship between OD, a categorical variable, and age as a categorical (<50 years and ≥50 years using the mean age as the cut point) and numerical variable. The Chi-square test of independence and analysis of variance (ANOVA) were applied using the statistical software SPSS v.16. Results showed that of the patients <50 years of age 16.8% were opioid-dependent and of those ≥50 years of age 23.5% were opioid-dependent. Pearson Chi-square test of independence showed no relationship between OD and age (p=0.254). ANOVA showed no significant difference in age between the two OD groups (p=0.484). We concluded that, contrary to clinical lore, there is no significant difference in opioid dependence between older and younger pre-spine surgery patients.

Keywords: Opioid dependence, older patients, spine surgery, DSM-IV.

---

[*] **Correspondence**: M. Sami Walid, MD, PhD, Medical Center of Central Georgia, 840 Pine Street, Suite 880, Macon, GA 31201 United States. Tel: 478-743-7092 ex 266; Fax 478-7383834; E-mail: mswalid@yahoo.com

Introduction

Chronic back pain is prevalent among older Americans. Causes of back pain - osteoarthritis, disc degeneration, osteoporosis and spinal stenosis - increase with age and interfere with activities of daily living with negative impact on the quality of life in the years of retirement (1,2). Studies show that elderly patients, who are particularly subject to chronic back problems, are less likely to be adequately treated for their pain. Federman et al (3) found that in outpatient settings, elderly (≥75 years) patients with back or joint pain use non-steroidal anti-inflammatory drugs (NSAIDs) more often and opioids less often than younger patients, indicating that older patients are receiving a poorer quality of pain management. Underutilization of opioids is a major factor in poor pain management which can be attributed to poor assessment of pain in this age group; fear of the adverse effects of medications (opiophobia); and avoidance of opioids because of concerns about physical dependence, addiction and unfavorable outcomes reported in the literature (4). For example, Webster et al (5) reported a negative association between receipt of early opioids for acute low back pain and outcomes represented by disability duration, medical costs, "late opioid" use (≥5 prescriptions from 30 to 730 days), and surgery in the 2-year period following low back pain onset. They concluded that the use of opioids for the management of acute low back pain may be counterproductive to recovery.

Back pain due to degenerative spine disease is a growing problem in our aging society and these patients are among those highly exposed to prescription painkiller abuse and opioid-dependence (OD). Our data show that 50% of patients admitted for spine surgery are using opioids and of these 20% are opioid dependent (6,7). A lot of talk is being heard about higher prevalence of OD among elderly patients (8) despite some evidence to the contrary (9). In order to settle this question we conducted the following study to check for any relationship between age and OD in this high-risk category of patients.

Methods

After approval from the Institutional Review Board preoperative spine surgery patients were prospectively screened for opioid use and asked about their choice to participate in the study or not. They were given a questionnaire designed according to the WHO and DSMIV guidelines for the diagnosis of OD which defines "dependence" as the presence of at least three of six criteria—strong desire, binge use, withdrawal, tolerance, neglect and use despite harm (6,7,10,11).

The prevalence of OD was calculated based on the questionnaire results. We evaluated the relationship between OD, a categorical variable, and age as a categorical (<50 years and ≥50 years using the mean age as the cutpoint) and numerical variable. The Chi-Square Test of Independence and Analysis of Variance (ANOVA) were applied using the statistical software SPSS v.16.

Results

By the end of the study, 186 questionnaires were filled. Of the 186 preoperative spine surgery patients [56 lumbar diskectomy (LMD), 71 cervical decompression and fusion (CDF) and 59 lumbar decompression and fusion (LDF)] on opioids (hydrocodone, Acetaminophen + Hydrocodone, Acetaminophen + Oxycodone, Hydromophone), 37 (20%) met the criteria for the diagnosis of OD. These participants were 23-87 years of age with the mean age, 50 years. They were 52% female and 75% Caucasian and were diagnosed with herniated nucleus pulposus or spinal stenosis. Of patients <50 years of age 16.8% were opioid-dependent and of those ≥50 years of age 23.5% were opioid-dependent (see table 1).

Table 1. Crosstabulation of OD and age showing the percentage of opioid dependent patients in each age group

			Age <50 yr	Age ≥50 yr
OD	No	Count	84	65
		Column N %	83.2%	76.5%
	Yes	Count	17	20
		Column N %	16.8%	23.5%

We evaluated the relationship between OD and age as categorical variables. After crosstabulation of OD (OD and No OD) and age (<50 years and ≥50 years) we applied Pearson Chi-Square Test of Independence which showed no relationship between OD and age (p=0.254).

Categorizing the sample according to OD, we applied ANOVA where age was the dependent numerical variable and OD the grouping factor (OD and No OD). Analysis showed no significant difference in age between the two OD groups (p=0.484).

Discussion

Older Americans, who make the fastest growing sector of the population, consume approximately one-third of all medications prescribed in the nation (12). They sometimes receive long-term and multiple prescriptions, which can lead to inappropriate use. These medications can interact with each other and cause serious side effects due to changes in drug metabolism, decreased renal clearance capacity, increased sensitivity to toxic effects, and higher rates of comorbidities. For example, if an elderly patient takes an opioid medication for back pain then adds a benzodiazepine for sleep or anxiety the synergistic effect of both medications can be so dangerous leading to respiratory failure and death. The adverse effects from opioid use and complications of opioid dependence make physicians very wary about prescribing these medications to elderly patients.

Fear of addiction remains a barrier to adequate pain control in the elderly population. Patients, families, the public and healthcare professionals continue to have misconceptions regarding addiction and the use of opioids to control pain (13). In addition, the media keeps concentrating on the negative uses of opioids which has only enhanced misconceptions concerning opioid use and addiction. In 2004, the International Narcotics Control Board (INCB) has called attention to the inadequate treatment of pain due, in part, to overly restrictive laws and regulations that impede the adequate availability and medical use of opioids (14). Before that, in 1999, the American Pain Society surveyed 805 people who had chronic pain regarding the adequacy of treatment received from their physicians. Only 26% of respondents who had "very severe" pain reported taking opioids at the time of survey (15).

In addition to undertreatment of pain, elderly patients are sometimes reluctant to report pain-related symptoms. This reluctance may be due to the belief that pain is a obligatory part of aging, concern about being negatively treated for complaining about pain, or the expectation that the clinician will give a low priority to pain, compared with other medical problems. They may also be afraid of involuntary hospitalization or subjection to invasive procedures if they report pain. Moreover, elderly patients are often misinformed about the senescence process and may see pain as a sign of serious illness or approaching death. Sengstaken and King (16) found that 66% of geriatric nursing home residents had chronic pain, but in 34% of cases it was not detected by the treating physician.

Our research was aimed at studying the relationship between age and OD in pre-spine-surgery patients who are thought to be highly predisposed to OD. In our study, 16.8% of patients <50 years of age and 23.5% of patients ≥50 years of age were opioid-dependent. There seemed to be a notable difference; however, Chi-Square showed no relationship between OD and age as categorical variables. When we used age as a numerical variable and applied ANOVA, there was also no significant difference in age between the two OD groups. This meant that the first impression was false and the perceived difference was most likely due to chance.

OD can start at any age, but problems associated with opioid use are usually first observed in the late teens or early twenties. Increasing age is associated with a decrease in the prevalence of OD (11). This tendency for dependence to remit generally begins after age 40 and is known as "maturing out" (11). On the other side, starting drug abuse after age 50 has been reported (17). Just because a patient is in the geriatric age-group does not mean that they need not be screened for substance abuse, especially when there are symptoms such as insomnia, anxiety, and depression.

Conclusions

Elderly patients are particularly subject to chronic pain but not to opioid dependence. There is no significant difference in opioid dependence between older and younger pre-spine surgery patients. Therefore, we need to fight opiophobia and overcome the barriers to opioid usage in the elderly population. We recommend regular pain assessments, utilisation of new-generation opioids (buprenorphine) and sustained release preparations, including transdermal forms (fentanyl and buprenorphine-fentanyl), and avoidance of inappropriate opioids (methadone, propoxyphene, meperidine, morphine, oral fentanyl) as advocated in the recently released consensus statement of an international expert panel (18). Actually, the latest guidelines of the American Geriatric Society advise doctors to have their patients avoid NSAIDs and COX-2 inhibitors and consider the use of low-dose opioid therapy instead because of the associated risks of cardiovascular, renal and gastrointestinal disorders which usually outweigh their benefits (19). It is also important to educate the physicians about the influence of psychological factors on pain experience, the rational prescribing of opioid medications, and managing adverse effects. A reason- and knowledge-based approach to the use of opioids in the treatment of chronic back pain in the elderly population will correct the current problems with poor management in this age-group. This can have important public health implications, as the proportion of elderly people will increase considerably in the coming years as in most industrialized societies.

References

[1] Wepner U. Controlling pain effectively in the elderly. Age is not an analgesic. MMW Fortschr Med 2006;148(19):12-3.
[2] Dionne CE, Dunn KM, Croft PR. Does back pain prevalence really decrease with increasing age? A systematic review. Age Ageing 2006;35(3):229-34.
[3] Federman AD, Litke A, Morrison RS. Association of age with analgesic use for back and joint disorders in outpatient settings. Am J Geriatr Pharmacother 2006;4(4):306-15.
[4] Auret K, Schug SA. Underutilisation of opioids in elderly patients with chronic pain: approaches to correcting the problem. Drugs Aging 2005;22(8):641–54.
[5] Webster BS, Verma SK, Gatchel RJ. Relationship between early opioid prescribing for acute occupational low back pain and disability duration, medical costs, subsequent surgery and late opioid use. Spine 2007;32(19):2127-32.
[6] Walid MS, Hyer LA, Ajjan M, Barth ACM, Robinson JS. Prevalence of opioid-dependence in spine surgery patients and correlation with length of stay. J Opioid Management 2007;3(3):127-8,130-2.
[7] Walid MS, Barth ACM, Ajjan M, Hyer LA, Robinson JS. Does opioid dependence impact length of stay. AANS Neurosurgeon 2008;17(2):19-23.
[8] Clarke T. America's elderly face growing drug addiction problem. Reuters. May 17, 2006.
[9] Ives TJ, Chelminski PR, Hammett-Stabler CA, Malone RM, Perhac JS, Potisek NM, Shilliday BB, DeWalt DA, Pignone MP. Predictors of opioid misuse in patients with chronic pain: a prospective cohort study. BMC Health Serv Res 2006;6:46.
[10] WHO Expert Committee on Addiction-Producing Drugs. Thirteenth report of the WHO expert committee. Geneva, World Health Organization, 1964.
[11] American Psychiatric Association Task Force on DSM-IV. Diagnostic and statistical manual of mental disorders. Washington, DC: Am Psychiatr Assoc, 2000.
[12] Statement of Nora D. Volkow Director, National Institute on Drug Abuse, National Institute of Health. Committee on House Government Reform Subcommittee on Criminal Justice, Drug Policy, and Human Resources. Accessed 2008 Jul 18. URL: http://www.drugabuse.gov/Testimony/7-26-06Testimony.html
[13] Forman WB. Opioid analgesic drugs in the elderly. Clin Geriatr Med. 1996 Aug;12(3):489-500.
[14] Use of essential narcotic drugs to treat pain is inadequate, especially in developing countries. Vienna: Intl Narcotics Control Board (INCB), Annual Report, 2004.
[15] Portenoy RK. What should we tell the public to do. APS Bulletin 1999;9(5).
[16] Sengstaken EA, King SA. The problems of pain and its detection among geriatric nursing home residents. J Am Geriatrics Soc 1993;41:541-4.
[17] Busko M. Study of older veterans sheds light on cocaine use. Am Assoc Geriatr Psychiatry, 21st Ann Meet, Poster 60, 2007 Mar 14-17. URL: http://www.medscape.com/viewarticle/571603

[18] Pergolizzi J, Böger RH, Budd K, Dahan A, Erdine S, et al. Opioids and the management of chronic severe pain in the elderly: Consensus statement of an International Expert Panel with focus on the six clinically most often used World Health Organization step III opioids (buprenorphine, fentanyl, hydromorphone, methadone, morphine, oxycodone). Pain Pract 2008;8(4):287-313.

[19] Rauscher M. Opioids recommended for elderly with chronic pain. Reuters. May 6, 2009.

In: Pain Management Yearbook 2009
Editor: Joav Merrick

ISBN: 978-1-61209-666-7
©2012 Nova Science Publishers, Inc.

Chapter 13

COMBINATION OF EVIDENCE-BASED MEDICATIONS FOR NEUROPATHIC PAIN: PROPOSAL OF A SIMPLE THREE-STEP THERAPEUTIC LADDER

Katsuyuki Moriwaki[*], MD, PhD, Kazuhisa Shiroyama, MD, PhD, Mikako Sanuki, MD, Minoru Tajima, MD, Tomoaki Miki, MD, Akihiko Sakai, MD and Ken Hashimoto, MD, PhD

Department of Anesthesiology, Critical Care and Pain Medicine, National Hospital Organization, Kure-Medical Center, Chugoku Cancer Center, Kure, Hiroshima, Japan

Abstract

Recent systematic reviews have identified tricyclic antidepressants (TCA), anticonvulsants (AC) and opioids (OP) as the first-line medications for the treatment of neuropathic pain. We proposed a simple three-step ladder as an algorithm to administer those evidence-based medications, where TCA or AC is the first, combination of TCA and AC is the second, and OP combined with both TCA and AC, or either one of them is the third step. Our early experience of the ladder's efficacy in the 32 patients with peripheral (n=26) and central (n=6) neuropathic pain showed that 69% of patients with peripheral, and 67% of patients with central neuropathic pain obtained more than 30% pain relief, and 46% patients with peripheral and 33% with central neuropathic pain experienced more than 50% excellent pain relief. Our three-step approach appears simple and feasible to treat patients experiencing both peripheral and central neuropathic pain.

Keywords: Neuropathic pain, tricyclic antidepressant, anticonvulsant, opioid.

---

[*] **Correspondence:** Katsuyuki Moriwaki, MD, PhD, Department of Anesthesiology, Critical Care and pain Medicine, National Hospital Organization, Kure-Medical Center, Chugoku Cancer Center, 3-1, Aoyama-cho, Kure, Hiroshima, 737-0023 Japan. Tel: +82-823-22-3111or +82-823-21-7100-7571(ext); E-mail: moriwaki@kure-nh.go.jp

Introduction

Recent systematic reviews (1,2) have identified antidepressants and anticonvulsants (AC) as the first-line medications for neuropathic pain, whereas opioids (OP) are also considered for first-line use in selected clinical circumstances (2). The number needed to treat (NNT) for neuropathic pain is lowest for tricyclic antidepressants (NNT=2-3), followed by opioids (NNT=2.5-3.9) and the anticonvulsant calcium channel alpha-2 ligands such as gabapentin (NTT=3.8-5.1) and pregabalin (NNT=4.2) (1). The aim of our present paper is to propose a simple three-step ladder in order to administer evidence-based medications in a particular step-by-step combination of these listed medications herein. We provide results of our early experience of the ladder's efficacy in patients diagnosed with peripheral and central neuropathic pain.

Proposal of a three-step ladder

Recommendations for pharmacological treatment of neuropathic pain have been proposed according to the results of systematic reviews and consensus of authorized special interest groups (1,2). One treatment algorithm proposed by Finnerup et al (1) for peripheral neuropathic pain is a logic flowchart using evidence-based medications including the lidocaine patch, and oral TCA, gabapentin, pregabalin, tramadol and oxycodone. Dworkins' group (2) has classified medications used for neuropathic pain into the first to the third line medications, and recommended treating patients with a stepwise pharmacological management strategy using those medications. These previous algorithms have significant impact on the practice of neuropathic pain management. However, from a clinical point of view, simpler therapeutic strategies to address treatments of all types of neuropathic pain conditions would be preferable. Therefore, we have proposed a simple three-step therapeutic ladder, with modifications for recommendations and algorithms, using reliable first line medications.

Our simple three-step ladder is depicted in figure 1. Briefly, in the first step (STEP1), TCA alone is given initially, or AC alone is given if TCA is contraindicated. In the second step (STEP2), TCA is administered in combination with AC. If combination medications in STEP2 have failed to alleviate the neuropathic pain, OP is added to STEP2 medications in the next step if it is not contraindicated. In STEP3, OP is used in combination with both of TCA and AC, or either of them. The candidates for STEP3 treatment are strictly selected according to a guideline on opioid usage proposed by Portenoy (see reference in the legend of figure 1) to avoid misuse or abuse of opioids.

Methods

We applied the three-step ladder to consecutive patients with neuropathic pain referred to our secondary pain clinic. We prescribed amitriptyline as TCA, gabapentin with or without clonazepam as an anticonvulsant. Morphine, pentazocine or oxycodone was given as an OP. Amitriptyline was prescribed only before sleep. The ladder-based medications were administered for at least a three-month period in the recruited patients. The efficacy of the ladder-based medications was assessed by reduction in the numerical rating scale (NRS). Reduction of NRS by more than 30%, or 50% after treatments, was considered effective and excellent, respectively. Medications and their detailed prescriptions used in the present case series are described in table 1.

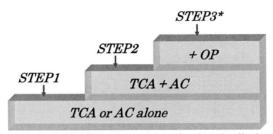

Figure 1. A three-step therapeutic ladder for neuropathic pain. See details in the text. TCA = tricyclic antidepressant, AC = anticonvulsant, OP = opioids. * The candidates for STEP3 should be selected according the guidelines on opioid usage such as Portenoy's (Portenoy RK. Opioid therapy for chronic nonmalignant pain. Current status. In: Fields HL, Liebeskind JC, eds. Progress in pain research and management, Seattle, WA: IASP Press, 1994:274).

Table 1. Medications employed to construct the ladder

Medications	Prescriptions
TCA (tricyclic anti-depressant)	*amitriptyline* 10-40mg (p.o.) h.s.
AC (anti-convulsant)	*gabapentin* 200-400 mg (p.o.) t.i.d. / q.i.d. with or without *clonazepam* 0.2-0.4 mg t.i.d/ q.i.d
OP (opioids)	*morphine* 10-30 mg (p.o.), *pentazocine* 25-50mg (p.o.), or *oxycodone* 5-30 mg (p.o.) d.i.d.

Clinical patient information

A total of 32 patients (age mean +/- SD = 62.8 +/- 16.0), 13 females and 19 males were recruited for the treatment algorithm. Neuropathic pain was diagnosed as peripheral in 26, and central in 6 patients. Details of the patients' characteristics are shown in table 2. Causes of the neuropathic pain, final therapeutic steps and details of treatments other than oral medications, if any, are also shown in table 2.

Table 2. Clinical information of patients and efficacy of the therapeutic ladder

A. Patients with peripheral neuropathic pain

1) ZAP/PHN

Tx Steps	Age	Sex	NRS(initial)	NRS(outcome)	%Pain relief	Note
1	61	M	8	0	100.0	
1	56	M	3	1	66.7	
2	71	F	6	0	100.0	Hunt syndrome
2	76	F	8	1	87.5	
2	81	F	8	2	75.0	
2	48	M	4	1	75.0	
2	56	M	5	3	40.0	
2	74	M	6	4	33.3	
2	67	M	10	7	30.0	
2	80	F	8	6	25.0	ICNB, Tpinj

2) Traumatic/operative peripheral nerve injury

Tx Steps	Age	Sex	NRS(initial)	NRS(outcome)	%Pain relief	Note
1	60	M	4	4	0.0	PTPS, psychiatric
2	62	M	7	1	85.7	
2	76	M	6	2	66.7	
2	66	F	8	4	50.0	
2	41	F	6	4	33.3	
2	47	F	7	7	0.0	

3) Spinal radicular pain

Tx Steps	Age	Sex	NRS(initial)	NRS(outcome)	%Pain relief	Note
1	39	M	4	2	50.0	TPInj
2	84	F	6	4	33.3	
2	64	M	6	5	16.7	MOBsynd
3	80	M	8	6	25.0	

4) Trigeminal neuralgia

Tx Steps	Age	Sex	NRS(initial)	NRS(outcome)	%Pain relief	Note
1	84	F	4	4	0.0	intorelance
2	60	F	4	1	75.0	

5) Diabetic peripheral neuropathy

Tx Steps	Age	Sex	NRS(initial)	NRS(outcome)	%Pain relief	Note
2	60	M	6	2	66.7	
3	69	M	8	3	62.5	

6) Cancer associated pain

Tx Steps	Age	Sex	NRS(initial)	NRS(outcome)	%Pain relief	Note
1*	72	M	4	2	50.0	Dx.Methothelioma chemoTx, *removed
3	16	M	7	3	57.1	

B. Patients with central neuropathic pain

1) Poststroke pain syndrome

Tx Steps	Age	Sex	NRS(initial)	NRS(outcome)	%Pain relief	Note
2	62	F	7	2	71.4	
2	53	M	6	4	33.3	
2	75	F	7	7	0.0	

2) Spinal cord injury

Tx Steps	Age	Sex	NRS(initial)	NRS(outcome)	%Pain relief	Note
2	64	F	8	2	75.0	RA, LSCS
2	28	M	8	4	50.0	
2	76	M	6	5	16.7	

See details in the text. ZAP=zoster-associated pain; PHN=post-herpetic neuralgia; ICNB= intercostal nerve block; TPinj=trigger point injection; PTPS=post-thoracotomy pain syndrome; MOBsynd=multiple operative back syndrome; Dx=diagnosed; Tx=therapy, therapeutic; RA= rheumatoid arthritis; LSCS=lumbar spinal column stenosis.

Results

Among patients experiencing peripheral neuropathic pain, 12 patients (46%) experienced more than 50% pain relief with the STEP1 (n=2), STEP2 (n=8), and STEP3 (n=2) treatments, respectively. Alleviation of pain by equal or less than 50% but more than 30% was observed for six patients with STEP2 (n=5) and STEP3 (n=1) treatment. Seven of the peripheral patients were removed from the ladder algorithm due to intolerance, unresponsiveness to the medications and indication of other treatments such as psychiatric and chemotherapy. One patient with spinal radicular pain was kept treated on STEP3, although the pain relief was reported less than 30%.

Among patients with central neuropathic pain, two patients (33%) experienced more than 50% pain relief with the STEP2 treatment. Alleviation of pain by equal or less than 50% but more than 30% was observed for two patients with STEP2 treatment. Another two patients were removed from the ladder algorithm on STEP2 due to intolerability and unresponsiveness to the medications.

Discussion

In our case series, 69% patients with peripheral and 67% with central neuropathic pain obtained effective (more than 30%) pain relief from our three-step ladder approach. Among these two groups, 46% patients with peripheral, and 33% with central neuropathic pain experienced greater than 50% excellent pain relief. Our results indicated that our three-step approach is feasible to treat patients experiencing peripheral as well as central neuropathic pain.

Because of heterogeneity across treatments of different neuropathic pain conditions, it is generally considered that algorithms need to be tailored to specific disease or disease categories (2). However, it may be useful to establish a fundamental generalized algorithm for the treatment of neuropathic pain. Such a strategy may be advantageous among practitioners who are not specialized in pain medicine. Our present three-step ladder is easy to remember and reminiscent of the WHO three-step ladder approach for cancer pain relief (see website: http://www.who.int/cancer/
palliative/painladder/en/index.html).

Our three-step ladder approach can emphasize the difference in treatment options for neuropathic pain and nociceptive pain. In the published WHO ladder, which is aimed at the management of nociceptive cancer pain, TCA and AC are considered as adjuncts for such cancer pain. However, these two medications are not adjuncts but rather principal medications for neuropathic pain (1,2). Importance and relevance of utilizing TCA and AC has been recognized when cancer patients present neuropathic pain components (3). Twycross has introduced a five-step ladder for cancer-related neuropathic pain: steroids for the first step; TCA or AC for the second step; combination of TCA and AC for the third step; N-methyl-D-aspartic acid (NMDA) receptor antagonists for the forth step; and, spinal analgesia for the fifth step (3). The second and third steps in Twycross' approach are the same as the STEP1 and STEP2 in our three-step approach. A similar strategy of either single or combination usage of TCA and AC is also recommended in the stepwise approach, published by Dworkin's group (2). Therefore, single and subsequent combination usage of TCA and AC in our three-step ladder seems to be a reasonable approach for neuropathic pain management.

Opioid is placed on the top of the step (STEP3) in our ladder and used in combination with both TCA and AC, or either one of these medications. One randomized controlled study has clearly shown that the combination of morphine and gabapentin achieved better analgesia at lower doses of each drug than either as a single agent for neuropathic pain (4). However, opioid adverse events are not rare when they are used for chronic non-malignant pain (5). Use of oral opioid produced higher rates of adverse events including dry mouth, nausea and constipation compared to a placebo (1, 2, 5). Misuse or abuse of opioid is also major problem when it is applied to the management of chronic non-cancer pain (5). Therefore, it seems reasonable to put opioid on the top of the ladder to avoid those opioid-related problems if at all possible.

Some of the first-line medications for neuropathic pain used in North American and European countries are not available in Japan (i.e. oral tramadol), thus were not included in the present medications tested (Table 1). Tramadol may be added in the STEP3 medications (1,2). The mixed serotonin noradrenaline reuptake inhibitors (SNRIs) may be also used to replace TCA to avoid their side effects (1,2). Each step of the three-step ladder may be modified by using pharmacologically compatible, first-line medications, according to their availability in each country.

In conclusion, we proposed a simple three-step therapeutic ladder for alleviating neuropathic pain. The results of our early test experiences seem to indicate that the ladder approach is feasible for the pharmacological management of neuropathic pain. However, the number of patients used to test the ladder was small. Studies of a larger sample size are needed to evaluate the efficacy of the three-step ladder approach for neuropathic pain.

References

[1] Finnerup NB, Otto M, McQuary HJ, Jensen TS, Sindrup SH. Algorithm for neuropathic pain treatment: An evidence based proposal. Pain 2005;118:285-305.

[2] Dworkin RH, O'Connor AB, Backonja M, Farrar JT, Finnerup NB, et al. Pharmacologic management of neuropathic pain: evidence-based recommendations. Pain 2007;132:237-51.

[3] Twycross RG, Wilcock A. Symptom management in advanced cancer. Oxford: Radcliffe Med Press, 2001:53-5.

[4] Gilron I, Bailey JM, Tu D, Holden RR, Weaver DF, Houlden RL. Morphine , gabapentin, or their combination for neuropathic pain. N Engl J Med 2005;352:1324-34

[5] Moore RA, Henry J, McQuay HJ. Prevalence of opioid adverse events in chronic non-malignant pain: systematic review of randomised trials of oral opioids. Arthritis Res Ther 2005;7:R1046-51.

In: Pain Management Yearbook 2009
Editor: Joav Merrick

ISBN: 978-1-61209-666-7
©2012 Nova Science Publishers, Inc.

Chapter 14

PSYCHOSOCIAL PREDICTORS OF HEALTH STATUS IN FIBROMYALGIA: A COMPARATIVE STUDY WITH RHEUMATOID ARTHRITIS

Paula Oliveira[*], *PhD and Maria Emília Costa, PhD*

Psychology Centre of University of Porto; Faculty of Psychology and Educational Sciences, University of Porto, Portugal

Abstract

Objective was to compare perceived health status as measured by the MOS 36-item Short Form Health Survey (SF-36) in fibromyalgia (FM) and rheumatoid arthritis (RA) patients; and, to identify psychosocial predictors of perceived physical and mental health status in both groups. Study group: 120 female patients who met the American College of Rheumatology (ACR) criteria for the classification of FM ($n = 68$) or RA ($n = 52$) were recruited. Methods: Patients completed a set of questionnaires assessing perceived physical and mental health status (SF-36v.2), emotional distress (BSI), active and passive coping strategies with chronic pain (PCI) and, negative and positive affect (PANAS). Results: FM patients reported greater impairment along physical and mental dimensions. Standard multiple regression analyses revealed that a model including emotional distress, passive coping, and negative affect was able to explain 23% of the variance in physical health status of FM patients ($p < .001$) and 24% in RA patients ($p < .05$). Passive coping made the largest unique contribution in FM patients ($\beta = -.29, p < .05$) and positive affect in RA patients ($\beta = .28, p < .05$). A model including emotional distress, passive coping, negative affect, and positive affect explained 44% of the variance in mental health status of FM patients ($p < .001$) and 68% in RA patients ($p < .001$). Emotional distress made the largest unique contribution both in FM ($\beta = -.60, p < .001$) and RA patients ($\beta = -.52, p < .001$). Conclusions: Our findings support the adoption of a biopsychosocial model for understanding the determinants of perceived physical and mental health status in both groups of patients.

---

[*] **Correspondence:** Paula Oliveira, PhD, Faculdade de Psicologia e de Ciências da Educação da Universidade do Porto, Instituto de Consulta Psicológica, Formação e Desenvolvimento, Rua Dr. Manuel Pereira da Silva, 4200-392 Porto, Portugal. E-mail: pjoliveira@fpce.up.pt

Keywords: Health status, fibromyalgia, rheumatoid arthritis.

Introduction

Fibromyalgia (FM) is a musculoskeletal chronic pain syndrome of unknown etiology and cure, which affects mostly women (1). One epidemiological study has shown a prevalence of 2% to 7% of FM in the general population of Europe; specifically in Portugal, a prevalence of 3.7% was found (2). FM is presently defined by the 1990 American College of Rheumatology (ACR) classification criteria, in which an individual is required to have both a history of chronic widespread pain and the presence of, at least, 11 of 18 tender points (3). In addition, patients could also present symptoms such as fatigue, morning stiffness, disturbed sleep, and emotional distress (1,3).

Research indicates that there is a widespread impact of rheumatic diseases on physical, psychological, and social factors in affected individuals, and thus, outcome measures that encompass multiple aspects of quality of life are needed (4,5). A widely used multidimensional generic health status measure is the Medical Outcomes Study 36-item Short Form Health Survey (SF-36). The measure includes eight subscales (physical function, physical role, bodily pain, general health, vitality, social function, emotional role, and mental health) which can be summarized along two dimensions to yield a physical health component score (PHC) and a mental health component score (MHC).

Empirical studies, using SF-36, have suggested that physical health status subscales (principally bodily pain subscale) tend to be significantly impaired in patients with FM compared to patients with myofascial pain (6), systemic lupus erythematosus (7), widespread chronic pain (8), and rheumatoid arthritis (RA) (9-11). However, Birtane et al. (12) did not find significant differences between FM and RA patients concerning physical health status subscales. Concerning mental health status subscales, FM patients tend to show significantly lower scores compared to controls particularly in the vitality subscale (6,7,8), but also in emotional role (6,7) and social function (7,8). Relating to mental health subscale, some studies reveal significant differences (9,11,12) but others not (6,7,8). So, it is still unclear whether aspects of health status are more affected in FM patients compared to patients with other chronic illnesses.

In accordance with a biopsychosocial perspective, it is relevant to identify psychosocial predictors of perceived health status given that patients' subjective status is an important factor to be considered when planning and evaluating therapeutic interventions (4). Even though studies have found associations between health status and psychosocial variables in FM patients (6-8,10,13,14), few of them have investigated the role of psychosocial predictors on health status. To date, studies point out the predictor role of anxiety (14), emotional distress (13), and coping with chronic pain (7) in predicting perceived health status of FM patients.

Concerning emotional distress, previous studies have shown that a high lifetime and/or current prevalence of both depression and anxiety are quite common in FM patients (11,14). Furthermore this symptomatology has been associated with pain and functional impairment (8,14).

Coping with chronic pain refers to cognitive and behavioral reactions to pain and can be classified into general active strategies for relieving, controlling, or functioning with pain and general passive strategies that include withdrawal, avoidance, and negative self-statements about pain (15). Research has shown positive associations between passive coping and higher levels of pain, functional disability, and psychological maladjustment (15,16). Associations between active coping and individual adjustment have been debated with divergent results found in empirical research (17).

As regards the negative affect and positive affect these are conceptualized as personality traits which can be helpful in understanding processes associated with health status. In fact, the negative affect has been related to subjective health complaints in non-clinical samples (18,19). On the other hand, positive affect has shown associations with lower levels of pain and has been viewed as a source of resilience to cope with chronic pain and interpersonal stress in FM patients (20).

In this study we intended to compare perceived health status in female patients with FM and RA using the Medical Outcomes Study 36-item Short Form Health Survey (SF-36). RA was chosen as comparison group because both conditions are characterized by pain, fatigue, chronicity, difficulties with the activities of daily living, and the affected quality of life. Despite their similarities, RA has a clear pathophysiology with a range of clinical measures being able to indicate its presence, contrary to FM. Acknowledging the disproportional gender prevalence of FM and RA, only female patients were included in order to control gender-related variables. A final goal was to identify psychosocial predictors of perceived physical and mental health status in both groups of patients.

Methods

Female patients who met the ACR criteria for the classification of FM ($n = 68$) (3) and RA ($n = 52$) (21) were included in the sample. Additional inclusion criteria included age at least 18 years and no major cognitive or psychiatric disturbances that would preclude questionnaire completion.

Procedures

Patients with FM were recruited from three Outpatients Hospital Departments in the Porto, Aveiro and Coimbra City areas (Hospital Geral de Santo António, Hospital Distrital de Oliveira de Azeméis, Hospitais da Universidade de Coimbra), as well as from an Association for FM patients (Myos Association). RA patients were recruited from the Department of Rheumatology of two Hospitals located in the Porto and Coimbra City areas (Hospital de São João, and Hospitais da Universidade de Coimbra). At all the Hospitals, patients were selected by their physicians to participate in the study in accordance with ACR criteria. In the Myos Association the participants were required to supply a standardized document from their physicians confirming that they met the FM ACR classification criteria. The study was approved by the Hospital Ethics Committees, as well as the Direction of *Myos* Association. All the participants gave their written informed consent after having received detailed information about the study. Then, participants completed a set of self-report questionnaires.

Variables and measures

Socio-demographic variables: Patients completed a questionnaire assessing age, marital status, employment status, and education level, as well as duration of symptoms.

Health status: The Portuguese Second Version of Medical Outcomes Study 36-item Short Form Health Survey - SF-36v2 (22) was used to measure perception of participants about their health status. SF-36v2, which was previously studied for its validity and reliability in the Portuguese language, questions 36 issues which are categorized under eight subscales: physical function (ten items), physical role (four items), bodily pain (two items), general health (five items), vitality (four items), social function (two items), emotional role (three items), and mental health (five items). The subscales may also be gathered in two large groups, the physical and mental components. The physical health component is composed of physical function, physical role, bodily pain, and general health. The mental health component is composed of vitality, social function, emotional role, and mental health. Each subscale and components are scored between 0 and 100 (standardized scores), and higher scores reflect a better perceived health status. The pattern of Pearson correlations between the eight subscales and the two health components fell within acceptable ranges, supporting the physical and mental health distinction. Good levels of validity and reliability of SF-36 are well-documented in clinical and non-clinical samples (23). In the present sample, as far as the Cronbach alpha coefficient is concerned it was $\alpha=0.89$ for the physical health component, and $\alpha=0.88$ for the mental health component.

Emotional distress: Emotional distress was measured by the Portuguese version of the Brief Symptom Inventory - BSI (24), a validated, 53-item self-report measure that assesses a variety of minor psychopathological symptoms that individuals have experienced during the previous week on a five-point Likert scale from 0 (never) to 4 (very often). Nine symptom dimensions are assessed including somatization, obsessive–compulsive, interpersonal sensitivity, depression, anxiety, hostility, phobic anxiety, paranoid ideation, and psychoticism. A summary score is derived by combining the items to create a global severity index (emotional distress) which has shown good internal consistency in the current study with a Cronbach alpha coefficient of $\alpha=0.97$.

Coping with chronic pain: Active and passive strategies for coping with chronic pain were assessed with the Portuguese version of the Pain Coping Inventory – PCI (15) a 33-item, six subscales, self-report questionnaire. Active coping was assessed by items of Pain transformation, Distraction, and Reducing demands subscales which reflect the patients' cognitive and behavioral efforts to distract themselves from the pain or to function in spite of pain. Passive coping was measured by items of Retreating, Worrying, and Resting subscales which represent behavioral tendencies to restrict functioning and to worry. Respondents were asked to indicate how frequently they used the coping strategies using a four-point scale ranging from 1 (hardly ever) to 4 (almost always). Active and passive coping scores are derived by calculating means of item responses. Kraaimaat and Evers (15) have supported the validity and reliability of PCI in assessing responses to chronic pain. In the present study PCI has been found to have acceptable internal consistency, with Cronbach alphas of $\alpha=0.74$ (active coping) and $\alpha=0.88$ (passive coping).

Positive affect and negative affect: Positive affect and negative affect were measured using the Portuguese version of the 20-item Positive Affect and Negative Affect Schedule - PANAS (25). Participants were asked to specify on a five-point Likert scale from 1 (very slightly or not at all) to 5 (extremely) the extent to which they describe themselves in terms of affects. The positive affect scale included items such as "interested", "excited", and "proud", and the negative affect scale included items such as "anxious", "fearful", and "irritable". Positive affect and negative affect scores were obtained by computing the mean for the 10 items in each scale. Good reliabilities of PANAS in rheumatic patients are well described in previous research (20) and in the present study Cronbach's alpha was α=0.86 for the positive affect scale and α=0.85 for the negative affect scale.

Data analyses

Statistical analyses were performed using the Statistical Package for Social Sciences (SPSS) for Windows version 13.0. Descriptive statistics including means and standard-deviations were computed for all key measures. Between-group t tests and chi-squared tests were carried out to compare groups on relevant variables. A Pearson correlation matrix was performed for each group to evaluate bivariate correlations between outcome variables (physical and mental health status) and potential psychosocial predictors. Finally, two standard multiple regressions were performed in each group to determine the psychosocial predictors of both physical and mental health status.

Results

Concerning the differences between groups in respect of socio-demographic variables, FM patients were significantly younger than RA patients (46.50 ± 9.33 vs 50.63 ± 10.08 years; $t = -2.32$, $df = 118$; $p < .05$). No significant differences were found regarding to education level ($X^2 = 2.51$; $df = 4$; ns).

The most prevalent education level within each group was elementary school (30.9% for FM and 40.4% for RA patients). 83.8% of FM patients were married, as well as 84.6% of RA patients without significant differences between groups ($X^2 = 9.18$; $df = 4$; ns). Significant differences were found with respect to employment status ($X^2 = 19.84$; $df = 5$; $p < .01$) with a high percentage of retired RA patients compared to FM patients (40.4% vs 13.2 %). Percentages of employed patients were 33.8% in FM patients and 34.6% in RA patients. Concerning the time lapsed since the appearance of first symptoms, there were no significant differences between FM and RA groups (11.47 ± 10.18 vs 13.37 ± 11.41 years; $t = -0.96$; $df = 118$; ns).

Differences between groups on psychosocial variables

Table 1 shows results from psychosocial self-report instruments. No significant differences between groups were found concerning active coping and positive affect. Significantly higher levels of emotional distress, passive coping, and negative affect were found in FM patients, compared to RA patients.

Table 1. Group comparisons on psychosocial variables in patients with FM and RA

	FM (n = 68) Mean (SD)	RA (n = 52) Mean (SD)	t (118)
Emotional Distress (BSI)	1.62 (0.75)	1.01 (0.52)	5.03***
Active Coping (PCI)	2.72 (0.44)	2.62 (0.51)	1.16[ns]
Passive Coping (PCI)	2.68 (0.48)	2.40 (0.52)	3.07**
Positive Affect (PANAS)	2.91 (0.68)	3.07 (0.68)	- 1.26[ns]
Negative Affect (PANAS)	2.80 (0.74)	2.41 (0.71)	2.96**

Note. N = 120; Clinical groups: FM (Fibromyalgia), RA (Rheumatoid arthritis);
* $p < .05$; ** $p < .01$; *** $p < .001$; ns – not significant.

Table 2. Group comparisons on SF-36 subscales and components

Variables	FM (n = 68) Mean (SD)	RA (n = 52) Mean (SD)	t (118)
Physical function	37.65 (18.40)	50.67 (20.51)	- 3.66*
Physical role	35.39 (19.72)	51.08 (24.96)	- 3.85*
Bodily pain	25.90 (15.88)	38.38 (17.84)	- 4.05*
General health	26.56 (14.62)	34.13 (15.80)	- 2.72[ns]
Vitality	24.36 (13.36)	40.62 (18.34)	- 5.62*
Social function	49.45 (22.59)	67.07 (19.65)	- 4.48*
Emotional role	49.14 (26.16)	66.02 (26.14)	- 3.50*
Mental health	44.56 (18.44)	55.10 (21.43)	- 2.89*
Physical health component	31.37 (13.18)	43.57 (14.58)	- 4.80*
Mental health component	41.88 (14.98)	57.20 (15.61)	- 5.45*

Note. N = 120; Clinical groups: FM (Fibromyalgia), RA (Rheumatoid arthritis);
* $p < .005$ (Bonferroni correction); ns – not significant.

Differences between groups on health status

Means and standard deviations of SF-36 subscales and components are shown in table 2, as well as between group t tests. Bonferroni correction was applied to reduce the probability of Type 1 error which can occur with multiple testing. Thus the significant *p* value was set at < .005.

FM patients reported significantly lower levels of perceived health status in seven subscales (physical function, physical role, bodily pain, vitality, social function, emotional role, and mental health). No significant differences were found in the general health subscale. Both physical and mental health components scores were significantly lower in the FM group compared with the RA group.

Health status predictors

To establish psychosocial predictors of physical and mental health status in each group of patients, correlation coefficients among variables were performed at first. In light of sample size constraints, and in order to both reduce the potential of Type 1 error (associated with multiple independent tests) and enhance data interpretation, only composite scores on the physical and mental health status subscales were considered in our subsequent analyses.

Better physical health status in the FM group was associated with lower scores of emotional distress, and passive coping, and higher scores of positive affect. The same pattern of results was found in the group of RA patients. Better mental health status for patients with FM and RA was inversely associated with emotional distress, passive coping, negative affect, and positively associated with positive affect.

Table 3. Correlates of physical and mental health status in FM and RA patients

	PHC		MHC	
Variable	FM	RA	FM	RA
Age	-.22^{ns}	-.06^{ns}	-.12^{ns}	.14^{ns}
Symptom duration	-.14^{ns}	-.12^{ns}	-.04^{ns}	.001^{ns}
Emotional distress	-.37**	-.37**	-.65***	-.74***
Active coping	-.07^{ns}	-.08^{ns}	-.02^{ns}	-.02^{ns}
Passive coping	-.42***	-.32*	-.38**	-.55***
Positive affect	.30*	.31*	.31*	.29*
Negative affect	-.09^{ns}	-.14^{ns}	-.40**	-.52***

Note. N = 120; PHC: Physical Health Component; MHC: Mental Health Component.
Clinical groups: FM (Fibromyalgia), RA (Rheumatoid arthritis); * $p < .05$; ** $p < .01$; *** $p < .001$; ns – not significant.

Table 4. Standard multiple regression: Predictors of physical health status in FM and RA patients

	FM ($n = 68$)			RA ($n = 52$)		
	B	SE B	β	B	SE B	β
Emotional distress	-3.36	2.20	-.19^{ns}	-7.40	3.93	-.26^{ns}
Passive coping	-7.87	3.40	-.29*	-5.24	3.92	-.19^{ns}
Positive affect	2.73	2.32	.14^{ns}	5.96	2.72	.28*

Note. N = 120; Clinical groups: FM (Fibromyalgia), RA (Rheumatoid arthritis);
* $p < .05$; ** $p < .01$; *** $p < .001$; ns – not significant.

Table 5. Standard multiple regression: Predictors of mental health status in FM and RA patients

	FM ($n = 68$)			RA ($n = 52$)		
	B	SE B	β	B	SE B	β
Emotional distress	-12.03	2.68	-.60***	-15.70	3.51	-.52***
Passive coping	-3.06	3.37	-.10^{ns}	-7.58	2.79	-.25**
Positive affect	1.62	2.32	.07^{ns}	5.98	2.01	.26**
Negative affect	0.59	2.55	.03^{ns}	-3.00	2.51	-.14^{ns}

Note. N = 120; Clinical groups: FM (Fibromyalgia), RA (Rheumatoid arthritis);
* $p < .05$; ** $p < .01$; *** $p < .001$; ns – not significant.

After that, variables which have shown significant correlations with both physical and mental health status, were included as independent ones in standard multiple regression analyses. So, significant predictors of physical and mental health status could be estimated in FM and RA patients. The results of standard multiple regression analyses examining factors related to physical health status in each group have shown that a model including emotional distress, passive coping, and positive affect was able to explain 23% of the variance in physical health status of FM patients ($p < .01$) and 24% of variance in physical health status of RA patients ($p < .01$). Of these variables passive coping makes the largest unique contribution in FM patients ($\beta = -.29, p < .05$) and positive affect in RA patients ($\beta = .28, p < .05$).

The results of standard multiple regression analyses examining factors related to mental health status have shown that a model including emotional distress, passive coping, positive affect, and negative affect explained 44% of the variance in the mental health status of FM patients ($p < .001$) and 68% of the variance in the mental health status of RA patients ($p < .001$). Emotional distress makes the largest unique contribution both in FM patients ($\beta = -.60, p < .001$) and RA patients ($\beta = -.52, p < .001$).

Discussion

Physical health status

Fibromyalgia (FM) patients reported more impairment in physical function, physical role, bodily pain, and the overall physical component summary score. No significant differences were found in the general health subscale. Da Costa et al (7) have found similar results when comparing patients with FM and systemic lupus erythematosus. Our findings suggest that FM patients perceive their symptoms as having a greater impact on their physical well-being compared to RA patients. This difference between groups could be explained by the absence of objective signs associated to FM which has been associated with a difficulty in acceptance of this syndrome as a medical disorder, even among health care providers. Thus, patients could accentuate physical complaints in order to try to get adequate medical assistance and comprehension among members of their social network. Moreover, FM patients showed significantly higher levels of negative affect compared to RA patients. In fact, individuals with high levels of negative affect could be more predisposed to noticing and attending to normal body sensations and minor discomfort (19). Thus, the perceptual style of FM patients could be responsible for their enhanced somatic complaining.

In the univariate analyses, worse physical health was correlated with more emotional distress, more passive coping, and less positive affect for FM patients. However, only passive coping emerged as a significant predictor of worse physical health status in the multivariate model. Passive coping represents a behavioral tendency to restrict functioning and to worry when individuals deal with pain (15) and seems to have an important role in the physical health status of FM patients. In fact, beyond inverse associations between passive coping and physical health status, FM patients are especially prone to showing this coping strategy compared to RA patients. So, cognitive-behavioral therapy could be relevant in order to reduce passive coping with chronic pain in FM patients.

On the other hand, positive affect was the most relevant predictor of physical health status in RA patients. These data support the role of positive affect as a source of resilience

(20) in coping with diseases symptoms. The propensity to experience feelings of joy and happiness (positive affect) could be improved with techniques of mindfulness meditation which promote individuals' ability to process affect with greater complexity, especially during times of pain and stress (26).

The amount of variance explained in the physical health status of each group suggest that other physical and psychosocial factors should be further considered in order to improve knowledge of variables associated with physical health perceptions.

Mental health status

Fibromyalgia (FM) patients reported more impairment in vitality, social function, emotional role, mental health, and the overall mental component summary score. Quartilho (9) and Walker et al (11) have found similar results when comparing FM and RA patients. These findings suggest that FM symptoms have a greater impact on the mental well-being of patients compared to RA patients. The significantly higher levels of emotional distress found among FM patients could explain, in part, such impact. Actually, emotional distress could be seen as a reaction to facing a chronic pain experience due to the burden and stressful consequences of a poorly understood pain condition. Another theoretical view states that FM pain and emotional distress could share similar pathophysiological roots even though this position does not have a sufficient amount of empirical support (9).

The amount of variance explained in mental health status by a model including emotional distress, passive coping, positive affect, and negative affect, support the fact that a psychosocial perspective is particularly useful in understanding this health status dimension. In FM patients, only emotional distress emerged as a significant predictor of worse mental health status. Otherwise in RA patients, more passive coping, and less positive affect also had an important predictor role, but emotional distress made the largest contribution to the prediction of worse mental health status. Thus, emotional distress was the most important predictor of mental health status, both in FM and RA patients. Consequently, when individuals show high levels of emotional distress, intervention should target them to improve the mental health status of these patients.

Limitations

This study has some limitations, such as the small size of the sample. Thus it is possible that there was insufficient power to detect a significant effect of psychosocial variables on multivariate models. Moreover, causal inferences between variables were precluded by the cross sectional design of the study.

Conclusion

Our findings support the adoption of a bio-psycho-social model for understanding determinants of perceived physical and mental health status among FM and RA patients, considering the distinctiveness of each group. Clinical interventions must approach specific psychosocial factors in order to improve individuals' health related quality of life, particularly in FM patients who report greater impairment on several health status dimensions.

Acknowledgments

This research was supported by a grant from the Portuguese Foundation for Science and Technology, SFRH/BD/18455/2004. We thank Dr. José Romão, sponsor of the preliminary presentation of this work at the 12th World Congress on Pain, Glasgow, 2008 organized by International Association for the Study of Pain.

References

[1] Blotman F, Branco J. Fibromyalgia: Daily aches and pain. Toulouse: Éditions Privat, 2007.
[2] Branco J, Saraiva F, Cerinic M, Bannwarth B, Failde I, Abello J, et al. Prevalência da fibromialgia na Europa [Fibromyalgia prevalence in Europe]. Poster presented at XIV Congresso Português de Reumatologia [XIV Portuguese Congress of Rheumatology], Vilamoura, Portugal, 2008, April.
[3] Wolfe F, Smythe H, Yunus M, Bennett R, Bombardier C, Goldenberg D, et al. The American College of Rheumatology 1990 criteria for the classification of fibromyalgia: report of the multicenter criteria committee. Arthritis Rheum 1990;33(2):160-72.
[4] Strömbeck B, Ekdahl C, Manthorpe R, Wikström I, Jacobsson L. Health-related quality of life in primary Sjörgen's syndrome, rheumatoid arthritis and fibromyalgia compared to normal population data using SF-36. Scand J Rheumatol 2000;29:20-8.
[5] Walker J, Littlejohn G. Measuring quality of life in rheumatic conditions. Clin Rheumatol 2007;26:671-3.
[6] Tüzün E, Albayrak G, Eker L, Sözay S, Daskapan A. A comparison study of quality of life in women with fibromyalgia and myofascial pain syndrome. Disabil Rehabil 2004;26(4):198-202.
[7] Da Costa D, Dobkin P, Fitzcharles M, Fortin P, Beaulieu A, Zummer M, et al. Determinants of health status in fibromyalgia: A comparative study with systemic lupus erythematosus. J Rheumatol 2000;27:365-72.
[8] Neumann L, Berzak A, Buskila D. Measuring health status in Israeli patients with fibromyalgia syndrome and widespread pain and healthy individuals: Utility of the Short Form 36-Item Health Survey (SF-36). Semin Arthritis Rheum 2000;29(6):400-8.
[9] Quartilho M. Fibromyalgia and somatization [dissertation]. Portugal, Coimbra: Faculty Med, Univ Coimbra, 1999.
[10] Tander B, Cengiz K, Alayli G, Ilhanli I, Canbaz S, Canturk F. A comparative evaluation of health related quality of life and depression in patients with fibromyalgia syndrome and rheumatoid arthritis. Rheumatol Int 2008;28(9):859-65.
[11] Walker E, Keegan D, Gardner G, Sullivan M, Katon M, Bernstein D. Psychosocial factors in fibromyalgia compared with rheumatoid arthritis: I. Psychiatric diagnoses and functional disability. Psychosom Med 1997;59(6):565-71.
[12] Birtane M, Uzunca K, Tastekin N, Tuna H. The evaluation of quality of life in fibromyalgia syndrome: A comparison with rheumatoid arthritis by using SF-36 Health Survey. Clin Rheumatol 2007;26:679-84.

[13] Dobkin P, De Civita M, Abrahamowicz M, Baron M, Bernatsky S. Predictors of health status in women with fibromyalgia: A prospective study. Int J Behav Med 2006;13(2):101-8.
[14] Epstein S, Kay G, Claw D, Heaton R, Klein D, Krupp L, et al. Psychiatric disorders in patients with fibromyalgia. A multicenter investigation. Psychosomatics 1999;40(1):57-63.
[15] Kraaimaat F, Evers A. Pain-coping strategies in chronic pain patients: Psychometric characteristics of the Pain-Coping Inventory (PCI). Int J Behav Med 2003;10(4):343-63.
[16] Davis M, Zautra A, Reich J. Vulnerability to stress among women in chronic pain from fibromyalgia and osteoarthritis. Ann Behav Med 2001;23(3): 215-26.
[17] Boothby J, Thorn B, Stroud M, Jensen M. Coping with pain. In RJ Gatchel, DC Turk (Eds.), Psychosocial factors in pain: Critical perspectives. New York: Guilford, 1999:343-59.
[18] Feeney J, Ryan S. Attachment style and affect regulation: Relationships with health behavior and family experiences of illness in a student sample. Health Psychol 1994;13(4):334-45.
[19] Watson D, Pennebaker J. Health complaints, stress and distress: Exploring the central role of negative affectivity. Psychol Rev 1989;96(2):234-54.
[20] Zautra A, Johnson L, Davis, M. Positive affect as a source of resilience for women in chronic pain. J Consult Clin Psychol 2005;73(2):212-20.
[21] Arnett F, Edworthy S, Bloch D, McShane D, Fries J, Cooper N, et al. The American Rheumatism Association 1987 revised criteria for the classification of rheumatoid arthritis. Arthritis Rheum 1988;31:315-24.
[22] Centre for Health Studies and Research (UC). Portuguese Second Version of Medical Outcomes Study 36-item Short Form Health (SF-36V.2). Portugal, Coimbra: Centre Health Stud Res, 1997.
[23] Ware J. SF-36 Health Survey Update. Spine 2000;25(24):3130-9.
[24] Canavarro MC. Inventário de sintomas psicopatológicos – BSI [Brief Symptom Inventory – BSI]. In: MR Simões, MM Gonçalves, LS Almeida, eds. Testes e provas psicológicas em Portugal [Psychological tests in Portugal] (Vol.2). Braga: APPORT/SHO, 1999:95-109.
[25] Watson D, Clark L, Tellegen A. Development and validation of brief measures of positive and negative affect: The PANAS scales. J Pers Soc Psychol 1988; 54(6):1063-70.
[26] Davis M, Zautra A, Smith B. Chronic pain, stress, and the dynamics of affective differentiation. J Pers 2004;72(6):1133-60.

In: Pain Management Yearbook 2009
Editor: Joav Merrick

ISBN: 978-1-61209-666-7
©2012 Nova Science Publishers, Inc.

Chapter 15

PAIN MANAGEMENT IN A NEONATAL INTENSIVE CARE UNIT

Edna Aparecida Bussotti, RN*
and Eliseth Ribeiro Leão, RN, PhD

Hospital Santa Helena Saúde, São Bernardo do Campo, Brazil and Hospital Samaritano, São Paulo, Brazil

Abstract

The aim investigation was to characterize the painful procedures performed by nursing team in Neonatal Intensive Care Unit (NICU) and to verify the pain management implemented. Methods: Descriptive and exploratory study conducted in private hospital in São Paulo city, Brazil. All hospitalized neonates were examined in the last quarter of 2007. The painful procedures were identified, counted and characterized according to type and pain intensity. The pain assessment was done using the Neonatal Infant Pain Scale (NIPS) and classified as to the type of therapeutic intervention applied: only pharmacological therapy (PT), only non pharmacological therapy (NPT), both pharmacological and non pharmacological therapy (PNPT) and no therapy (NT). Results: Thirty five neonates were included in this study, 31 (88%) gestational age >37 weeks and 4 (12%) gestational age < 37 weeks. Average length in NICU was 8.7 days and the average of procedures for neonates for day was 1.1. Three hundred thirty nine painful procedures were analyzed: heel lancet 128 (37%), venipuncture 99 (29%), arterial puncture 56 (17%), intramuscular injection 28 (9%), catheterization gastric tract 18 (5%), puncture for peripherally insertion central catheter 7 (2%) and catheterization urinary tract 3 (1%). Average procedures for neonate was 9.6 (range 1-48). Interventions adopted were classified according: PT 2 (1%), NPT 305 (89%), PNPT 25 (8%) and NT 7 (2%). Conclusions: Non pharmacological therapy appears to facilitate pain relief, but scarcity of publications regarding pain management in the NICU warrant the development of research and interventions to help this population when in distress.

---

* **Correspondence:** Edna Aparecida Bussotti, RN, Assistant Professor, Rua Ernesto dos Santos, 247. Jardim Independência. CEP 03225-000, São Paulo, SP Brasil. E-mail: edna.bussotti@ig.com.br

Keywords: Nursing, neonatal nursing, pain management, pain assessment.

Introduction

The effective evaluation and handling of pain in pediatrics constitute a challenge for the health professionals, especially pre-verbal children, who depend on the professional's interpretation for evaluation and interpretation of the painful pronouncement (1).

The Brazilian Society for Study of Pain, Brazilian chapter of the International Association for Study of Pain (IASP), adopted the IASP definition of pain as: "an unpleasant sensory and emotional experience associated with actual or potential tissue damage, or described in terms of such damage". However, it is important to highlight that we need an addition to the definition, so that individuals prevented from communicating orally are contemplated. In they definition non-verbal children and those with a clinically serious status or those with some neurological impairment should be noted and included. The note specifies that: "the inability to communicate verbally does not negate the possibility that an individual is experiencing pain and is in need of appropriate pain-relieving treatment." (2).

Studies showed that as of the seventh week of the gestational period, the human embryo presents sensorial receptors in the perioral region, evolving throughout all the corporeal surface until the 20th gestational week. Thus, both the term newborn and the premature newborn have anatomical and neurochemical structures capable of making the nociceptive impulse perception possible. Nevertheless, the modulatory mechanisms of the transmission system of the painful phenomenon mature more belatedly. In this regard, the term newborn and, especially the premature newborn, have an exaggerated response to the painful impulse, which results in a greater behavioral disorder (3). Therefore, the painful perception of term newborn, premature and young infant differs from the older children and that of the adults, a relevant fact to be known by the assistant team for the development of specific strategies for this age group as regards evaluation, prevention, treatment and reevaluation of the painful process (4).

During the hospitalization period, especially in an Intensive Care Unit (ICU), the child may be submitted to procedures and handlings that can be painful and the assistant team must offer the treatment, which is most appropriate to the situation.

Some studies have disclosed non-appropriate treatment of pain for ICU children, even when submitted to painful procedures or to small surgical procedures (5). The predetermining factor for such situation is the unpreparedness of the health team in relation to the following aspects: knowledge of the painful process in the child, the methods for evaluating the pain, knowledge of pharmacological and non-pharmacological measures for relief of the pain, influence of personal beliefs and reasonings of the health professionals and comprehension of the results of the pain, which is not treated for the child's future. In order to contribute towards a better evaluation of the pain in a child it is recommended to use valid and objective instruments for assessment (6). With involvement of the professionals it is possible to guide care of the newborn infant, as regards prevention, evaluation, treatment and reevaluation of the pain, safely and effectively, which will result in a positive impact in the family's satisfaction. In order to evaluate the care provided to the newborn and to his/her family, concerning the painful process, indicators for the management of pain are recommended. The indicators allow for verifying whether the strategies of pain evaluation and treatment are effective (7).

Due to scarcity of publications regarding pain management indicators in the Neonatal Intensive Care Unit (NICU), we found it relevant to contribute with our experience and the objective of this study was to characterize the painful procedures performed by nursing team in the NICU and to verify the pain management implemented.

Methods

It is an exploratory and descriptive and retrospective analysis study of the medical records carried out in a private hospital, Sao Paulo, Brazil, during October to December, 2007. The sample was characterized according to gestational age, clinical specialty and time of stay in the NICU. The painful procedures were quantified and characterized per type and painful intensity, measured by Neonatal Infant Pain Scale (NIPS) (8). The pain management was classified by the type of therapy used: only pharmacological therapy (PT), only non-pharmacological therapy (NPT), association of both therapies (PNPT) or no therapy (NT). The project was approved by the Institutional Review Board.

Results and discussion

The NICU has six beds and there is no arrangement for level of severity. The newborn infants who need ICU, regardless of severity, remain in the same physical space. Since 2003 the pain evaluation is carried out in a systematical way, considering the non-provoked pain (clinical condition of the newborn infant) and the provoked pain (needed painful procedures). As of 2007 we have used this procedure as an indicator of care quality.

Thirty five neonates were included in the study, out of whom 31 (88%) with gestational age >37 weeks and four (12%) with gestational age lower than 37 weeks. As to specialty, 29 (82%) were clinical and six (18%) surgical and out of these 100% were submitted for cardiac surgery. The average stay was 8.7 days and the average procedures per neonates/day was 1.1. There was a variation from 1 to 48 procedures per neonates in total with the average of 9.6. Since the institution serves high, medium, and low severity neonates in the same physical space, the results lower than those presented in the study, on the average of procedures per neonate, is justified.

Simons et al (5) evaluated 151 neonates over the first 14 days of NICU and verified on average, that each neonate was submitted to 14 painful procedures per day. In table 1, the 339 painful procedures are listed and we can note that more than 90% of the procedures carried out by the nursing department are related to some kind of punishment. Such procedure has an invasive and potentially painful character (3,9).

The therapies used upon execution of potentially painful procedures were classified in Pharmacological Therapy (PT), Non-Pharmacological Therapy (NPT), association of both Pharmacological and Non-Pharmacological Therapies (PNPT) and No Therapy (NT), as shown in table 2.

Among the NPT the following were used: non-nutritive sucking, swaddling (gently involve the neonate in a cotton cloth maintaining the members flexed towards the medium line of the body), containment (maintain neonate with members flexed towards medium line of his/her body, in the bed and involved by his/her nest), warm dressing and music. Such therapies were used in isolation or in association among them and were carried out upon evaluation and prescription of the nurse.

Table 1. Classification of the potentially painful procedures in a NICU during the period from October to December, 2007

Procedures	N°	%
Heel lancet	128	37
Venous puncture	99	29
Arterial puncture	56	17
Intramuscular puncture	28	9
Peptic probing	18	5
Puncture for central catheter of peripheral insertion	7	2
Vesical probing of delay	3	1
Total	339	100

Table 2. Therapy adopted upon execution of potentially painful procedures in neonates hospitalized in the NICU during the period from October to December, 2007

Therapy Adopted	N°	%
Pharmacological	02	0.5
Non-Pharmacological	305	90
Association of Pharmacological and Non-Pharmacological	25	7.5
No Therapy	7	2
Total	339	100

Table 3. Classification of the painful intensity upon execution of invasive procedures and the therapies adopted for the neonates hospitalized in NICU from October to December, 2007

Score NIPS	N (%)	PT	NPT	PNPT	NT
0	61 (18%)	-	54 (89%)	-	7 (11%)
1 - 3	118 (35%)	2 (2%)	102 (86%)	14 (12%)	-
4 - 5	135 (40%)	-	128 (94%)	7 (6%)	-
6 - 7	25 (7%)	-	21 (84%)	4 (16%)	-

During execution of the procedure the pain evaluation NIPS scale was used which is composed of five categories and the rate ranges from 0 to 7, where 0 is an indication of absence of pain and 7 is considered as the greatest painful intensity. The pain scores in relation to the 339 procedures were classified in a didactic manner, as follows: score 0 – absence of pain; score from 1 to 3 – light pain; score from 4 to 5 – moderate pain and score from 6 to 7 – intense pain.

Table 3 presents classification of the scores, number of the procedure upon pain scores and the therapies adopted.

The data from table 3 shows that strategies for relief of the neonate pain upon potentially painful procedures is needed. Low use of analgesics upon potentially painful procedures also calls to attention, possibly due to the erroneous idea that a simple (required) puncture does not cause greater sequela for the neonate. The study shows that there is also a scarce availability of effective and safe pharmacological therapeutic options for treating the neonate.

Usage of the EMLA® for lanceting of the heel bone, which is a very common procedure in the NICU, is also found in our results (see table 1) and seems not to be effective for the relief of pain. For venous, arterial and intramuscular punctures it is necessary to obtain better results with controlled and well designed studies so as to have a safe recommendation for the neonate (9).

Taking into account the importance of pain control for the neonate, the assistant team made use of NPT when feasible, as shown by the data in table 3, but in more than 80% of the procedures the action was only followed by NPT. Studies point out to effectiveness of some NPT for the relief of pain in neonate, such as usage of sucrose solutions with and without non-nutritive sucking (pacifiers) (10), the non-nutritive sucking (11) and the association of swaddling and music as the previously mentioned therapies (12-14).

Conclusions

The nursing staff carries out painful procedures in newborn infants, when they are hospitalized in the NICU and there is a need for interventions that can lower the neonate distress. The non-pharmacological therapy was the most used in this study and seems to have contributed towards a lower pain intensity. Scarcity of publications regarding pain management in the NICU warrant the development of research and interventions to help this population when in distress.

References

[1] Guinsburg R, et al. Reliability of two behavioral tools to assess pain in preterm neonates. Sao Paulo Med J 2003;121(2):72-7.
[2] International Association for the Study of Pain. Pain terminology. Available: <http://www.iasp-pain.org.> Accessed 2008 Oct 15.
[3] Anand KJ, Phil D, Hickey PR. Pain and its effects in the human neonate and fetus. New Engl J Med 1987;317(21):1321-9.
[4] Mitchell A, Boss BJ. Adverse effects of pain on the nervous systems of newborns and young children: a review of the literature. J Neurosci Nurs 2002;34(5):228-36.
[5] Simons SHP, et al. Do we still hurt newborn babies? A prospective study of procedural pain and analgesia in neonates. Arch Pediatr Adolesc Med 2003;157:1058-64.
[6] Merkel SI, Voepel-Lewis T, Shayevitz JR, Malviya S. The FLACC: a behavioral scale for scoring postoperative pain in young children. Pediatr Nurs 1997;23(3):293-7.
[7] Lacey SR, Smith JB, Cox KS, Dunton NE. Developing measures of pediatric nursing quality. J Nurs Care Quality 2006;21(3):210-20.

[8] Lawrence J, et al. The development of a tool to assess neonatal pain. Neonatal Netw 1993;12(6):59-66.
[9] Anand KJ, Phil D. Consensus statement for the prevention and management of pain in the newborn. Arch Pediatr Adolesc Med 2001;155:173-80.
[10] Stevens B, Yamada J, Ohlsson A. Sucrose for analgesia in newborn infants undergoing painful procedures. Cochrane Database Syst Rev 2004;(3):CD001069.
[11] Pinelli J, Symington A. Non-nutritive sucking for promoting physiologic stability and nutrition in preterm infants Cochrane Database Syst Rev. 2005 Oct 19;(4):CD001071.
[12] Whipple J. The effect of parent training in music and multimodal stimulus on parent-neonate interactions in the neonatal care unit. J Music Ther 2000;37(4):250-68.
[13] Satndley JM. The effect of music-reinforced nonnutritive sucking on feeding rate of premature infants. J Pediatr Nurs 2003;18(3):169-17.
[14] Huang Chin-Mei, Tung Wan-Shu, Kuo Li-Lin, Chang Ying-Ju. Comparison of pain responses of premature infants to the heelstick between containment and swaddling. J Nurs Res 2004;12(1):31-9.

In: Pain Management Yearbook 2009
Editor: Joav Merrick

ISBN: 978-1-61209-666-7
©2012 Nova Science Publishers, Inc.

Chapter 16

SEX DIFFERENCES IN ANXIETY SENSITIVITY AMONG CHILDREN WITH CHRONIC PAIN AND NON-CLINICAL CHILDREN

Jennie CI Tsao, PhD[*1], *Subhadra Evans, PhD*[1], *Marcia Meldrum, PhD*[2] *and Lonnie K Zeltzer, MD*[1]

[1]Pediatric Pain Program, Department of Pediatrics, David Geffen School of Medicine at UCLA. Los Angeles and [2]John C. Liebeskind History of Pain Collection, Louise M Darling Biomedical Library, UCLA, Los Angeles, California, United States of America

Abstract

Although sex differences in anxiety sensitivity or the specific tendency to fear anxiety-related sensations have been reported in adults with clinical pain, there is a dearth of relevant research among children. This study examined sex differences in anxiety sensitivity across unselected samples of 187 children with chronic pain (71.7% girls; mean age = 14.5) and 202 non-clinical children (52% girls; mean age = 13.6). Girls in the chronic pain and non-clinical samples reported elevated anxiety sensitivity relative to boys irrespective of clinical status. Girls with chronic pain also reported heightened fears of the physical consequences of anxiety compared to non-clinical girls but there were no such differences for psychological or social concerns. Among boys, anxiety sensitivity did not differ between the chronic pain and non-clinical groups. Future longitudinal research may examine whether specific fears of anxiety-related somatic sensations constitutes a sex-based vulnerability factor in the development of chronic pain.

Keywords: Chronic pain, children, anxiety sensitivity, anxiety, sex differences.

---

[*] **Correspondence:** Jennie CI Tsao, PhD, Pediatric Pain Program, Department of Pediatrics, David Geffen School of Medicine at UCLA, 10940 Wilshire Blvd., Suite 810, Los Angeles, California 90024 United States. E-mail: jtsao@mednet.ucla.edu

Introduction

Increasing evidence supports a robust association between chronic pain and anxiety disorders among adults (1,2) and children (3-6). Epidemiological findings indicate that adult women are at higher risk of developing chronic pain disorders (7,8), as well as anxiety disorders (9-11). However, this female predominance is less clear among younger populations. Studies of children's clinical pain generally show no sex differences until adolescence (12-16). Longitudinal research in the anxiety disorders similarly points to sex differences in separation anxiety (17) and generalized anxiety disorder (18) that emerge around 11-13 years of age. These findings suggest that there may be latent vulnerability factors in girls that emerge with age or pubertal maturity that lead to greater risk for development of chronic pain and anxiety disorders in adolescence that persist into adulthood.

It has been suggested that anxiety sensitivity (AS), or the specific tendency to view anxiety sensations as dangerous (19,20) may constitute a key dispositional construct that influences the development and maintenance of clinical anxiety (20) and chronic pain (21,22). In longitudinal work, AS has been found to predict the experience of panic attacks in adolescents over a four year period (23), indicating that AS is a vulnerability factor for the experience of severe anxiety. Relatively few studies have examined AS in children with chronic pain. One report found elevated AS in pediatric patients with noncardiac chest pain compared to controls (24).

Higher AS among females compared to males has been widely reported in non-clinical samples of adults (25) and children (26-29). The factor structure of AS however, appears similar across male and female adults (25) and children (27,29). The AS factor structure consists of a higher order global factor and inter-related lower order factors including physical concerns, psychological concerns, and social concerns (see (30) for review). Research examining the lower order factors points to a particularly pronounced sex difference for AS physical concerns among adults (25) and children (26,29), suggesting that fears of physical sensations associated with anxious arousal may be particularly salient for females. Despite the potential importance of AS in understanding the female predominance in chronic pain, there have been few relevant investigations in clinical pain samples. An adult study found that women with chest pain reported elevated global AS compared to men; sex differences in the AS lower order factors were not tested (31).

Not only is there a paucity of research on sex differences in AS among children with chronic pain, to the authors' knowledge, no existing work has directly tested the magnitude of sex differentiation in AS across chronic pain and non-clinical samples. Such research may assist in the identification of sex-specific vulnerability factors for the development of chronic pain. To address this gap in the literature, the current study tested the following hypotheses in a sample of children with chronic pain and a comparison sample of non-clinical children: 1) Girls will report higher levels of global AS and AS physical concerns compared to boys across the pain and non-pain groups; 2) The pain group will report higher levels of global AS and AS physical concerns compared to the non-pain group across sex. These primary hypotheses focused on global AS and AS physical concerns since these constructs have demonstrated the strongest sex differences in previous research. Exploratory analyses examined sex differences in AS psychological concerns and AS social concerns across the pain and non-pain samples.

Methods

The chronic pain sample consisted of 225 children (159 girls, 70.7%) presenting for treatment at a multidisciplinary, tertiary clinic specializing in pediatric chronic pain. From this larger sample, the present study included 187 children (age range = 9-18 years; M = 14.5, SD = 2.4) with complete data on the main measure of interest, i.e., the Childhood Anxiety Sensitivity Index (CASI; see detailed description below). Demographic information for the chronic pain sample is shown in table 1.

Pain diagnoses for the chronic pain sample are displayed in table 2. The non-clinical sample was drawn from a larger study on laboratory pain that included 244 children without chronic pain (124 girls; 50.8%; age range = 8 to 18 years; M = 13.6, SD = 2.6) (32,33). From this larger sample, 202 non-clinical children in the same age range as the chronic pain sample were included in the present study. Demographic data for the non-pain sample are displayed in table 1. The UCLA Institutional Review Board approved the study. Written informed consent forms were completed by parents, and children provided written assent.

Procedure

For the chronic pain sample, detailed description of the procedures for the administration of the questionnaire data examined in the current study is available elsewhere (34,35).

Table 1. Demographic data for the chronic pain and non-pain samples

	Pain Sample		Non-Pain Sample	
	M	*SD*	*M*	*SD*
Mean Age (years ± SD)	14.5	2.4	13.6	2.6
	n	%	*n*	%
Sex:				
Girls	133	71.1	105	52.0
Boys	54	28.9	97	48.0
Race/Ethnicity:				
Caucasian	127	68.3	79	39.1
African-American	5	2.7	29	14.4
Latino/Hispanic	26	14.0	51	25.2
Asian-American/Pacific Islander	3	1.6	21	10.4
Other	25	13.4	22	10.9
Parent Education:				
< 8th grade	4	2.2	6	3.1
< High School diploma	3	1.6	7	3.7
High School diploma	9	4.9	20	10.4
Some college/Associate's degree	67	36.1	55	28.5
College degree	44	23.8	50	25.9
Post-graduate degree	58	31.4	55	28.5

Table 2. Clinical characteristics of the chronic pain sample by sex and for the total sample

	Girls		Boys		Total Patient Sample	
	n	%	*n*	%	*n*	%
Pain Diagnosis						
Headaches	61	46.9	26	50.0	87	47.8
FNPD	47	36.2	17	32.7	64	35.2
Myofascial	49	37.7	19	36.5	68	37.4
Fibromyalgia	17	13.1	2	3.8	19	10.4
CRPS	12	9.2	1	1.9	13	7.1
Arthritis	2	1.5	1	1.9	3	1.6
Multiple Pain Diagnosis	41	31.5	12	23.1	53	29.1
Pain Duration	*Months*	*SD*	*Months*	*SD*	*Months*	*SD*
	35.0	41.0	44.6	45.2	37.8	42.3

Note: Frequencies for pain diagnoses sum to more than 100% due to multiple pain diagnoses. FNPD = functional neurovisceral pain disorder; CRPS = complex regional pain syndrome, type 1 or type 2; Duration of pain symptoms: range = 1 – 213 months.

Briefly, prior to patients' initial clinic evaluation, two questionnaire packets, one for the child and one for a parent, were mailed to the home following verbal consent from a parent obtained via telephone. Written informed consent from parents and written assent from children were obtained either at the initial clinic evaluation or prior to an in-home qualitative interview for those families who agreed to be interviewed. The qualitative interview focused on the effect of chronic pain on the child's self-perceptions and on the child's and family's daily functioning. The questionnaire packets contained instructions that parents and children were to complete them separately, without consulting each other. A research assistant reviewed the questionnaires with parents and children at the initial clinic evaluation to clarify ambiguous or missing responses. The questionnaires assessed demographic and general health information including measures of the child's pain, anxiety and functioning. Only those measures relevant to the present study are discussed below.

Recruitment and study procedures for the non-pain sample and the laboratory pain study are described in detail elsewhere (32,36). In brief, participants were recruited through mass mailing, posted advertisements, and children's classroom presentations. Advertisements were posted around the UCLA campus and other sites (e.g., community centers) in the greater Los Angeles area to enhance enrollment of children from low-income and minority neighborhoods. After confirmation of eligibility and verbal consent from a parent by telephone, written informed parental consent and child assent forms were mailed for review and signature. On the day of the laboratory session, participants completed questionnaires in a quiet room prior to undergoing experimental pain procedures. Only questionnaires relevant to the present study are discussed below. Participants received a $30 gift certificate and a T-shirt for participation.

Questionnaire measures

Demographics: Locally developed questionnaires completed by the parent assessed demographic information for children and parents including age, sex, race/ethnicity, and education.

The Childhood Anxiety Sensitivity Index (CASI) (37) is an 18-item instrument that assesses the specific tendency to view anxiety sensations as dangerous (e.g., "It scares me when my heart beats fast"). Items are scored on a 3-point scale (none = 1, some = 2, a lot = 3); total scores are calculated by summing all items. The CASI has demonstrated good internal consistency (Cronbach's alpha = .87) and adequate test-retest reliability (range = .62 - .78 over two weeks) (37). The CASI correlates well with measures of trait anxiety (r's = .55 - .69) but also explains variance in fear that is not attributable to trait anxiety (38). Cronbach's alpha for the CASI total scores in the pain group were 0.88, 0.81, and 0.87 for girls, boys, and the total sample, respectively. Cronbach's alpha for the CASI total scores in the non-pain group were 0.82, 0.72, and 0.78 for girls, boys, and the total sample, respectively.

Although there is controversy regarding the precise number of CASI lower order factors (27,39-41), the subscale scores pertaining to the three lower order factors identified in prior research, i.e., physical concerns, psychological concerns, social concerns, were used to be consistent with prior work on sex differences in the CASI dimensions (28). Cronbach's alpha in the pain group for the CASI physical concerns subscale were 0.86, 0.84, 0.86 for girls, boys, and the total sample respectively. Cronbach's alpha in the non-pain group for the CASI physical concerns subscale were 0.81, 0.71, 0.77 for girls, boys, and the total sample respectively. Cronbach's alpha in the pain group for the CASI psychological concerns subscale were 0.72, 0.77, 0.73 for girls, boys, and the total sample respectively. Cronbach's alpha in the non-pain group for the CASI psychological concerns subscale were 0.63, 0.48, 0.57 for girls, boys, and the total sample respectively. Cronbach's alpha in the pain group for the CASI social concerns subscale were 0.65, 0.76, 0.69 for girls, boys, and the total sample respectively. Cronbach's alpha in the non-pain group for the CASI social concerns subscale were 0.54, 0.55, 0.55 for girls, boys, and the total sample respectively.

Results

Independent t-tests and chi-square tests for continuous and categorical data, respectively, were used to preliminarily examine sex differences in demographic characteristics across the pain and non-pain groups, as well as sex differences in clinical characteristics in the pain group. Pooled-variance t-tests were employed if Levene's tests indicated unequal variance across groups. To examine sex differences in AS, total CASI and CASI subscale scores were compared using a series of 2 (group: non-pain, pain) x 2 (sex: girls, boys) ANCOVAs, controlling for child age and race/ethnicity (Caucasian vs. non-Caucasian). Following detection of significant interaction effects, simple-effects analyses were conducted on adjusted means. For the primary hypotheses of sex differences in global AS and AS physical concerns, a Bonferroni correction was used to protect against inflation of Type I error. To evaluate the two sets of hypotheses, alpha was set at .025 (two-tailed). For exploratory analyses of AS psychological and social concerns, as well as the preliminary analyses of sex differences in demographic and clinical characteristics described above, a standard probability level of .05 (two-tailed) was used.

Following established procedures for the detection of outliers (42), 2 outliers (1 girl in the non-pain group and 1 boy in the pain group) were identified and excluded. These outliers reported total CASI scores greater than three standard deviations above the mean for their sex. Thus, the analyses were conducted on a final sample of 186 pain patients (132 female; 70.6%) and 201 non-pain participants (104 female; 51.7%). Because cell sizes were unequal with more girls than boys in the pain group compared to the non-pain group (χ^2_1 = 15.20, p < .001), potential violations of assumptions were carefully investigated. To ensure robustness of ANCOVA results with unequal sample sizes for two-tailed tests, the recommended ratio of the largest to smallest cell size should not exceed 4:1 and the ratio of the largest to smallest variance should not exceed 10:1 (42); page 328). For the current analyses, these ratios were 2.4:1 and 2.6:1, respectively.

Sex differences in clinical and demographic characteristics-chronic pain group

Table 2 displays the presenting pain diagnoses, presence of multiple pain disorders (yes/no), as well as average duration of pain symptoms for girls, boys, and the total pain group. Pain diagnoses were categorized as follows: headaches (migraines; myofascial, vascular, tension, stress-related or other type of headaches), functional neurovisceral pain disorder (functional bowel, uterine, or bladder disorder), myofascial pain (of any part of the body excluding headaches), fibromyalgia, complex regional pain syndrome, type 1 or type 2 (CRPS-I; CRPS-II), and arthritis. As shown in table 2, over 30% of the patient sample presented with more than one pain diagnosis. In the pain group, there were no sex differences on the following demographic variables: child age, child race/ethnicity (Caucasian vs. non-Caucasian), or parent education. Similarly, no sex differences were found for the presence of multiple pain disorders. However, girls reported significantly shorter pain duration compared to boys ($t_{95.8}$= 2.10, p < .05). There were no sex differences in the presence of any individual pain disorders except fibromyalgia (χ^2_1 = 4.83, p < .03); girls were more likely to present with this condition than boys.

Sex differences in demographic characteristics-non-pain group

There were no sex differences in the non-pain group on any of the following demographic variables: child age, child ethnicity (Caucasian vs. non-Caucasian), or parents' education. Comparisons on demographic characteristics between the non-pain and pain groups indicated the following: the mean age of the non-pain group was significantly lower than that of the pain group (t_{420} = -3.72, p < .001), despite that fact that both groups were comprised of children in the same age range. In addition, there were significantly more non-Caucasian children in the non-pain group (60.9%) compared to the pain group (35.0%) (χ^2_1= 27.90, p < .001). Thus, child age and child race/ethnicity were used as covariates in the multivariate analyses examining sex differences in CASI scores across the two groups.

Table 3. Means and standard deviations for the CASI total and subscale scores in the chronic pain and non-pain groups by sex and for the total samples

	Chronic Pain							Non-Pain							Complete Sample						
	Girls (n = 133)		Boys (n = 54)		Total (n = 187)			Girls (n = 105)		Boys (n = 97)		Total (n = 202)			Girls (n = 238)		Boys (n = 151)		Total (n = 389)	
	M	SD	M	SD	M	SD		M	SD	M	SD	M	SD		M	SD	M	SD	M	SD
Total CASI	29.2	7.2	26.5	6.0	28.4	7.0		27.9	5.6	26.8	4.4	27.4	5.1		28.6	6.6	26.7	5.1	27.9	6.1
Physical	19.4	5.3	16.9	4.6	18.6	5.2		17.8	4.3	16.8	3.3	17.3	3.9		18.6	5.0	16.9	3.8	18.0	4.6
Psychological	4.1	1.5	3.8	1.3	4.0	1.4		3.9	1.3	3.8	1.0	3.9	1.1		4.0	1.4	3.8	1.2	3.9	1.3
Social	5.9	1.7	5.8	1.9	5.8	1.7		6.2	1.4	6.0	1.4	6.1	1.4		6.0	1.5	5.9	1.6	6.0	1.6

Note: Physical = CASI physical concerns subscale; Psychological = CASI psychological concerns subscale; Social = CASI social concerns subscale.

Sex differences in CASI scores-chronic pain vs. non-pain groups

Frequencies for the CASI total and CASI subscale scores for boys, girls, and the total sample for the pain and non-pain groups are displayed in table 3. Analyses comparing total CASI scores across the pain and non-pain groups indicated a significant main effect for sex ($F_{1,380} = 10.73$, $p < .01$), such that across groups, girls exhibited higher total scores than boys. There was no main effect of group ($F_{1,380} = .82$, $p = .37$). The group by sex interaction did not reach significance ($F_{1,380} = 3.82$, $p = .052$). Inspection of the total CASI scores indicated that girls in the pain group tended to score higher than non-pain girls whereas boys in the pain group tended to score similarly to non-pain boys.

Results for AS physical concerns subscale indicated a significant main effect for sex ($F_{1,378} = 10.73$, $p < .01$, $?2 = .04$), such that girls reported higher scores than boys. In addition, there was a significant group by sex interaction ($F_{1,378} = 5.31$, $p = .022$). This interaction is illustrated in Figure 1. Simple effects analysis indicated that girls in the pain group scored significantly higher on AS physical concerns compared to girls in the non-pain group ($F_{1,231} = 7.00$, $p < .01$), but there was no such difference among boys. There was no main effect of group for AS physical concerns ($F_{1,378} = 2.78$, $p = .10$). Exploratory analyses of the AS social and AS psychological concerns subscales indicated no significant main effects of sex or group and no interaction effects.

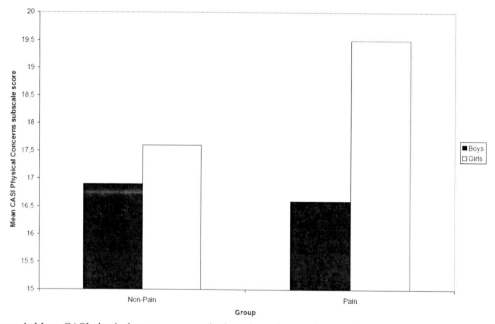

Figure 1. Mean CASI physical concerns scores in the pain and non-pain group by sex.

Discussion

Consistent with our first main hypothesis, girls in both the chronic pain and non-clinical groups reported elevated global AS and AS physical concerns relative to their male counterparts. These findings of sex differences irrespective of clinical status held after controlling for child age and child race/ethnicity (Caucasian vs. non-Caucasian). Contrary to our second main hypothesis, children with chronic pain did not report higher global AS or AS physical concerns relative to non-clinical children. However, these findings were qualified by a significant group by sex interaction effect which indicated that girls with chronic pain reported elevated AS physical concerns relative to non-clinical girls but no such group differences for boys (see figure 1). This interaction did not reach significance for global AS and the results of the exploratory analysis of AS social and psychological concerns did not indicate any differences based on sex or group, nor any interaction effects. Taken together, these findings indicate that AS physical concerns reflect the most salient aspect of sex-based differentiation in AS for chronic pediatric pain. Thus, girls with chronic pain evidenced greater fears of the physical consequences of anxious arousal compared to girls without chronic pain but these differences did not extend to fears of the social or psychological consequences of anxiety sensations. Boys with chronic pain did not differ from non-clinical boys with respect to any such fears of anxious arousal.

To our knowledge, this is the first study that has specifically investigated sex differences in AS among children with chronic pain and a comparison sample of non-clinical children. One prior study that did not compare boys and girls found that children with noncardiac chest pain endorsed heightened global AS as well as elevated AS physical and psychological (but not social) concerns compared to controls (24). Our findings of elevated global AS in non-clinical girls relative to non-clinical boys agree with the results of four previous studies with non-clinical children (26-29). In an earlier report, with a subset of roughly half the current non-clinical sample, we found no sex differences in global AS (36) but this may have been due to restricted sample size or the inclusion of younger children (i.e., aged 8 years). Similarly, in a previous study in a subset of less than half the present chronic pain sample (N = 87), we did not find any sex differences in global AS (43), possibly due to low power. It should be noted however, that neither of our prior analyses explicitly tested for sex differences in AS physical concerns and this subscale has revealed the strongest sex-based differences in previous research (25,26,29) as well as in the current study. It is unclear why our findings of heightened fears of anxiety-related somatic sensations in chronic pain vs. non-clinical girls were not evident among boys. Analyses of the clinical characteristics in the pain sample indicated that girls reported shorter duration of pain than boys, suggesting that in this respect, boys were more severely impacted than girls. On the other hand, there were no differences between boys and girls in the presence of multiple pain diagnoses or any individual pain diagnosis with the exception of fibromyalgia. Girls were more likely to present with fibromyalgia than boys and it is possible that this condition is more strongly linked with heightened AS. Fibromyalgia involves widespread pain and numerous tender points throughout the body as well as fatigue and disruptions in sleep, mood and cognition. Recent population-based estimates indicate that women are 1.64 times more likely than men to have fibromyalgia (95% CI = 1.59-1.69)(44). It is possible that fibromyalgia, because of its diffuse nature, demonstrates a more robust association with fears of physical sensations related to anxious arousal compared to pain conditions with a more discrete focus (e.g., headaches; abdominal pain). This possibility is speculative and requires further study. Because approximately 30% of our pain sample presented with more than one pain diagnosis, comparisons between individual diagnoses on AS were not conducted.

Reasons for the observed sex differences in AS are not well-understood. One possibility is that girls are more willing to report fears compared to boys (45). Research in twins indicates that AS is heritable in women but not in men (46) suggesting that genetic susceptibility to AS in females may be a factor. A recent report (47) found that for women, the more severe the AS, the more strongly it was influenced by genetic factors. In women, each of the three AS dimensions was influenced by both genetic and environmental factors. Among men, the AS dimensions were influenced by environmental but not genetic factors. Thus, the authors concluded that AS dimensions appear to arise from both dimension-specific and non-specific etiologic factors, the salience of which varied as a function of sex and severity. In accord, we recently found evidence for possible sex differentiation in routes of transgenerational transmission for AS in two studies conducted with a subset of the non-clinical sample included in this report. In the first study, we found that whereas parent AS was significantly positively associated with child AS in girls, no such parent-child AS relationship existed for boys (48). In the second study, we found that in girls only, parent AS was positively linked with child AS, which in turn positively predicted children's experimental pain intensity (49). These findings are consistent with the view that parent AS may operate via girls' own fear of anxious arousal to influence their responses to pain. One limitation of these findings is that the majority of parents in the two studies were mothers and an important consideration for future research is the examination of possible differences in father-daughter/son vs. mother-daughter/son AS and pain associations.

Limitations to the present findings should be mentioned. The cross-sectional nature of this work precludes any conclusions regarding causality. The current study relied on a self-report measure of AS; corroboration of the findings with behavioral measures of AS (e.g., laboratory stress tasks of anxious arousal) would increase confidence in the results. It has been reported that children with chronic pain endorse levels of anxious symptomatology comparable to that of children with clinical anxiety (4). Thus, it is possible that the findings of sex differences in the pain sample could have been due to higher levels of anxious symptoms among girls with chronic pain. Although we did not include a measure of anxiety symptoms, additional analyses of the chronic pain sample indicated that our findings held even after we controlled for the presence of possible anxiety disorder as assessed by a clinical psychologist or child psychiatrist during the initial clinic evaluation. Although formal clinical assessment of anxiety disorder(s) was not conducted, the possible presence of an anxiety disorder was noted on the patients' chart by the evaluating psychologist or psychiatrist. Notably, there were no sex differences in the frequency of possible anxiety disorder in our pain sample. Future studies of AS in chronic pain samples should include established measures of anxious symptomatology and/or formal clinical assessment of anxiety disorders. Nevertheless, research on vulnerability characteristics for chronic pain among children is still nascent (45) and few modifiable risk factors have been identified for the development of chronic pain and pain-related disability. Given that AS is a potentially modifiable risk factor that appears to be particularly salient among girls, these findings may point the way to sex-specific interventions targeting AS in vulnerable populations.

Conclusions

In sum, the findings point to heightened global fears of anxious arousal as well as elevated specific fears of the negative physical consequences of such arousal in girls with chronic pain and non-clinical girls relative to their male counterparts. Moreover, girls with chronic pain reported increased specific fears of anxiety-related physical sensations compared to non-clinical girls whereas such differences were not apparent among boys. These results indicate that specific aspects of AS focused on physical concerns are associated with the experience of chronic pain in girls but not in boys. Longitudinal studies are warranted to examine the extent to which AS may predict the development of chronic pain problems in a sex-dependent manner across adolescence and adulthood. Additional work may also examine whether interventions aimed at reducing AS prevents the development of chronic pain and/or reduces acute pain sensitivity among girls. Research on sex-specific childhood learning experiences may also shed light on the role of AS and related factors in the development of the adult female predominance in chronic pain.

Acknowledgments

This study was supported by R01MH063779, awarded by the National Institute of Mental Health (PI: Margaret C. Jacob), by 2R01DE012754, awarded by the National Institute of Dental and Craniofacial Research (PI: Lonnie K. Zeltzer), and by UCLA General Clinical Research Center Grant MO1-RR-00865 (PI: Lonnie K. Zeltzer).

References

[1] McWilliams LA, Goodwin RD, Cox BJ. Depression and anxiety associated with three pain conditions: results from a nationally representative sample. Pain 2004;111:77-83.
[2] Tsao JCI, Dobalian A, Naliboff BD. Panic disorder and pain in a national sample of persons living with HIV. Pain 2004;109:172-80.
[3] Beidel DC, Christ MG, Long PJ. Somatic complaints in anxious children. J Abnorm Child Psychol 1991;19:659-70.
[4] Dorn LD, et al. Psychological comorbidity and stress reactivity in children and adolescents with recurrent abdominal pain and anxiety disorders. J Am Acad Child Adolesc Psychiatry 2003;42:66-75.
[5] Hofflich SA, Hughes AA, Kendall PC. Somatic complaints and childhood anxiety disorders. Int J Clin Health Psychol 2006;6:229-42.
[6] Mulvaney S, Lambert EW, Garber J, Walker LS. Trajectories of symptoms and impairment for pediatric patients with functional abdominal pain: a 5-year longitudinal study. J Am Acad Child Adolesc Psychiatry 2006;45:737-44.
[7] Berkley KJ. Sex differences in pain. Behav Brain Sci 1997;20:371-80.
[8] Unruh AM. Gender variations in clinical pain experience. Pain 1996;65:123-67.
[9] Kessler RC, et al. Lifetime and 12-month prevalence of DSM-III-R psychiatric disorders in the United States. Results from the national comorbidity survey. Arch Gen Psychiatry 1994;51:8-19.
[10] Kessler RC, Sonnega A, Bromet E, Hughes M, Nelson CB. Posttraumatic stress disorder in the national comorbidity survey. Arch Gen Psychiatry 1995;52:1048-60.
[11] Weissman MM, Merikangas KR. The epidemiology of anxiety and panic disorders: an update. J Clin Psychiatry 1986;47(Suppl):11-7.
[12] El-Metwally A, Salminen JJ, Auvinen A, Kautiainen H, Mikkelsson M. Prognosis of non-specific musculoskeletal pain in preadolescents: a prospective 4-year follow-up study till adolescence. Pain 2004;110:550-9.

[13] Goodman JE, McGrath PJ. The epidemiology of pain in children and adolescents: a review. Pain 1991;46:247-64.
[14] Munoz M, et al. Prevalence of headache in a representative sample of the population in a French department (haute-vienne-limousin). Headache 1993;33:521-3.
[15] Perquin CW, et al. Pain in children and adolescents: a common experience. Pain 2000;87:51-8.
[16] Stahl M, Mikkelsson M, Kautiainen H, Hakkinen A, Ylinen J, Salminen JJ. Neck pain in adolescence. A 4-year follow-up of pain-free preadolescents. Pain 2004;110:427-31.
[17] Poulton R, Milne BJ, Craske MG, Menzies RG. A longitudinal study of the etiology of separation anxiety. Behav Res Ther 2001;39:1395-410.
[18] Velez CN, Johnson J, Cohen P. A longitudinal analysis of selected risk factors for childhood psychopathology. J Am Acad Child Adolesc Psychiatry 1989;28:861-4.
[19] Reiss S, Peterson RA, Gursky DM, McNally RJ. Anxiety sensitivity, anxiety frequency and the predictions of fearfulness. Behav Res Ther 1986;24:1-8.
[20] Taylor S, editor. Anxiety sensitivity: theory, research, and treatment of the fear of anxiety. London: Erlbaum, 1999.
[21] Asmundson GJG. Anxiety sensitivity and chronic pain: empirical findings, clinical implications, and future directions. In: Taylor S. Anxiety sensitivity: theory, research and treatment of the fear of anxiety. London: Erlbaum, 1999:269-85.
[22] Norton PJ, Asmundson GJG. Anxiety sensitivity, fear, and avoidance behavior in headache pain. Pain 2004;111:218-23.
[23] Weems CF, Hayward C, Killen J, Taylor CB. A longitudinal investigation of anxiety sensitivity in adolescence. J Abnorm Psychol 2002;111:471-7.
[24] Lipsitz JD, et al. Anxiety and depressive symptoms and anxiety sensitivity in youngsters with noncardiac chest pain and benign heart murmurs. J Pediatr Psychol 2004;29:607-12.
[25] Stewart SH, Taylor S, Baker JM. Gender differences in dimensions of anxiety sensitivity. J Anxiety Disord 1997;11:179-200.
[26] Deacon BJ, Valentiner DP, Gutierrez PM, Blacker D. The anxiety sensitivity index for children: factor structure and relation to panic symptoms in an adolescent sample. Behav Res Ther 2002;40:839-52.
[27] Muris P, Schmidt H, Merckelbach H, Schouten E. Anxiety sensitivity in adolescents: factor structure and relationships to trait anxiety and symptoms of anxiety disorders and depression. Behav Res Ther 2001;39:89-100.
[28] van Widenfelt BM, Siebelink BM, Goedhart AW, Treffers PD. The Dutch childhood anxiety sensitivity index: psychometric properties and factor structure. J Clin Child Adolesc Psychol 2002;31:90-100.
[29] Walsh TM, Stewart SH, McLaughlin E, Comeau N. Gender differences in childhood anxiety sensitivity index (CASI) dimensions. J Anxiety Disord 2004;18:695-706.
[30] Zinbarg RE, Mohlman J, Hong NN. Dimensions of anxiety sensitivity. In: Taylor S. Anxiety sensitivity: theory, research, and treatment of the fear of anxiety. London: Erlbaum, 1999:83-114.
[31] Keogh E, Hamid R, Hamid S, Ellery D. Investigating the effect of anxiety sensitivity, gender and negative interpretative bias on the perception of chest pain. Pain 2004;111:209-17.
[32] Lu Q, Zeltzer LK, Tsao JCI, Kim SC, Turk N, Naliboff BD. Heart rate mediation of sex differences in pain tolerance in children. Pain 2005;118:185-93.
[33] Tsao JCI, Lu Q, Kim SC, Zeltzer LK. Relationships among anxious symptomatology, anxiety sensitivity and laboratory pain responsivity in children. Cogn Behav Ther 2006;35:207-15.
[34] Bursch B, Tsao JCI, Meldrum M, Zeltzer LK. Preliminary validation of a self-efficacy scale for child functioning despite chronic pain (child and parent versions). Pain 2006;125:35-42.
[35] Tsao JCI, Meldrum M, Bursch B, Jacob MC, Kim SC, Zeltzer LK. Treatment expectations for CAM interventions in pediatric chronic pain patients and their parents. Evid Based Complement Alternat Med 2005;2:521-7.

[36] Tsao JCI, Myers CD, Craske MG, Bursch B, Kim SC, Zeltzer LK. Role of anticipatory anxiety and anxiety sensitivity in children's and adolescents' laboratory pain responses. J Pediatr Psychol 2004;29:379-88.

[37] Silverman WK, Fleisig W, Rabian B, Peterson RA. Child anxiety sensitivity index. J Clin Child Adolesc Psychol 1991;20:162-8.

[38] Weems CF, Hammond-Laurence K, Silverman WK, Ginsburg GS. Testing the utility of the anxiety sensitivity construct in children and adolescents referred for anxiety disorders. J Clin Child Adolesc Psychol 1998;27:69-77.

[39] Chorpita BF, Daleiden EL. Properties of the childhood anxiety sensitivity index in children with anxiety disorders: autonomic and nonautonomic factors. Behav Ther 2000;31:327-49.

[40] Silverman WK, Ginsburg GS, Goedhart AW. Factor structure of the childhood anxiety sensitivity index. Behav Res Ther 1999;37:903-17.

[41] Silverman WK, Goedhart AW, Barrett P. The facets of anxiety sensitivity represented in the childhood anxiety sensitivity index: confirmatory analyses of factor models from past studies. J Abnorm Psychol 2003;112:364-74.

[42] Tabachnick BG, Fidell LS. Using Multivariate Statistics. 3rd ed. New York: Harper Collins, 1996.

[43] Tsao JCI, Meldrum M, Kim SC, Zeltzer LK. Anxiety sensitivity and health-related quality of life in children with chronic pain. J Pain 2007;8:814-23.

[44] Weir PT, et al. The incidence of fibromyalgia and its associated comorbidities: a population-based retrospective cohort study based on International Classification of Diseases, 9th Revision codes. J Clin Rheumatol 2006;12:124-8.

[45] Martin A, McGrath PA, Brown SC, Katz J. Anxiety sensitivity, fear of pain and pain-related disability in children and adolescents with chronic pain. Pain Res Manag 2007;12:267-72.

[46] Jang KL, Stein MB, Taylor S, Livesley WJ. Gender differences in etiology of anxiety sensitivity: a twin study. Gend Med 1999;2:39-44.

[47] Taylor S, Jang KL, Stewart SH, Stein MB. Etiology of the dimensions of anxiety sensitivity: A behavioralgenetic analysis. J Anxiety Disord 2008;22:899-914.

[48] Tsao JCI, Myers CD, Craske MG, Bursch B, Kim SC, Zeltzer LK. Parent and child anxiety sensitivity: relationship in a non-clinical sample. J Psychopathol Behav Assess 2005;27:259-68.

[49] Tsao JCI, Lu Q, Myers CD, Turk N, Kim SC, Zeltzer LK. Parent and child anxiety sensitivity: Relationship to children's experimental pain responsivity. J Pain 2006;7:319-26.

In: Pain Management Yearbook 2009
Editor: Joav Merrick

ISBN: 978-1-61209-666-7
©2012 Nova Science Publishers, Inc.

Chapter 17

NURSING QUALITY: PAIN MANAGEMENT IN THE EMERGENCY ROOM

Rafaela Aparecida Marques Caliman[*], RN,
Maria Fernanda Zorzi Gatti[#], RN, MSc
and Eliseth Ribeiro Leão[°], RN, PhD

Hospital Samaritano, São Paulo, Brazil

Abstract

Acute pain treatment represents a major issue for the health area. In the emergency room, handling of pain is frequently neglected, which results in additional suffering for patients. Therefore, the monitoring of such nursing process is required. Our objective was to characterize management of pain in adult patients nursed in the observation area of the emergency room and efficacy of such nursing procedure from a nurse point of view. Methods: A descriptive exploratory study was carried out from October 2007 to October 2008. Data were obtained from 1,221 medical records considering the following variables: the index for evaluation of the pain, prevalence of measured pain, type of pain, pharmacological treatment, pain score in the hospital discharge and in transfer to other units as well as evaluation of the pain management procedure. Results: Pain prevalence was 50.8%, out of which 49.2% was visceral pain, 22.4% muscular-skeletal pain, 23.1% other types of pain, 4.7% neuropathic pain and 0.6% oncologic pain. 40.8% of the patients received pharmacological treatment. Upon transfer to other units 80.4% of the patients did not present pain, 9.2% presented a slight pain, 8.2% a moderate pain and 2.2% intense pain. At discharge from hospital 81% of the patients did not present pain, 11.2% a slight pain, 6.9% moderate pain and 0.9% intense pain. Pain management was considered effective in 91.8% of the cases. Conclusion: Pain management reflects a nursing quality indicator and has to be effective.

---

[*] **Correspondence:** Rafaela Aparecida Marques Caliman, RN, Hospital Samaritano, Rua Aragão 290, São Paulo, Brazil, CEP 02308-000. Tel: 55 11 3821 5650. E-mail: rafaela.caliman@samaritano.org.br
[#] Maria Fernanda Zorzi Gatti, RN, MSc, Hospital Samaritano, São Paulo, Brazil, maria.gatti@samaritano.org.br, Rua Conselheiro Brotero 1486, São Paulo, Brazil, CEP 01232-010, Phone: 55 11 3821 5650.
[°] Eliseth Ribeiro Leão ,RN, PhD, Hospital Samaritano, São Paulo, Brazil, eliseth.leao@samaritano.org.br, Rua Conselheiro Brotero 1486, São Paulo, Brazil, CEP 01232-010, Phone: 55 11 3821 5891.

Keywords: Pain, emergency room, nursing, quality.

Introduction

Treatment of acute pain represents a major issue for the health professional. The emergency room is prominent in such a context, since it is the place where pain is the main cause leading the individual to look for treatment. Acute or acute chronic, pain symptom, indicating or not the severity potential, is responsible for the need for immediate medical service.

Acute pain is related to the appearance of an inflammatory injury, whether infectious or traumatic, and is very well delimited in the time-space relation, it has neural-vegetative responses such as the arterial hypertension, tachycardia, tachypnea, diaphoresis, as well as psychic and motor agitation, tenseness and anxiety. It is generally related to intensity of the nociceptive stimulus and habitually, it is reduced as the concentration of tissue algiogenic substances is dissipated, therefore, remission is expected after cure of the primary injury (1).

Treatment of pain in the emergency room is not always evaluated as a priority (2). In addition to considering the risk of life in an emergent form, the fact that the possibility of pain relief makes difficult or even masks diagnosis causes professionals to prefer monitoring of the pain evolution instead of relieving it, until the medical diagnosis is known (3). This may result in sub-treatment of pain, although some studies showed that analgesia in acute conditions does not interfere with the evaluation of the individual (1). It can even facilitate the physical examination and diagnostic conclusion (1).

Deficiency of knowledge – by physicians and nurses – in relation to the physiological and pharmacological effects of the drugs also seems to contribute (2,4). Lack of evaluation and priorities of the individual in pain was observed in a study with 249 nurses from several hospitals in Taiwan, a fact that indicated the need for differentiated training on the subject with the inclusion of protocols to guide professionals (5). Another major aspect to be considered is the large diversity of invasive and painful procedures for diagnostic and therapeutic purposes, such as the tracheal intubation, venous dissection, arterial puncture, reduction of fractures and many others, resulting in a greater concern for prevention and relief of pain.

Investigation of pain in the emergency room requires a fast and objective systematization, which is the reason that the one-dimensional instruments are more used in order to provide a fast assessment of intensity of the pain and distress of the individual allowing for the service prioritization. One study (6) showed that usage of the visual analogical scale provided management of pain, which reduced time between the initial service and analgesia (6) and there are protocols for the purpose of guiding immediate service for individuals who are victims of traumas.

PHTLS (Prehospital Trauma Life Support) presents some restrictions when handling the pain, mainly around the side effects of drugs, such as depression of the respiratory system, aggravation of preexisting hypoxia and increase of vasodilatation with complication of hypotension and chock. Pre-hospital control of pain is not usual, but there is a consensus in the treatment of pain in individuals with isolated injuries of extremities and in the prolonged transportation of patients with no signs of ventilatory commitment or chock (7).

According to ATLS (Advanced Trauma Life Support) one of the basic principles is treating first the greater threat to life and further continued reevaluation of the individual and only treatment of pain as per specificity of the injury (8).

The protocol of ACLS (Advanced Cardiology Life Support) states the importance of relieving the pain in the cardiac individual, since production and perception of the pain involve local neuronal channels, spinal, thalamic and cortical, adversely increasing the determining factors for consumption of oxygen of the myocardium. A situation that may be difficult with preexisting ischemia and prejudice a conterminal hemodynamics (9).

In the protocol of PALS (Pediatric Advanced Life Support) (10) analgesia and sedation are treated in a separate chapter, due to the specific aspects of treatment of the infant and the child in an emergency situation.

It is clear that the usage of medicines to individuals in life threatening situations should be given with care and here it is paramount that the team in the emergency room should have knowledge of pain physiopathology, pharmacology and non-invasive analgesic techniques. In this situation the evaluation instruments is important in order to assess the pain with greater precision so that treatment can be initiated already in the primary evaluation (11,12).

In this context the Joint Commission on Accreditation of Healthcare Organizations, an entity that carries out quality certification in health care service facilities, recommend that each individual must be questioned on his/her admission to a hospital as to the presence of pain and the health institution must be responsible for the effective treatment, which should also involve the family (13). In an interview study (14) of 200 patients in the emergency room, 20% were not satisfied with treatment of pain and considered it not effective.

This study was conducted at the Samaritano Hospital of Sao Paulo in Brazil in order to characterize pain management for adult patients served in the observation area of the emergency room and study the efficacy of such assistance procedure from a nurse point of view.

Methods

An exploratory descriptive study was carried out with selection of the patients served in the observation area of the adult emergency room at the Samaritano Hospital of Sao Paulo in Brazil from October 2007 to October 2008. The representative sample was estimated from the previous statistical analysis of the number of patients served monthly by the service.

The data was obtained from 1,221 medical records and we considered the following variables for inclusion in the study: the index for evaluation of pain, the prevalence of pain measured by means of usage of the verbal numeric scale (0-10), the type of pain, the evidence of pharmacological treatment (medical prescription), the pain score in the hospital discharge and when transferred to other units the evaluation of the pain management process. The study was approved by the Institutional Review Board.

Results and discussion

From the 1,221 medical records analyzed, 1,203 patients were evaluated in relation to the pain (98.5%). The patients that were not evaluated (1.5%) were in the emergency observation area for execution of small procedures, such as exchange of gastrostomy botton and enteral washing. Despite the fact that we consider the absence of evaluation as a failure in the pain management procedure, we could verify that such procedures were resolutive and these patients received discharge from hospital as soon as they were finalized.

The average age of the evaluated patients was 56.6 years with variation from 12 to 99 years. 43.9% of the patients were male and 56.1% were female. The pain prevalence was 50.8%. Due to the fact that we did not consider the evaluations and the treatment of pain previous to sending the patient to the observation area, we could infer that the remaining population (49.2%) did not have pain or had pain, but could have been medicated and admitted to the observation sector already cured.

As seen in figure 1, the visceral pain mainly constituted by the cases of pain and thoracic pain represented the greatest complaint of pain in the investigated population, followed by the muscular-skeletal pain (very common in the orthopedic cases), from other types of pain (thus classified in the cases of cephalalgia and vascular pain), from the neuropathic and oncologic pain. Patients received pharmacological treatment with analgesics and anti-inflamatories in 40.8% of the cases.

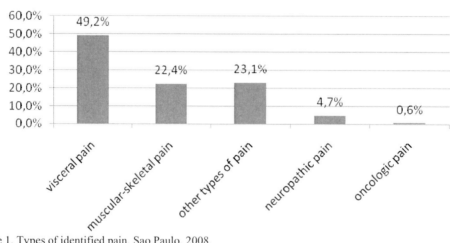

Figure 1. Types of identified pain. Sao Paulo, 2008.

In figure 2 it can be seen that 19.6% of the patients were transferred to other units with some type of pain, which is somewhat expected. The time for effect to take place of a medicine administered is variable, but we believe this is not a reason for concern, since the continuity of the treatment is assured by means of the information provided and documented in the medical record.

In discharge from hospital, absence of pain was documented for the majority of patients, as seen in fugure 3. Continuity of treatment at home is encouraged and guidance in writing was provided to the regular physician, the patient and family.

In a previous study, we evaluated whether patients that are discharged from hospital with moderate to intense score of pain return to the emergency room in the period of seven days with the same complaint. In that study we identified that 27% of the patients returned in the first 72 hours and the cases were characterized as chronic cases with a severity of the pain symptoms (15).

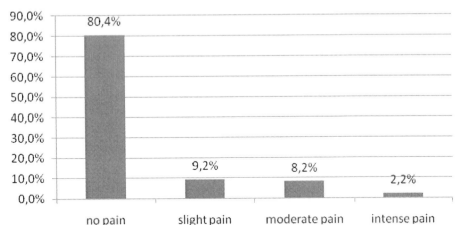
Figure 2. Prevalence of pain upon transfer to internment units. Sao Paulo, 2008.

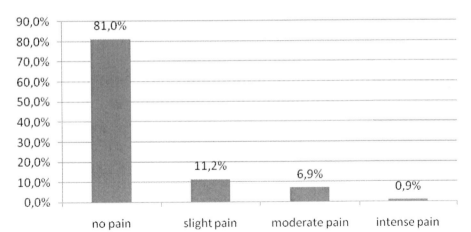
Figure 3. Prevalence of pain upon discharge from hospital. Sao Paulo, 2008.

Conclusions

Pain management was considered effective in 91.8% of the cases, which seemed to be corroborated by the fact that the majority of patients (81%) refered absence of pain in the discharge from hospital. Pain is a very prevalent phenomenon in the emergency room with predominance of cases related to visceral pain. Most of the patients referred had pharmacological treatment prescribed and by discharge or at transfer to other units presented appropriate control of the pain.

References

[1] Teixeira MJ, Valverde Filho J. Dor aguda. In: Teixeira MJ, ed. Dor: Contexto interdisciplinar, 1th ed. Curitiba: Maio, 2003:241-65.
[2] Tanabe P, Buschmann MB. Emergency nurse's knowledge of pain management principles. J Emerg Nurs 2000;26:299-305.
[3] Lenehan GP. On making pain a nursing priority. J Emerg Nurs 1992; 18:91-2.
[4] Teixeira MJ, Shibata MK, Pimenta CAM, Corrêa CF. Dor no Brasil: estado atual e perspectivas. São Paulo: Limay, 1995.
[5] Tsai FC, Tsai YF, Chien CC, Lin CC. Emergency nurses' knowledge of perceived barriers in pain management in Taiwan. J Clin Nurs 2007;16(11):2088-95.
[6] Stalnikowicz R, Mahamid R, Kaspi S, Brezis M. Undertreatment of acute pain in the emergency department: a challenge. Int J Qual Health Care 2005;17(2):173-6.
[7] PHTLS basic and advanced prehospital trauma life support, 5th ed. St. Louis MI: Natl Assoc Emerg Med Tech (NAEMT), 2003.
[8] Advanced trauma life support instructor manual. Chicago, IL: Am Coll Surgeons, 1997.
[9] American Heart Association. Suporte avançado de vida em cardiologia. Accessed 2008 Nov 20. http://www.americanheart.org/presenter.jhtml?identifier=3057944
[10] American Academy of Pediatrics. Suporte avançado de vida em pediatria. Accessed 2008 Nov 20. http://www.saj.med.br/uploaded/File/novos_artigos/155.pdf
[11] Holleran RS. The problem of pain in emergency care. Nurs Clin North Am 2002;37(1):67-78.
[12] Johnston MS. Are we effectively managing acute pain in the ED trauma patient? J Emerg Nurs 1999;25:163-4.
[13] Joint Commission on Accreditation of Healthcare Organizations. Pain standards for 2001. Accessed 2008 Nov 20. http://www.jcaho.org
[14] Muntlin A, Gunningberg L, Carlsson M. Patients' perceptions of quality of care at an emergency department and identification of areas for quality improvement. J Clin Nurs 2006;15(8):1045-56.
[15] Caliman RAM, Sereia DS, Gatti MFZ. O retorno do paciente com dor como indicador de qualidade da assistência. In: Anais do I Simpósio Internacional de Enfermagem Hospital Samaritano São Paulo. São Paulo: Hospital Samaritano, 2008:17-20.

In: Pain Management Yearbook 2009
Editor: Joav Merrick

ISBN: 978-1-61209-666-7
©2012 Nova Science Publishers, Inc.

Chapter 18

A COGNITIVE-BEHAVIOURAL GROUP INTERVENTION FOR CHRONIC PAIN PATIENTS: FIRST FINDINGS

Maaike J de Boer*, MSc, Gerbrig J Versteegen, PhD and Theo K Bouman, PhD

Pain Expertise Center, Department of Anaesthesiology, University Medical Center Groningen and Department of Clinical and Developmental Psychology, University of Groningen, the Netherlands

Abstract

Catastrophizing and inadequate coping strategies are associated with the development and maintenance of chronic pain. These can be targeted in a structured cognitive-behavioural group intervention. *Objective:* Evaluation of the effectiveness and feasibility of a 6-session structured cognitive-behavioural group intervention for chronic pain patients. *Study group*: Participants were 27 chronic pain patients of the Pain Center of the University Medical Center Groningen. *Methods:* An uncontrolled pilot study. *Results:* Results demonstrated that this cognitive-behavioural group intervention leads to positive change in catastrophizing and locus of control.
Conclusions: It is concluded that a structured cognitive-behavioural group intervention of short duration is a much promising treatment for patients with chronic pain at relatively lows costs. The present results can be seen as an indication that a psychological approach has potential as a useful intervention for chronic pain patients.

Keywords: Chronic pain, cognitive-behavioural therapy, group intervention, treatment evaluation.

---

* **Correspondence:** Maaike J de Boer, MSc, Pain Expertise Center, department of Anaesthesiology, University Medical Center Groningen, University of Groningen, PO Box 30.001, 9700 RB Groningen, The Netherlands. Tel: +31 50 3614886; Fax: +31 50 3619317; E-mail: m.de.boer@anest.umcg.nl

Introduction

Psychological factors have been found to play an important role in the development and maintenance of chronic pain. Inadequate coping strategies and negative cognitions about pain are identified as contributing factors (1).

With regard to coping, passive coping strategies, such as avoidance behaviour, seem to be of particular importance. In recent years it has become clear that the opposite of avoidance, which is prolonged activity, can also be held responsible for the development and maintenance of chronic pain conditions. This phenomenon is called 'ergomania' (2) or 'overuse' (3), and can in the long run result in an increase in pain and physical limitations.

With respect to attributions, it is often stressed that catastrophizing is an important factor in the development and maintenance of chronic pain (4). Catastrophizing can be defined as an excessively negative way of thinking (5). It involves the amplification of pain symptoms, rumination about pain, pessimism about the consequences of pain and experienced helplessness (6). Catastrophizing is related to pain intensity, limitations due to pain, pain behaviour, health care utilization, duration of hospital admissions and use of pain medication (5). In addition, thoughts about the (in)ability to control one's pain (locus of control or internal/external pain control) also seem to be important. A study by Keefe et al (7) showed that patients who considered themselves highly capable of controlling their pain (internal locus of control) experienced less pain and demonstrated fewer psychological complaints than their counterparts who reported that they were unable to exert any influence over their pain. Patients with an external locus of control feel that they are subjected to the pain. They do not experience the feeling of having control over their pain and as a result feelings of negativity, passivity and helplessness are amplified. In contrast, an internal locus of control will lead the patient to perceive him/herself as an active participant in dealing with the pain. This will lead to the use of active coping strategies, which will make it possible for the patient to exert some degree of influence on their pain. Jensen et al (8) reported that patients who believe in their own ability to control their pain (internal locus of control) and who do not catastrophize about their complaints function more adequately than those who tend to catastrophize and who have the feeling of being subjected to their pain.

Treatment

Pain coping, catastrophizing and locus of control are important issues in the cognitive-behavioural treatment of patients with chronic pain (9). A treatment programme based on a cognitive-behavioural approach is directed at helping the patient adapt to the pain that remains after medical interventions have been completed. A cognitive-behavioural intervention offers a valuable addition to pharmacological, physical or surgical treatment and should be directed towards modifying pain-related cognitions, catastrophizing and pain-related coping strategies (10). Pain reduction is not the primary goal of this type of intervention, but may be a secondary 'side effect'.

Recent years have seen the development and evaluation of a range of cognitive-behavioural programmes. In the literature these interventions are referred to as for example cognitive-behavioural programme, cognitive behaviour therapy, multi-modal biopsychosocial programme, self-management group intervention and psycho-educational group programme. Unfortunately, in many cases these programmes lack detailed description, which makes it hard to compare the various effect studies.

What these programmes have in common is the combination of cognitive-behavioural intervention techniques and psycho-education concerning chronic pain and the contributing factors to chronic pain. These programmes are aimed at learning to better cope with pain complaints. They concern monodisciplinary interventions, often within a multidisciplinary treatment approach, implemented by psychologists or sometimes by the nursing staff.

Cognitive-behavioural group programmes have proven to be effective in patients with chronic headache (11,12), chronic low back pain and other musculoskeletal pain (13), non-specific chronic pain (14-16) and (rheumatoid) arthritis (17,18). Interventions specifically aimed at adolescents (19) and elderly people (20) also appeared to be effective. Research into these interventions reported positive results on among others pain complaints, use of medication, quality of life, self-efficacy, limitations, depression, pain coping and fatigue. The effects of cognitive-behavioural group interventions for chronic pain do not differ significantly from the effects of comparable individual treatments (12,21). However, group interventions have a number of important advantages, such as cost and time effectiveness for the facilitator and the fact that participants are given the opportunity to share experiences and feel acknowledged by fellow sufferers. Chronic pain sufferers often have a sense of isolation because of their ongoing struggle in living with pain. By participating in a group programme participants realize that they are not the only ones with chronic pain and that they can learn from each other. A course or training of short duration is seen as 'low threshold' compared to individual (psychological) treatment. A beneficial side-effect is that participants are no longer addressed as patients but rather as active participants who are learning to cope with pain. The target is therefore for patients to treat themselves instead of being treated.

Research question

The present study aims to describe and evaluate a structured cognitive-behavioural psycho-educational course of short duration for persons with chronic pain. This exploratory study was conducted to examine the feasibility of a cognitive-behavioural group intervention in a patient group (characterized by long-standing pain complaints and serious limitations) of a university pain center. Patients' participation in the group programme is expected to effect positive changes in catastrophizing, pain coping and locus of control. Because of the exploratory nature, no waiting list control group was used in this pilot study.

Methods

Participants

Participants were patients of the Pain Center of the University Medical Center Groningen, who fulfilled specified inclusion and exclusion criteria and were advised to take part in the course after interdisciplinary evaluation. All new patients of the Pain Center are subjected to an interdisciplinary evaluation in which they are evaluated by a physician (anaesthesiologist), physical therapist and psychologist. Patients with non-specific chronic pain (defined as pain which has persisted beyond the normal tissue healing time of three months (22)) who are advised to take part in the course receive an additional introductory interview and are asked to complete a few questionnaires, after which they can participate in the course.

The following inclusion criteria applied: a) having non-specific, medically unexplained chronic pain complaints and/or chronic pain complaints for which no (longer) somatic treatment could be offered, b) minimum age of 18 years, c) motivated for a cognitive-behavioural approach and d) prepared to actively participate in the course. Exclusion criteria were a) severe psychopathology (as measured by psychodiagnostic interview and scores on the Symptom Checklist 90 (cut-off score of 224 (23)) and b) limited intelligence (highest education level achieved less than primary education).

Thirty patients entered the course, which was presented in six groups of 4-6 participants. During the course three participants dropped out on account of an increase in psychological or physical complaints. The biographical and clinical data concerning the 27 completers are shown in table 1.

Remarkable features of our sample are the relatively high mean age of the participants, the overrepresentation of women and the relatively long duration of pain complaints. The age and sex distribution found in this group do not differ significantly from those found in a previous study among patients of our Pain Center (24). When asked about the nature of their pain complaints nearly half of the participants reported diffuse pain complaints (extensive pain in various parts of the body) explained by various reasons.

Instruments

Repeated measurements took place at the start of the course (T0), directly after the 6-week course (T1) and at the booster session 2 months after the last session (T2).

VAS-scores (Visual Analogue Scale, with scores from 0 = 'not al all', to 10 = 'extremely') were used at three time points to measure (a) the extent of pain, (b) the extent of fatigue, (c) the extent of impairment because of the pain, and (d) the extent to which a person was able to relax.

The Pain Coping and Cognitions List (25) is a questionnaire for the overall measurement of pain coping, locus of control and pain cognitions. It consists of 42 items and comprises the subscales Catastrophizing (negative thoughts about the catastrophical consequences of pain), Pain Coping (ways of coping with pain, either active or passive), Internal Pain Management (the extent to which a person thinks he/she is able to manage or control the pain) and External Pain Management (the extent to which a person believes that other persons or powers (e.g. God) are able to manage or control the pain).

The subscales Catastrophizing, Pain Coping and Internal Management of this Dutch questionnaire show high internal consistency. The internal consistency of the subscale External Pain Management is somewhat lower, but still sufficient.

Table 1. Characteristics of the participants (n = 27)

		N	%
Age			
	Mean ± SD (Range)	46.6 ± 12.3 (24-69)	
Duration of symptoms (years)			
	Mean ± SD (Range)	9.5 ± 6.3 (2-25)	
Gender			
	Male	9	33.3
	Female	18	66.7
Education			
	Primary education	3	11.1
	Lower secondary education	10	37.0
	Higher secondary education	10	37.0
	Tertiary education	4	14.8
Marital status			
	Married	16	59.3
	Divorced	4	14.8
	Widow/ widower	1	3.7
	Not married/ living with partner	1	3.7
	Single	5	18.5
Job status			
	Employed	9	33.3
	Homemaker	3	11.1
	Unemployed	3	11.1
	Retired	1	3.7
	On disability	8	29.6
	Other benefit than disability	1	3.7
	Other	2	7.4
Pain location			
	Head/ neck	5	18.5
	Back	1	3.7
	Arm/ shoulder	3	11.1
	Hand/ wrist	1	3.7
	Leg/ hip/ knee	1	3.7
	Ankle/ foot	2	7.4

Table 1. (Continued)

		N	%
	Stomach	1	3.7
	Diffuse pain	12	44.4
	Other	1	3.7
Cause of pain			
	Accident	7	25.9
	Pregnancy	1	3.7
	Strain	2	7.4
	No clear cause	9	33.3
	Other cause	8	29.6

The Tampa Scale of Kinesiophobia (26-28) is a questionnaire for measuring fear of injury due to physical activity in patients with chronic pain in the motor apparatus. The questionnaire comprises 17 items. The total score measures fear of movement/kinesiophobia. Its internal consistency and test-retest reliability of the Dutch version of the TSK have found to be good (29).

After completing the course participants were asked to fill in a short questionnaire to evaluate the course. They were asked to what extent they felt they had improved or worsened and which components of the course they had found useful. In addition, they were asked to rate the course as a whole on a scale from 1 ('very bad') to 10 ('excellent'). At the booster session they were once again asked about their subjective improvement/ deterioration and to what extent they had been able to proceed with the course instructions afterwards.

The course

The course 'Learning to live with pain in a relaxed way' consists of 6 sessions of two hours each and a booster session that takes place two months after the last course session. The group is a closed entity; no new participants are admitted once the group has started. The course is supervised by two facilitators. For the groups in this study it concerned a psychologist and a trainee psychologist or a psychologist and a social worker. The psychologist of the course facilitator team was the same in all groups. A structured protocol was used (30), which was based on a psycho-educational group approach for hypochondriasis (31). Use of the protocol ensured a standardized administration of the course. In the first session participants are given a 25 page course book containing background information and relevant material for the homework assignments. Central to the course is the cognitive-behavioural model in the format of a pain circle. This pain circle (see figure 1) is based on the circle for hypochondriasis (31) and was adapted for chronic pain. Pivotal to the model of hypochondriasis is the catastrophic misinterpretation of bodily sensations, leading to anxiety, anxiety-reducing behaviour and selective attention to bodily symptoms. A vicious circle of bodily sensations, thoughts/interpretations, feelings, behaviour and selective attention is central to cognitive-behaviour therapy in general and also for chronic pain. During each session of the course the emphasis is on one particular aspect of the pain circle. Medical issues are not discussed in the course.

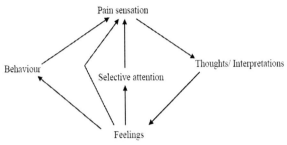

Figure 1. A cognitive-behavioural model of pain.

The sessions consist of brief lectures explaining the theory of pain, group exercises, focused group discussion and discussing of homework. Audio-visual aids are used. Session 1 focuses on the introduction of the course and the question 'What is chronic pain'. Session 2 is dedicated to pain and activities with a focus on pacing/ graded activity. Sessions 3 focuses on pain and stress. In this sessions relaxation techniques are taught. In session 4 the theme 'pain and thoughts' is discussed. Techniques from cognitive therapy are explained and practiced. The subject of session 5 is 'pain and attention to your body', with various exercises to learn to focus and switch one's own attention. Session 6 is dedicated to recapitulation and integration of all subjects discussed during the course. Session 7, which takes place two months after session 6, is a booster session containing a short refresher course and discussion of how to proceed on one's own after the course.

Statistical analysis

Due to the small sample size and non-normal distribution of the scale scores, nonparametric tests were used. The Friedman test was used to compare the scores at three time points and the Wilcoxon Signed Ranks test (comparison of two time points) was used for post-hoc contrasts. Cohen's d values were calculated as measures of effect size. An exploratory approach was pursued.

Results

As can be seen in table 2, three of the four subscales of the PCCL (i.e. catastrophizing, internal pain management and external pain management) show a significant overall effect. Posthoc analyses on these three scales (see table 3) show a significant improvement ($p<.05$) between pre-assessment and both post-assessments on the subscales Catastrophizing and Internal Pain Management. The effect sizes of these differences are of medium magnitude (see table 3). Compared to the pre-assessment situation participants reported fewer catastrophizing thoughts about their pain directly after the course and even more so at the booster session. After the course participants felt that they had more control over their pain and this improvement was even stronger at the booster session two months later. A significant decrease can be seen on the subscale External Pain Management between pre-assessment and first post-assessment. This means that directly after the course participants were less convinced that other people or higher powers could control their pain. At the two month follow-up this improvement was no longer significant. The Visual Analogue Scale shows a significant improvement of medium effect size between pre-assessment and first post-assessment with regard to the extent to which participants were able to relax.

Table 2. Means and standard deviations of the questionnaire scores and results of the Friedman test on three time points

		T0 M	T0 SD	T1 M	T1 SD	T2 M	T2 SD	χ^2	p
VAS	Pain	5.8	2.1	6.0	2.2	5.4	2.1	3.42	0.181
	Impairment	6.1	2.3	6.0	2.4	5.7	2.3	2.95	0.229
	Fatigue	6.3	2.6	6.4	2.1	6.6	2.6	4.07	0.131
	Relaxation	6.0	2.5	5.2	2.1	5.0	2.0	6.38	0.041*
PCCL	Catastrophizing	3.4	0.9	3.0	1.1	2.9	1.0	18.46	0.000*
	Pain Coping	3.6	0.9	3.7	0.7	3.8	0.8	1.03	0.597
	Int. Pain Management	3.6	0.8	4.0	0.9	4.1	1.0	9.52	0.009*
	Ext. Pain Management	2.7	1.0	2.3	0.9	2.5	1.0	6.02	0.049*
TSK		34.2	6.0	33.4	7.5	31.8	6.8	3.66	0.160

Note: T0: Pre-assessment; T1: Post-assessment after 6 sessions; T2: Post-assessment at 2 month follow-up; VAS: Visual Analogue Scale; PCCL: Pain Coping and Cognition List, TSK: Tampa Scale of Kinesiophobia, χ^2: Chi-square; p: level of significance of Friedman test.

The TSK (see table 3) shows no differences between the three measurements. No improvement can be seen in fear of movement. It should be noted that participants formed a heterogeneous group with regard to the location of their pain and that a number of participants experienced no fear of movement at all. The mean score on the TSK is low (at pre-assessment in decile 3 in comparison with the norm group of chronic patients and around the second decile at follow-up) (27).

Course evaluation

Participant rated the course on average as 7 out of 10 (1= 'very bad', 10= 'excellent'). This means they were satisfied with the course. When asked about useful themes all participants (100%) indicated that they found the sessions on 'Behaviour' and 'Relaxation' useful. The subject 'What is chronic pain?' was experienced as useful by 95.9% of the participants. Selective attention was found useful by 91.3% and 87.2% of the participants found

'Thoughts' a useful subject. At the follow-up 37.6% of the participants indicated that they were very well or well capable of applying the course instructions in their daily lives. Fifty-six percent managed reasonably well and only 6.3% reported that they were unable to apply the material from the course.

Table 3. Posthoc analyses at successive time points

			Z	p	ES
VAS					
	Relaxation	T0 - T1	-2.07	0.038*	0.35
		T0 - T2	-1.81	0.070	0.44
		T1 - T2	-0.31	0.755	0.10
PCCL					
	Catastrophizing	T0 - T1	-2.52	0.012*	0.40
		T0 - T2	-3.45	0.001*	0.53
		T1 - T2	-1.53	0.125	0.10
	Internal Pain Management	T0 - T1	-3.27	0.001*	0.47
		T0 - T2	-2.96	0.003*	0.55
		T1 - T2	-0.66	0.511	0.11
	External Pain Management	T0 - T1	-2.79	0.005*	0.42
		T0 - T2	-1.53	0.126	0.20
		T1 - T2	-1.77	0.076	0.21

Note: T0: Pre-assessment; T1: Post-assessment after 6 sessions; T2: Post-assessment at 2 month follow-up; Z: Wilcoxen Z; p: level of significance of Wilcoxen Signed Ranks test; ES: effect sizes (Cohen's d).

Drop-outs and attendance

Three of the 30 participants dropped out of the course. This was due to an increase in psychological complaints and worsening of physical complaints. Biographical and clinical variables of the three drop-outs hardly differ from those of the completers. At pre-assessment drop-outs experienced significantly more pain on the VAS ($M_{drop-outs}=7.5$; $M_{completers}=5.9$; Mann-Whitney $U=11.5$; $p=0.041$).

Of the 27 participants who completed the course, 55.5% attended all sessions, while 37.0% missed one session and 7.5% missed two sessions. Compared to other studies in a similar area the attendance rate is quite satisfactory.

Discussion

The aim of the present study was to evaluate our recently developed cognitive-behavioural course for chronic pain patients and to evaluate its application in a university hospital pain center. Based on the results of the present study it can be concluded that a cognitive-behavioural group programme has potential as a useful intervention for chronic pain patients.

The results of this pilot study confirm the assumption that the intervention would effect positive changes in the areas of catastrophizing and locus of control. After the intervention participants experienced fewer negative thoughts and felt that they were more in control of their pain. However, no improvement could be observed with regard to pain coping. This may be explained by the fact that a change in cognitions comes prior to and is possibly a prerequisite for a change in coping behaviour. This assumption is supported by the findings of Prochaska and DiClemente (32) that a change in behaviour is hard to achieve and that it takes time before newly learned behaviour can actually be incorporated. In the relatively short period of time between pre-assessment and follow-up a change in cognitions may have been effected, but a longer period of time may be needed before a change in coping behaviour can be demonstrated.

The results from this pilot study are preliminary since it concerns an uncontrolled study with a relatively brief follow-up period. Future studies including a waiting list control group are needed to control for potential spontaneous improvement. In addition, alternative explanations for positive changes should also be taken into account in future studies. Because of the uncontrolled nature of the study, non-specific therapy effects can not be ruled out. A factor to consider may be the non-specific positive effect of the contact with fellow sufferers. When evaluating the course participants reported that this course had given them the opportunity to share feelings and concerns with group members. However, there is also a negative side to this contact with fellow sufferers. Some participants find it difficult to listen to other people talking about their problems. Another consequence may be that participants tend to amplify each other's dysfunctional pain cognitions. Therefore course facilitators should be directive in their approach.

Our participants formed a relatively severe and chronic group of pain patients. At the onset of the course the mean duration of pain complaints was 9.5 years, ranging from a minimum of 2 years to a maximum of 25 years. Compared to other studies (14,16) this mean duration of pain can be considered a long time. It would be interesting to examine the effects of the group intervention in patients with a shorter history of pain complaints, in for example a general hospital or a psychologists' private practice. Patients with a shorter illness duration may be better able to change their way of dealing with their pain complaints. Cognitive-behavioural group interventions have shown to be effective in persons with pain complaints who have not yet sought medical treatment for their complaints (non-patients). A preventive cognitive-behavioural group intervention has been shown to have a positive effect on limitations experienced and work leave in a group of non-patients with neck and back complaints (33).

Earlier intervention can also be recommended for our patient group. It is our experience that participants in this course are rather stuck in their own way of coping with pain. This can hardly be called surprising considering their longstanding chronic complaints and the limited effectiveness of (medical or psychological) interventions. A cognitive-behavioural intervention at an earlier stage may prevent extreme chronicity.

The attendance rate and drop-out were quite satisfactory. Patients who start with the course are in general inclined to complete the course and miss few sessions. They seem motivated to attend all sessions. In the cases that participants did miss sessions, the severity of the pain complaints may have played a role. Travelling to the hospital is a strenuous undertaking for chronic pain patients, especially for those who have to cover a great distance to the hospital. It can therefore be recommended to start future courses in different places within the region in order to reduce participants' travel distance. Obstacles like having to travel to the hospital can also be overcome by the development of internet interventions. Cognitive-behavioural internet-based interventions have shown to be effective in patients with chronic back pain (34) and chronic headache (35,36).

From the perspective of cost-effectiveness it is also recommended to provide cognitive-behavioural interventions to chronic pain patients. Based on their research Turk and Burwinkle (37) conclude that a cognitive-behavioural intervention is 10.6 times more cost-effective than spinal cord stimulation, 12 times more cost-effective than standard medical care and 26 times more cost-effective than a surgical intervention. Although this study is based on the American situation it is probably comparable to the Dutch situation. As to the cost-effectiveness of the current study, cost reduction is expected to be even greater since the course is considerably briefer and a lot less labour intensive than the one described in the study by Turk and Burwinkle (37).

It can be concluded that a cognitive group intervention is a much promising treatment for patients with chronic pain complaints. Based on the current research the intervention has proved to effect positive changes in catastrophizing and locus of control at relatively low costs. Further controlled study however is needed.

Acknowledgments

An earlier version of this study has been published in Dutch (De Boer MJ, Versteegen GJ. Een cognitief gedragsmatige groepsinterventie voor pijnpatiënten: eerste bevindingen. Gedragstherapie 2006; 39(3):157-69).

References

[1] Hasenbring M, Hallner D, Klasen B. Psychological mechanisms in the transition from acute to chronic pain. Schmerz 2001;15(6):442-7.
[2] Van Houdenhove B, Neerinckx E. Is "ergomania" a predisposing factor to chronic pain and fatigue? Psychosomatics 1999;40(6):529-30.
[3] Vlaeyen JW, Morley S. Active despite pain: the putative role of stop-rules and current mood. Pain 2004;110(3):512-6.
[4] Buer N, Linton SJ. Fear-avoidance beliefs and catastrophizing: occurrence and risk factor in back pain and ADL in the general population. Pain 2002;99(3):485-91.
[5] Sullivan MJ, Thorn B, Haythornthwaite JA, Keefe F, Martin M, Bradley LA, et al. Theoretical perspectives on the relation between catastrophizing and pain. Clin J Pain 2001;17(1):52-64.
[6] Edwards RR, Bingham CO, III, Bathon J, Haythornthwaite JA. Catastrophizing and pain in arthritis, fibromyalgia, and other rheumatic diseases. Arthritis Rheum 2006;55(2):325-32.
[7] Keefe FJ, Caldwell DS, Martinez S, Nunley J, Beckham J, Williams DA. Analyzing pain in rheumatoid arthritis patients. Pain coping strategies in patients who have had knee replacement surgery. Pain 1991;46(2):153-60.
[8] Jensen MP, Turner JA, Romano JM, Karoly P. Coping with chronic pain: a critical review of the literature. Pain 1991;47(3):249-83.
[9] Turk DC. Cognitive-behavioral approach to the treatment of chronic pain patients. Reg Anesth Pain Med 2003;28(6):573-9.

[10] Turner JA, Jensen MP, Romano JM. Do beliefs, coping, and catastrophizing independently predict functioning in patients with chronic pain? Pain 2000;85(1-2):115-25.
[11] Nash JM, Park ER, Walker BB, Gordon N, Nicholson RA. Cognitive-behavioral group treatment for disabling headache. Pain Med 2004;5(2):178-86.
[12] Johnson PR, Thorn BE. Cognitive behavioral treatment of chronic headache: group versus individual treatment format. Headache 1989;29(6):358-65.
[13] Nielson WR, Weir R. Biopsychosocial approaches to the treatment of chronic pain. Clin J Pain 2001;17(Suppl 4):S114-S127.
[14] Cole J. Psychotherapy with the chronic pain patient using coping skills development: Outcome study. J Occupat Health Psychol 1998;3(3):217-26.
[15] LeFort S, Gray-Donald K, Rowat K, Jeans M. Randomized controlled trial of a community-based psychoeducation program for the self-management of chronic pain. Pain 1998;74(2):297-306.
[16] Flik CE, Van Der Kloot WA, Koers H. Can a pain-control course help patients to fixate less on physical pain and become more aware of their psychological and emotional problems? Tijdschrift Psychiatrie 2005;47(2):63-73.
[17] Leibing E, Pfingsten M, Bartmann U, Rueger U, Schuessler G. Cognitive-behavioral treatment in unselected rheumatoid arthritis outpatients. Clin J Pain 1999;15(1):58-66.
[18] Barlow J, Turner AP, Wright CC. Sharing, caring and learning to take control: Self-management training for people with arthritis. Psychol Health Med 1998;3(4):387-93.
[19] Merlijn VP, Hunfeld JA, van der Wouden JC, Hazebroek-Kampschreur AA, Suijlekom-Smit LW, Koes BW, et al. A cognitive-behavioural program for adolescents with chronic pain-a pilot study. Patient Educ Couns 2005;59(2):126-34.
[20] Ersek M, Turner JA, McCurry SM, Gibbons L, Kraybill BM. Efficacy of a self-management group intervention for elderly persons with chronic pain. Clin J Pain 2003;19(3):156-67.
[21] Turner-Stokes L, Erkeller-Yuksel F, Miles A, Pincus T, Shipley M, Pearce S. Outpatient cognitive behavioral pain management programs: a randomized comparison of a group-based multidisciplinary versus an individual therapy model. Arch Phys Med Rehabil 2003;84(6):781-8.
[22] International Association for the Study of Pain. Classification of chronic pain. Pain 1986;(Suppl 3):S1-S226.
[23] Groenman NH, Rober IM, Reitsma B, Tuymelaar Koldenhof CTH, Lousberg R. Patients with chronic benign pain: further psychometric research with the SCL-90. NVBPijnbulletin 1993;13:9-12.
[24] Reitsma B, Meijler WJ. Pain and patienthood. Clin J Pain 1997;13:9-21.
[25] De Gier M, Vlaeyen JW, Van Breukelen G, Stomp SGM, Ter Kuile M, Kole-Snijders AM. Pain coping and cognition list. Validation and norms. Maastricht: Pain Manage Res Center, Univ Hosp Maastricht, 2004.
[26] Vlaeyen JW, Kole-Snijders AM, Boeren RG, Van Eek H. Fear of movement/(re)injury in chronic low back pain and its relation to behavioral performance. Pain 1995;62(3):363-72.
[27] Kori SH, Miller RP, Todd DD. Kinisophobia: a new view of chronic pain behavior. Pain Manag 1990;5(1):35-43.
[28] Goubert L, Crombez G, Vlaeyen J, Van Damme S, Van den Broeck A, Van Houdenhove B. The Tampa Scale for Kinesiophobia: psychometric chracteristics and norms. Gedrag und Gezondheid: Tijdschrift Psychol Gezondheid 2000;28(2):54-62.
[29] Peters ML, Vlaeyen JW, Köke AJA, Patijn J. Measurements of chronic pain. Pain-related fear and catastrophizing. Maastricht: Pain Manage Res Center, Univ Hosp Maastricht, 2004.
[30] De Boer MJ. Treatment protocol 'Learning to live with pain in a relaxed way'. Groningen: Pain Expertise Center, Univ Med Center Groningen, 2004.
[31] Bouman TK. A community based psychoeducational group approach to hypochondriasis. Psychother Psychosom 2002;71:326-32.

[32] Prochaska JO, DiClemente CC. Stages of change in the modification of problem behaviors. Prog Behav Modif 1992;28:183-218.

[33] Linton SJ, Ryberg M. A cognitive-behavioral group intervention as prevention for persistent neck and back pain in a non-patient population: a randomized controlled trial. Pain 2001;90(1-2):83-90.

[34] Buhrman M, Faltenhag S, Strom L, Andersson G. Controlled trial of Internet-based treatment with telephone support for chronic back pain. Pain 2004;111(3):368-77.

[35] Devineni T, Blanchard EB. A randomized controlled trial of an internet-based treatment for chronic headache. Behav Res Ther 2005;43(3):277-92.

[36] Strom L, Pettersson R, Andersson G. A controlled trial of self-help treatment of recurrent headache conducted via the Internet. J Consult Clin Psychol 2000;68(4):722-7.

[37] Turk D, Burwinkle T. Clinical outcomes, cost-effectiveness, and the role of psychology in treatments for chronic pain sufferers. Prof Psychol Res Pr 2005;36(6):602-10.

In: Pain Management Yearbook 2009
Editor: Joav Merrick

ISBN: 978-1-61209-666-7
©2012 Nova Science Publishers, Inc.

Chapter 19

CHRONIC PAIN IN INJURED WORKERS

Policarpo Rebolledo, MD[*1], *Alonso Mújica, MD*[2],
Luis Guzmán, MD[3], *Verónica Herrera, MD*[4]
and Ricardo Acuña, LLB[5]

[1]Department of Mental Health, [2]Department of Rehabilitation and [3]Department of Orthopedics, Hospital del Trabajador de Santiago, [4]Department of Health and [5]Legal Department, Asociación Chilena de Seguridad, Santiago, Chile

Abstract

Chronic pain is a frequent sequelae in patients, who have suffered a work-related injury. The aim of the present investigation was to assess the frequency of chronic pain in different kinds of injuries suffered by patients with a work-related accident and assessed by a Medical Disability Evaluation Committee once treatment had concluded. 614 patients were evaluated during 2007. Clinical records were reviewed and final outcome assessed by a thorough physical examination. Demographic data, diagnosis and sequelae were registered. Classical statistical measures were used for data analysis. In the total sample, 543 patients were male (88%), average age 43.6 years (range 17-82). 276 patients were blue collar workers (44.9%), 228 patients suffered chronic pain (37,1% of the sample). Demographic data of patients in pain were similar to the total sample. Depending on the type of injury, chronic pain appeared more frequently in different kinds of fractures, head injuries, burns and low back pain post lumbar surgery. It is important to note that from 202 fractures, 97 (48%) remained in chronic pain and from 78 head injuries, 36 (46.2%) remained with post traumatic headache. From 22 burns, 12 (54.5%) continued in pain. Chronic pain is a frequent sequelae in patients after a work injury. Depending on the type of injury, some patients experience more chronic pain than others. This fact should be taken into account in order to take appropriate actions and corresponding medical measures.

Keywords: Chronic pain, injured worker, incidence, disability.

---

* **Correspondence:** Policarpo Rebolledo, MD, Department of Mental Health, Hospital del Trabajador de Santiago, Vicuña Mackenna 200, 3rd floor, Santiago, Chile. Tel: +56(2) 6853723; Fax: +56(2) 2441670; E-mail: prebolledo@achs.cl or policarpo@vtr.net

Introduction

Work related injuries can inflict direct and indirect losses to workers, their families, employers, health system and society, as well as to their quality of life (1-5). Asociación Chilena de Seguridad (ACHS) is a private, non-profit organization, which administers compensation insurance, based upon Chilean Law 16.744 concerned with work accidents and occupational diseases. ACHS is a mutual insurance company that provides for workers and insured companies the following benefits: comprehensive occupational risk prevention, medical care, compensations and pensions. Its goal is to promote healthy habits, behaviors and improve quality of life for all workers of affiliated companies. The accidents suffered while going home from work or vice versa are covered as well (in-itinere accidents).

When a worker suffers a work-related accident, this institution provides complete free medical care which includes: diagnostic examination, hospitalization, surgery, all needed drugs, transportation services, rehabilitation, prothesis/orthesis and economic benefits until return to work is possible (6). If the patient losses part of his/her productivity capacity, because of any sequelaes, e.g. amputees, spinal cord injuries, head injury and others, he/she receives a one time economic or a pension until legal retirement age, depending on their disability degree.

Besides physical or mental impairments, injured workers can also present with chronic pain as a sequeale. According to the International Association for the Study of Pain (IASP) pain can be defined as an unpleasant sensory and emotional experience associated with actual or potential tissue damage, or described in term of such damage. There is no universal agreed definition of chronic pain. Our definition was based on the International Association for the Study of Pain's definition (7). When patients experience chronic pain, it often causes difficulties to return to work, because it alters the global functioning and health status of workers (8).

Since chronic pain is a frequent sequelae in patients who have suffered a work-related accident (9), the aim of this investigation was to assess the frequency of chronic pain in different patients, who had a work-related accident and assessed by a Medical Disability Evaluation Committee once treatment has concluded.

Methods

This is a descriptive study. The study consisted of 614 patients who were evaluated during 2007 by a Medical Disability Evaluation Committee once treatment was concluded to determine their level of disability. When the treatment was concluded, patients were examined by a physiatrist and an occupational therapist to assess their capacity and loss of work productivity in their job according to their status before the accident. Then, they were seen by the Medical Disability Evaluation Committee, which determined the final loss of work productivity in terms of percentage of function loss.

The Medical Disability Evaluation Committee is a group of physicians (physiatrist, orthopedic surgeon, occupational physician and psychiatrist) and a lawyer who helps with legal issues. Clinical records of these patients were reviewed and the final outcome assessed by a thorough medical interview and physical examination. Demographic data, diagnosis, sequelae and level of disability were registered.

The information was described by absolute and relative frequencies for categorical variables; for those continuous variables mean, median, standard deviation and limits are presented. For the analysis of association chi-square was used for qualitative variables and Wilcoxon test for independent samples for quantitative variables. All tests were conducted in the program SAS JMP 5.1.

Results

The Hospital del Trabajador de Santiago provides medical attention to persons who suffer a work-related accident. During 2007, 103,417 patients were admitted for work-related accidents (11). These patients have different kinds of injuries with different levels of severity. When the treatment is finished, some of them present with sequelaes, which need to be evaluated by the Medical Disability Evaluation Committee in order to provide for their legal economic compensation. Demographic data of the total sample is shown in table 1. In the total sample, 543 patients were men (88,6%) and 71 were women (11,4%), average age is 43.6 years (range 17-82). 407 patients (66,2%) were blue collar workers.

Table 1. Demographic data (N=614)

	Men	Women	Total
Gender	543 (88,4%)	71 (11,6%)	614 (100%)
Average Age	31,5 (17-82)	44.0 (22-62)	43,6 (17-82)
Occupation:			
Professional	5 (0,9%)	7 (9,8%)	12 (1,9%)
Technician	29 (5,3%)	5 (7.0%)	34 (5.5%)
Service Sector	15 (2,7%)	3 (4,2%)	18 (2,9%)
Administrative	125 (23,0%)	18 (25,3%)	143 (23,2%)
Blue collar skilled worker	125 (23,0%)	6 (8,4%)	131 (21,3%)
Blue collar unskilled worker	244 (44.0%)	32 (45.0%)	276 (44,9%)

From these 614 patients evaluated during 2007 by the Medical Disability Evaluation Committee, 228 presented with chronic pain among other sequelae. Table 2 shows demographic data of 228 patients who suffered from chronic pain at the time of their evaluation and physical examination. This number represents 37.1% of the total sample.

By comparing the group with chronic pain with those without, we observed significant differences related to age and gender: chronic pain appeared more frequently in women and older patients (see tables 2A and 2B). There was no observed significant differences related to occupational level (see table 2C). Chronic pain appeared more frequently in the following injuries: Fractures, traumatic brain injury, herniated lumbar disc, amputations and burns (see table 3, figure 1).

Table 2. Demographic data for patients in chronic pain (N=228)

	Men	Women	Total
Gender	190 (83,1%)	38 (16,8%)	228 (100%)
Average Age	56 (17-82)	44.0 (22-62)	45.9 (17-82)
Occupation:			
Professional	1 (1,0%)	4 (10,5%)	5 (2,6%)
Technician	12 (6,3%)	3 (7.8%)	15 (6,6%)
Service Sector	7 (37%)	2 (5,2%)	9 (3,9%)
Administrative	40 (21,2%)	12 (31,5%)	52 (23,0%)
Blue collar skilled worker	44 (23,4%)	3 (7,8%)	47 (20,7%)
Blue collar unskilled worker	86 (44.1%)	14 (36,8%)	100 (42,9%)

Figure 2 shows the location of pain caused by fractures according to body segment. In this study, chronic pain was more frequent in lower limbs and includes feet, ankle, knee, shin, calf and thighs. Figure 3 compares total number of injuries with patients with chronic pain. It is important to notice that out of 202 fractures in the total sample, 97 (48.%) remained in chronic pain. From 78 head injuries of the total sample, 36 (46.2%) remained with post traumatic headache and from 22 burns, 12 (54.5%) continued in pain.

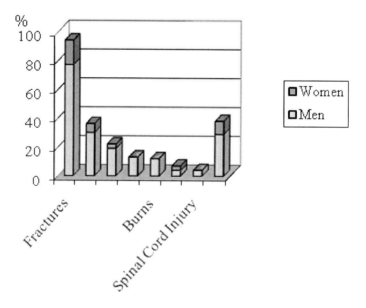

Figure 1. Primary injury. Patients with chronic pain (N=228).

Discussion

In this study, the sample represented all patients with sequelaes after having suffered a work-related accident and treated in Hospital del Trabajador de Santiago during 2007 (10). Asociación Chilena de Seguridad (ACHS) is an institution with national presence and there are other patients treated in other health centers, which are not included in this study. It is relevant to notice that one third of the 103,417 patients, who requested assistance because of a work related accident, presented minor injuries, which did not require lost working days (11). We observed that chronic pain was a frequent sequelae in patients after a work injury. Biological, psychological and social changes after a work related accident may be experienced differently by the two genders and in this study, older patients and females ppeared more frequently with chronic pain, findings coincident with international medical literature (12,13).

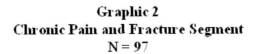

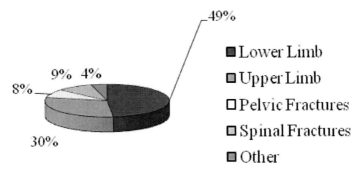

Figure 2. Chronic pain and fracture segment (N=97).

Table 2A. Demographic Data. Patients with chronic pain and age (N=228)

	Without Pain Group	Pain Group	Total
N	386	228	614
Mean	42,3	45,9	43,6
SD	13,1	11,3	12,6
Median	41,0	47,0	44,0
Limits	17 - 82	21 - 79	17 - 82

p value: 0,002.

Table 2B. Demographic data. Patients with chronic pain and gender (N=228)

	Without Pain Group		Pain Group		Total	
	N	%	n	%	n	%
Men	353	91,5	190	83,3	543	88,4
Women	33	8,5	38	16,7	71	11,6
Total	386	100	228	100	614	100

p value : 0,002.

Table 2C. Demographic data. Patients with chronic pain and occupational level (N=228)

	Without Pain Group		Pain Group		Total	
	n	%	n	%	n	%
Professional	7	1,8	5	2,2	12	2,0
Technician	19	4,9	15	6,6	34	5,5
Service Sector	9	2,3	9	3,9	18	2,9
Administrative	91	23,6	52	22,8	143	23,3
Blue collar skilled Worker	84	21,8	47	20,6	131	21,3
Blue collar unskilled Worker	176	45,6	100	43,9	276	45,0
Total	386	100	228	100	614	100

p value : 0,804.

Table 3. Primary injury. Patients in chronic pain (N=228)

Primary Injury	Men	Women	Total	%
Fractures	80	17	97	42,5
Traumatic Brain Injury	29	6	35	15,4
Herniated Lumbar Disc	19	3	22	9,6
Amputations	13	0	13	5,7
Burns	12	0	12	5,3
Sprains	4	3	7	3,1
Spinal Cord Injury	4	0	4	1,8
Others	29	9	38	16,7
TOTAL	190	38	228	100,0

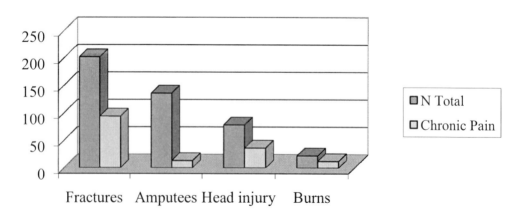

Figure 3. Type of injury and chronic pain (N = 614).

Depending on the type of injury, some patients experienced chronic pain longer than others and in our study, nearly half of the patients with fractures in different segments of the body presented chronic pain, especially in lower limbs.

Workers who have suffered traumatic brain injuries, remained with post traumatic headache as a sequelae. In case of patients with herniated lumbar disc, they experienced chronic pain even after undergoing laminectomy. Patients with any type of amputation can present pain in the amputation trunnion, pain that is due to neuroma or phantom pain.

In our opinion, chronic pain has a high incidence as a sequelae in patients who have suffered a work-related accident. This fact should be taken into account, especially by different medical teams (14) in order to take appropriate actions and corresponding medical measures not only after treatment, but also in the early stages of it.

References

[1] Concha-Barrientos M, Nelson DI, Fingerhut M, Driscoll T, Leigh J. The global burden due to occupational injury. Am J Ind Med 2005;48(6):470-81.
[2] Nelson DI, Concha-Barrientos M, Driscoll T, Steenland K, Fingerhut M, et al. The global burden of selected occupational diseases and injury risks: Methodology and summary.. Am J Ind Med 2005;48(6):400-18.
[3] McGovern P, Kochevar L, Lohman W, Zaidman B, Gerberich SG, et al. The cost of work-related physical assaults in Minnesota. Health Serv Res 2000;35(3):663-86.
[4] Waehrer G, Leigh JP, Cassady D, Miller TR Costs of occupational injury and illness across states. J Occup Environ Med 2004;46(10):1084-95.
[5] Schulte PA. Characterizing the burden of occupational injury and disease. J Occup Environ Med 2005:47(6):607-22.
[6] Asociación Chilena de Seguridad. Normas legales sobre accidentes del trabajo y enfermedades profesionales. Santiago de Chile, ACHS, 2002. 245 p.
[7] Merskey H, Bogduk N. Taxonomy of chronic pain. Seattle, WA: IASP Press, 1994.
[8] Xu YW, Chan CC, Lam CS, Li-Tsang CW, Lo-Hui KY, Gatchel RJ. Rehabilitation of injured workers with chronic pain: a stage of change phenomenon. J Occup Rehabil 2007;17(4):727-42.
[9] Correa G. Dolor crónico y trauma músculo esquelético: discapacidad e impacto económico. Rev. Iberoamericana del Dolor, 2007 N° 4: 9-16.
[10] Statistics of rehabilitation. Santiago: Rehabilitation Department, HTS, 2007.
[11] General statistics summary. Santiago: Occupational Safety Health Department, ACHS, 2006.
[12] LeResche L. Epidemiologic perspectives on sex differences in pain. In: Fillingim R, ed. Sex, gender and pain. Seattle, WA: IASP Press, 2000:233-49.
[13] Farrell MJ, Gibson SJ Psychosocial aspects on pain in older people. In: Dworkin RH, Breitbart WS, eds. Psychosocial aspects on pain. Seattle, WA: IASP Press, 2004:495-518.
[14] Turner J, Franklin G, Turk D. Predictors of chronic disability in injured worker: A systematic literature synthesis. Am J Ind Med 2000;38:707-32.

Chapter 20

INVASIVE PAIN MANAGEMENT PROCEDURES: HIGH EXPECTATIONS LEAD TO PERCEIVED POOR OUTCOMES

Carol Campbell[*], BSc (Hons), MAEd, PhD
College of Arts and Sciences, Zayed University, Abu Dhabi, United Arab Emirates

Abstract

Despite the recent shift toward rehabilitative pain management for people who live with and experience chronic pain, minor invasive treatments with local anaesthetic combinations continue to be indicated and performed for both diagnostic and therapeutic purposes. Method: An opportunity sample of 46 patients undergoing invasive procedures for chronic pain management participated. Participants were asked pre-injection to describe the site and duration of pain; provide a current pain rating; state whether they had experienced any previous injection therapy; how much pain relief they expected to experience; and whether they expected any long-term effect from the injection. Four weeks after the injection the participants were contacted by telephone and asked to rate their current pain; state whether the injection met their expectations; how long the effect of the injection had lasted and whether they expected to have the injection repeated. Results: Significant difference between mean number of days of expected pain relief and the actual length of time that the injection was perceived as efficacious (F=4.1502; df (12,33) p<0.001). Significant difference between the expected amount pain relief and actual pain ratings post-injection (F=20.8513 df(1,44) p<0.001). Conclusion: Expectations were unrealistic insofar as they expected significant pain relief post-injection and expected relief to last for considerable time despite the fact that the injections were diagnostic purposes only. Receiving an injection fosters the desire for repeat injections, which may promote patient dependence on health care system. Perceived poor outcomes may be fuelled by pre-injection high expectations and may be counter-productive to current pain management strategies.

Keywords: Invasive pain management; patient expectations; pre- and post-quasi-experimental design.

---

[*] **Correspondence:** Carol Campbell BSc (Hons), MAEd, PhD, College of Arts and Sciences, Zayed University, PO Box 4783, Abu Dhabi, United Arab Emirates. Tel: 00 9712 4079761; Fax: 00 9712 4434847; E-mail: carol.campbell@zu.ac.ae

Introduction

Why one injury completely resolves without residual pain or functional impairment and another produces chronic pain or long-term disability is not at all clear (1) and poses a great challenge to the whole of the health care system. Compared with acute pain, chronic pain is complex and multi-factorial in nature and the growing number of individuals who suffer from chronic pain together with the resultant disability experienced, bears witness to the limitations of medical management of these patients (2). The dominant biomedical model is not always appropriate for managing chronic illness because it implies that through a process of investigation, a diagnosis will be made and the problem resolved with appropriate medical treatment. However, most individuals with chronic pain have usually spent a great deal of time in the traditional medical system yet little clinical improvement is noted. Despite this, many people maintain their attachment to the medical system which they believe will eventually provide a 'magic bullet' and their search for cure (provided by physicians) continues (3).

In recognition of the above limitations, treatment for individuals with a chronic pain problem has shifted emphasis in the recent past toward more rehabilitative treatments that aim towards behaviour change and related coping (4). Nevertheless, for some patients (e.g. those with low back pain and sympathetically maintained pain) minor invasive treatments with local anaesthetic combinations continue to be indicated for both diagnostic and therapeutic purposes. Local and regional analgesia, achieved by injecting a local anesthetic into tissues, or in proximity to certain parts of the peripheral nervous system to relieve pain has been used for nearly a century (5). A large body of literature supports the efficacy of invasive injection interventions for diagnostic purposes and the relief of pain (6-9).

Irrespective of whether patients undergo conventional or rehabilitative treatments their beliefs and expectations about chronic pain have been shown to be critical cognitive facilitators or impediments to the recovery process. DeGood and Kiernon (10) suggested that these specific cognitions influence responses to and subsequent outcomes of treatment. Expectations emerge repeatedly as having a fundamental role in expressions of satisfaction; indeed it has been suggested (11) that patient expectations are the key to understanding the reason for expressed dissatisfaction with delivered care. Therefore, meeting patient expectations or changing unrealistic expectations should assist in achieving patient satisfaction with all types of treatment undertaken. Mayou and Sharpe (12) proposed that there is often a mismatch between the expressed hopes and unrealistically high expectations of a patient and the care the physicians can offer and this demonstrates a shortfall in the provision of effective psychological and social interventions. Examining chronic pain, expectations and invasive pain relieving procedures, Galer et al (13) specifically explored the relationships between patient and physician pre-treatment expectations of pain relief and subsequent pain relief reported by chronic pain patients immediately after treatment. They proposed that physicians were better predictors than patients to the likely responses following pain-relieving procedures, and/or that physicians somehow communicate their expectations to the patients during the procedure, and the expectations ultimately influence patient response. They concluded that patient pre-treatment expectations may not always play a significant role in non-specific treatment effects.

Since medical treatment for chronic pain is not invariably followed by clinical improvement, exploration of current practice to ensure that delivered treatment has a positive outcome is crucial. As the research studies cited above in relation to patient expectations indicate, assessment of outcomes must include not only physiological effects of medical interventions but also patient-perceived health outcomes. Outcomes are regarded as the most important aspect of the evaluation of quality of care (14); this is not simply a measure of health, well-being, or any other state, rather it is a change in a patient's current and future health status that can be confidently attributed to antecedent care. Pickering (15) also suggested that to assess quality care properly, we should maintain a patient-centered approach and ask, "Did the patient benefit from medical intervention, did they not, or were they made worse?" (p.380).

However, the studies discussed earlier concerning the efficacy of invasive pain-relieving procedures did not include information about patient outcome so were unable to consider whether the injections were perceived by patients as being beneficial. Furthermore by omitting post-intervention perceptions of pain relief the studies fail to consider whether pre-procedural expectations were actually realized. Instead, the focus tends to be on the technical success of the procedure, whether pain was relieved and, if so, for how long. While the resulting pain relief may be welcomed by many patients, through limiting the research criteria to largely physiological outcomes the impact of the psychosocial context of the treatment process may be underestimated. For example, it has been suggested that in those patients who derive secondary or tertiary gains (e.g. relief from financial responsibilities, being excused from interpersonal functions) (2), the realization that the pain could be permanently eliminated may be alarming. Other studies suggest that invasive therapies may create patient dependence on physicians and related medical interventions and should therefore be used judiciously (16, 17), other researchers propose that they are ineffective in terms of pain relief (18, 19) and Steal et al (20) suggested that there is limited evidence to support the use of injection therapy for sub-acute and chronic low back pain.

The research literature exploring the perceived efficacy of invasive procedures therefore demonstrates variable results in terms of physiological outcomes. In relation to assessment outcomes it has neglected to elicit the patient-perspective which, it has been argued, is central to a comprehensive understanding of quality of care. Furthermore, while the exploration of patient expectations has been investigated, such data is of little value without the critical post-intervention perception data to compare it with.

To develop a more comprehensive assessment of patient outcome additional factors are worthy of consideration. Firstly, there needs to be some consideration of the potential that diversity across both patient expectations and outcomes is mediated by psychological processes. Secondly, in anesthesia or pharmacological treatment of pain in male and female patients, there are no absolute differential drug use recommendations (21). This stems from the predominant paternalistic policy to exclude women from clinical drug trials due to the fear of teratogenic effects (22). Therefore, female patients may inadvertently be receiving too little or too much of a drug because little attention is paid to the woman's hormone cycle and the effect this may have on their metabolism and resultant efficacy of some treatments. Ciccone and Holdcroft (21) suggested that sex-specific effects should be considered to enable changes in the type or dose of the drug to be made. Whether local anaesthetic preparations are affected the same way is unknown.

In order to address the disparities within the literature, this study aimed to ascertain whether patients attending one pain clinic in the North East of England for minor invasive interventions for chronic pain perceived a reduction in pain relief thereafter. One additional aim was to explore whether there were any patient perceived benefits from the interventions. The study therefore explored the following three research questions:

- How are pre-procedure expectations of treatment efficacy rated and are the expectations realised post-injection?
- What, if any, is the expected duration of pain relief and is this realised post-injection?
- Are sex differences evident in any of the dependent variables measured?

Methods

A pre- and post-quasi experimental research design was employed. An opportunity sample of 46 consecutive patients undergoing an invasive injection procedure for chronic non-malignant pain at one pain clinic in the North East of England gave informed consent to participate in the study. There were 21 male and 25 female participants. Ages ranged from 29 – 86 years of age, the median age was 51.5 years. The majority (n=30, 65.2%) of the invasive procedures were undertaken for diagnostic purposes.

Following ethical approval from the local National Research Ethics review board and host university ethics committee patients attending the Surgical Day Unit (SDU) were approached by the researcher in the waiting area of the SDU and asked to participate in the study. A study information leaflet was provided explaining the procedure for participation. Informed consent was obtained and documented from those patients willing to participate. Each participant was then asked to describe the site and duration of their pain; to provide a rating of their pain using a Visual Analogue Scale (VAS); whether they had undergone any previous invasive pain-relieving procedure; how much pain relief, if any, that they expected from the injection, scored using a VAS; how long they expected any relief to last (in days); and whether they held any expectations as to the long term outcomes following the procedure (e.g. did they expect the procedure to cure their pain).

Four weeks after the injection was performed all of the participants were contacted by telephone and asked to rate their current pain using a VAS; whether the injection had lived up to their expectations via a simple yes or no response; how long the effect of the injection had lasted; and whether they expected to have the injection repeated. Participants were then provided with a study debrief.

Analysis

Analysis of variance (ANOVA) was used to explore the differences between expectations and perceptions of pain relief, pain scores pre- and post- procedure, and gender. Pearson Product-Moment Correlation Coefficients were also calculated. In all cases $p<0.05$ was considered significant.

Results

Descriptive statistics showed that local injections were performed most frequently and this was generally for pain originating in the back. More injections were performed on female patients when the pain site was to the back (n=16) and the lower leg (n=8), whereas injections to sites of the upper limb, neck and torso were solely performed on male patients. These data are shown in table 1.

Previous injection treatment had been given to 28 patients (60.9%). At the follow-up period, 20 participants expected to have the injection repeated, 10 did not and 16 were undecided. Of the 20 individuals (43.5%) who expected to have the injection repeated, 4 rated their pain unchanged, five rated their pain higher and 11 rated their pain as improved. As indicated in table 2 those individuals with prior experience of injection treatment were more likely to expect further injections.

At the four week follow up, 16 participants rated their pain higher, 10 rated their pain unchanged and 20 rated their pain as lower. Fourteen participants stated that they continued to experience pain relief. As shown in table 3, of those 16 individuals who rated their pain as higher, 14 felt that their expectations were not met, with 3 expecting the injection to be repeated. Of the 10 individuals who rated their pain the same, eight stated their expectations were not met and three expected to have a repeat injection. Overall, from the total sample, 20 participants felt that the injection lived up to their expectations. Of these, half had undergone previous injection treatment and eight expected the injection to be repeated.

Female participants had experienced pain longer (mean= 89 months) than the male participants (mean= 77 months). The mean number of days of expected relief following the injection were 290 for males and 297 for females. Male participants perceived the injection to have been effective for a mean number of 10 days whereas female participants perceived this to be longer with a mean of 15 days. Additionally more female participants expected to have the injection repeated (n=13) compared with only seven male participants.

The first inferential analyses were concerned with exploring the perceived efficacy of the invasive procedure, and whether patient expectations were realised. Mean VAS scores were calculated as pre-injection 7, and post-injection 6. In terms of exploring expectations and outcome perception a significant difference was found between the expected amount of pain relief and the actual pain ratings post injection (F=20.8513 df(1,44) $p<0.001$). A significant difference was also observed between how long the patients expected the effect of the injection to last for (mean =293 days) and the actual length of time (mean =13 days) that the injection was perceived as efficacious (F=4.1502; df (12,33) $p<0.001$).

Further analyses investigated whether the injection had lived up to individual expectations and how long the effect of the injection had lasted. A significant difference was observed (F=170.737 df (1,44) $p<0.001$). Patient expectations prior to the injection were rooted in the belief that they would experience a substantial reduction in pain from the injection and a prolonged period of pain relief thereafter, however, both of these expected outcomes were not realised.

A significant negative association was also found between individuals who had undergone previous injection treatment and whether there was an expectation that the injection would be repeated r = -0.376 (p <0.01).

Table 1. Distribution of male/female patients by treatment type and treatment site

Treatment	Back M	Back F	Lower limb M F	Upper limb M F	Neck M	Neck F	Torso M	Torso F
Local	7	12	1	6	2	1	2	
Neurolytic	3	1	3	2	1			
Thermo-coagulation	1	3						
Total	11	16	4	8	3	1	2	

Table 2. Numbers of patients who had received previous injections and the numbers who expected injection to be repeated

Previous Injections	Do you expect to have injection repeated?		
	Yes	No	Don't Know
Yes	13	1	4
No	7	9	12
Total	20	10	16

Table 3. Distribution of responses in relation to expectations and pain perception

	Pain higher	Pain same	Pain lower	Total
Expectations met	2	2	16	20
Expectations not met	14	8	4	26
Expect repeat injection	3	3	14	20

Discussion

This study has offered important insights relating to the assessment of outcome efficacy from a patient-centred perspective in relation to invasive pain management procedures. It particularly highlights the need to consider perceptions, both prior to and following the intervention, to gain a meaningful account of patient evaluations, the latter assessment having been absent from the literature to date. The results outlined above suggest that patients' expectations of invasive pain-relieving treatments for chronic non-malignant pain are unrealistic, insofar as patients were expecting significant pain relief, and for pain relief to last for a great deal longer, than was actually realised. This finding coupled with the fact that over half of the patients in the study reported no reduction in their pain, or worse pain, may indicate that patients were dissatisfied with the treatment despite the majority of the procedures being undertaken for diagnostic purposes. However, a substantial number of patients, and significantly those patients who had previously undergone an invasive procedure expected to have the injection repeated which may indicate their endorsement of the procedure. The association between previous injection treatment and the expectation of repeated treatment appears to support previous research findings (16,17) that showed injection treatments and invasive interventions promoted patient dependence. The potential for patient dependence to be created through the provision of injection treatments appears to be evident as expectations of treatment efficacy were unrealistically high, despite injection outcome being perceived as particularly disappointing. The dependency claim is also consistent with the view that patients remain entrenched within the biomedical model through which, despite outcomes to the contrary, they believe physical interventions will provide a cure.

The 26 individuals who perceived no difference to their pain, or that their pain was worse, four weeks following injection treatment raise cause for concern. The duration of pain relief stated by those patients who reported an efficacious effect was also particularly low. When these poor physical outcome assessments are coupled with low patient-perspective evaluations (where only 20 patients felt the injection lived up to their expectations) the overall quality of care cannot be judged to be satisfactory. For no benefit to be noted by these patients suggests that greater detailed investigation (or pre-procedural) information relating to the injection procedure and possible outcomes should be provided. For example, if injections are to be performed as a diagnostic measure in an attempt to ascertain the type and nature of the pain and, therefore, pain relief is not necessarily to be expected, this should be communicated cogently to the patient to bring pre-procedure expectations in line with probable outcomes. If, however, the injection is to be performed for therapeutic purposes, a realistic range of outcomes should be promoted prior to the procedure, to prevent expectations being unwittingly heightened. The need for clear, practical and relevant information would enable greater patient involvement in treatment decisions and may forestall the cycle of dependency as mentioned above. Changing the provision of relevant and appropriate patient information demands a 'de-medicalising' of symptoms and likely outcomes in recognition that chronic pain is multifactorial in nature (19).

The outcomes observed in this study differ from those reported elsewhere (13). Other researchers have suggested that non-specific (placebo) treatment effects may be responsible for enhanced active treatment effects; that the perspective of the physician may predict pain relief; or that the doctor-patient relationship may influence patient responses to treatment. The fact that the majority of patients did not experience any pain reduction following treatment in this study counters the non-specific and physician perspective claims. Furthermore, the research evidence discussing doctor-patient relationships (23) and the tendency of patients to play down poor outcomes when talking with doctors appears to be overlooked as an explanation in the Galer et al paper (13). However, in the study reported here, patients were in the comfort of their own home talking over the telephone and not face to face with their doctor when describing the perceived outcomes of the procedure. It may have been that once the balance of power was restored to the patient, they felt more able to give an accurate account of their outcome.

One other area to consider in the interpretation of these findings is that of anxiety about treatment. Although participants were fully briefed about the procedural aspects of injections, they may not have been psychologically prepared for the discomfort experienced both during and after the therapeutic procedure. While anxiety was not systematically investigated through this study, medical staff involved in this procedure commonly observe that patients report anxiety prior to the administration of these injections. Similar findings have been reported by others (24,25). Maier and Watkins (26) have also documented the relationship between increased anxiety and heightened pain perception. The lack of perceived efficacy in relation to injection treatment demonstrated by high pain ratings post injection in this study could well imply that the procedure itself is disempowering to patients.

Although statistically significant differences were not found in relation to gender, several interesting trends did emerge. Female participants had experienced chronic pain for longer than their male counterparts; they also expected the effect of the injection to last longer; but nevertheless did perceive greater pain relief from the invasive treatments than the male participants. These findings may provide some support for Ciccone and Holdcroft (21), who argued that gender differences must be considered in the design of treatments. However, before firm conclusions can be drawn on this matter further investigation is required.

In conclusion, this study raises questions about the outcome efficacy of injection treatments and about previous research designs that have neglected to consider pre and post intervention perceptions and patient-centred assessments. On measures of outcome efficacy, invasive interventions were not judged to be beneficial by patients. Furthermore, given the costs associated with administering this procedure and the discomfort experienced by patients the effectiveness of this intervention as a treatment strategy is also compromised. Nevertheless, if current practice is to continue, the disparities between patient expectations and reported outcomes indicate that more attention needs to be devoted to the psychological preparation of patients. The findings lead to concurrence with other researchers (11,12) that tackling patient expectations are key to this process. Patients begin their treatment holding unrealistically high expectations in relation to both the amount of pain relief and the duration of this relief. Furthermore, post-intervention, they also expect the treatment to be repeated. If expectations are not modified this is likely to mean that patients will remain 'trapped' within the medical system, both searching for a cure and yet continuing to be dissatisfied with their treatment.

References

[1] Chaplin ER. Chronic pain: A sociobiological problem. Phys Med Rehabil 1991;5(1):1-47.
[2] Potter RG. The prevention of chronic pain. In: Carter B, ed. Perspectives on pain: Mapping the territory. London: Arnold, 1998.
[3] McCracken LM. Learning to live with the pain: acceptance of pain predicts adjustment in persons with chronic pain. Pain 1998;74(1): 21-7.
[4] Main CJ, Parker H. Pain management programmes. In: Roland M, Jenner J, eds. Back pain: New approaches to rehabilitation and education. Manchester, UK: Manchester Univ Press, 1989.
[5] Bonica JJ, Butler SH. Local anaesthesia and regional blocks. In: Wall PD, Melzack R, eds. Textbook of pain, 3rd ed. New York: Churchill Livingstone, 1994.
[6] Boas RA. Sympathetic nerve blocks: In search of a role. Reg Anesth Pain Med 1998;23(3):292–305.
[7] Bowman SJ, Wedderburn L, Whaley A, et al. Outcome assessment after epidural corticosteroid injection for low back pain and sciatica. Spine 1993;18(10):1345-50.
[8] Davies HTO, Crombie IK, Macrae WA. Back pain in the pain clinic: nature and management. Pain Clinic 1995;8(2):191-9.
[9] Fischer HBJ. Peripheral nerve blockade in the treatment of pain. Pain Rev1998;5:183-202.
[10] DeGood DE, Kiernon B. Perception of fault in patients with chronic pain. Pain 1996;64:153-9.
[11] Williams B. Patient satisfaction: a valid concept? Soc Sci Med 1994;38:509-19.
[12] Mayou R, Sharpe M. Diagnosis, illness and disease. Quart J Med 1995;88(11):827-31.

[13] Galer BS, Shwartz L, Turner JA. Do patient and physician expectations predict response to pain-relieving procedures? Clin J Pain 1997;13(4):348-51.
[14] Donabedian A. The definition of quality and approaches to its mangement, volume 1: Explorations in quality assessment and monitoring. Ann Arbor, MI: Health Adm Press, 1980.
[15] Pickering WG. Does medical treatment mean patient benefit? Lancet 1996;347:379-80.
[16] Russo CM, Brose WG. Chronic pain. Ann Rev Med 1998;49:123-33.
[17] Milligan KA, Atkinson RE. The "two week syndrome" associated with injection treatment for chronic pain--fact or fiction? Pain 1991;44(2):165-6.
[18] Chaplin ER. Chronic pain: A sociobiological problem. Rehabilitation of chronic pain. State Art Review 1991;5(1):1-47.
[19] Kouyanou K, Pither CE, Wessely S. Iatrogenic factors and chronic pain. Psychosom Med 1997;59(6):597-604.
[20] Staal JB, de Bie R, de Vet HC, Hildebrandt J, Nelemans P. Injection therapy for subacute and chronic low back pain. Cochrane Database Syst Rev 2008;3:CD001824.
[21] Ciccone GK, Holdcroft A. Drugs and sex differences: a review of drugs relating to anaesthesia. Br J Anaesthesia 1999;82:255-65.
[22] Holdcroft A. Females and their variability. Anaesthesia 1997;52: 931-4.
[23] Hall JA, Roter DL, Katz NR. Meta-analysis of correlates of provider behavior in medical encounters. Med Care 1998;26(7):657-75.
[24] Anderson KO, Masur FT. Psychological preparation for invasive medical and dental procedures. J Behav Med 1993;6(1):1-40.
[25] King NJ, Murphy GC. Contributions from health psychology: preparing patients for aversive medical procedures. NZ Nurs J 1993;76(2):9-11.
[26] Maier SF, Watkins LR. Stressor controllability, anxiety and serotonin. Cogn Ther Res 1998;22:595-613.

In: Pain Management Yearbook 2009
Editor: Joav Merrick

ISBN: 978-1-61209-666-7
©2012 Nova Science Publishers, Inc.

Chapter 21

CHILDREN'S DRAWINGS OF PAIN FACES: A COMPARISON OF TWO CULTURES

Jacqueline A Ellis RN, PhD[*1], *Eufemia Jacob, RN, PhD*[2] *and Bryan Maycock, MA*[3]

[1]School of Nursing, University of Ottawa, Ottawa, Ontario, Canada, [2]UCLA School of Nursing, Los Angeles, California, United States and [3]Foundation Studies, NSCAD University, Halifax, Nova Scotia, Canada

Abstract

Young children that experience difficulty using number scales to rate pain intensity are often able to use faces scales. Controversy exists over whether the validity of a faces scale is affected by the expressions on the faces, especially in the anchor positions. The aim of this study was to understand how children from two cultural groups draw faces portraying pain. Study group: Thirty-nine Chinese and 46 Inuit children from 5 to 13 years of age participated in the study. Methods: In face-to-face interviews children were asked to draw a face that represented the amount of hurt indicated by each of the six pain descriptors in the Wong- Baker FACES pain assessment scale. Results: The shape of the mouth was the feature that most clearly distinguished the different levels of pain. The 'no hurt' face was almost exclusively drawn with a smile in the Inuit children's drawings (96%) and in the Chinese children's drawings it was divided between a smile (59%) and an O-shaped mouth (21%). As pain increased, children drew a straight-line mouth and then a frowning mouth. The presence of tears was also a distinguishing feature associated with increasing levels of pain. In addition, a small number of Chinese children (13%) drew sweat from the forehead to indicate severe pain. Conclusion: Similar to the Wong Baker FACES scale, smiles, frowns, and tears emerged from our data as the defining features of pain faces. The cultural variations were interesting and congruent with much of the developmental literature on how children draw and how culture influences children's drawings.

Keywords: Pain faces, children's pain drawings, cross cultural pain drawings.

---

* **Correspondence:** Jacqueline A Ellis, RN, PhD, School of Nursing, University of Ottawa, 451 Smyth Road, Ottawa, ON, Canada K1H 8M5. Tel: 613 562 5800 x 8440; Fax: 613 562 5443; E-mail: jellis@uottawa.ca

Introduction

Pain is a purely subjective phenomenon that can only be communicated through verbal or behavioral mechanisms. The "gold standard" for measuring pain is an individual's self report. (1) Measurements of pain represent a blend of the strength of the pain and the person's emotional response to it. (1) Typically, sensory and intensity dimensions of pain are assessed by asking the individual to choose words that describe their pain experience and to quantify the intensity with numbers, line length, color, or pictures.(2) Pain measurement in children is complicated by their limited use and understanding of pain-related language and, for young children, their inability to understand the concept of order, which is essential for numerical rating scales.(3) Despite these limitations a number of pain scales have been developed over the past two decades that can be used by children to describe pain intensity.

The Wong-Baker FACES scale (4) has been used successfully with young children from a number of cultural groups and has been translated into a number of languages. (5) The scale was developed in 1988 with the help of school-aged children that were asked to draw faces that portrayed increasing pain levels. (4) A professional artist captured the commonalities in the drawings and developed the cartoon facial scale that is illustrated in figure 1.

The scale has undergone psychometric testing with a number of cultural groups including three Asian groups (Chinese, Japanese, and Thai). (5) As part of that psychometric study, Chinese children were asked to complete a pain drawing task using the same methods that were used in the original scale development study. The Wong-Baker FACES scale was adapted for use with Inuktitut speaking individuals in Alaska and the Baffin region of the Canadian arctic. (6,7) The FACES Scale was redesigned to fit a northern context, and as part of a study to establish the psychometrics of the revised scale, the Inuit children completed the same pain drawing task as the Chinese children mentioned above. The two sets of drawings were analyzed and compared as part of a cross-cultural examination of children's pain drawings.

The aim of this study was to understand how children from two cultural groups draw faces portraying pain. More specifically, it was to determine the extent to which features such as the eyebrows, eyes, mouth and nose may be varied to depict levels of pain. A second aim was to determine if the faces depict increasing levels of pain consistent with the Wong-Baker FACES scale descriptors of 'no hurt' to 'hurts worst'.

McGrath (2) suggests a pain measure should be reliable in that it provides consistent scores for the same pain, regardless of the child's age, sex, or cognitive level. It must also be bias free, and provide the same information irrespective of who administers the measure, and it must be versatile and practical for use in a variety of medical, dental and home settings. Children, starting at about 3-4 years of age, can use simple pictures or object scales to rank order painful events and describe clinical pain with some degree of consistency. (8) Younger children tend to use the anchors of the scale more reliably then the middle range indicators and tend to rate a pain experience as more intense than older children. (9-11) Children over five years of age are generally able to use numerical rating scales reliably to describe pain intensity. (12)

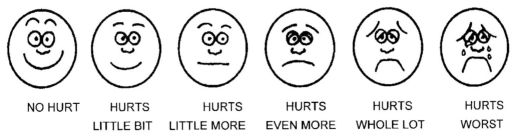

Wong-Baker FACES Pain Rating Scale from Hockenberry MJ, Wilson D: Wong's Nursing Care of Infants and Children, ed 8, St. Louis, p.1876. Used with permission. ©Elsevier/Mosby

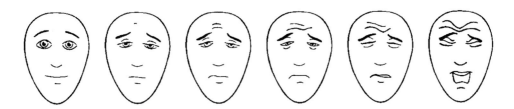

Faces Pain Scale-Revised International Association for the Study of Pain (IASP) © 2001

Figure 1. Wong-Baker FACES Scale and the Faces Pain Scale-Revised.

Young children that experience difficulty using number scales to rate pain intensity are often able to use faces scales to describe their pain. (13) Faces scales typically consist of a series of line drawings or photographs of facial expressions that depict increasing amounts of pain. The child is asked to match their pain experience with that depicted in the facial expression of the scale faces. For the purposes of scoring, each face is numbered. Controversy exists over whether the validity of a faces scale is affected by the expressions on the faces in the anchor positions. (14) For example, a smiling face at the 'no hurt' position and a frowning face with tears at the 'hurts worst' position are the anchors for the Wong-Baker FACES scale. (4) In the Faces scale developed by Bieri and colleagues (15,16) the faces are drawn with a straight-line mouth at the 'no pain' position and an open mouth and no tears at the 'most pain' anchor. See figure 1.

Chambers and Craig (9) examined the impact of a smiling or neutral anchor and concluded that pain ratings vary according to the affective tone of the anchors and a smiling-face as the 'no pain' anchor is associated with higher pain ratings. They suggest that smiles and tears at the anchor positions confounds pain and affect. Wong and Baker, (14) argue that there is no evidence indicating that the straight line mouth in the Faces (15,16) scale is actually perceived by children as neutral and is not confounded with negative affect. The Faces scale (15,16) and the Wong-Baker FACES scale (4) were developed from actual drawings produced by children and both scales have good reliability and validity and are highly correlated with each other (17,18).

Methods

Design. A descriptive design with face-to-face interviews was used to collect data. Both the Chinese Pain Drawing Task and the Inuit Pain Drawing Task were part of larger studies to determine the psychometrics of pain scales. Prior to data collection ethical approval for the study protocol was obtained from the ethical review board at the University of Ottawa and the Nunavut Research Institute.

The study took place in Pangnirtung, Nunavut and Tianjin, China. Pangnirtung is located in the Canadian arctic on the east side of Baffin Island. Tianjin is located in northern China on the Pacific coast. Chinese and Inuit children from 5 to 13 years of age participated in the study. The Chinese children were recruited from the pediatric ward of a general hospital in Tianjin, China. The Inuit children were recruited from the primary school in Pangnirtung, Nunavut.

Appropriate consent was obtained from the parents and assent from the children prior to data collection. The procedures for the Tianjin data collection varied slightly from the Pangnirtung procedures and both will be described. The Inuit children were given an 11 x 17 inch piece of white paper with six empty circles arranged horizontally and spaced equidistant to each other. Pain descriptors from the Wong-Baker FACES scale were translated into Inuktitut and placed beneath the appropriate circle. The Chinese children were given a blank 8 by 11 inch piece of white paper and were shown the descriptors for the Wong-Baker FACES scale which were translated into Mandarin. The descriptors were read to the children and available for them to refer to as they were drawing but they were not on the same page as the drawings.

Since no standardized instructions existed for eliciting children's pain drawings, a composite of instructions reported by Wong and Baker (4) and Bieri et al. were used (15). To avoid the problem of confounding positive or negative emotions with the pain faces, only pain information was presented and descriptions referring to the child in pain as happy or sad were avoided.

Each group of the six faces drawn by the children was evaluated by three research personnel. Coding schemes were created specifically for the study based on the features that were present in the drawings. The codes were assigned when 100% consensus was reached by the three research personnel on the following features of the faces: 1) eyebrow presence and shape; 2) eye shape, position, and presence or absence of tears and 3) shape of the mouth. Each set of 6 faces was also evaluated to determine whether there was a change in the features indicative of increasing levels of pain.

Results

Forty-six Inuit children, 5 to 13 years (mean age 11.1 ± 2.1 years), and 39 Chinese children, 5 to 12 years (mean age 8.2 ± 2.7 years), participated in the study. One Inuk child completed only one of the six faces and was deleted from the analyses. Tables 1 and 2 summarize the most frequent features that were included in the two sets of drawings for each of the six faces.

Children's drawings of pain faces: A comparison of two cultures   229

Table 1. A summary of facial features in Inuit children's pain drawings.

FACES

	0	1	2	3	4	5
Eyebrows						
No Eyebrows	54.3%	51.1%	51.1%	57.8%	53.3%	55.6%
Arched	34.8%	33.3%	34.4%	30.0%	32.2%	30.0%
Eyebrows Other	11%	15.6%	14.5%	12.2%	14.5%	14.4%
Eye Shape						
Round	43.5%	42.2%	42.2%	44.4%	40.0%	37.8%
Almond	32.6%	31.1%	31.1%	31.1%	31.1%	33.3%
Dot	19.6%	22.2%	22.2%	20.0%	24.4%	22.2%
Eye Position						
Open	95.7%	95.6%	95.6%	95.6%	95.6%	93.3%
Closed	4.3%	4.4%	4.4%	4.4%	4.4%	6.7%
Tears						
Present	0	0	6.7%	20.0%	33.3%	55.6%
Nose						
Present	69.6%	71.1%	71.1%	71.1%	71.1%	68.9%
Mouth Shape						
Downward	0%	26.7%	55.6%	82.2%	80.0%	91.1%
Straight Line	4.3%	37.8%	40.0%	13.3%	15.6%	4.4%
Upward	95.7%	33.3%	4.4%	2.2%	2.2%	4.4%

Table 2. A summary of facial features in Chinese children's pain drawings

FACES

	0	1	2	3	4	5
Eyebrows						
No Eyebrows	15.0%	7.7%	10.3%	12.8%	15.4%	15.4%
Arched Downward	67.7%	43.6%	33.3%	23.1%	30.8%	30.8%
Curved Upward	0%	7.7%	10.3%	5.1%	15.4%	10.3%
Straight Line	12.8%	25.6%	23.1%	28.2%	12.8%	9%
Slanted Downward	2.8%	15.4%	23%	30.8%	25.6%	34.5%
Eye Shape						
Round	23.1%	20.5%	23.1%	17.9%	17.9%	15.4%
Almond	38.5%	48.7%	41.0%	46.2%	35.9%	35.9%
Dots	6.1%	5.1%	10.3%	7.7%	7.7%	7.7%
Slit line	30.8%	25.6%	25.6%	28.2%	38.5%	41.1%
Eye Position						
Open	66.7%	74.4%	76.9%	71.8%	64.1%	59.0%
Closed	30.8%	25.6%	23.1%	28.2%	35.9%	41.0%
Tears						
Present	0%	0%	2.6%	7.7%	23.1%	59.0%
Nose						
Present	87.2%	87.2%	84.6%	87.2%	87.2%	87.2%
Mouth Shape						
Downward	4.6%	15.4%	25.6%	30.8%	30.8%	30.8%
Straight Line	13.8%	59.0%	41.0%	7.7%	7.7%	7.7%
Upward	59.0%	12.8%	5.1%	30.8%	30.8%	5.1%
O-Shaped	20.5%	12.8%	28.2%	30.8%	30.8%	56.4%

Distinguishing features. The shape of the mouth was a feature that most clearly distinguished the different levels of pain. The 'no hurt' face (face 0) was almost exclusively drawn with a smile in the Inuit children's drawings (96%) and in the Chinese children's drawings it was divided between a smile (59%) and an open or O-shaped mouth (21%). As pain levels increased, children drew a straight-line mouth and then a more downward-curved or frowning mouth. The straight-line mouth was present in face 1 (38%) and face 2 (44%) of the Inuit children's drawings, and in face 1 (59%) and face 2 (41%) of the Chinese children's drawings. In faces 3 to 5, some variation of a frown predominated in both sets of drawings. The anchor face with the descriptor 'hurts worst' (face 5) was portrayed with a frown in 91% of the Inuit children's drawings and 31% of the Chinese children's drawings. Chinese children tended to favor an O-shaped mouth to portray the most severe pain (56%). See figure 2 for examples of mouth shapes.

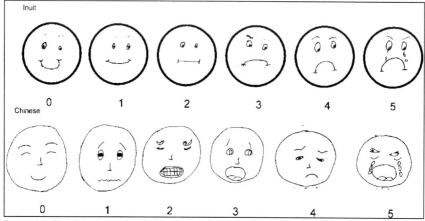

Figure 2. Example of smiles, frowns and O-shaped mouth.

The presence of tears was also a distinguishing feature that was associated with increasing levels of pain. In addition, a small number of Chinese children (13%) drew sweat from the forehead to indicate severe pain. In 56% of the Inuit drawings and in 59% of the Chinese drawings tears were present in face 5 to indicate 'hurts worst'. Figure 2 shows examples of tears and figure 3 shows examples of sweat droplets to indicate increasing pain.

Cultural variations. There were many commonalities among the two sets of drawings and a few differences with respect to the shapes used to define the features. For example the eye shapes in the Inuit children's drawings varied among round, almond-shaped or dot, which was similar to the Chinese children's drawings with the addition of a line by the Chinese children to represent the eye. Approximately 26 to 41 % of the eyes in the Chinese faces were drawn with a horizontal line. The mouth was also a feature that showed variation by culture. The three mouth shapes common to both sets of drawings were a line that was drawn with an upward, horizontal or downward orientation. In addition, a portion of the Chinese faces were drawn with a round or O-shaped mouth that was consistent across the six faces. This shape was not seen in any of the Inuit children's drawings. Generally, the amount and type of detail varied in the Inuit and Chinese drawings, and as we examined the drawings from the perspective of 'general impressions', differences emerged. The Chinese children typically drew more detailed and complex faces with a range of eye shapes, ears, hairstyles and even hats. It was interesting to note that there were 15 sets of faces drawn by 5 to 6 year old children and all the drawings had a similar cartoon style and features (see figure 4). The Inuit children were consistent in drawing facial features relatively simplistically and only a few of the drawings had details like hair or eyelashes.

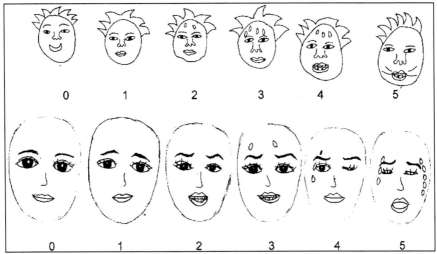

Figure 3. Example of sweat droplets in Chinese children's drawings to portray increasing pain.

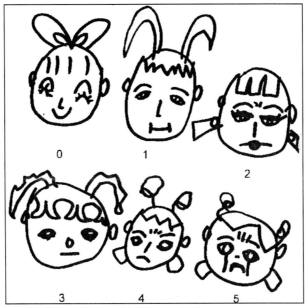

Figure 4. Example of cartoon schema, 6 years old Chinese child.

Gradation. We were interested in comparing sequentially among the six faces to determine the extent that the children varied the facial features to portray increasing pain intensity. The majority of drawings from both cultures consistently showed evidence of increasing levels of pain over the six faces (Inuit drawings = 78% and Chinese drawings = 77%).

Discussion

In this study we replicated the drawing task that children completed during the initial phase of the development of the Wong-Baker FACES scale. The FACES scale is the first pain scale to be based on children's representational drawings of pain faces. Ours is the first study to examine cultural variations in children's drawings of pain faces. As we undertook to interpret the two sets of drawings it became increasingly evident that the literature about children's art would provide a reasonable context to understand the drawings.

See figure 5 for examples of gradation. However, in 22 to 23 % of the drawings, there was no consistent pattern or change in facial features that suggested increasing pain severity.

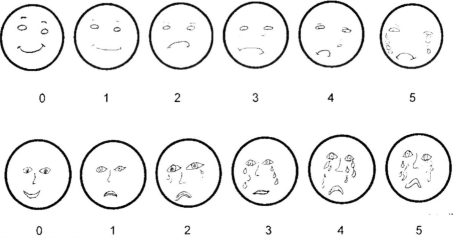

Figure 5. Inuit children's drawings portraying increasing pain levels.

There are a number of authors that have examined children's drawings from a developmental and a cultural perspective. Kellogg (19) has collected and analyzed thousands of preschool children's drawings over a thirty-year time span. She has developed a typology of scribbles that characterize children's developmental progression related to drawing. Around the age of three years, children combine basic scribbles that include lines, arcs, circles and rectangles to form what Kellogg describes as an 'aggregate face' (p.95). She pays particular attention to the 'Mandala', which is the Sanskrit word for circle, and how this shape is used to define the face as a simple, usually round object. This face is refined and becomes more representational as the child develops both physically and cognitively (19). The shapes of the mouths in the drawings depicted by Kellogg in her collection (p.109) are similar to the drawings by the Chinese and Inuit children. Arcs, lines and circles predominate and these are the mouth shapes that the children in our study varied to express changing pain levels.

Cox (20) suggested that children draw objects from an internal model which contains central or defining characteristics or facts about the object. When drawing the 'canonical view' of the object it is portrayed in such a way as to be clearly recognizable (p. 90). The aim of the artist is to depict the most important and typical characteristics so the drawing clearly represents what it is intended to be. Freeman (21) suggested that children attach great importance to these defining features. For example: a picture of a lion must have a mane and a tiger must have stripes (21). In our study, the task that we set for the children was to draw faces that clearly portrayed varying pain levels. In essence, we asked them to draw the 'canonical view' of a pain face. The defining features of the scale anchors in both the Chinese and Inuit drawings replicated the smile, frown, and tears in the Wong-Baker FACES scale. Virtually all of the Inuit children and greater than half of the Chinese children depicted the 'no hurt' face with a smile, and greater than half of both sets of drawings depicted tears and a frown in the 'most hurt' face. In addition, the Chinese and Inuit children varied theses features to clearly depict increasing levels of pain in the six faces. The data from our study supports the construct validity of the Wong-Baker FACES scale in that the features portrayed in the scale are consistent with the child's view of a pain face. This is important given that the scale was initially developed 'by children, for children'.

The notion of the 'canonical view' of an object or picture may explain, in part, why children, when asked their preference for pain faces, most frequently choose the Wong Baker FACES scale instead of a scale with a more realistic face such as the scale developed by Bieri and colleagues (i.e. Faces scale) (15-18). The Wong-Baker scale features the Mandala shape in the round head, is clearly cartoon-like, with drawings that are simple and direct. The viewer immediately understands its purpose. In the Faces scale, (15,16) the head is somewhat 'unfamiliar' for, while the oval shape alludes to a more sophisticated and therefore more realistic representation, placement of the features is not in proportion to a normal head. The addition of ears and hair would remedy this. But, perhaps the result would be too complex for this purpose: in effect, too realistic. And repositioning the features without the addition of ears and hair would result in an even more alien image where empathy with the face experiencing pain may be even less likely.

Images that appear to attempt reality but fall short, usually for reasons of accuracy, are less 'satisfying' than images that are clearly abstract or clearly real. The Faces scale (15,16) is not clearly a cartoon image or a realistic image of a face. It seems to straddle both 'camps' and this may add to the viewers discomfort with the images. An example of the struggle to produce a drawing that 'looks right' is observed with novice drawing students, who often see the world one piece at a time and without much subtlety. As they gain experience, more detail is seen in their drawings but still in relative isolation of each part to the whole. It is only when the subtlety of the particular is read and reproduced within the whole that the drawing 'looks right'. Eisner suggests that teaching in the arts is very much concerned with helping students learn how to see the interactions among the qualities constituting the whole. (22)

A criticism of the smile, frown and tears in the Wong Baker FACES scale is that these features potentially confound pain and emotion (9,14). The argument is that the child might not choose the 'no hurt' smiling face if he/she did not feel happy or the 'most hurt' tearful face if he/she did not feel sad. To prevent linking pain and emotion, words such as 'happy' or 'sad' were avoided when providing instruction to the children about the drawing task. Our data supports the view that a pain face, for young children, includes smiles, frowns, and tears.

Interestingly, children are able to accurately use both the realistic and the cartoon scale to rate pain intensity and the two scales are highly correlated ($r = 0.91$) (17,18). However, when asked to choose their preference, the children seem most comfortable with the faces that clearly and unambiguously, albeit from their perspective, depict pain. There has been limited research asking children to describe what they like or dislike about a pain scale; and when asked young children have a limited range of vocabulary to describe their preferences. In a previous study, we asked children why they liked the Wong-Baker scale and the answers were simple statements. "Because its fun". "It's a cartoon face."

There were characteristics of the Chinese children's drawings that were consistent with the descriptions of a number of authors that examined cultural differences related to how children draw. Cox (20) suggests that "even average children in China reach a very high level of drawing ability and do so at a remarkably early age" (p.183). Winner (23) observed children in a classroom in China and described the importance placed on drawing and calligraphy. Children were exposed to a uniform art curriculum and perfected basic drawing skills at a relatively young age. Allande (24) examined how children draw and use color in a cross-cultural field study among six cultural groups of children. He described the Chinese children's drawings as detailed, dense with markings and polychromatic. This is in contrast, for example, to children from Ponape, an island in Micronesia, These children's drawings tended to be monochromatic and sparsely constructed with substantial unfilled space on the page (24).

Consistent with the cross-cultural research presented above, we noted that the Chinese children in our study tended to draw richly detailed faces that included a variety of hairstyles, hats, ear shapes and characteristics that suggested the gender of the face. There was rich variation among the sets of drawings and sometimes even among the six faces in a single drawing.

Some of the drawings stylistically represented a real face and others were clearly a cartoon image. The similarities among the drawings of the 5 to 6 year old children were striking. They were all cartoon images and many had similar round eyes with large pupils and large round ears. The children were likely exposed to a cartoon schema through television, books, or art instruction in school that included drawing cartoon characters.

The Inuit children's drawings, generally, were less detailed than the Chinese drawings with less variation in the features and less sophistication. The O-shaped mouth that was common in the Chinese drawings was not used at all in the Inuit drawings. The presence of sweat was unique to a small subset of the Chinese drawings.

Conclusions

Children from both cultures were skilled at varying facial features to clearly depict increasing pain intensity over the six faces. Similar to the Wong Baker FACES scale, smiles, frowns, and tears emerged from our data as the defining features of pain faces for these children. The cultural variations were interesting and congruent with much of the developmental literature on how children draw and how culture influences artistic expression.

Acknowledgments

We would like to thank Tanya Gaffney for her help with the data analysis. This research was supported by the Canadian Institute of Health Research, Institute of Aboriginal People's Health and ACADRE-CIET.

References

[1] McDowell I, Newell C. Measuring health A guide to rating scales and questionnaires. New York: Oxford Univ Press, 1987.
[2] McGrath PA. Pain in children nature assessment and treatment. New York: Guilford Press, 1990.
[3] Beyer JE, Knapp TR. Methodological issues in the measurement of children's pain. Children's Health Care 1986;14(4):233-41.
[4] Wong DL, Baker CM. Pain in children: Comparison of assessment scales. Pediatr Nurs 1988;14(1):9-17.
[5] Wong D, DeVito-Thomas P. Multicultural study of FACES pain rating scale. 2003, Unpublished manuscript.
[6] DeCourtney C A, Jones K, Merriman M P, Heavener N, Branch K P. Establishing a culturally sensitive palliative care program in rural Alaska Native American communities. J Palliat Med 2003:6(3):501-11.
[7] Ellis J, Ootoova A, Blouin R, Rowley B, Taylor M, DeCourtney C, Joyce M, Greenley W. Establishing the psychometric properties and preferences for the Northern Pain Scale 2007, Unpublished manuscript.
[8] Lehman H P, Bendebba M, DeAngelis C. The consistency of young children's assessment of remembered painful events. J Dev Behav Pediatrics 1990;11:128-34.
[9] Chambers CT, Craig KD. An intrusive impact of anchors in children's faces pain scales. Pain 1998;78:27-37.
[10] Chambers CT, Johnston C. Developmental differences in children's use of rating scales. J Pediatr Psychol 2002;27(1):27-36.
[11] Goodenough B, Kampel L, Champion GD, Laubreaux L, Nicholas MK, Zeigler JB, McInerney M. An investigation of the placebo effect and age-related factors in the report of needle pain from venapuncture in children. Pain 1997;72:383-91.
[12] McGrath PA. An assessment of children's pain: a review of behavioral, physiological and direct scaling techniques. Pain 1987; 31:147-76.
[13] Kuttner L, LePage T. Faces scales for the assessment of pediatric pain: a critical review. Can J Behav Sci 1989;21:198-209.
[14] Wong DL, Baker CM. Smiling face as anchor for pain intensity scales. Pain 2001;89(2-3):295-7.
[15] Bieri D, Reeve RA, Champion GD, Addicoat L, Ziegler JB. The faces pain scale for the self-assessment of the severity of pain experienced by children: development, initial validation, and preliminary investigation for ratio scale properties. Pain 1990;41: 139-50.
[16] Hicks CL, von Baeyer CL, Spafford P, van Korlaar I, Goodenough B. The Faces Pain Scale - Revised: Toward a common metric in pediatric pain measurement. Pain 2001;93:173-83.
[17] Chambers CT, Giesbrecht K, Craig K, Bennett S M, Huntsman E. A comparison of faces scales for the measurement of pediatric pain: children's and parents' ratings Pain1999;83:25-35.
[18] Chambers CT, Hardial J, Craig KD, Court C, Montgomery C. Faces scales for the measurement of postoperative pain intensity in children following minor surgery. Clin J Pain 2005;21(3):277-85.
[19] Kellogg R. Analyzing children's art. California: Mayfield Publ, 1970.
[20] Cox M. Children's drawings. London: Penguin Books 1992.
[21] Freeman NH. Process and product in children's drawing. Percept 1972;1:123-40.
[22] Eisner EW. The arts and the creation of mind. New Haven: Yale Univ Press, 2002.
[23] Winner E. How can Chinese children draw so well? J Aesthetic Educ 1989;22:41-63.
[24] Alland A.xPlaying with form children draw in six cultures. New York: Columbia Univ Press, 1983.

In: Pain Management Yearbook 2009
Editor: Joav Merrick

ISBN: 978-1-61209-666-7
©2012 Nova Science Publishers, Inc.

Chapter 22

CATASTROPHIZING WAYS OF COPING AND PAIN BELIEFS IN RELATION TO PAIN INTENSITY AND PAIN-RELATED DISABILITY

Christina Knussen[*]*, PhD and Joanna L McParland, PhD*
Division of Psychology, Glasgow Caledonian University, Glasgow, United Kingdom

Abstract

While catastrophizing has been found to be related to self-reported pain intensity and disability, there is debate as to its theoretical meaning or role. The main aim of this analysis was to consider the roles of catastrophizing, ways of coping (from the Coping Strategies Questionnaire), and pain beliefs (from the Survey of Pain Attitudes) in the context of the Lazarus model of stress. Pain intensity (from the Chronic Pain Grade) was identified as the potential source of stress, and two variables were identified as indicative of the outcome of the stress process: pain-related disability (Roland-Morris Disability Scale) and psychological distress (GHQ), each residualized for the other. This was a secondary analysis of an existing cross-sectional database. The sample consisted of 95 members of support groups for people with chronic pain in Central Scotland, 86 of whom were female. Ages ranged from 43 to 93 years (M = 66 years). Measures were taken from self-report questionnaires. Catastrophizing was found to moderate, but not mediate, the Pain Intensity-Disability relationship, such that the relationship was no longer significant when catastrophizing scores were high. The relationships between catastrophizing, pain intensity and pain-related disability remained significant when psychological distress was controlled for. It was concluded that catastrophizing was conceptually distinct from distress. The results were to some extent consistent with a construction of catastrophizing as secondary appraisal. Further research at the within-person level is required to fully understand the transactional roles of catastrophizing, beliefs and ways of coping in the stress process over time.

Keywords: Chronic pain, catastrophizing, coping, pain beliefs, stress.

---

[*]**Correspondence:** Christina Knussen, Division of Psychology, Glasgow Caledonian University, 70 Cowcaddens Road, Glasgow, G4 0BA, United Kingdom. Tel: +44 (0) 141 331 3497; Fax: +44 (0) 141 331 3636; E-ail: c.knussen@gcal.ac.uk

Introduction

The construct of catastrophizing has been an enduring focus of interest in pain research in recent years (1,2). In part, the degree of interest is due to the finding that those who tend to catastrophize also tend to report more symptoms of pain and disability (1); however, interest has also been fuelled by the debate concerning the definition or meaning of catastrophizing, and its position within various theoretical perspectives (1-3). The aim of this paper, based on a secondary analysis of an existing cross-sectional database (4), is to contribute to this debate by considering the nature of the relationships among catastrophizing, ways of coping, and pain beliefs, in the context of the model of stress and coping described by Lazarus and colleagues (5,6). In this analysis, pain intensity was identified as the potential source of stress, and two variables were identified as indicative of the outcome of the stress process: pain-related disability and psychological distress.

Elements common to most definitions of catastrophizing include the feeling of helplessness in the face of pain, a negative evaluation of one's own ability to cope with the pain, negative appraisal or magnification of the symptoms of pain, and rumination (1-3). As noted above, greater use of catastrophizing has been found to be significantly associated with poorer outcome, both physical and psychological (1,7). Catastrophizing has also been found to be related to such factors as neuroticism, negative affectivity, anxiety, and depression (3), to the extent that questions relating to the redundancy of the construct of catastrophizing have been raised (1-3). However, there is evidence to suggest that catastrophizing is related to measures of pain when measures of depression are controlled for (1,8). Although in the current analysis pain intensity was identified as the potential source of stress rather than as an outcome variable, this point was addressed by examining the relationship between pain intensity and catastrophizing when psychological distress had been controlled for, and also by controlling for psychological distress when examining the relationship between catastrophizing and pain-related disability.

It could be argued that the relationship between catastrophizing and outcome is more important than the exact meaning of the construct at a theoretical level (9), and the various theoretical frameworks that could explain the meaning clearly overlap (1). However, when data analysis is guided by theory, the position of a construct with regard to other elements of the model becomes relevant. Catastrophizing had originally been construed as a way of coping (10), and may serve a coping function by eliciting supportive or solicitous responses from others (1). However, Lawson et al (11), through confirmatory factor analysis of the Coping Strategies Questionnaire (CSQ; 10), concluded that catastrophizing was distinct from all but one of the other CSQ coping scales (the other exception being increasing behavioural activity). Recent constructions of catastrophizing tend to centre on belief or appraisal (12,13), in line with the Lazarus model of stress and coping (5,6). Briefly, this model centres on three processes: primary appraisal, or the extent to which a potential source of stress (such as pain) is seen as harmful, threatening or a loss; secondary appraisal, during which the individual considers his or her options for dealing with the source of stress; and coping, or the cognitive and behavioural strategies used to address the source of stress, irrespective of the success or failure of those strategies. The deployment of coping strategies is dependent upon the way in which the potential source of stress is appraised, the options perceived to be open to the individual, and the available coping resources. Coping resources can be broadly categorized as follows (6): material, or the resources associated with finances, employment and socioeconomic status; physical, such as health, strength, fitness and mobility; psychological, including values, beliefs, attitudes, and personality; and social, or sources of practical and emotional social support. Beliefs about pain, a focus of the current analysis, would therefore be conceptualized as indicators of psychological resources. Both forms of appraisal, particularly secondary appraisal, are likely to be influenced by such coping resources.

Within this model, catastrophizing could function as an aspect of secondary appraisal (that the pain is overwhelming and little or nothing can be done), or as a psychological coping resource (a belief, cognition or stable aspect of personality that influences the choice of coping strategies). If it is to be considered as an aspect of secondary appraisal, then one would expect relationships between catastrophizing and outcome measures to be at least partly mediated or explained by coping resources (in this case, beliefs about pain) and ways of coping: for example, appraising the pain as beyond control could trigger the belief that further activity would cause damage, and inactivity as a way of coping. In addition, it would be reasonable to assume that catastrophizing could moderate the relationship between pain intensity (the potential source of stress) and outcome, in line with recent findings noted by Wolff et al (8): the impact of pain intensity on outcome could interact with the appraisal that the pain is too intense to be borne or is beyond control. However, this moderating role might also be expected if catastrophizing were to be construed as a coping resource (that is, as a relatively stable belief or cognition), as would mediation of the relationship between catastrophizing and outcome by ways of coping. For example, the belief that pain is overwhelming could lead to ignoring the pain as a way of coping, such that the strategy rather than the belief influences outcome.

A problem arises when considering the extent to which beliefs and ways of coping might mediate relationships between pain intensity and outcome, or ways of coping mediate relationships between beliefs and outcome. While a number of authors have noted significant relationships between various beliefs and ways of coping (12), there is evidence to suggest that the relationships between beliefs and outcome are not significantly mediated by ways of coping (1,2,13). While such findings might appear to challenge the utility of the Lazarus model in the field of chronic pain, alternative explanations are worthy of consideration. First, it is possible that certain beliefs are associated with stable individual differences, such as negative affectivity or neuroticism; if this were the case, we would not expect the relationship between a belief and psychological outcome to be mediated by ways of coping. This argument is also relevant to the consideration of the role of catastrophizing (1,3), and was addressed in the current analysis by controlling for psychological distress in the analysis of disability (physical outcome) through residualization: this approach was taken to help clarify the extent to which the relationship between catastrophizing and pain-related disability was influenced by distress. Second, it is notoriously difficult to measure ways of coping with complete accuracy, particularly retrospectively (14). In particular, summed scores on self-report retrospective measures of coping may mask the potential influence of proportional use of coping strategies. For example, the outcome of coping by ignoring the pain may vary according to whether or not the individual is also coping through activity. Relative or proportional scores on coping subscales (the proportion of total endorsements of strategies falling within each subscale) not only take account of individual differences in the extent to which items are endorsed (15), but may also give an indication of the pattern of coping responses used (14). This scoring technique was adopted in the current analysis.

With relatively few exceptions, most studies of the psychological aspects of chronic pain have used clinical samples to the exclusion of community samples (7). The current sample was drawn from community support groups for those experiencing pain, and the study therefore provided the opportunity to explore beliefs and ways of coping in the community context. In summary, two outcome measures were identified for the current analysis: the General Health Questionnaire (GHQ-28; 16), and the Roland-Morris Disability Scale (17); each was residualized for the other prior to analysis. The main aim of the analysis was to explore the potential role of catastrophizing within the model of stress and coping (i.e., as secondary appraisal and/or as a psychological coping resource), while the second aim was to explore the relationships of pain beliefs and ways of coping with the outcome variables. Specifically, the analysis focused on whether catastrophizing would mediate or moderate any relationship between pain intensity and outcome (disability and distress); and whether beliefs and ways of coping would mediate or moderate any relationship between catastrophizing and outcome.

Methods

The design of the study was cross-sectional. Initially, all four of the national chronic pain organizations with support group representation in the Central Scotland region were approached to ask if they would be willing to co-operate with recruitment, and two (for people with arthritis and fibromyalgia) agreed. These two organizations hosted 15 support groups in the region: four for people with fibromyalgia and 11 for people with arthritis, each with between 20 and 40 members. The functions of these groups were social and educational, and to provide sources of advice and support from relevant health professionals. The principal researcher and research assistant each attended one different monthly meeting for each group to explain the aims of the study and to invite participation.

Questionnaire packs (containing study information, questionnaires and return envelopes) were distributed in two ways: by the researchers in person to those who expressed interest at the meetings they attended, and by group leaders to those who expressed interest at the end of the meeting or at subsequent meetings. In total, 405 questionnaire packs were distributed in these two ways. One hundred and seven completed packs were returned either by post or through collection at the next meeting. It is impossible to calculate an accurate response rate because there is no guarantee that all group members received or intended to complete a questionnaire pack. However, given the large number of groups adequate representation of these chronic pain support group members might be expected. Twelve of the returned questionnaires (11.2%) were markedly incomplete (i.e. over 50% of items had been omitted) and these were excluded from the analysis. The final sample therefore consisted of 95 participants. The only inclusion criterion of the study, apart from membership of a targeted support group, was that participants should be aged 18 years or over.

Measures

Distress. This was measured using the 28-item General Health Questionnaire (GHQ-28) (16). The scale contains four subscales, each with seven items, that examine somatic symptoms, anxiety and insomnia, social dysfunction and severe depression experienced in the previous few weeks; however, two items relating to thoughts of suicide were removed from the depression section for ethical reasons. A 4-point response scale is provided for each item, the wording of which varies according to the item. In the current analysis, each item was scored as 0,1,2, or 3, with a higher score indicating a poorer outcome. The total score for the 26 items was used in the analysis.

Disability. Disability arising from pain was assessed using the 24-item Roland-Morris Disability Scale (RM Disability; 17): e.g., "I stay at home most of the time because of my pain". Response options are "yes" and "no", awarded scores of 1 and 0 respectively, and the total score was obtained by summing the number of "yes" responses, allowing up to three missing responses.

Pain intensity. This was envisaged as an indication of the source of stress, and was measured using the first three items (of seven) of the Chronic Pain Grade (18), the full version of which was presented to participants. The items used to assess pain intensity were as follows: "How would you rate your pain on a 0-10 scale, at the present time, that is right now, where 0 is 'no pain' and 10 is 'pain as bad as could be'?"; "In the past six months, how intense was your worst pain rated on a 0-10 scale, where 0 is 'no pain' and 10 is 'pain as bad as could be'?"; and "In the past six months, on average, how intense was your pain rated on a 0-10 scale, where 0 is 'no pain' and 10 is 'pain as bad as could be? (That is, your usual pain at times you were experiencing pain.)". Mean scores were taken of the responses to these items, allowing one missing value.

Pain beliefs. Participants completed the 57-item Survey of Pain Attitudes (SOPA) questionnaire (19). This includes seven subscales that address beliefs in the following areas: having control over the pain (Control, 10 items); inability to function because of pain (Disability, 10 items); that pain signifies damage and activity will cause further harm (Harm, 8 items); that emotions influence the experience of pain (Emotion, 8 items); that medication is an appropriate treatment for chronic pain (Medication, 6 items); that others should respond sympathetically (Solicitude, 6 items); and that doctors can provide a cure (Medical Cure, 9 items). Each item was scored on a 5-point scale, from 0 ("This is very untrue for me") to 4 ("This is very true for me"). Scores on the subscales were derived from the mean of contributing items, allowing up to two missing values.

Ways of coping and catastrophizing. Participants completed the Coping Strategies Questionnaire (CSQ; 10). This consists of 50 items. Six of these are "filler" items and not scored, and two reflect control. The remaining 42 items contribute to seven subscales (six items to each subscale), one of which is catastrophizing (e.g., "It is terrible and I feel it is never going to get any better"). The remaining subscales include diverting attention from the pain (e.g., "I try to think of something pleasant"); reinterpreting pain sensations (e.g., "I don't think of it as pain but rather as a dull, warm feeling"); coping self-statements, or exhortations to oneself to overcome the pain (e.g., "I tell myself to be brave and carry on despite the pain"); ignoring the pain sensations (e.g., "I don't think about the pain"); praying or hoping (e.g., "I pray for the pain to stop"); and increasing behavioural activity (e.g., "I try to be around other people"). For each item, participants were presented with a 7-point scale, from 0

("Never do that") to 6 ("Always do that"), through the mid-point, 3 ("Sometimes do that"). For the calculation of raw scores, the mean of contributing items was taken, allowing one missing value.

Other measures. Participants were asked to give their age in years; sex; marital status (married, co-habiting, separated, widowed, single, divorced); current employment status (employed, unemployed, retired, homemaker, student); and whether or not they would say that they were a religious person (yes/no). They were also asked in open-ended questions to indicate the type of pain they had, and how long they had had the pain.

Treatment of data and main statistical analyses

The analysis was conducted using SPSS 16.0 for Mac. Descriptive statistics for each scale or subscale were calculated and square-root transformations were conducted to correct for skew (Catastrophizing and Reinterpretation of Pain). The intercorrelations among raw CSQ scores were examined, and proportional scores were then calculated. To calculate proportional scores, raw scores on the contributing subscales were summed, and each individual subscale score was divided by this sum. Thus, for each participant, the sum of the proportional scores on the contributing subscales was 1 (although the following proportional scores were subsequently subjected to square-root transformation to correct for skew: Self-statements, Ignoring Pain, and Increasing Activity).

Two new outcome variables were calculated, by residualizing GHQ for RM Disability, and RM Disability for GHQ. Prior to the examination of mediation and moderation, all variables were centred. The procedure for examining mediation was that proposed by Baron and Kenny (20). Thus it was necessary to show that both the target variable and the potential mediator were significantly related to the outcome, and also to each other, before any test of mediation could be used. In the examination of moderation, interaction terms based on centred variables were computed, and entered into a regression equation after the main variables.

Results

Of the 95 participants, 86 were female. The mean age of participants was 66 years (M = 66.23, SD = 11.44), ranging from 43 to 93 years. Thirty-eight participants were married, 36 were widowed and 21 indicated that they were single, divorced or separated. As would be expected, most of the participants (n = 79, 84%) described themselves as retired from employment; of the remainder, nine indicated that they were unemployed, four that they were homemakers and two that they were employed. Seventy-two participants gave a positive response to the question of whether they would say that they were religious, while 22 participants gave a negative response.

Participants were asked to indicate the type of pain they had, and the length of time they had had that pain (both open-ended questions): 43 participants reported that their pain was related to a form of arthritis, 15 participants related the pain to fibromyalgia, 10 reported back pain, and 15 participants named both arthritis and fibromyalgia (joint/muscular pain). Twelve participants did not indicate the type of pain (although seven of these provided information on the length of time). The mean length of time that the pain had been experienced was 16 years (M = 16.21, SD = 14.66), although this ranged from six months to 68 years. Eighteen participants failed to indicate length of time of having the pain.

Descriptive statistics and zero-order relationships

Descriptive statistics for the scales are shown in table 1. All coefficients of internal consistency were acceptable, except that for the SOPA Medical Cure scale ($\alpha = 0.48$), which was therefore excluded from further analysis. GHQ and RM Disability scores were significantly correlated (r = 0.51, p < 0.001). Each was residualized for the other, and these residual scores were used in further analysis.

Table 1. Descriptive statistics for main continuous variables

Variable	Mean (SD)	Range	Cronbach's alpha
Distress (GHQ)	24.62 (11.75)	6-53	0.94
Pain disability (RM Disability)	0.61 (0.25)	0-1	0.91
Pain Intensity (CPG)	6.84 (2.12)	0-10	0.88
Pain beliefs (SOPA)			
Control	2.10 (0.81)	0-4	0.80
Disability	2.29 (0.85)	0.4-4	0.77
Harm	2.08 (0.70)	0.38-3.75	0.62
Emotion	1.93 (0.81)	0.38-3.50	0.71
Medication	3.00 (0.82)	0.5-4	0.73
Solicitude	1.39 (1.10)	0-3.83	0.87
Medical cure	1.67 (0.62)	0.22-2.89	0.48
Ways of coping (CSQ): raw scores			
Catastrophizing	1.92 (1.50)	0-6	0.87
Diverting attention	2.74 (1.45)	0-6	0.87
Reinterpretation of pain	1.34 (1.33)	0-5	0.85
Self-statements	3.56 (1.38)	0.17-6	0.82
Ignoring pain	2.43 (1.44)	0-6	0.85
Praying/hoping	2.61 (1.58)	0-6	0.79
Increasing activity	3.28 (1.29)	0.33-6	0.81

First the intercorrelations among the raw CSQ scales, including Catastrophizing, were examined. These are shown in table 2 (upper right). Excluding Catastrophizing, all of the coping scores were significantly and positively correlated with one another, with coefficients ranging between 0.29 and 0.72. In other words, those who scored highly on one scale tended to score highly on all of the others. Catastrophizing was significantly and positively related to Reinterpretation of Pain and Praying/hoping, but not to the other coping scales. It appeared therefore that Catastrophizing was different from the other coping scales, and that there were grounds for treating it as separate variable (11). In addition, the results suggested that the use of proportional coping scores was justified, since this would control for the variation in the number of strategies endorsed by each participant, variation which could account for the uniformly positive intercorrelations. The intercorrelations among the proportional coping scores, and the relationship of each with Catastrophizing (raw score), are shown in table 2 (lower left). Given that negative intercorrelations are to be expected with proportional scores (because a higher proportional score on one scale implies a lower proportional score on another scale), the two positive intercorrelations are noteworthy: between Diverting Attention and Reinterpretation of Pain, and between Self-statements and Increasing Activity. With regard to Catastrophizing, higher scores were related to higher proportional use of Reinterpretation of Pain, and a lower proportional use of Self-statements and Ignoring Pain.

Table 2. Intercorrelations of CSQ scores (including Catastrophizing): raw scores, upper right; proportional scores, lower left

	Catastrophizing	Diverting attention	Reinterpretation of pain	Self-statements	Ignoring pain	Praying/ hoping	Increase activity
Catastrophizing	-	.14	.30**	.04	.04	.29**	.15
Diverting attention	-.01	-	.71***	.64***	.64***	.51***	.61***
Reinterpretation of pain	.26*	.21*	-	.57***	.66***	.59***	.44***
Self-statements	-.28**	-.20	-.35***	-	.72***	.38***	.72***
Ignoring pain	-.21*	-.11	.01	.08	-	.40***	.56***
Praying/hoping	.19	-.29**	-.04	-.44***	-.19	-	.29**
Increase activity	-.01	-.05	-.36***	.22*	-.48***	-.34***	-

*p < 0.05; ** p < 0.01; ***p < 0.001.

Table 3. Zero-order correlations: Pain Intensity and the residualized outcome variables (GHQ and RM Disability), with SOPA pain beliefs, Catastrophizing, and proportional ways of coping

Variable	Pain Intensity	GHQ (residualized for RM Disability)	RM Disability (residualized for GHQ)
Pain intensity	-	.07	.51***
SOPA control	-.28**	-.21	-.10
SOPA disability	.31**	.09	.44***
SOPA harm	.26*	.16	.18
SOPA emotion	.21*	.08	.29**
SOPA medication	.30**	.13	.19
SOPA solicitude	.36***	.15	.33**
Catastrophizing	.50***	.24*	.41***
Diverting Attention (prop)	.03	.05	.14
Reinterpretation of Pain (prop)	.22*	.01	.24*
Self-statements (prop)	-.18	-.08	-.19
Ignoring Pain (prop)	-.16	-.04	-.12
Praying/hoping (prop)	.08	.11	.08
Increasing Activity (prop)	.19	-.09	.09

* p < 0.05; ** p < 0.01; *** p < 0.001.
prop = proportional scores.

Zero-order correlation coefficients between Pain Intensity, the residualized outcome variables and the belief and proportional coping scales are displayed in table 3. The identified source of stress, Pain Intensity, was significantly related to residualized RM Disability but not GHQ. Catastrophizing was significantly related to Pain Intensity (r_{12} = 0.50, $p < 0.001$); the effect size was reduced but remained significant when unresidualized GHQ scores were partialled out ($r_{12.3}$ = 0.39, $p < 0.001$). Catastrophizing was also significantly related to both residualized outcome variables, particularly RM Disability. These results suggested that the relationships among Pain Intensity, Catastrophizing and RM Disability were not solely due to the influence of psychological distress. Given that Pain Intensity was not related to GHQ when RM Disability was controlled for, GHQ was not treated as an outcome variable in further analysis.

All of the SOPA belief scores were significantly related to Pain Intensity, and those with higher scores on the SOPA Disability, Emotion and Solicitude scales gained higher scores on residualized RM Disability. With regard to proportional coping scores, those with higher proportional Reinterpretation of Pain scores gained higher Pain Intensity and higher RM Disability scores.

The relationships among Catastrophizing, ways of coping and the SOPA beliefs are shown in table 4. Catastrophizing was significantly related to all of the SOPA belief scores, particularly Solicitude, Disability, and Control. With regard to ways of coping, those with higher proportional scores on Diverting Attention had higher scores on the SOPA Disability and Emotion scales; those with higher proportional Reinterpretation of Pain scores gained higher scores on the SOPA Emotion scale; those with higher proportional Self-statement scores had lower scores on the SOPA Disability and Harm scales; and those with higher proportional Increasing Activity scores gained lower scores on the SOPA Emotion scale.

Table 4. Zero-order correlations: Catastrophizing and proportional ways of coping with SOPA pain beliefs

Variable	Catastro-phizing	Diverting Attention (prop)	Reinter-pretation of Pain (prop)	Self-state-ments (prop)	Ignor-ing Pain (prop)	Praying/ hoping (prop)	Increas-ing Activity (prop)
SOPA control	-.35***	.10	.09	.09	.14	-.19	-.13
SOPA disability	.40***	.24*	-.01	-.29**	-.20	.15	.07
SOPA harm	.27**	.10	.09	-.23*	-.19	.15	.03
SOPA emotion	.21*	.29**	.25*	-.16	.02	.07	-.22*
SOPA medication	.21*	.19	.03	.08	.13	-.05	-.01
SOPA solicitude	.56***	.13	.18	-.18	.01	.08	-.04

* $p < 0.05$; ** $p < 0.01$; *** $p < 0.001$.
prop = proportional scores.

The potential roles of demographic and descriptor variables were then considered. Age was related to a number of variables (but not to Pain Intensity, residualized GHQ or RM Disability scores). Older participants gained lower Catastrophizing scores (r = -0.21, p < 0.05), and lower scores on the SOPA Disability (r = -0.39, p < 0.001), Harm (r = -0.21, p < 0.05) and Emotion (r = -0.29, p < 0.01) scales. They also gained lower proportional scores on Diverting Attention (r = -0.21, p < 0.05). Those who were widowed, and those who described themselves as religious, also gained lower scores on the SOPA Disability scale, but these relationships were found to be mediated by age. As might be expected, those who described themselves as religious gained higher proportional scores on Praying/hoping (t (89) = 3.22, p < 0.01), and this difference remained significant when age was controlled for. No significant differences were found on any of the variables according to type of pain. One variable was found to be related to duration of pain: the longer the duration, the lower the score on the SOPA Solicitude scale (r = -0.26, p < 0.05). This relationship remained significant when age was controlled for.

Mediation

An analysis was conducted to determine whether Catastrophizing mediated the relationship between Pain Intensity and residualized RM Disability. The conditions for the analysis were met (20), given that Pain Intensity and Disability were significantly related to each other, and Catastrophizing was significantly related to both. Residualized RM Disability was then regressed on Pain Intensity and Catastrophizing. No evidence was found to suggest that Catastrophizing mediated the Pain Intensity-RM Disability relationship. Pain Intensity remained significantly related to RM Disability when Catastrophizing was controlled for: B = 0.20, SE B = 0.05, β = 0.44, t = 4.02, p < 0.001, and Catastrophizing lost significance: B = 0.26, SE B = 0.17, β = 0.17, t = 1.53, ns.

Three SOPA belief scales (Disability, Emotion and Solicitude) and one way of coping (Reinterpretation of Pain) were also considered as possible mediators of the Pain Intensity-RM Disability relationship. No evidence of mediation was found with any of these variables: Pain Intensity remained significantly related to RM Disability in every analysis, and all but SOPA Disability lost significance in the analysis when Pain Intensity was controlled for.

The same four variables (SOPA Disability, Emotion and Solicitude, and Reinterpretation of Pain) also satisfied the conditions of potential mediators of the Catastrophizing-RM Disability relationship. No evidence was found to suggest that any of these variables mediated this relationship: Catastrophizing remained significantly related to RM Disability in every analysis, and all but SOPA Disability lost significance when Catastrophizing was controlled for.

Moderation

To determine whether Catastrophizing significantly moderated the relationship between Pain Intensity and RM Disability, a hierarchical regression analysis was conducted, with residualized RM Disability as the dependent variable. The Pain Intensity X Catastrophizing interaction term was entered after the two independent variables. The interaction term made a significant contribution to the variance: B = -0.19, SE B = 0.07, β = -0.26, t = -2.67, p = 0.009. A simple slope analysis was then conducted (21), to examine the relationship between Pain Intensity and residualized RM Disability at two levels of Catastrophizing (one standard deviation above and below the mean). No other variables were included in this analysis. When Catastrophizing scores were low (one standard deviation below the mean), the relationship between Pain Intensity and residualized RM Disability scores was significant: B = 0.27, SE B = 0.06, β= 0.58, t = 4.93, p < 0.001. However, when Catastrophizing scores were high, the Pain Intensity-RM Disability relationship was no longer significant: B = 0.03, SE B = 0.08, β = 0.07, t = 0.41, ns.

Two further analyses were conducted. It had been noted that SOPA Disability made a significant contribution to the variance of residualized RM Disability scores when either Pain Intensity or Catastrophizing was statistically controlled, although no evidence was found to suggest that this belief filled a mediating role. It was therefore decided to determine whether SOPA Disability moderated the relationships between RM Disability and either Pain Intensity or Catastrophizing. No evidence of moderation was found in either case. Finally, residualized RM Disability was regressed on the following variables: age, Pain Intensity, Catastrophizing, SOPA Disability, and the Pain Intensity X Catastrophizing interaction term. The results are shown in table 5: F (5, 78) = 12.08, p < 0.001. SOPA Disability made a significant contribution to the variance of RM Disability, as did the Pain Intensity X Catastrophizing interaction term.

Table 5. Results of multiple regression analysis, with residualized RM Disability as the dependent variable

Step	Variable	R^2	ΔR^2	B	SE B	β	t
1	(Constant)	.36	.36	-.62	.53		-1.17
	Age			.01	.01	.13	1.42
	Pain Intensity			.12	.05	.26	2.38*
	Catastrophizing			.18	,17	.11	1.09
	SOPA Disability			.42	.12	.34	3.44***
2	Pain Intensity X Catastrophizing	.44	.08	-.22	.07	-.31	-3.27**

Discussion

The main aim of the current analysis was to examine the roles of catastrophizing, pain beliefs and ways of coping in the context of the model of stress and coping described by Lazarus and colleagues (5,6). The potential source of stress identified in the analysis, Pain Intensity, was found to be significantly related to scores on the residualized RM Disability scale (i.e., RM Disability scores controlled for GHQ), and a number of the variables of interest were significantly related to both: Catastrophizing, SOPA Disability, SOPA Emotion, SOPA Solicitude, and the proportional Reinterpretation of Pain coping scale. However, none of these variables was found to mediate, or account for, the relationship between Pain Intensity and residualized RM Disability. Thus, there was no evidence to suggest that greater pain intensity was associated with greater pain-related disability because of catastrophizing, or of holding certain beliefs about pain, or because of using a greater proportion of coping strategies aimed at reinterpreting the pain sensations. Catastrophizing was found to interact with, or moderate, Pain Intensity in its relationship with residualized RM Disability scores: the Pain Intensity-RM Disability relationship was no longer significant when Catastrophizing scores were high. One further finding of note was that SOPA Disability scores made an independent contribution to the variance of residualized RM Disability scores, such that those who held a stronger belief that pain would result in disability experienced more pain-related disability, irrespective of the intensity of the pain.

The failure to find evidence of mediation, noted also by a number of other authors in the field (1,2,8,13), may result in part from reliance on a cross-sectional between-persons analysis. In addition, it should be noted that the source of stress would have been chronic for most participants in this study, such that the transactional nature of the stress process would have been brought to the fore. For example, many of the participants could have been in a cycle or spiral of pain-related stress, such that the consequences of pain — pain-related disability and distress — had become sources of stress in their own right. In fact, there would be grounds for treating intensity of pain as an outcome variable rather than as a source of stress (3,8). The hypothesis that secondary appraisal, coping resources and ways of coping mediate the stressor-outcome relationship assumes a sequence of relatively distinct processes, which may not be captured by a single cross-sectional data collection (22). An additional explanation for lack of mediation may be found in the treatment of the data, particularly the two potential outcome variables of the stress process. The statistical control of symptoms of distress when considering pain-related disability as an outcome addressed an important aspect of the role of catastrophizing, but may have resulted in a model that lacked ecological validity, in that distress may be an integral part of disability in the real world. Further, in common with most of the research in this area, the analysis lacked a positive outcome variable, or a variable representing the result of "successful" coping, such as contentment or wellbeing, rather than merely the absence of symptoms.

With these points in mind, we turn to a consideration of catastrophizing. Those who had higher Catastrophizing scores gained higher scores on the measures of Pain Intensity and RM Disability, whether or not GHQ scores were controlled or partialled out; further, the correlation between Catastrophizing and residualized RM Disability was stronger than that between Catastrophizing and residualized GHQ. These findings suggest that, in the present study at least, Catastrophizing was not merely a reflection of distress, and thus support the conclusion reached by Sullivan et al (1) on this point. Catastrophizing did not explain the relationship between Pain Intensity and residualized RM Disability, but it did moderate the relationship, such that the Pain Intensity-RM Disability relationship was no longer significant when Catastrophizing levels were high. It was perhaps the case that those with a tendency to magnify their experience of pain, and to feel that it was beyond their control, experienced disability irrespective of the intensity of their pain, an explanation consistent with the conceptualization of catastrophizing as secondary appraisal. Taking the transactional nature of stress into account, the results might also suggest that the experience of pain-related disability increased any tendency to catastrophize the pain, contributing in turn to the exacerbation of the interpretation of pain. Alternatively, the interaction could be interpreted in the context of the "communal coping" model of catastrophizing (1), which suggests that people who catastrophize may cope with the aim of eliciting social support, by overtly displaying distress. Low levels of catastrophizing, failing to bring any level of support from others, may have resulted in high levels of pain-related disability, while high levels may have elicited the support required to prevent disability. This explanation must remain tentative, given that no measure of coping through social support was included in the analysis, and although a significant relationship was found between Catastrophizing and the SOPA Solicitude scale, Solicitude did not explain the Catastrophizing-RM Disability relationship.

Higher residualized RM Disability scores were positively related to beliefs that pain leads to disability, that pain can be increased by emotion, and that solicitude should be expected; further, all of the SOPA belief scales were significantly related to Pain Intensity and Catastrophizing. The findings are therefore reasonably consistent with those reported elsewhere (12,13). One belief in particular – that pain leads to disability - appeared to play an independent role in the explanation of residualized RM Disability scores. The most parsimonious explanation of this finding is that pain-related disability enhanced the belief that pain leads to disability, rather than that the disability resulted from the belief. However, it could also signal that this belief is central to the spiral of stress. Overall, the results suggest that further research on the impact of changing specific beliefs about pain could be beneficial (12,13).

The decision to treat Catastrophizing as distinct from ways of coping was made a priori, in line with the recommendations of other authors in the field (11,13). Although the alternative model was not fully explored in the current analysis, this decision was consistent with the pattern of associations noted between Catastrophizing and the other CSQ scales. The use of proportional scores on the coping scales proved useful, given that there was a wide variation in the number of strategies used by participants; those who used more strategies in one category also tended to use more in the other categories (14,15). However, it is acknowledged that a greater emphasis on within-person analysis of the relationships between ways of coping and outcome is needed to increase our understanding of the process (22). In the present analysis, those using a greater proportion of strategies associated with reinterpreting the pain were found to have higher residualized RM Disability scores, residualized GHQ scores, and higher Pain Intensity and Catastrophizing scores. No other proportional coping scores were related to the outcome or stressor variables. Although no evidence of mediation was found, the results suggested that using a high proportion of strategies aimed at reinterpreting pain sensations (for example, trying to imagine it as numbness) was not beneficial for the participants in the present study, a conclusion also reached by Newman et al (23) using a sample of participants with rheumatoid arthritis. Those who used a higher proportion of such strategies also tended to use a higher proportion of strategies aimed at diverting attention from the pain. It may be that such a pattern of coping with pain sensations, associated with avoiding engagement with, or acknowledgement of, the pain, interferes with the adoption of more beneficial strategies. However, given the cross-sectional nature of the analysis, it is possible that the tendency to reinterpret the pain sensations resulted from the experience of pain-related disability and the associated distress, perhaps because prior experience suggested that the use of other coping strategies made little difference. The relationships between ways of coping and pain beliefs noted in the analysis, and the pattern of those relationships, suggested that further research into the nature of these relationships would be warranted. For example, those who used proportionately more strategies directed at reinterpreting the pain also held a stronger belief that pain could be exacerbated by emotion; the aim of such a coping strategy may therefore be to "damp down" the emotion rather than to avoid disability per se. Again, only within-person analysis can provide the means of testing such hypotheses (22).

The problems associated with reliance on cross-sectional data have already been mentioned, but the study was also limited in a number of other ways. The sample did not vary a great deal with regard to their demographic characteristics or source of pain, and thus it was not possible to take full account of the roles of such factors within the stress process (1); the results may therefore not be generalizable to the wider population of people experiencing chronic pain. Age was found to be related to a number of variables, such that older adults, while not experiencing less pain or pain-related disability, were less likely to catastrophize and to hold beliefs that pain leads to disability or harm, or that emotion plays a role in the experience of pain. Such findings are consistent with the conclusion reached by Turk et al (24), that older people may be more accepting of pain and disability as part of the natural aging process. However, the age range of the current sample was too limited to investigate this further.

In conclusion, the results of the current analysis were consistent with the construction of catastrophizing as secondary appraisal within the transactional model of stress and coping. The measure of catastrophizing was strongly related to both the measures of pain intensity and pain-related disability when psychological distress was controlled for, adding weight to the conclusion reached by Sullivan et al (1), that catastrophizing can be distinguished from distress, both conceptually and in measurement. However, further research, at the within-person level, is required to fully understand the transactional roles of catastrophizing, pain beliefs and ways of coping in the stress process over time.

Acknowledgments

This research was funded by Glasgow Caledonian University. Dr Anne Whyte played an important role in the design and conduct of the study, and her contribution is gratefully acknowledged. Thanks are also due to Emily Smith for help with data collection and data entry.

References

[1] Sullivan MJL, Thorn B, Haythornthwaite JA, Keefe F, Martin M, Bradley LA, Lefebvre JC. Theoretical perspectives on the relation between catastrophizing and pain. Clin J Pain 2001;17:52-64.
[2] Turner JA, Aaron, LA. Pain-related catastrophizing: What is it? Clin J Pain 2001;17:65-71.
[3] Hirsh AT, George SZ, Riley JL III, Robinson ME. An evaluation of the measurement of pain catastrophizing by the coping strategies questionnaire. Eur J Pain 2007;11:75-81.
[4] McParland JL, Knussen C. Just world beliefs moderate the relationship of pain intensity and disability with psychological distress in chronic pain support group members. Eur J Pain, in press.
[5] Lazarus RS. Theory-based stress measurement. Psychol Inq 1990;1:3-13.

[6] Folkman S. Personal control and stress and coping processes: A theoretical analysis. J Pers Soc Psychol 1984;46:839-52.
[7] Keefe FJ, Rumble ME, Scipio CD, Giordano LA, Perri LM. Psychological aspects of persistent pain: Current state of the science. J Pain 2004;5:195–211.
[8] Wolff B, Burns JW, Quartana PJ, Lofland K, Bruehl S, Chung OY. Pain catastrophizing, physiological indexes, and chronic pain severity: tests of mediation and moderation models. J Behav Med 2008;31:105-14.
[9] Boothby JL, Thorn BE, Stroud MW, Jensen MP. Coping with pain. In: Gatchel RJ, Turk DC, eds. Psychosocial factors in pain: Critical perspectives. London: Guilford, 1999:343-59.
[10] Rosenstiel AK, Keefe FJ. The use of coping strategies in chronic low back pain patients: relationship to patient characteristics and current adjustment. Pain 1983;17:33-44.
[11] Lawson K, Reesor KA, Keefe FJ, Turner JA. Dimensions of pain-related cognitive coping: cross-validation of the factor structure of the Coping Strategy Questionnaire. Pain 1990;43:195-204.
[12] Gatchel RJ, Peng YB, Peters ML, Fuchs PN, Turk DC. The biopsychosocial approach to chronic pain: Scientific advances and future directions. Psychol Bull 2007;133:581-624.
[13] Turner JA, Jensen MP, Romano JM. Do beliefs, coping and catastrophizing independently predict functioning in patients with chronic pain? Pain 2000;85:115-25.
[14] Knussen C, Tolson D, Brogan CA, Swan IRC, Stott DJ, Sullivan F. Family caregivers of older relatives: Ways of coping and change in distress. Psychol Health Med 2008;13:274-90.
[15] Vitaliano PP, Maiuro RD, Russo J, Becker J. Raw versus relative scores in the assessment of coping strategies. J Behav Med 1987;10:1-18.
[16] Goldberg DP, Hillier VF. A scaled version of the General Health Questionnaire. Psychol Med 1979;9:139-45.
[17] Roland M, Morris R. A study of the natural history of back pain. Part 1: Development of a reliable and sensitive measure of disability in low back pain. Spine 1983;8:141-4.
[18] Von Korff M, Ormel J, Keefe FJ, Dworkin, SF. Grading the severity of chronic pain. Pain 1992;50:133-49.
[19] Jensen MP, Turner JA, Romano JM, Lawler BK. Relationship of pain specific beliefs to chronic pain adjustment. Pain 1994;57:301-9.
[20] Baron RM, Kenny DA. The moderator-mediator variable distinction in social psychological research: Conceptual, strategic and statistical considerations. J Pers Soc Psychol 1986;51:1173-82.
[21] Preacher KJ. A primer on interaction effects in multiple linear regression. University of Kansas, 2003. [Retrieved December, 2008]. Available from: http://www.people.ku.edu/~preacher/interact/ interactions.htm
[22] Keefe FJ, Affleck G, Lefebvre JC, Starr K, Caldwell DS, Tennen H. Pain coping strategies and coping efficacy in rheumatoid arthritis: a daily process analysis. Pain 1997;69:35-42.
[23] Newman SP, Fitzpatrick R, Lamb R, Shipley M. Patterns of coping in rheumatoid arthritis. Psychol Health 1990;4:187-200.
[24] Turk DC, Okifuji A, Scharff L. Chronic pain and depression: Role of perceived impact and perceived control in different age cohorts. Pain 1995;61:93-101.

Section Three - Brain Stimulation and Pain

In: Pain Management Yearbook 2009
Editor: Joav Merrick

ISBN: 978-1-61209-666-7
©2012 Nova Science Publishers, Inc.

Chapter 23

BRAIN CHANGES RELATED TO CHRONIC PAIN: IMPLICATIONS FOR STIMULATION TREATMENT

Herta Flor[*], *PhD*

Department of Cognitive and Clinical Neuroscience, Central Institute of Mental Health, University of Heidelberg, Mannheim, Germany

Abstract

In this paper the evidence supporting plastic functional and structural changes in the primary sensory and motor areas as well as areas involved in affective and cognitive processing in states of chronic pain, specifically neuropathic pain and musculoskeletal pain is reviewed. These plastic changes are viewed as implicit memory traces that may – over time – become associated with a large number of antecedents and consequences of pain that now add to a chronic pain network in the brain and are instrumental in the maintenance of chronic pain. The reason why stimulation treatments might be effective in extinguishing these memory traces related to pain is discussed and suggestions made on how stimulation treatments should be applied.

Keywords: Cortical plasticity, learning, chronic pain, reorganization, behavioral.

Introduction

Recent scientific evidence shows that chronic pain is accompanied by plastic changes on multiple levels of the nervous system (1). This review will focus on brain changes related to the experience of chronic pain in humans and will elucidate consequences for the stimulatory

---

[*] **Correspondence:** Herta Flor, PhD, Department of Cognitive and Clinical Neuroscience, Central Institute of Mental Health, University of Heidelberg, J5, 68159 Mannheim, Germany, phone: +4962117036302; FAX +4962117036305; E-mail: herta.flor@zi-mannheim.de

treatment of chronic pain. Advanced imaging methods have made it possible to study brain changes in response to pain and to determine how alterations in the brain might contribute to the experience of chronic pain.

Neuropathic pain

Deafferentation leads to a loss of sensory input into the brain and evokes changes in the primary sensory and motor areas. For example, in patients with amputations, the map in primary somatosensory cortex changes in a manner that input from neighboring areas occupies the region that formerly received input from the now amputated limb (2-4). These changes are mirrored in motor cortex (5-8). Interestingly, reorganizational changes were only found in amputees with phantom limb pain after amputation but not in amputees without pain. This suggests that pain may contribute to the changes observed and that the persisting pain might also be a consequence of the plastic changes that occur. In several studies in human upper extremity amputees, displacement of the lip representation in the primary motor and somatosensory cortex was positively correlated with the intensity of phantom limb pain, and was not present in pain-free amputees or healthy controls. Also, in the patients with phantom limb pain, but not the pain free amputees, imagined movement of the phantom hand activated the neighboring face area (8). The co-activation occurs probably due to the high overlap of the hand, arm and mouth representations. These changes occur already very early after amputation (9) and are maintained over time (10).

Similar observations were made in patients with complex regional pain syndrome (CRPS). In these patients the representation of the affected hand tended to be smaller compared to that of the unaffected hand and the individual digit representations had moved closer together (11-16). The extent of the pathological changes in the cortical representations correlated with the intensity of pain but was also related to a degradation of sensibility in the affected hand (11-13).

In addition to cortical reorganization, general cortical hyperexcitability has been observed in chronic neuropathic pain syndromes (5,11,17-22). For example, Larbig et al (18) presented pain-relevant and pain-irrelevant words and found enhanced late visual potential amplitudes of the electroencephalogram in the amputees with pain but not the amputees without phantom limb pain or healthy controls. Karl et al (19) found significantly higher P300 amplitudes in amputees with pain compared to amputees without pain and healthy controls in a visual oddball paradigm suggesting a higher magnitude of non-specific cortical excitability in amputees with pain and a reduced excitability in amputees without pain. Schwenkreis et al (17) observed a significant reduction of intracortical inhibition in both hemispheres in CRPS patients compared to healthy control subjects. In upper- and lower- limb amputees, transcranial magnetic stimulation studies demonstrated elevated excitability of the motor system at the site ipsilateral to the stump (5, 22). Motor evoked potentials were elicited at lower intensities in muscles immediately proximal to the site of amputation compared to the homologous muscle on the unaffected side. Transcranial magnetic stimulation also recruited a higher percentage of the motorneuron pool in the muscle on the side on the stump then on the unaffected side. These results suggested that the excitability of the motor system projecting to the muscle immediately above the amputation was increased. Cortical hyperexcitability and reorganization of cortical maps was also reported in patients with trigeminal neuralgia (23, 24).

Some studies have also focused on the affective and cognitive processing of pain and how this might be related to map changes and changes in associative areas in the brain (25). For example, a study by Witting et al (26) examined the brain correlates of allodynia in patients with allodynia related to neuropathic pain. In this positron emission tomography study the authors observed that allodynia was correlated with enhanced ipsilateral insular and more orbitofrontal activation as well as a lack of contralateral SI activation, which the authors explained in terms of a stronger emotional load and higher computational demands in the processing of a mixed sensation of brush and pain. The orbitofrontal activation is probably related to mechanisms of descending pain modulation but it might also be involved in anticipatory anxiety related to pain. Similarly, in trigeminal neuralgia, allodynia activated not only areas in the primary sensory pathway but also the basal ganglia and the frontal cortex (24). Schweinhardt et al (27) also observed a relationship of allodynia and caudal insular activity in pain patients. In CRPS patients hyperalgesia was associated with enhanced activation in all pain-relevant areas including SI and SII.

In amputees, Willoch et al (28) used hypnosis to induce painful phantom sensations and observed activation in areas such as the insula and the anterior cingulate cortex, regions that have been identified as important in the processing of affective pain components. However, the influence of the effort to create the specific sensation in the hypnotic condition can not be controlled in this type of study. In a study that varied both acute and chronic pain intensity simultaneously it was observed that chronic pain intensity covaried with prefrontal activation whereas acute pain intensity changes covaried with insular activation suggesting different processing modes for acute and habitual pain (29). These changes were, however, observed in musculoskelatal pain (see below).

In addition to functional changes structural and biochemical abnormalities have also been reported in several types of neuropathic pain (30) and it has also been found that structural and functional abnormalities are often colocalized (31). In addition, changes in the resting activation of the brain, the so-called default mode have been observed [e.g., 32]. It is, however, still not clear if these abnormalities precede the onset of chronic pain and are thus a vulnerability factor or if they are a consequence of the chronic pain state.

Musculoskelatal pain syndromes

Not only decreased input related to deafferentation but also increased behaviorally relevant input related to non-neuropathic pain leads to changes in the cortical map (33-37). For example, Flor et al (33) reported a close association between pain chronicity and enhanced excitability and map expansion of the back representation in primary somatosensory cortex in patients with non-neuropathic back pain. The back representation had expanded and shifted towards the leg representation the longer the pain had persisted. Similar changes were reported by Giesecke et al (34) using functional magnetic resonance imaging. Recently, Tsao et al (35) observed a close interaction between changes in motor cortex and postural control in patients with chronic back pain suggesting an intricate interaction between peripheral and central traces of plastic changes related to chronic pain.

Greatly enhanced representations of painful stimulation were also found in patients with fibromyalgia who showed more areas of the brain responding to painful stimulation of a standard value and also higher activation intensities (36). These changes were present in cortical activation maps as well as in areas involved in the affective and cognitive processing of pain (37). In addition to changes in functional activation structural and biochemical changes and changes in brain connectivity have also been reported for musculoskeletal pain syndromes (38).

Potential mechanisms underlying plastic changes of the brain in pain

Potential mechanisms of plasticity related to pain are the unmasking of previously present but inactive excitatory synapses and growth of new connections (sprouting). Immediate plasticity could be shown in humans and suggests that reorganization of sensory pathways occurs very soon after amputation, potentially due to the unmasking of ordinarily silent inputs or dendritic sprouting rather than sprouting of new axon terminals (39,40). Unmasking of latent excitatory synapses can be caused by increased release of excitatory neurotransmitters, increased density of postsynaptic receptors, changes in conductance of neuronal membrane, decreased inhibitory inputs or removing inhibition from excitatory input (41,42), but the evidence up to date is pointing at removal of inhibition from excitatory synapses as the major contributor. The crucial element in this process is the decrease in inhibition induced by gamma-butyric acid (GABA). GABA is the most important inhibitory neurotransmitter in the brain, and GABAergic neurons represent about one third of the neuronal population in the motor cortex. Alterations in GABAergic inhibition can induce rapid changes in cortical excitability. It is of interest that drugs that enhance GABAergic inhibition (e.g. Lorazepam) increase intracortical inhibition (42,43), but do not affect motor threshold suggesting that the reduced intracortical inhibition described was most likely mediated by GABA, while changes in the motor threshold had another underlying mechanism. As proposed by Chen et al (44) the reduction of motor threshold might involve enhancement of cortico-cortical connections. Since drugs that block voltage-gated sodium channels increase the motor threshold, it is possible that the proposed enhancement in cortical connections could be mediated by voltage-gated sodium channels. In fact, in models of spinal cord injury Waxman and Hains (45) reported a substantial calcium-channel mediated upregulation of activity in supraspinal pathways. Structural changes as revealed by voxel-based morphometry (46) and magnetic resonance spectroscopy (47,48) suggest neuronal loss and cell death to be induced in chronic pain. However, the relationship of these changes to pain severity has not yet been documented. Birbaumer et al (49) used regional anesthesia in upper limb amputees to treat phantom limb pain and observed a very rapid reversal of somatosensory cortical reorganization in those who experienced substantial pain relief but not in those whose pain remained unchanged. This suggest that rapid modulation of cortical plasticity and pain is possible even in long-term chronic pain states.

Plastic changes in the brain and learning and memory processes

Plastic changes in the brain are greatly determined by learning processes that are related to pain. A fundamental distinction of memory mechanism is that of implicit or non-declarative and explicit or declarative memory processes. Implicit memory processes refer to often non-conscious changes in behavior as a consequence of experience and involve nonassociative learning such as habituation and sensitization but also associative processes such as operant and respondent conditioning. Explicit learning usually refers to semantic and episodic memory processes that rely on the conscious reproduction of an encoded memory item. These memory processes also involve different brain structures and neuronal networks and may be differentially interacting in health and disease. For example, explicit memory depends heavily on intact hippocampal structures whereas some types of implicit emotional memory require an intact amygdala or striatum. Although both types of learning and memory processes are important in chronic pain (for a review on explicit memory see, for example, (50)) we have proposed that implicit learning processes may be more pronounced in chronic pain since pain has a high biological relevance suggesting that fast automatic processes may be important, and since implicit learning processes change behavior without the person knowing about it and they may therefore be especially difficult to extinguish (51).

For example, operant conditioning of pain by verbal reinforcement persists in patients with chronic pain on both the verbal and the cortical levels, whereas persons who do not suffer from chronic pain quickly extinguish acquired pain expressions and concomitant physiological changes (52). The role of changes in pain as reinforcers is currently being explored (53) and may be especially important for chronic pain. Pavlovian conditioning of peripheral and central changes is also enhanced in chronic pain (54) and seems to involve somatosensory cortex as do other pain-specific memory traces (55,56). Nonassociative learning such as sensitization seems to be especially enhanced in chronic pain (57).

Much of the current evidence suggests that these pain memory traces are stable over time and do not easily extinguish. Whereas the acquisition of conditioned responses is fairly generalized the extinction is confined to the specific extinction context thus implying that extinction requires more extensive learning. We therefore assume that the extinction or „unlearning" rather than the acquisition of pain memories is the main problem in chronic pain. In addition, central and peripheral memories are closely interwoven and both need to be addressed, and treatment can be viewed as extinction and relearning and needs to be based on learning principles.

Extinction as the basis of brain stimulation treatments

If ongoing pain is associated with abnormal crosstalk from other brain regions as well as enhanced peripheral input, then alterations of the respective brain region or the peripheral input should alter the brain map and also pain. Stimulation treatment can thus involve peripheral stimulation such as prosthesis training or sensory discrimination training but can also be based on invasive or noninvasive brain stimulation or some intermediate form of stimulation. Since the various stimulation approaches to pain will be discussed in the companion articles we will focus on guidelines for stimulation based on the research on learning, memory and brain plasticity in chronic pain.

Treatments should be site-specific. Much of the older research on brain stimulation did not determine the cortical representation of the body site affected by pain. Since much of the research on cortical representation of pain and on pain-related changes shows great site-specificity (33,59) it should be determined to what extent site-specific versus more general stimulation methods are effective.

Treatments should enhance inhibition and reduce overactivation. In addition to site-specific changes general hyperreactivity of central nervous system structures seems to be an important factor in chronic states of pain. Thus a reduction of neuronal excitability and an enhancement of inhibition are important additional targets of stimulation treatment. A general lack of cortical control and inhibitory capacity might be a problem in chronic pain since it has been shown that frontal areas important for cognitive control processes are especially affected by structural changes in chronic pain (60).

Treatments should be massed and should cover several contexts. Since extinction is context-specific, training as many varied behaviors as possible, training in many different environments, and the use of stress and pain episodes to train relapse prevention are important parts of this training.

Treatments that combine stimulation with behavioral and pharmacological interventions might be more effective. Behavioral treatments that focus on the extinction of pain behaviors and the acquisition of healthy behaviors can also alter brain processes related to pain and could be combined with stimulation approaches. In addition, pharmacological substances that enhance plasticity and learning might also be useful. In anxiety disorders it has been shown that exposure with or without additional pharmacological intervention can alter brain processes related to stimuli that are relevant for the disorder (61). The partial NMDA receptor agonist d-cycloserine has been found to be effective in enhancing extinction of aversive memories and has been used as an effective adjunct to exposure treatment in two studies (62,63). In addition, cannabinoids have been identified as important modulators of extinction (64,65) and might be interesting compounds for extinction training.

Cognitive and emotional aspects of pain need to be targeted. Imaging studies have shown that pain is not only accompanied by map changes in the primary somtosensory and motor areas but also affects cognitive and affective processing. In addition, comorbidity of chronic pain with mental disorders such as anxiety or depression is frequent. Therefore stimulation methods that target emotional and motivational processing and methods that enhance adaptive cognitive processing may be useful.

Treatment outcome measures need to be multidimensional. Most studies on stimulation treatment of chronic pain have so far relied excusively on pain ratings. However, pain-related interference, pain-related behaviors and affective distress may often be more meaningful variables of change and need to be considered (66).

Conclusions

Although recent scientific evidence has shown that chronic pain leads to changes in many brain regions the responsiveness of pain to plastic changes also opens the door for new intervention methods, which rely on stimulation, behavioral training or pharmacological interventions that prevent maladaptive memory formation or enhance extinction.

References

[1] Price DD, Verne GN, Schwartz JM. Plasticity in brain processing and modulation of pain. Prog Brain Res 2006;157:333-52.
[2] Elbert T, Flor H, Birbaumer N, et al. Extensive reorganization of the somatosensory cortex in adult humans after nervous system injury. NeuroReport 1994;5:2593-7.
[3] Yang TT, Gallen C, Ramachandran V, et al. Magnetoencephalographic evidence for massive cortical reorganization in the adult human somatosensory system. Nature 1994;368:592-3.
[4] Flor H, Elbert T, Knecht S, et al. Phantom limb pain as a perceptual correlate of massive cortical reorganization in upper extremity amputees. Nature 1995;357:482-4.
[5] Cohen LG, Bandinelli S, Findley TW, et al. Motor reorganization after upper limb amputation in man. Brain 1991;114:615-27.
[6] Kew JJ, Ridding MC, Rothwell JC, et al. Reorganization of cortical blood flow and transcranial magnetic stimulation maps in human subjects after upper limb amputation. J Neurophysiol 1994;72:2517-24.
[7] Karl A, Birbaumer N, Lutzenberger W, et al. Reorganization of motor and somatosensory cortex in upper extremity amputees with phantom limb pain. J Neurosci 2001;21:3609-18.
[8] Lotze M, Flor H, Grodd W, et al. Phantom movements and pain: An fMRI study in upper limb amputees. Brain 2001;2268-77.
[9] Borsook D, Becerra L, Fishman S, Edwards A, Jennings CL, Stojanovic M, et al. Acute plasticity in the human somatosensory cortex following amputation. Neuroreport 1998;9:1013-7.
[10] Hunter JP, Katz J, Davis KD. Stability of phantom limb phenomena after upper limb amputation: A longitudinal study. Neuroscience 2008;156:939-49.
[11] Juottonen K, Gockel M, Silen T, et al. Altered central sensorimotor processing in patients with complex regional pain syndrome. Pain 2002;98:315-23.
[12] Pleger B, Ragert P, Schwenkreis P, Forster AF, Wilimzig C, Dinse H, et al. Patterns of cortical reorganization parallel impaired tactile discrimination and pain intensity in complex regional pain syndrome. Neuroimage 2006;32:503-10.
[13] Pleger B, Tegenthoff M, Ragert P, et al. Sensorimotor retuning in complex regional pain syndrome parallels pain reduction. Ann Neurol 2005;57:425-429.
[14] Maihofner C, Handwerker HO, Neundorfer B, et al. Patterns of cortical reorganization in complex regional pain syndrome. Neurology 2003;61:1717-25.
[15] Maihöfner C, Handwerker HO, Birklein F. Functional imaging of allodynia in complex regional pain syndrome. Neurology 2006;66:711–7.
[16] Maihöfner CCA, Handwerker HO, Neundorfer B, et al. Cortical reorganization during recovery from complex regional pain syndrome. Neurology 2004;63:693-701.
[17] Schwenkreis P, Maier C, Tegenthoff M. Motor cortex disinhibition in complex regional pain syndrome (CRPS)-a unilateral or bilateral phenomenon? Pain 2005;115:219-20.
[18] Larbig W, Montoya P, Flor H, et al. Evidence for a change in neural processing in phantom limb pain patients. Pain 1996;67:275-83.
[19] Karl A, Diers M, Flor H. P300-amplitudes in upper limb amputees with and without phantom limb pain in a visual oddball paradigm. Pain 2004;110:40-8.
[20] Krause P, Foerderreuther S, Straube A. Bilateral motor cortex disinhibition in complex regional pain syndrome (CRPS) type I of the hand. Neurology 2004;62:1654-5.

[21] Eisenberg E, Chistyakov AV, Yudashkin M, et al. Evidence for cortical hyperexcitability of the affected limb representation area in CRPS: a psychophysical and transcranial magnetic stimulation study. Pain 2005;113:99-105.
[22] Hall EJ, Flament D, Fraser C, et al. Non-invasive brain stimulation reveals reorganized cortical outputs in amputees. Neurosci Lett 1990;116:379-86.
[23] Tinazzi M, Valeriani M, Moretto G, et al. Plastic interactions between hand and face cortical representations in patients with trigeminal neuralgia: a somatosensory-evoked potentials study. Neurosci 2004;127:769-76.
[24] Becerra L, Morris S, Bazes S, et al. Trigeminal neuropathic pain alters responses in CNS circuits to mechanical (brush) and thermal (cold and heat) stimuli. J Neurosci 2006;26:10646-57.
[25] Apkarian AV, Baliki MN, Geha PY. Towards a theory of chronic pain. Prog Neurobiol 2009;87:81-97.
[26] Witting N, Kupers RC, Svensson P, et al. A PET activation study of brush-evoked allodynia in patients with nerve injury pain. Pain 2006;120:145-54.
[27] Schweinhardt P, Glynn C, Brooks J, et al. An fMRI study of cerebral processing of brush-evoked allodynia in neuropathic pain patients. Neuroimage 2006;32:256-65.
[28] Willoch F, Rosen G, Tolle TR, et al. Phantom limb pain in the human brain: unraveling neural circuitries of phantom limb sensations using positron emission tomography. Ann Neurol 2000;48:842-9.
[29] Baliki MN, Chialvo DR, Geha PY, et al. Chronic pain and the emotional brain: specific brain activity associated with spontaneous fluctuations of intensity of chronic back pain. J Neurosci 2006;26:12165-73.
[30] Seifert F, Maihofner C. Central mechanisms of experimental and chronic neuropathic pain: findings from functional imaging studies. Cell Mol Life Sci 2009;66:375-90.
[31] DaSilva AF, Becerra L, Pendse G, Chizh B, Tully S, Borsook D. Colocalized structural and functional changes in the cortex of patients with trigeminal neuropathic pain. PLoS ONE 2008;3:e3396.
[32] Cauda F, Sacco K, Duca S, Cocito D, D'Agata F, Geminiani GC, et al. Altered resting state in diabetic neuropathic pain. PLoS ONE 2009;4:e4542.
[33] Flor H, Braun C, Elbert T, et al. Extensive reorganization of primary somatosensory cortex in chronic back pain patients. Neurosci Lett 1997;224:5-8.
[34] Giesecke T, Gracely RH, Grant MA, et al. Evidence of augmented central pain processing in idiopathic chronic low back pain. Arthritis Rheum 2004;50:613-23.
[35] Tsao H, Galea MP, Hodges PW. Reorganization of the motor cortex is associated with postural control deficits in recurrent low back pain. Brain 2008;131:2161-71.
[36] Gracely RH, Petzke F, Wolf JM, et al. Functional magnetic resonance imaging evidence of augmented pain processing in fibromyalgia. Arthritis Rheum 2002;46:1333-43.
[37] Burgmer M, Pogatzki-Zahn E, Gaubitz M, Wessoleck E, Heuft G, Pfleiderer B. Altered brain activity during pain processing in fibromyalgia. Neuroimage 2009;44:502-8.
[38] Staud R, Spaeth M. Psychophysical and neurochemical abnormalities of pain processing in fibromyalgia. CNS Spectr 2008;13:12-7.
[39] Churchill JD, Tharp JA, Wellman CL, et al. Morphological correlates of injury-induced reorganization in primate somatosensory cortex. BMC Neurosci 2004;5:43.
[40] Kaas JH. Plasticity of sensory and motor maps in adult mammals. Annu Rev Neurosci 1991;14:137-67.
[41] Kaas JH, Florence SL. Mechanisms of reorganization in sensory systems of primates after peripheral nerve injury. Adv Neurol 1997;73:147-58.
[42] Ziemann U, Lonnecker S, Steinhoff BJ, et al. The effect of lorazepam on the motor cortical excitability in man. Exp Brain Res 1996;109:127-35.
[43] Ziemann U, Rothwell JC, Ridding MC. Interaction between intracortical inhibition and facilitation in human motor cortex. J Physiol 1996;496:873-81.

[44] Chen R, Cohen LG, Hallett M. Nervous system reorganization following injury. Neuroscience 2002;111:761-73.
[45] Waxman SG, Hains BC. Fire and phantoms after spinal cord injury: Na(+) channels and central pain. Trends Neurosci 2006;29:207-15.
[46] Draganski B, Moser T, Lummel N, et al. Decrease of thalamic gray matter following limb amputation. Neuroimage 2006;31:951-7.
[47] Grachev ID, Fredrickson BE, Apkarian AV. Abnormal brain chemistry in chronic back pain: an in vivo proton magnetic resonance spectroscopy study. Pain 2000;89:7-18.
[48] Grachev ID, Thomas PS, Ramachandran TS. Decreased levels of N-acetyl aspartate in dorsolateral prefrontal cortex in a case of intractable severe sympathetically mediated chronic pain (complex regional pain syndrome, type I). Brain Cogn 2002;49:102-13.
[49] Birbaumer N, Lutzenberger W, Montoya P, et al. Effects of regional anesthesia on phantom limb pain are mirrored in changes in cortical reorganization. J Neurosci 1997;17:5503-8.
[50] Erskine A, Morley S, Pearce S. Memory for pain: a review. Pain 1990;41:255-65.
[51] Flor H. Maladaptive plasticity, memory for pain and phantom limb pain: review and suggestions for new therapies. Expert Rev Neurother 2008;8:809-8
[52] Flor H, Knost B, Birbaumer N. The role of operant conditioning in chronic pain: an experimental investigation. Pain 2002;95:111-8.
[53] Becker S, Kleinbohl D, Klossika I, Holzl R. Operant conditioning of enhanced pain sensitivity by heat-pain titration. Pain 2008;140:104-14.
[54] Schneider C, Palomba D, Flor H. Pavlovian conditioning of muscular responses in chronic pain patients: central and peripheral correlates. Pain 2004;112:239-47.
[55] Diesch E, Flor H. Alteration in the response properties of primary somatosensory cortex related to differential aversive Pavlovian conditioning. Pain 2007;131:171-80.
[56] Albanese MC, Duerden EG, Rainville P, et al. Memory traces of pain in human cortex. J Neurosci 2007;27:4612-20.
[57] Kleinbohl D, Holzl R, Moltner A, Rommel C, Weber C, Osswald PM. Psychophysical measures of sensitization to tonic heat discriminate chronic pain patients. Pain 1999;81:35-43.
[58] Staud R, Craggs JG, Perlstein WM, Robinson ME, Price DD. Brain activity associated with slow temporal summation of C-fiber evoked pain in fibromyalgia patients and healthy controls. Eur J Pain 2008;12:1078-89.
[59] Avenanti A, Bueti D, Galati G, Aglioti SM. Transcranial magnetic stimulation highlights the sensorimotor side of empathy for pain. Nat Neurosci 2005;8:955-60.
[60] Luerding R, Weigand T, Bogdahn U, Schmidt-Wilcke T. Working memory performance is correlated with local brain morphology in the medial frontal and anterior cingulate cortex in fibromyalgia patients: structural correlates of pain-cognition interaction. Brain 2008;131:3222-31.
[61] Flor H. Maladaptive plasticity, memory for pain and phantom limb pain: review and suggestions for new therapies. Expert Rev Neurother 2008;8:809-18.
[62] Ressler KJ, Rothbaum BO, Tannenbaum L, et al. Cognitive enhancers as adjuncts to psychotherapy: use of D-cycloserine in phobic individuals to facilitate extinction of fear. Arch Gen Psychiatry 2004;61:1136-44.
[63] Hofmann SG, Pollack MH, Otto MW. Augmentation treatment of psychotherapy for anxiety disorders with D-cycloserine. CNS Drug Rev 2006;12:208-17.
[64] Marsicano G, Wotjak CT, Azad SC, et al. The endogenous cannabinoid system controls extinction of aversive memories. Nature 2002;418:530-4.
[65] Wotjak CT. Role of endogenous cannabinoids in cognition and emotionality. Mini Rev Med Chem 2005 Jul;5:659-70.
[66] Dworkin RH, Turk DC, Farrar JT, Haythornthwaite JA, Jensen MP, Katz NP, et al. Core outcome measures for chronic pain clinical trials: IMMPACT recommendations. Pain 2005;113:9-19.

In: Pain Management Yearbook 2009
Editor: Joav Merrick

ISBN: 978-1-61209-666-7
©2012 Nova Science Publishers, Inc.

Chapter 24

INTRODUCTION TO ELECTROTHERAPY TECHNOLOGY

Marom Bikson[*], PhD, Abhishek Datta, MS, Maged Elwassif, MS, Varun Bansal and Angel V Peterchev, PhD

Department of Biomedical Engineering, City College of New York of CUNY, New York and Division of Brain Stimulation and Therapeutic Modulation, Department of Psychiatry, Columbia University, New York, United States of America

Abstract

Electrotherapy involves electric or magnetic stimulation of the human body in a range of therapeutic applications including pain alleviation. A wide spectrum of electrotherapy paradigms have been deployed in pain treatment, illustrating the inherent flexibility of this technology, but also the fundamental challenge of determining an optimal strategy. The effective and safe application of electrotherapy requires an understanding of the basic components of electrotherapy technology, as well as how to control electrotherapy dose. These topics are introduced in this review, along with related comments on the general mechanisms of electrotherapy, as well as an overview of various electrotherapy paradigms.

Keywords: Electrotherapy, pain, functional electrical stimulation, electrical, magnetic, stimulation, magnetotherapy.

---

[*] **Correspondence:** Marom Bikson, PhD, Department of Biomedical Engineering, City College of New York of CUNY, T-403B Steinman Hall, 160 Convent Avenue, New York, NY 10031 United States. Tel: 212-650-6791; Fax: 212-650-6727; E-mail: bikson@ccny.cuny.edu

Introduction

Electrotherapy is the application of electricity to the human body for therapeutic purposes, including the alleviation of acute or chronic pain states. Here we briefly introduce the basic technology of electrotherapy, as it relates to practical decisions made by clinicians in determining a therapeutic strategy. A basic understanding of electrotherapy technology must inform effective and safe clinical treatment, and is therefore important for all practitioners of electrotherapy.

Electrotherapy device components

It is convenient to understand electrotherapy devices, including implanted and non-invasive (surface) devices, as made out of only two distinct functional components with additional support accessories. The first functional component is the stimulator device which generates the electrical signal. What electrical signal is generated is selectable by the operator from a set provided by the manufacturer. How this electrical signal changes over time is called the waveform of the electrical signal and can be described by features such as pulse shape, width, amplitude, polarity and frequency. The second functional component of electrotherapy devices are the electrodes. An electrode is where the metal conductor contacts the tissue or skin; for skin stimulation a sponge or gel may be placed between the metal and skin. At the electrodes, the electrical signal generated by the stimulator enters and then exits the body; for this reason there must always be at least two electrodes. The user positions the electrodes near the direct target of stimulation. For implanted devices, the stimulator device casing can serve as one electrode.

Whereas for non-invasive devices the stimulation waveform is adjusted by controls (e.g., knobs or keyboard) directly on the stimulator device, for implanted stimulation systems a telemetry system is used to adjust the stimulation waveform. Some devices use measurements from sensors, such as electrical potential recordings, to change stimulation waveform in real time using automatic feedback control.

Most electrical stimulator devices are either voltage-controlled or current-controlled. In a voltage-controlled device, the user specifies peak device output in units of volts, and the voltage output waveform of the device is regulated. For current-controlled devices, the user specifies peak device output in units of amperes, and the current output waveform of the device is regulated. However, all stimulators output both a voltage and a current. For example, a current-controlled device changes its output voltage to achieve a desired current level. Finally, it should be noted that the voltage and current waveforms do *not* necessarily have the same shape, due to capacitive behavior of tissues and the electrode-tissue interface (1).

For magnetic stimulation, the electrodes are replaced with coils that are positioned on the body over the direct target. It appears that pulsed magnetic fields are not therapeutic in themselves, but rather, the magnetic fields produce tissue stimulation by inducing electrical currents in the body. Therefore, we consider electrotherapy inclusive of pulsed magnetic therapy. Analogously to electrical stimulation, in magnetic therapy, the electrical signal generated by the stimulator determines the waveform of the electrical currents in the body.

However, unlike electrical stimulation, in magnetic stimulation there is no current entering or exiting the body. Rather, the electric currents induced by the magnetic field circulate within the body.

Additional hardware of electrotherapy devices can be considered accessories which largely serve mechanical and safety purposes rather than directly determine therapeutic efficacy. For example, for convenience the stimulator is often at some distance from the electrodes or magnetic coil, therefore insulated wires connect the stimulator to the electrodes/coil. The non-conducting mechanical support around implanted electrodes is referred to as leads. Surface electrodes accessories may include some form of position support (adhesive, cap, or straps). For high intensity TMS, accessories such as air compressors, and water or oil circulation systems are used to cool the coil. Still additional accessories are used to position electrodes during implantation or around the cranium, as well as calibrate device output. Finally, all electrotherapy devices need a power source such as a battery or a line-connected power supply.

Electrotherapy paradigm classification

A number of electrotherapy devices and paradigms have been introduced over the years and given names that are generally descriptive of the electrode or coil positions and/or the stimulation waveforms. Some examples of electrotherapy paradigms for cranial stimulation are illustrated in figure 1. For instance, Transcutaneous Electrical Nerve Stimulation (TENS) refers to electrical therapy with superficial skin electrodes placed anywhere on the body including the cranium, with stimulation signals of repeated pulses (2-4). Electroacupuncture is similar to TENS, but uses needle electrodes that penetrate the skin (5). If one or more electrodes, or the stimulating coil, is placed on the head to target the brain, the stimulation paradigm is typically referred to as "transcranial" or "cranial", such as in Transcranial Electrical Stimulation (TES) (6-8). For example, transcranial Direct Current Stimulation (tDCS) employs superficial skin electrodes, with at least one placed on the cranium and stimulation signal that is direct current (DC) (9-, 11). The same electrode configurations can be used with alternating currents—transcranial alternating current stimulation (tACS) (12). Similarly, Cranial Electrical (or Electrotherapy) Stimulation (CES) uses superficial cranial electrodes, but the stimulation signals are square waves modulated at various frequencies (13). High-density Transcanial Electrical Stimulation (HD-TES) incorporates arrays of surface cranial electrodes to increase focality (14). High-density transcanial Direct Current Stimulation (HD-tDCS) similarly employs arrays of cranial electrodes and use DC current.

For more targeted and chronic stimulation, the electrodes can be implanted intracranially. For example, Deep Brain Stimulation (DBS) employs electrodes implanted proximal to deep brain structures and stimulation with pulse trains (15). A less invasive form of intracranial stimulation uses epidural or subdural electrodes to stimulate a specific superficial cortical area such as motor cortex (e.g., epidural cortical stimulation (ECS), motor cortex stimulation (MCS)) (16-18). Implanted electrodes can also be used for chronic extracranial nerve stimulation. For example, Vagus Nerve Stimulation (VNS) and Spinal Cord Stimulation (SCS) involve chronic stimulation with electrodes implanted around the vagus nerve and the spinal cord, respectively (19-22).

Finally, electrical stimulation can also be induced by pulsed magnetic fields. Transcranial Magnetic Stimulation (TMS) encompasses treatments using a magnetic stimulation coil placed over the head inducing brief electrical current pulses in the brain (6,18). Therapeutic TMS applications typically apply stimulation with pulse trains (repetitive TMS (rTMS)). Low-frequency rTMS is administered in continuous trains at 0.2-1 Hz, whereas high-frequency rTMS is administered as intermittent pulse trains of 5-20 Hz (18). A number of novel TMS paradigms that aim to increase the neuromodulatory effectiveness and selectivity of rTMS have been introduced recently, including theta burst stimulation (TBS), repetitive monophasic pulse stimulation, paired- and quadri-pulse stimulation, paired associative stimulation, controllable pulse shape TMS (cTMS), and deep-brain TMS (12).

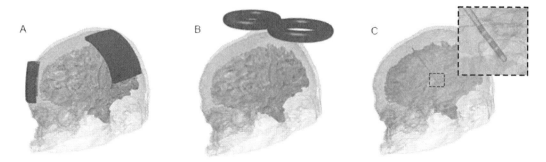

Figure 1. Illustration of some brain stimulation paradigms. Stimulation with surface electrodes is called transcutaneous stimulation. When the electrodes are placed on the scalp to target the brain, the paradigm is referred to as cranial or transcranial stimulation (A). Magnetic stimulation employs coils of wire wound in specific patterns (e.g., "figure of 8"). When the coil is positioned on the head, the paradigm is called Transcranial Magnetic Simulation (TMS) (B). Electrotherapies using implanted electrodes are generally classified by the target anatomical structure near the electrodes such as Spinal Chord Stimulation, Vagus Nerve Stimulation, or Deep Brain Stimulation (C).

The above examples indicate that the electrotherapy paradigm classification usually involves a description of the electrodes/coil position and/or the stimulation signal generated. It should be emphasized that each of these classifications typically covers a wide parameter set. For example, TENS encompasses a range of stimulation amplitudes and frequencies (4,23). Moreover, simply because two distinct electrotherapies fall under the same umbrella classification does not mean that those therapies share a common mechanism of action or therapeutic outcome. This point is particularly important from the perspective of controlling and reproducing electrotherapy dose. For example, the fact that two medical devices share the same label (e.g., TENS) does not mean that they generate stimulation with identical parameters. Therefore, indicating only the therapy classification (e.g., TENS) in a report does not provide enough information for the therapy to be reproduced. Rather, it is necessary to fully account for and report the electrode or coil type and positions, and the stimulator waveform parameters (pulse shape, width, amplitude, polarity, frequency, train duration, etc.). Typically, the stimulation paradigm can be fully described by providing the manufacturer name and a unique model or part number (P/N) of the stimulator device and the electrodes or coil, as well as the settings of the user-selectable stimulation parameters used in the treatment.

In summary, from the perspective of therapeutic efficacy, what makes each electrical therapy different is 1) the waveform generated by the stimulator, and 2) the electrodes/coil type and location. Thus, when considering an appropriate electrical therapy, the decisions that a clinician must make can be conceptually reduced to selecting electrode/coil types and positions, and the stimulation waveform (24). The former can be conceived of as spatial targeting of the stimulation, whereas the latter amounts to controlling the magnitude and waveform of the stimulation.

Rational electrotherapy design

The combination of electrode/coil type and positions, and stimulator output waveform determine electrotherapy dose. Clinicians must integrate both factors together in determining an electrotherapy strategy, however, it is also useful to conceptually consider each independently. As emphasized above, clinicians must fully account for and report stimulation dose for therapies to be reproducible (24). When stimulation is administered repeatedly, the dose may change between sessions, for example, as the clinician optimizes stimulation parameters. Any changes of the electrotherapy dose during the course of treatment should be accounted for and reported as well.

The decision of where to place the electrodes or the coil is pivotal to electrotherapy outcome. Neuronal tissue near the electrodes/coil will be preferentially directly activated by stimulation. When considering the focality of electrical stimulation, to a first approximation, one can picture current entering the tissue at one electrode and travelling in a diffuse line toward the other electrode. Thus, the further apart the electrodes are, the longer and more diffuse the tissue region of current flow is. This is one reason why two closely implanted electrodes may generate more focal stimulation, compared to two surface electrodes on opposite sides of the head. For magnetic stimulation, the induced electrical currents follow roughly the shape of the stimulation coil. For example, a circular TMS coil will induce circular currents under the circumference of the coil. In this manner, one can grossly estimate where in the brain or peripheral nerves the current will flow, based on electrode/coil type and position.

There has been a continued effort to make the spatial targeting and dosing of stimulation paradigms more precise. For example, DBS electrodes are implanted using stereotactic guidance systems (25) and TMS applications are increasingly adopting stereotactic coil positioning based on individual MRI and fMRI scans (26). Further, recent technical innovations in stimulation hardware are aiming to improve spatial targeting as well. For example the use of "ring" electrode configurations in High-Density Transcranial Electrical Stimulation is intended to enhance the focality of non-invasive cortical stimulation (27). Finally, setting of stimulation intensity relative to the subject's response threshold is frequently used to individualize the treatment dose, exemplified by the rTMS dose adjustment relative to the motor evoked potential (MEP) threshold (28).

The region of the brain or the peripheral nervous system where the stimulation current is flowing is directly affected by the electricity. The cells in the targeted region will be exposed to electricity and as a result their function may change. The waveform of the electrical currents experienced by the cells depends on the waveform generated by the stimulator. The decision of what waveform to apply is complicated for a number of interrelated reasons. First, the ability to design rational electrotherapies is limited by our incomplete understanding of brain function and the mechanisms leading to pathology. Second, the interaction of electricity with neural tissue is complex. Third, there is a very large set of possible stimulation paradigms, thus empirical determination of an optimal configuration for a particular application is daunting. Finally, inter-individual and intra-individual variability of response to stimulation often precludes effective use of a standard stimulation configuration in all patients, requiring steps to individualize the treatment.

Regions of the brain that are functionally connected to the direct target of stimulation may be indirectly modulated by electrical and magnetic stimulation. For example, cortical stimulation may activate, inhibit, or otherwise modulate activity of various cortico-subcortical networks (18). Electrotherapies with direct targets in the peripheral nervous system, such as VNS, are particularly based on indirect actions.

The cells in the nervous system (neurons) use electrical signals to process and transmit information. Because the nervous system is an electrical organ, it is sensitive to electricity. At the cellular level, the effect of applied electricity can be considered on three inter-related scales (see figure 2). First, the stimulating electrical currents may change the electrical state of the neurons (e.g., triggering of action potentials or blocking of firing). Second, changes in neuronal electrical state may lead to changes in neuromodulator or neurotransmitter activity (e.g., endogenous opioids and GABA). Third, the electrical activity on a network of neurons may be concomitantly altered (e.g., brain oscillations and gate control). To be therapeutically relevant, these electrical and chemical changes at cellular and network level must manifest as changes in behavior and/or cognition. Various basic cellular mechanisms of electrical stimulation have been elucidated (1,29-32), however, relating cellular modulation to behavioral or cognitive changes remains a fundamental challenge. As a result, clinical determination of electrotherapy dose is currently driven largely by empirical considerations and patient-specific titration.

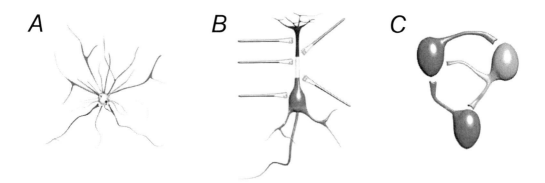

Figure 2. Schematic of the various levels of neural modulation induced by electrical stimulation. A) Individual neurons process information through changes in trans-membrane electrical potentials, including action potentials in axons. Applied electrical stimulation will modulate the electrical properties of single cells. B) Neuronal communication at synapses is itself an electrically driven phenomenon which will be modulated by applied electricity. C) Groups of neurons organize in neuronal networks which often generate coherent electrical signals such as electric fields oscillations (e.g. gamma oscillations). This network electrical activity may be modulated by applied electricity. The effects of applied electricity on single neurons, neurotransmitters, and neuronal networks can be quantified with biomarkers and in animal studies. However, relating these cellular and network level changes to complex behavioral and cognitive outcomes remains a fundamental challenge toward developing rational electrotherapy paradigms.

Due to the complexity and heterogeneity of strategies for empirical determination of electrotherapy dose, we limit ourselves to some general cautions here. First, the therapeutic/behavioral outcome of electrotherapy is not necessarily a monotonic function of any waveform parameter. For example, increasing stimulation frequency may first increase efficacy while further frequency increase may reduce efficacy. Nor is it necessarily possible to optimize each waveform parameter independently. For example, at stimulation frequency X the optimal amplitude may be determined as A, but at frequency Y the optimal amplitude may be B. Further, it is important to distinguish the acute (during stimulation) and plastic (lasting after stimulation) outcomes of stimulation. It is not necessarily the case that an electrotherapy optimized for acute changes will be similarly effective for plastic change, and vice versa.

Inter-individual variability relates to difference in anatomy, physiology, and disease etiology across individuals that may fundamentally affect stimulation outcomes. For example, pain can arise from a myriad of tissues and be transmitted through distinct neurological pathways. Because of inter-individual variability, the same stimulation dose applied to two patients may have fundamentally different outcomes (33,34). Intra-individual variability relates to the dependence of electrotherapy on the current physiological state on the patient, including physical and mental states. For this reason, it may be necessary to adjust dose for the same patient across sessions or as the patient's response to stimulation changes.

For practitioners optimizing electrotherapy dose, there is generally a large set of possible parameter settings within the limits of each commercial device, in combination with an infinite set of possible electrode and coil positions. This flexibility should not be viewed as a limitation of electrotherapy, compared to, for example, pharmacological approaches where dosing is limited to far fewer parameters. The ability to change stimulation parameters (e.g., by the turn of a knob) and then iteratively optimize therapy in a patient-specific manner is a fundamental advantage of electrotherapy.

Safety of electrotherapy

As with any therapeutic approach, in selecting electrotherapy technology and dose, safety and efficacy considerations must often be balanced. For example, the use of implanted electrodes allows focal stimulation of regions inaccessible with surface electrodes, but is associated with potential surgical complications. Surface electrodes and coils are non-invasive, but are at some distance from the target, resulting in less focal stimulation that could induce unintended modulation of regions around the target.

In the context of waveform selection, commercial stimulation devices generally add safety features such as the limitations of stimulation intensity, ramping on/off of stimulation intensity, or automatic waveform controls such as the use of charge-balanced pulses. These limits are generally predetermined by the manufacturer and are not necessarily apparent to the clinician programming the device. However, even though automatic waveform changes may not be transparent to the clinician, they may still impact efficacy.

Electrotherapy within safety guidelines established by clinicians and manufacturers is generally well tolerated in the majority of patients (28,35). None-the-less, fundamental unknowns about the reaction of tissue to electrical stimulation, combined with the desire by clinicians to explore new stimulation targets and protocols, warrants continued vigilance on the part of clinicians and researchers. There are specific safety concerns for each technology. For example, seizure risk is the major safety concern in rTMS (28). On the other hand, electrochemical damage is not a factor in TMS, whereas it is of paramount concern for stimulation with implanted electrodes. Moreover, there are distinct safety concerns for voltage-controlled and current-controlled stimulation (1). Both potential tissue damage, and cognitive or behavioral changes induced by stimulation need to be addressed for each stimulation technology and dose. Even for FDA approved treatments (and especially for technologies that are "grandfathered" without FDA evaluation), there are lingering and emerging concerns about potential damage of tissue during normal operation and under unexpected conditions (36,37).

Conclusions

Electric and magnetic stimulation (electrotherapy) can confer therapeutic benefit by inducing electrical currents in neural tissue. Electrotherapy paradigms can be conceptually reduced to two functional components: 1) electrode or coil type and position, and 2) stimulation waveform. Stimulation paradigms are often classified based on the electrode/coil location and/or waveform parameters. For each electrotherapy technology, there is a balance of efficacy and safety factors. Basic knowledge of the biophysics of neural stimulation is necessary for rational determination of electrotherapy dose, however, the present lack of full understanding of the mechanisms of electrotherapy necessitates empirical optimization of treatment dose. For this reason, we expect that the full potential of electrotherapy has yet to be realized. Basic research on the mechanisms of electrotherapy may thus manifestly improve electrotherapy outcomes. For specialized discussion on these issues we refer the reader to more specialized literature reviews (6,28,38) and to the articles in this issue.

Acknowledgments

This work was supported in part by NIH (41341-03, 41595-00), PSC-CUNY, and the Andrew Grove Foundation.

References

[1] Merrill DR, Bikson M, Jefferys JG. Electrical stimulation of excitable tissue: design of efficacious and safe protocols. J Neurosci Methods 2005;141:171-98.
[2] Nolan M F. Selected problems in the use of transcutaneous electrical nerve stimulation for pain control: An appraisal with proposed solutions. A special communication. Phys Ther 1988;68:1694-8.
[3] Milne S, Welch V, Brosseau L, Saginur M, Shea B, Tugwell P, et al. Transcutaneous electrical nerve stimulation (TENS) for chronic low back pain. Cochrane Data Base Syst Rev 2001;2:CD003008.

[4] Sluka KA, Walsh D. Transcutaneous electrical nerve stimulation: Basic science mechanisms and clinical effectiveness. J Pain 2003;4:109-21.
[5] Ulett GA, Han S, Han JS. Electroacupuncture: mechanisms and clinical application. Biol Psychiatry 1998;44(2):129-38.
[6] Rosen AC, Ramkumar M, Nguyen T, Hoeft F. Noninvasive transcranial brain stimulation and pain. Curr Pain Headache Rep 2009;13(1):12-7.
[7] Nekhendzy V, Fender CP, Davies MF, Lemmens HJ, Kim MS, Bouley DM, et al. The antinociceptive effect of transcranial electrostimulation with combined direct and alternating current in freely moving rats. Anesth Analg 2004;98(3):730-7.
[8] Marshall L, Helgadottir H, Molle M, Born J. Boosting slow oscillations during sleep potentiates memory. Nature 2006;444(7119):610-3.
[9] Nitsche MA, Paulus W. Excitability changes induced in the human motor cortex by weak transcranial direct current stimulation. J Physiol 2000;527:633-9.
[10] Fregni F, Boggio PS, Lima MC, Ferreira MJ, Wagner T, Rigonatti S P,et al. A sham-controlled, phase II trial of transcranial direct current stimulation for the treatment of central pain in traumatic spinal cord injury.Pain 2006;122:197-209.
[11] Priori A, Berardelli A, Rona S, Accornero N, Manfredi M. Polarization of the human motor cortex through the scalp. NeuroReport 1998;9:2257-60.
[12] Huang Y-Z, Sommer M, Thickbroom G, Hamada M, Pascual-Leone A, Paulus W, et al. Consensus:New Methodologies for brain stimulation. Brain Stimulation 2009;2:2-13.
[13] Schroeder MJ, Barr RE. Quantitative analysis of the electroencephalogram during cranial electrotherapy stimulation. Clin Neurophysiol 2001;112:2075-83.
[14] Datta A, Elwassif M, Battaglia F, Bikson M. Transcranial current focality using disc and ring electrode configurations:FEM analysis. J Neural Eng 2008;5:163-74.
[15] Kim HJ, Paek SH, Kim JY, Lee JY, Lim YH, Kim MR, et al. Chronic subthalamic deep brain stimulation improves pain in Parkinson disease. J Neurol 2008;255:1889-94.
[16] Henderson JM, Lad SP. Motor cortex stimulation and neuropathic facial pain. Neurosurg Focus 2006;21(6):E6.
[17] Canavero S, Bonicalzi V. Extradural cortical stimulation for central pain. Acta Neurochir Suppl 2007;97(2):27-36.
[18] Lefaucheur JP. Principles of therapeutic use of transcranial and epidural cortical stimulation. Clin Neurophysiol. 2008;119(10):2179-84.
[19] Cook AW, Weinstein SP. Chronic dorsal column stimulation in multiple sclerosis; preliminary report. NY State J Med 1973;73: 2868-72.
[20] Turner JA, Loeser JD, Bell KG. Spinal cord stimulation for chronic low back pain: A systematic literature synthesis. Neurosurgery 1995;37:1088-96.
[21] Meyerson BA, Linderoth B. Mechanisms of spinal cord stimulation in neuropathic pain. Neurol Res 2000;22:285-92.
[22] Multon S, Schoenen J. Pain control by vagus nerve stimulation: from animal to man...and back. Acta Neurol Belg. 2005;105(2):62-7.
[23] Wolf SL, Gersh MR, Rao VR. Examination of electrode placements and stimulating parameters in treating chronic pain with conventional transcutaneous electrical nerve stimulation (TENS). Pain 1981;11:37-47.
[24] Bikson M, Bulow P, Stiller JW, et al. Transcranial direct current stimulation for major depression: a general system for quantifying transcranial electrotherapy dosage. Curr Treat Options Neurol 2008; 10(5):377-385.
[25] Miocinovic S, Zhang J, Xu W, Russo GS, Vitek JL, McIntyre CC. Stereotactic neurosurgical planning,recording, and visualization for deep brain stimulation in non-human primates. J Neurosci Methods 2007;162:32-41.

[26] Neggers SF, Langerak TR, Schutter DJ, Mandl RC, Ramsey NF, Lemmens PJ, et al. A stereotactic method for image-guided transcranial magnetic stimulation validated with fMRI and motor-evoked potentials. Neuroimage. 2004;21(4):1805-17.
[27] Datta A, Bansal V, Diaz J, Patel J, Reato D, Bikson M. Gyri-precise head model of transcranial DC stimulation:Improved spatial focality using a ring electrode versus conventional rectangular pad. Brain Stimulation, in press.
[28] Wassermann EM. Risk and safety of repetitive transcranial magnetic stimulation: report and suggested guidelines from the International Workshop on the Safety of Repetitive Transcranial Magnetic Stimulation, June 5-7, 1996. Electroencephalogr Clin Neurophysiol. 1998;108(1):1-16.
[29] Moffitt MA, McIntyre CC, Grill WM. Prediction of myelinated nerve fiber stimulation thresholds:limitations of linear models. IEEE Trans Biomed Eng 2004;51:229-36.
[30] Bikson M, Durand D. Suppression and control of epileptiform acticity by electrical stimulation: A review Proceedings of the IEEE 2001;89:1065-82.
[31] Bikson M, Inoue M, Akiyama H, Deans JK, Fox JE, Miyakawa H, et al. Effects of uniform extracellular DC electric fields on excitability in rat hippocampal slices in vitro. J Physiol 2004;557:175-90.
[32] Holsheimer J. Computer modelling of spinal cord stimulation and its contribution to therapeutic efficacy. Spinal Cord 1998;36(8):531-40.
[33] Mannheimer JS.Electrode placements for transcutaneous electrical nerve stimulation. Phys Ther 1978;58:1455-62.
[34] Murphy DG, DeCarli C, Schapiro MB, Rapoport SI, Horwitz B. Age-related differences in volumes of subcortical nuclei, brain matter, and cerebrospinal fluid in healthy men as measured with magnetic resonance imaging. Arch Neurol 1992;49(8):839-45.
[35] Nitsche MA, Liebetanz D, Lang N, Antal A, Tergau F, Paulus W. Safety criteria for transcranial direct current stimulation (tDCS) in humans. Clin Neurophysiol 2003;114:2220-2.
[36] Datta A, Tarbell JM, Bikson M. Electroporation of endothelial cells by high frequency electric fields:implications for DBS. Bioengineering Conference 2007, NEBC'07. IEEE 33RD Annual Northeast, 2007:138-9.
[37] Elwassif MM, Kong Q, Vasquez M, Bikson M. Bio-heat transfer model of deep brain stimulation-induced temperature changes. J Neural Eng 2006;3:306-15.
[38] Wagner T, Valero-Cabre A, Pascual-Leone A. Noninvasive human brain stimulation. Annu Rev Biomed Eng. 2007;9:527-65.

In: Pain Management Yearbook 2009
Editor: Joav Merrick

ISBN: 978-1-61209-666-7
©2012 Nova Science Publishers, Inc.

Chapter 25

PRINCIPLES AND MECHANISMS OF TRANSCRANIAL MAGNETIC STIMULATION

Monica A Perez, PT, PhD[*1] *and Leonardo G Cohen, MD*[2]

[1]University of Pittsburgh, Department of Physical Medicine and Rehabilitation, Center for the Neural Basis of Cognition, Pittsburgh, Pennsylvania and [2]Human Cortical Physiology and Stroke Neurorehabilitation Section, NINDS, NIH, Bethesda, Maryland, United States of America

Abstract

More than 20 years ago transcranial magnetic stimulation (TMS) was introduced as a non-invasive method to stimulate the brain of intact conscious human subjects painlessly through the scalp. Since then, an increasing number of studies in the field of motor control have used TMS to gain understanding on different aspects of human cortical physiology. In this review we will discuss the mechanisms by which TMS excites cortical neurons and the available evidence on which neuronal elements are excited by TMS, the electrophysiological markers of motor cortical function that can be examined by TMS and the role of TMS in the study of brain plasticity and motor learning.

Keywords: Motor control, primary motor cortex, motor evoked potentials, plasticity, motor learning.

Introduction

Transcranial magnetic stimulation (TMS) has emerged as an important tool to investigate the contribution of the corticospinal tract to human motor control. It has been used most extensively in the corticospinal system, since the output of the primary motor cortex (M1) can be easily assessed in the form of a motor evoked potential (MEP) by using surface electromyographic (EMG) recording electrodes in humans (1). A large number of review

---

[*] **Correspondence:** Monica A Perez, Department of Physical Medicine and Rehabilitation, Center for the Neural Basis of Cognition, University of Pittsburgh, PA 15261 United States. Tel: (412) 383-6563; Fax: (412) 383-9061; E-mail: perezmo@pitt.edu

papers have addressed many aspects of TMS from mechanisms of action in health and disease to more complex interactions to address hemispheric specialization in motor and cognitive domains (2-12). This review will specifically address the neuronal elements that are excited by TMS and integrate this information into the larger framework of our knowledge on corticospinal tract function in humans. In the first section, we will discuss general principles of TMS actions in the human brain. We will describe how induction of a magnetic field by a TMS device serves as a "vehicle" for delivering currents focally onto target brain structures. This information provides the basis for discussing which neuronal elements are excited by TMS and the available techniques that are used to make these inferences. The combination of TMS with simultaneous recording of descending volleys in the spinal cord using epidural electrodes and pharmacological interventions has made it possible to study inhibitory/excitatory circuits in the human cerebral cortex. In the second section, we will focus on the description and discussion of some of the most widely used electrophysiological markers available to assess motor cortical function at rest and during different types of motor behavior in humans. In the third section, we will discuss the contribution of TMS to the understanding of the mechanisms underlying brain plasticity and motor learning.

Principles of TMS

Transcranial magnetic stimulation (TMS) is based on Faraday's principles of electromagnetic induction. A brief and high-current pulse is produced in a coil of wire, which is called the magnetic coil. A magnetic field is produced with lines of flux passing perpendicular to the plane of the coil. The magnetic field can reach up to about 1.5-2 Tesla depending on the specific device and usually lasts for about 100 μs. In terms, an electric field is induced perpendicularly to the magnetic field. While the voltage of the field itself may excite neurons, it induces currents that run parallel to the plane of the coil. There are several shapes of magnetic coils available but the ones most widely used are the circular and the figure-of-eight coil (13). The circular coil induces concentric current loops in the tissue whose amplitudes is zero on the axis of the coil, rise to a maximum approximately under the mean diameter of the wind and drop at greater distances from the axis. The figure-of-eight coil induces currents that rise to a maximum approximately under the intersection of both wings of the coil. Neuronal elements are activated by the induced electric field via two mechanisms. First, if the electrical field is parallel to the neuronal element, the field will be most effective where the intensity changes and become more diffuse with distance below the coil. Second, if the field is not completely parallel, activation will occur at bends of the axons. When the current amplitude, duration, and direction are appropriate, they will depolarize cortical neurons and generate action potentials (14). Therefore, the magnetic field serves as a "vehicle" for delivering currents focally in the brain. The induced electrical current is responsible for the excitation of the cortical neurons.

Neuronal elements activated by TMS

The primary motor cortex (M1) is one of the major sources of descending pyramidal tract neurons originated in layer V. There are two types of corticospinal tract neurons (CST). One type has axons terminating in the intermediate zone of the spinal cord, where they synapse with spinal interneurons. In turn, some of these interneurons make connections with alpha motoneurons and conduct the descending commands necessary for movement. A second type of CST neurons has axons that terminate in the ventral horn of the spinal cord, where they make monosynaptic connections with motoneurons (called corticomotoneuronal cells). The available data suggest that CST cells are involved in the generation and control of skilled motor behavior. In humans, TMS can induce movements involving specific muscles through the activation of monosynaptic CST neurons in both hand and arm (15-16) and leg (17-19). Electrophysiological studies support the view that with TMS we can assess monosynaptic CST connections by examining the effect of TMS on a) the probability of discharge of single motor units voluntarily preactivated (i.e. poststimulus time histograms, PSTHs) (15,17,20) and b) the amplitude of H-reflexes (21).

A suprathreshold TMS stimulus results in multiple descending waves as recorded from epidural electrodes positioned over the spinal cord and in a complex configuration of MEP as measured by single motor unit recordings with needle electrodes (22). A short latency direct wave (D-wave) is followed by several longer latency indirect waves (I-waves). The D-wave is thought to result from direct depolarisation of the initial axon segment of the CST neuron and is most effectively activated in human subjects by high intensity TMS or by transcranial electrical stimulation. I-waves, which follow the D-wave occur sequentially with a periodicity of approximately 1.5 ms and reflect the delay required for synaptic discharge. The reason for the periodicity is not completely understood at this time. It has been proposed that it may depend on reverberating activity of circuits within the cortex or, alternatively, on changes in the membrane properties of corticospinal neurons which cause it to fire repeatedly after the application of a synchronous depolarizing stimulus. The first I-wave (I1) is thought to be generated through the depolarization of an axon synapsing directly onto a corticospinal neuron (i.e. monosynaptically), and the following I-waves (I2 and later) may require local polysynaptic circuits.

Which functions can we access with TMS?

To address this question, first, we need to take into consideration the functions of the CST in humans and nonhuman primates. The CST originates in different cortical areas with rather different functions. In the macaque, there are corticospinal projections emerging from M1, dorsal premotor cortex or PMd, ventral premotor cortex or PMv, supplementary motor area or SMA, and cingulate motor areas (CMAv, CMAd, CMAr; 23).

TMS has been used extensively to assess corticospinal projections from M1, since the output of the M1 can be easily measured in the form of MEPs by using surface EMG recording electrodes in humans. However, previous evidence has suggested that TMS is also capable of stimulating non-primary cortical areas such as the PMd and the SMA (11) and secondarily influence M1. Two main approaches have been used to investigate the influence of PMd onto M1. The first approach involves the application of repetitive TMS (rTMS) over PMd. Different groups have used parameters of stimulation known to up- or down-regulate cortical excitability over PMd, and afterwards assess motor cortical excitability in M1 by using single pulse TMS. In these experiments the intensity used to stimulate PMd was based on the M1 resting motor threshold. Gerschlager and collaborators (2001) (24) demonstrated that application of subthreshold rTMS at 1 Hz over PMd resulted in a reduction of MEP amplitudes elicited from M1. In contrast, the use of an rTMS protocol that increases cortical activity (5 Hz at 90% AMT) over PMd had the opposite effects and increased MEP amplitudes elicited from M1(25). Together, these studies demonstrate that stimulation of PMd by rTMS can affect corticospinal excitability in M1, suggesting that it is possible to use TMS to make inferences about physiological effects of non primary motor areas over M1. The second approach has used two coils in a paired pulse protocol. For example, Civardi and collaborators (26) showed that a subthreshold stimulus pulse over PMd reduces the size of MEPs elicited by stimulation of the ipsilateral M1. The authors observed a maximum inhibitory effect at inter-stimulus intervals of around 6 ms. It was argued that this interaction involved conditioning PMd rather than acting via current spread to M1, on the basis of spatial separation (conditioning at an intermediate point produces no inhibition), temporal separation (a time course that is distinct from intracortical inhibition) and the effect of coil orientation (26).

Another approach involves the use of TMS to examine the effect of PMd stimulation of one hemisphere over the M1 in the opposite hemisphere. This paired pulse approach is used to investigate interhemispheric interactions between PMd and the contralateral M1. It has been demonstrated that at inter-stimulus intervals 8-10 ms and at stimulus intensities below (90%) and above (110%) of the resting motor threshold a single pulse over PMd inhibits a control response elicited from the contralateral M1 (27). An interhemispheric inhibitory effect between PMd-M1 has also been described at the longer interstimulus interval of 150 ms (28). The effect of PMd stimulation on the contralateral M1 seems to depend on the stimulation intensity and the position of the coil (29). A possible mechanism proposed for these intra and interhemispheric effects is the activation of projections from the PMd to ipsi- or contralateral M1. This is consistent with anatomical studies in primates showing dense connections between those areas (30-31).

TMS had been used to study connectivity between the SMA and M1. In contrast to the PMd, the SMA is a more difficult area to stimulate since it is located in the interhemispheric fissure, relatively unexposed to the surface of the hemisphere. As for PMd, two main approaches have been used to investigate the influence of SMA onto M1. Matsunaga and collaborators (2005) (32) used 5 Hz suprathreshold rTMS over the SMA to investigate the effect of this stimulation protocol on the size of MEPs elicited from M1. The authors demonstrated that rTMS increased the MEP amplitudes recorded in a finger muscle. Another approach involved the use of a paired pulse protocol (26). Civardi et al. (2001) (26) demonstrated that a conditioning stimulus interval applied to SMA around 6 ms preceding M1 stimulation reduced the size of MEPs. Overall, these results suggest that SMA stimulation by TMS can affect M1 excitability, most likely through anatomical connections between these two regions (30-31).

In summary, these studies demonstrate that it is possible to use TMS to make inferences about the influence of non-primary motor regions onto M1. However, since the effects of TMS over a non-primary motor region are based on stimulations parameters obtained from

M1 the interpretation of the results should take this information into consideration. It is still unclear, which parameters are needed to optimally stimulate a non-primary motor region by TMS in humans.

Neurophysiological measurements

Several TMS applications have been developed to examine the physiology of the human motor system. These range from simple measurements that are used in clinical practice such as the assessment of central motor conduction time to more complex examples that include the use of pairs of TMS stimuli or pairs of TMS and peripheral nerve stimuli, used to assess the excitability of corticospinal neurons, interneurons, and connected structures. Paired pulse TMS protocols have provided insight into the nature of the cortical circuitry that is activated by TMS. A variety of different methods exist to examine the connections within and between primary motor cortices. In this section we will discuss two of the most widely used paired pulse TMS protocols in humans: short interval intracortical inhibition (SICI) and interhemispheric inhibition (IHI). For both techniques, direct recordings of the effects on descending volleys have not only confirmed the mechanisms of these effects, but also revealed some degree of selectivity for different waves (D, I1, I2, etc.) of the response.

Short-interval intracortical inhibition (SICI)

SICI was first reported by Kujirai and collaborators in 1993 (33). The authors demonstrated that a conditioning TMS pulse of a subthreshold intensity decreased the size of an MEP elicited by a later suprathreshold test stimulus when applied over the M1. This effect was observed at conditioning time intervals between 1 and 5 ms. Two main phases of inhibition have been described, at conditioning time intervals of 1 ms and 2.5 ms (34-35). Since the intensity of the conditioning stimulus was below the active motor threshold, Kujirai et al (33) suggested that this effect was occurring at the cortical level and that the conditioning stimulus was suppressing the recruitment of descending volleys by the test stimulus. Later evidence provided by Di Lazzaro and collaborators (36) confirmed the cortical effect of SICI. They demonstrated that a subthreshold conditioning stimulus which itself did not evoke descending activity produced a clear suppression of late I-waves if the interval between the stimuli was between 1 and 5 ms. The I1-wave was nearly unaffected but the I3-wave and later volleys were the most sensitive to the stimulation. These results were supported by the study of Hanajima et al (37) who showed that a subthreshold conditioning stimulus given over M1 moderately suppresses I3 waves but did not affect I1 waves. The duration of suppression of the I3 waves supported the idea that this was an effect of GABAergic inhibition within the motor cortex. Kujirai et al (33) in the original paper suggested that SICI was GABAergic in origin. Later studies have shown that, administration of a single oral dose of lorazepam, an agonist at the GABAA receptor increases the amount of SICI and also increases the inhibition of later descending I-waves (38). Other studies have confirmed that GABAA agonists enhance SICI (39-40). It has been demonstrated that inhibition at a conditioning time interval of 1 ms does not depend on GABAA activity but that the inhibition observed at 2.5 ms is likely to be mediated by GABAergic inhibition at the intracortical level (34-35). At present, SICI is considered as one of the standard paired pulse TMS protocols used to examine intracortical function at rest and during voluntary movement in humans.

Interhemispheric inhibition (IHI)

Ferbert and collaborators (41) published the first extensive study that reveals powerful interhemispheric interactions between primary motor cortices in intact human subjects by using TMS. The authors demonstrated that a TMS suprathreshold pulse applied over of the motor cortex of one hemisphere can inhibit motor responses evoked in distal and proximal muscles by a magnetic stimulus given 6-30 ms later over the opposite hemisphere. Ferbert et al (41) suggested that the inhibition was produced at cortical level via a transcallosal route. Direct proof of the cortical origin of the inhibition was provided by Di Lazzaro et al (42) who recorded descending volleys produced by the test MEP alone and with and without a prior conditioning stimulus to the contralateral motor cortex. In the spinal recordings it was demonstrated that the inhibitory effect was present in the later I3-waves.

Motor cortical excitability, brain plasticity and motor learning

This section focuses on how TMS can be used to induce changes in motor cortical excitability, the potential mechanisms underlying these effects, and the usefulness of this knowledge to gain insight into motor learning mechanisms. rTMS is a novel, non-invasive and painless way to apply TMS to stimulate the human brain with the purpose of modulating function of the stimulated cortical region or interconnected areas. The use of repeated pulses can have prolonged effects on the brain. For example, the duration of the after-effects of rTMS over M1 are often between 15-60 min, but depend on stimulation parameters such as the number of pulses applied, the rate of application and the intensity of each stimulus.

rTMS

Several studies have examined the effects of rTMS on the excitability of the hand (43) and leg (44-45) motor representations in the M1. The nature of the after-effects of rTMS depends on the number, intensity and frequency of stimulation pulses. In some cases, the stimulus intensity used is below the threshold for evoking a muscle twitch in relaxed muscles, so that any effects observed could not be attributed to sensory input produced by movement. In this regard, stimulation of the M1 at a subthreshold intensity and at a frequency of 1 Hz for about 25 min (1,500 total stimuli) reduced the size of MEPs evoked in finger muscles for the next 30 min (46). A similar protocol also increased motor reaction times, demonstrating that rTMS can be used to interfere with processes that contribute to motor behaviors. Stimulation at frequencies higher than 1 Hz tends to increase rather than decrease cortical excitability. The after-effects of rTMS also depend on the pattern of the individual TMS pulses. For example, Huang and collaborators (47) used theta-burst stimulation (TBS), a protocol in which three 50

Hz pulses are applied regularly 5 times per second for 20-40s. In this protocol, low intensities of stimulation produces suppression of motor cortex excitability as measured by MEP size. However, if each TBS burst is applied for only 2 s followed by a pause of 8 s and repeated the after effect becomes facilitatory.

Mechanisms of the after-effects of rTMS

One of the important questions to address is if the after effects of rTMS are due to changes in cortical or spinal cord excitability or both. Several studies have documented that rTMS induces long lasting adaptations in cortical neuronal circuitries (43,48-50). For example, high-frequency subthreshold rTMS can reduce SICI in the stimulated motor cortex (43,51). Although, the cellular mechanisms of the aftereffects of rTMS are not yet understood some hypotheses have been postulated. It has been proposed that operating mechanisms include changes in the effectiveness of synapses between cortical neurons (long-term depression (LTD) and LTP of synaptic connections). Like LTP/LTD, there is evidence from pharmacological interventions that the after-effects of rTMS depend on the glutamatergic NMDA (N-methyl-D-aspartate) receptor, as they are blocked by a single dose of the NMDA-receptor antagonist dextromethorphan (52). Another example is the use of an NMDA-receptor antagonist, which can block the suppressive and facilitatory effect of some rTMS protocols (53). Importantly another study demonstrated that the after effects of rTMS on motor cortical excitability disappear when MEPs are tested in actively contracting muscle rather than at rest (54). In this study the authors suggested that rTMS was to some extent changing the level of excitability of the resting corticospinal system, rather than changing the effectiveness of transmission at synapses within the cortex. It is possible that both effects occur on different degrees depending on the parameters of rTMS.

In humans and primates, corticospinal cells exert modulation over a large group of spinal interneurones (55). Therefore, it is possible that activating corticospinal neurons by rTMS may also induce long-lasting changes in spinal neuronal circuitries. Indeed, H-reflex recording has been used to assess spinal motoneuronal excitability following rTMS (44,54, 56-58). Perez and collaborators (44) applied 15 trains of 20 pulses at 5 Hz at intensities between 75 to 120% of resting motor threshold of the tibialis anterior muscle and reported a decrease in the size of the soleus H-reflex at stimulus intensities ranging from 92% to 120% of the resting motor threshold. In this study the authors showed that rTMS increased the level of presynaptic inhibition at the terminals of Ia afferent fibers but did not change the level of disynaptic reciprocal Ia inhibition. These results suggest that rTMS-induced changes in spinal cord excitability are, at least in part, mediated by changes in presynaptic inhibition at the terminals of the Ia afferent fibers. At rTMS frequencies of 1 Hz different results have been reported. Valero-Cabré et al (57) applied 600 pulses of 1-Hz rTMS at 90% of resting motor threshold of the flexor carpi radialis (FCR) muscle and reported a lasting decrease in threshold and an increase in size of the FCR H-reflex. Touge et al (54) found no effect of rTMS on the size of the FCR H-reflex after 600 stimuli at 1 Hz and 95% of resting motor threshold of the FDI muscle. It seems likely that the difference in results is due to differences in the intensity of the rTMS.

TMS, rTMS and motor learning

It is well documented that learning of a motor task is accompanied by changes in M1 excitability. TMS has had a critical role in the characterization of those changes and in the understanding on the neuronal mechanism involved in human motor learning. We will describe in this section some protocols in which TMS and rTMS has been successfully used to demonstrate motor cortical plasticity associated with different types of motor learning.

Previous studies have reported focal changes in motor cortical excitability such as an increase in the size of MEP (specific to the trained muscle) and a decrease in intracortical inhibition which can be induced with as little as 30 min of training (59-62). In addition, evidence has demonstrated that the direction of a thumb movement in response to a single TMS pulse can be altered by training over a similar period, suggesting that motor practice can influence directional coding at the level of M1 (59). In this study, since changes identified with TMS were not present with transcranial electrical stimulation the authors suggested that cortical mechanisms might contributed to the observed results (59). Using a similar paradigm Butefisch et al (60) demonstrated that changes in motor cortical excitability were decreased by GABAergic agents also pointing to the view of a cortical mechanism contributing to the observed cortical plasticity. In another paradigm, TMS has been used to assess the involvement of the M1 in the consolidation of learning. Muellbacher et al (61) demonstrated that low frequency 1 Hz TMS applied to M1 immediately after practice resulted in disruption of improvement in motor performance in a pinch-grip task.

The disruptive effect was specific for M1 and was not found when stimulating the visual cortex indicating that M1 is involved in the early phase of motor consolidation. A recent paper demonstrated that a different form of stimulation, transcranial DC stimulation could actually facilitate acquisition of a new motor skill (63).

Recent studies have also use TMS to understand the neurophysiological mechanisms involved in the ability of individuals to transfer finger motor sequence learning to the contralateral hand which did not trained and remained at rest. In these studies, subjects were trained in the serial reaction time task by using the dominant right hand and the performance improvements were observed not only the trained hand but also the untrained hand.

The results points to a role for IHI in general aspects of motor performance in the untrained hand and to the involvement of the SMA in the transfer of sequence learning (62,64-65). rTMS applied over the SMA blocked intermanual transfer of sequence learning without affecting skill acquisition. These findings provide direct evidence for an SMA-based mechanism that supports intermanual transfer of motor-skill learning.

Conclusions

This review focused on the description of the basic physiological mechanisms by which TMS influences cortical excitability, motor function in general and cognitive functions like motor learning in particular. Additioanlly, TMS is a valuable tool investigate body part representations in the human motor cortex and other brain interactions. While it has been used most extensively in the evaluation of the CST system, it has also been applied over non-primary motor regions to assess their effect on M1 excitability. Although, some of these effects are indirect and the interpretation of the results must be cautions there is a growing of number studies providing insights into effective connectivity between cortical regions assessed by TMS.

The use of TMS during behavioral tests has made it possible to make inferences about cortical function during motor learning and a variety of other motor and cognitive processes.

More importantly, these studies have provided information that was crucial to the development of TMS as a technical tool to facilitate or to down regulate activity in target brain areas, an issue of crucial clinical importance.

References

[1] Barker AT, Jalinous R, Freeston IL. Non-invasive magnetic stimulation of human motor cortex. Lancet 1985;1:1106-07.
[2] Weber M, Eisen AA. Magnetic stimulation of the central and peripheral nervous systems. Muscle Nerve 2002;25:160-75.
[3] Walsh V, Cowey A. Transcranial magnetic stimulation and cognitive neuroscience. Nat Rev Neurosci 2000;1:73-9.
[4] Cantello R, Tarletti R, Civardi C. Transcranial magnetic stimulation and Parkinson's disease. Brain Res Brain Res Rev 2002;38:309-27.
[5] Lisanby SH, Luber B, Perera T, Sackeim HA. Transcranial magnetic stimulation: applications in basic neuroscience and neuropsychopharmacology. Int J Neuropsychopharmacol 2000; 3:259-73.
[6] Petersen NT, Pyndt HS, Nielsen JB. Investigating human motor control by transcranial magnetic stimulation. Exp Brain Res. 2003; 152:1-16.
[7] Hallett M. Transcranial magnetic stimulation and the human brain. Nature 2000;406:147-50.
[8] Bailey CJ, Karhu J, Ilmoniemi RJ. Transcranial magnetic stimulation as a tool for cognitive studies. Scand J Psychol 2001;42:297-305.
[9] Siebner HR, Rothwell J. Transcranial magnetic stimulation: new insights into representational cortical plasticity. Exp Brain Res 2003; 148:1-16.
[10] Ward NS, Cohen LG. Mechanisms underlying recovery of motor function after stroke. Arch Neurol 2004;61:1844-48.
[11] Reis J, Swayne OB, Vandermeeren Y, Camus M, Dimyan MA, et al. Contribution of transcranial magnetic stimulation to the understanding of cortical mechanisms involved in motor control. J Physiol 2008;586:325-51.
[12] Bestmann S. The physiological basis of transcranial magnetic stimulation.Trends Cogn Sci 2008;12:81-3.
[13] Roth BJ, Saypol JM, Hallett M, Cohen LG. A theoretical calculation of the electric field induced in the cortex during magnetic stimulation. Electroencephalogr Clin Neurophysiol 1991;81:47-56.
[14] Rothwell JC, Hallett M, Berardelli A, Eisen A, Rossini P, Paulus W. Magnetic stimulation: motor evoked potentials. The International Federation of Clinical Neurophysiology. Electroencephalogr Clin Neurophysiol 1999; 52(Suppl):97-103.
[15] Palmer E, Ashby P. Corticospinal projections to upper limb motoneurones in humans. J Physiol 1992;448:397-412.
[16] Baldissera F, Cavallari P. Short-latency subliminal effects of transcranial magnetic stimulation on forearm motoneurones. Exp Brain Res 1993;96:513-8.
[17] Brouwer B, Ashby P. Corticospinal projections to lower limb motoneurons in man. Exp Brain Res 1992;89:649-54.
[18] Rothwell JC, Thompson PD, Day BL, Boyd S, Marsden CD. Stimulation of the human motor cortex through the scalp. Exp Physiol 1991;76:159-200.

[19] Nielsen J, Petersen N, Ballegaard M. Latency of effects evoked by electrical and magnetic brain stimulation in lower limb motoneurons in man. J Physiol (Lond) 1995;484:791–802.
[20] Mills KR. Magnetic brain stimulation: a tool to explore the action of the motor cortex on single human spinal motoneurons. Trends Neurosci 1991;14:401-5.
[21] Petersen NT, Pyndt HS, Nielsen JB. Investigating human motor control by transcranial magnetic stimulation. Exp Brain Res 2003; 152:1-16.
[22] Amassian VE, Cracco RQ, Maccabee PJ. Focal stimulation of human cerebral cortex with the magnetic coil: a comparison with electrical stimulation. Electroencephalogr Clin Neurophysiol 1989;74:401-16.
[23] Strick PL, Dum RP, Picard N. Motor areas on the medial wall of the hemisphere. Novartis Found Symp 1998;218:64-75.
[24] Gerschlager W, Siebner HR, Rothwell JC. Decreased corticospinal excitability after subthreshold 1 Hz rTMS over lateral premotor cortex. Neurology 2001;57:449-55.
[25] Rizzo V, Siebner HR, Modugno N, Pesenti A, Munchau A, Gerschlager W, Webb RM, Rothwell JC. Shaping the excitability of human motor cortex with premotor rTMS. J Physiol 2004; 554:483-95.
[26] Civardi C, Cantello R, Asselman P, Rothwell JC. Transcranial magnetic stimulation can be used to test connections to primary motor areas from frontal and medial cortex in humans. Neuroimage 2001; 14:1444-53.
[27] Mochizuki H, Huang YZ, Rothwell JC. Interhemispheric interaction between human dorsal premotor and contralateral primary motor cortex. J Physiol 2004;561:331-8.
[28] Mochizuki H, Terao Y, Okabe S, Furubayashi T, Arai N, et al. Effects of motor cortical stimulation on the excitability of contralateral motor and sensory cortices. Exp Brain Res 2004;158:519-26.
[29] Baumer T, Bock F, Koch G, Lange R, Rothwell JC, Siebner HR, Munchau A. Magnetic stimulation of human premotor or motor cortex produces interhemispheric facilitation through distinct pathways. J Physiol 2006;572:857-68.
[30] Ghosh S, Porter R. Corticocortical synaptic influences on morphologically identified pyramidal neurons in the motor cortex of the monkey. J Physiol 1988;400:617-29.
[31] Tokuno H, Nambu A. Organization of nonprimary motor cortical inputs on pyramidal and nonpyramidal tract neurons of primary motor cortex: An electrophysiological study in the macaque monkey. Cereb Cortex 2000;10:58-68.
[32] Matsunaga K, Maruyama A, Fujiwara T, Nakanishi R, Tsuji S, Rothwell JC. Increased corticospinal excitability after 5 Hz rTMS over the human supplementary motor area. J Physiol 2005; 562:295-06.
[33] Kujirai T, Caramia MD, Rothwell JC, Day BL, Thompson PD, et al. Corticocortical inhibition in human motor cortex. J Physiol 1993; 471:501-19.
[34] Fisher RJ, Nakamura Y, Bestmann S, Rothwell JC, Bostock H. Two phases of intracortical inhibition revealed by transcranial magnetic threshold tracking. Exp Brain Res 2002;143:240-8.
[35] Roshan L, Paradiso GO, Chen R. Two phases of short-interval intracortical inhibition. Exp Brain Res 2003;151:330-37.
[36] DiLazzaro V, Restuccia D, Oliviero A, Profice P, Ferrara L, et al. Magnetic transcranial stimulation at intensities below active motor threshold activates intracortical inhibitory circuits. Exp Brain Res 1998;119:265-8.
[37] Hanajima R, Ugawa Y, Terao Y, Sakai K, Furubayashi T, Machii K, Kanazawa I. Paired-pulse magnetic stimulation of the human motor cortex: differences among I waves. J Physiol 1998;509:607-18.
[38] Di Lazzaro V, Oliviero A, Profice P, Pennisi MA, Di Giovanni S, Zito G, Tonali P, Rothwell JC. Muscarinic receptor blockade has differential effects on the excitability of intracortical circuits in the human motor cortex. Exp Brain Res 2000;135:455-61.

[39] Ziemann U, Lonnecker S, Steinhoff BJ, Paulus W. The effect of lorazepam on the motor cortical excitability in man. Exp Brain Res 1996;109:127-35.
[40] Ilic TV, Meintzschel F, Cleff U, Ruge D, Kessler KR, Ziemann U. Short-interval paired-pulse inhibition and facilitation of human motor cortex: the dimension of stimulus intensity. J Physiol 2002; 545:153-67.
[41] Ferbert A, Priori A, Rothwell JC, Day BL, Colebatch JG, Marsden CD. Interhemispheric inhibition of the human motor cortex. J Physiol 1992;453:525-46.
[42] Di Lazzaro V, Oliviero A, Profice P, Insola A, Mazzone P, Tonali P, Rothwell JC. Direct demonstration of interhemispheric inhibition of the human motor cortex produced by transcranial magnetic stimulation. Exp Brain Res 1999;124:520-4.
[43] Pascual-Leone A, Tormos JM, Keenan J, Tarazona F, Canete C, Catala MD. Study and modulation of human cortical excitability with transcranial magnetic stimulation. J Clin Neurophysiol 1998; 15:333-43.
[44] Perez MA, Lungholt BK and Nielsen JB. Short-term adaptations in spinal cord circuits evoked by repetitive transcranial magnetic stimulation: possible underlying mechanisms. Exp Brain Res 2005; 162:201-12.
[45] Zuur AT, Christensen MS, Sinkjaer T, Grey MJ, Nielsen JB. Tibialis anterior stretch reflex in early stance is suppressed by repetitive TMS. J Physiol 2009, in press.
[46] Chen R, Classen J, Gerloff C, Celnik P, Wassermann EM, Hallett M, Cohen LG. Depression of motor cortex excitability by low-frequency transcranial magnetic stimulation. Neurology 1997;48:1398-03.
[47] Huang YZ, Edwards MJ, Rounis E, Bhatia KP, Rothwell JC. Theta burst stimulation of the human motor cortex. Neuron 2005; 45:201-6.
[48] Di Lazzaro V, Oliviero A, Mazzone P, Pilato F, Saturno E, Dileone M, Insola A, Tonali PA, Rothwell JC. Short-term reduction of intracortical inhibition in the human motor cortex induced by repetitive transcranial magnetic stimulation. Exp Brain Res 2002; 147:108–13.
[49] Gilio F, Rizzo V, Siebner HR, Rothwell JC. Effects on the right motor hand-area excitability produced by low-frequency rTMS over human contralateral homologous cortex. J Physiol 2003;551:563-73.
[50] Kobayashi M, Hutchinson S, Theoret H, Schlaug G, Pascual-Leone A. Repetitive TMS of the motor cortex improves ipsilateral sequential simple finger movements. Neurology 2004;62:91-8.
[51] Peinemann A, Lehner C, Mentschel C, Munchau A, Conrad B, Siebner HR. Subthreshold 5-Hz repetitive transcranial magnetic stimulation of the human primary motor cortex reduces intracortical paired-pulse inhibition. Neurosci Lett 2000;296:21-4.
[52] Stefan, K., Kunesch, E., Benecke, R., Cohen, L. G. and Classen, J. Mechanisms of enhancement of human motor cortex excitability induced by interventional paired associative stimulation. J. Physiol (Lond) 2002;543:699-708.
[53] Huang YZ, Chen RS, Rothwell JC, Wen HY. The after-effect of human theta burst stimulation is NMDA receptor dependent. Clin Neurophysiol 2007;118:1028-32.
[54] Touge T, Gerschlager W, Brown P, Rothwell JC. Are the after-effects of low-frequency rTMS on motor cortex excitability due to changes in the efficacy of cortical synapses? Clin Neurophysiol 2001; 112:2138-45.
[55] Jankowska E. Interneuronal relay in spinal pathways from proprioceptors. Prog Neurobiol 1992;38:335-78.
[56] Berardelli A, Inghilleri M, Rothwell JC, Romeo S, Curra A, Gilio F, Modugno N, Manfredi M. Facilitation of muscle evoked responses after repetitive cortical stimulation in man. Exp Brain Res 1998; 122:79-4.
[57] Valero-Cabre A, Oliveri M, Gangitano M, Pascual-Leone A. Modulation of spinal cord excitability by subthreshold repetitive transcranial magnetic stimulation of the primary motor cortex in humans. Neuroreport 2001;12:3845-8.

[58] Modugno N, Nakamura Y, MacKinnon CD, Filipovic SR, Bestmann S, Berardelli A, Rothwell JC. Motor cortex excitability following short trains of repetitive magnetic stimuli. Exp Brain Res 2001; 140:453-9.

[59] Classen J, Liepert J, Wise SP, Hallett M, Cohen LG. Rapid plasticity of human cortical movement representation induced by practice. J Neurophysiol 1998;79:1117-23.

[60] Butefisch CM, Davis BC, Wise SP, Sawaki L, Kopylev L, Classen J, Cohen LG. Mechanisms of use-dependent plasticity in the human motor cortex. Proc Natl Acad Sci USA 2000;97:3661-65.

[61] Muellbacher W, Ziemann U, Boroojerdi B, Cohen L, Hallett M. Role of the human motor cortex in rapid motor learning. Exp Brain Res 2001;136:431-8.

[62] Perez MA, Wise SP, Willingham DT and Cohen LG. Neurophysiological mechanisms involved in transfer of procedural knowledge. J Neuroscience 2007;27:1045-53.

[63] Reis J, Schambra HM, Cohen LG, Buch ER, Fritsch B, Zarahn E, Celnik PA, Krakauer JW. Noninvasive cortical stimulation enhances motor skill acquisition over multiple days through an effect on consolidation. Proc Natl Acad Sci USA 2009;106:1590-5.

[64] Perez MA, Tanaka S, Wise SP, Sadato N, Tanabe HC, Willingham DT and Cohen LG. Neural substrates of intermanual transfer of a newly acquired motor skill. Current Biology 2007;17:1896-1902.

[65] Perez MA, Tanaka S, Wise SP, Willingham DT and Cohen LG. Time-specific contribution of the supplementary motor area to intermanual transfer of procedural knowledge. J Neuroscience 2008; 28:9664-9.

Principle and mechanisms of transcranial Direct Current Stimulation (tDCS)

Andrea Antal, PhD, Walter Paulus, MD and Michael A Nitsche, MD*
Department of Clinical Neurophysiology, University of Goettingen, Goettingen, Germany

Abstract

Brain stimulation with weak direct current was re-introduced about a decade ago as a method to elicit and modulate neuroplasticity of the human cerebral cortex. Transcranial direct current stimulation (tDCS) generates modulations of excitability during as well as up to hours after the end of stimulation, depending on the duration and intensity of stimulation. While anodal stimulation increases excitability, cathodal stimulation reduces it. During the last ten years tDCS has been demonstrated to modify perceptual, motor and cognitive functions reversibly in healthy subjects. Moreover, the results of clinical pilot studies suggest its efficacy as a treatment in neurological and psychiatric diseases. Increasing evidence shows that tDCS improves motor functions after stroke, reduces symptoms in chronic pain and depressed patients.

Keywords: Direct current stimulation, plasticity, NMDA-receptors.

Introduction

Brain stimulation techniques have generated renewed interest in recent decades as promising tools to explore human cortical functions and to treat neuropsychiatric diseases (1). Apart from invasive stimulation paradigms such as deep brain and vagal nerve stimulation, non-invasive tools, such as repetitive transcranial magnetic stimulation (rTMS) and transcranial direct current stimulation (tDCS) are attractive for use in humans, because they permit painless modulation of cortical activity and excitability through the intact skull (2). Indeed, brain stimulation with weak direct currents, although a relatively old method in strict terms (3), has recently been regaining increasing interest as a potentially valuable tool for inducing and modulating neuroplasticity. About 45 years ago it was demonstrated that in anesthetized rats weak direct currents, delivered by intracerebral or epidural electrodes, induce activity and excitability diminutions or enhancements of the sensorimotor cortex which can be stable for hours after the end of stimulation (4). A few years later it was demonstrated that also transcranial application of weak direct currents can induce an intracerebral current flow sufficiently large to achieve the intended effects. In monkeys, approximately 50% of the transcranially applied currents enter the brain through the skull (5) and these results have been replicated in humans (6). It was also found that this kind of stimulation changed EEG patterns and evoked potentials at the cortical level in humans (7). Apart from early clinical studies in which mainly depressive patients were treated with mixed results (for an overview see 8), anodal tDCS of the primary motor cortex (M1) was reported to optimise performance in a choice reaction time task in healthy subjects (9,10). In the following years, electrical stimulation of the human brain via transcranial application of weak direct currents as a tool to influence brain function was nearly forgotten. Nevertheless, in the last decade DC stimulation has been re-evaluated following the development of methods (TMS, functional magnetic resonance imaging - fMRI, positron emission tomography - PET) that allow probing its effects on a neurophysiological level. tDCS developed into a method that reliably induces and modulates neuroplasticity in the human cerebral cortex non-invasively, and painlessly in order to induce focal, prolonged - but yet reversible - shifts of cortical excitability (11-13). This review offers an overview of the basic and functional effects of weak tDCS, focussing mainly on TMS studies.

Technical aspects

For tDCS, direct currents are routinely delivered via a pair of surface conductive rubber electrodes covered with saline-soaked sponges (size between 16 and 35 cm^2 in different studies). A recently conducted study suggests that a medium NaCl concentration (between 15 and 140 mM) is optimally suited to minimize discomfort (14). Alternatively, the rubber electrodes can be spread with electrode cream and mounted directly on the head. The correct position of both electrodes is crucial for achieving the intended effects. The electrodes are connected with a stimulator. Since strength of current and not voltage determines the effects of electrical stimulation, a stimulator delivering constant current is needed. The current strength delivered varies between 1 and 2 mA in most studies. The resulting current densities are sufficient to achieve the desired excitability, perceptual and behavioural changes, and are regarded as safe with the currently used protocols, as shown by behavioural measures, EEG, serum neurone-specific enolase concentration, and diffusion-weighted and contrast-enhanced MRI measures (12,15,16). However, electrode positions above cranial foraminae and fissures should be avoided because these could increase effective current density, and thus safety of stimulation may no longer be guaranteed. Most subjects stimulated will perceive a slight itching sensation at the beginning of stimulation, which then fades. With certain electrode positions (especially frontopolar), retinal phosphenes can be perceived at the start and end of stimulation. These are eliminated by starting and terminating the stimulation gradually (ramping up and down for 8-20 sec).

Primary mechanism of action

The primary mechanism of DC stimulation of the cerebral cortex is a subthreshold modulation of neuronal resting membrane potential. In animal experiments anodal stimulation results in a subthreshold depolarisation, while cathodal stimulation hyperpolarises neuronal membranes (4,17). The situation in humans is probably identical, since blocking voltage-dependent ion channels pharmacologically abolishes any effect of anodal tDCS on cortical excitability, but does not influence the impact of cathodal tDCS (18). This modulation of resting membrane potential results in stimulation-polarity-dependent cortical excitability and activity changes. Generally, cathodal stimulation decreases cortical excitability, whereas anodal stimulation increases it.

Parameters shaping the effects of tDCS

In monkeys, approximately 50% of the transcranially-applied current enters the brain through the skull (5). These estimates were confirmed in humans (6). The relevant parameters determining efficacy and direction of the excitability changes induced by tDCS are the current density (i.e. current strength/stimulated area), the stimulation duration and the stimulation polarity.

It was observed that a current density of about 0.03 mA/cm^2 is sufficient to induce relevant excitability shifts in the human M1 (11). Increasing current density might increase efficacy of stimulation due to a larger membrane polarisation shift, but might also affect additional neuronal populations because of a greater efficacy of the electrical field in deeper cortical layers and additionally because of different sensitivities of specific neuronal populations to DC stimulation (18). Current density delivered has varied between 0.029 and 0.08 mA/cm^2 in most published studies (for a review see: 2). These limits will probably continue to expand with experience.

Stimulation duration has been shown to determine the occurrence and length of after-effects of DC stimulation in animals and humans. In humans, tDCS for less than 3 min induces cortical excitability shifts that do not outlast the stimulation period. Prolonged tDCS, however, induces after-effects which can last for about an hour or much longer under specific medication (see below) in humans. Importantly, there is a positive relationship between the duration of tDCS treatment and the duration of the after-effects (11-13). Therefore if repeated sessions of tDCS are performed and cumulative effects are not the goal of a given study, the inter-session interval has to be sufficiently long to avoid carry-over effects. The duration of this interval depends on the stimulation procedure (for short duration tDCS – 1 hour, for long duration – 1 week). However, if the aim is to induce more stable changes in cortical function, repeated daily tDCS sessions may be adequate.

Stimulation polarity determines the direction of cortical excitability changes elicited by tDCS. In humans and animals, anodal DC stimulation enhances excitability and activity, whereas cathodal stimulation results in reversed effects (11-13,19). However, not only the polarity of the electrode over the stimulated area seems to be relevant for the net effects on excitability, but also the direction of current flow: the respective current has to flow along the longitudinal axis of a given neuron to induce relevant effects on membrane polarity (20), and the polarisation of the soma and axon might determine the direction of the effects rather than dendritic polarisation. Consequently, the position of the reference electrode is critical for achieving the intended excitability shifts. Indeed, effects are reversed with reversal of current flow (11).

As it was summarized in a recent review (2), increasing focality of tDCS can be achieved by: (i) reducing electrode size while keeping current density constant, for the electrode which is intended to affect the underlying cortex; (ii) increasing the size, and thus reducing current density, of the electrode, which should not affect the underlying cortex; or (iii) using an extracephalic reference.

Mechanisms of action

Neurophysiological studies

The M1, especially the hand area of the M1 (), has been widely used as a model system in order to study cortical excitability in healthy subjects as well as in patients with different neuropsychiatric conditions. This is due to two facts (i) the M1 lies on the cortical convexity of the precentral gyrus with a minimal distance to the scalp surface and (ii) the MEP evoked by TMS is the most efficient tool for quantification of plastic cortical alterations. Within the past years several parameters have been developed to investigate cortical excitability with TMS in M1. First, by comparing the size of MEPs elicited by single pulse TMS with those evoked by transcranial electrical stimulation (TES), intracortical modifications (TMS) can be separated from direct effects on pyramidal tract neurons (TES). Responses to TES are dominated by direct stimulation of corticospinal axons, whereas those evoked by TMS are dominated by transsynaptic activation of corticospinal neurones (21). For the after-effects of tDCS, TES does not modify MEPs when applied at moderate intensity - in contrast to the effect on the TMS-generated MEP amplitudes (11,12), which implies a predominant intracortical effect of tDCS. However, in another study, a reduction of the TES-evoked MEP was reported for the after-effects of cathodal tDCS (22). Since low-intensity TES, as applied in this experiment, is thought to influence the proximal aspect of pyramidal tract axons, this might be an indication for an additional membrane effect of tDCS on corticospinal neurones. The intra-cortical effect of tDCS was explored by monitoring intracortical inhibition and facilitation via a TMS double-stimulation paradigm (23). Paired-pulse TMS with short (1-15 ms) or longer (50-200 ms) interstimulus-intervals can be used to differentially access inhibitory or facilitatory neuronal circuits in M1 (24,25), involving a variety of transmitter systems (25). In the above mentioned study, during tDCS intracortical facilitation was diminished and inhibition enhanced by cathodal tDCS, while anodal stimulation resulted in reversed effects.

tDCS can also modify the excitability of the visual cortex. Antal et al. (26) have published a pilot study giving evidence for the modulation of visual perception in human primary visual cortex (V1) in healthy volunteers. The study was based on the measurement of contrast threshold. They applied anodal and cathodal stimulation to the occipital cortex. Visual stimuli were Gabor patches (vertical Gaussian filtered black and white sinusoidal gratings). Binocular static (sCS) and dynamic contrast sensitivity (dCS) was measured. In this study the current was applied for 7 min with an intensity of 1 mA. Cathodal tDCS significantly diminished both the sCS and dCS during and immediately after stimulation. Anodal stimulation did not influence contrast sensitivity. This was the first human study revealing that the elementary visual functions can be transiently modified by tDCS.

The first electrophysiological evidence of a DC effect on the healthy human V1 was published in 2004 (27). The amplitude and latency of the N70 and P100 visual evoked potential (VEP) peaks were measured. Stimuli were high- and low-contrast sinusoidal luminance gratings. Significant DC after-effects were observed only on the VEP amplitudes using low-contrast stimuli. No significant effects were detected for the latency of the VEP components. The presentation of high-contrast stimuli did not modify VEP amplitudes. Anodal tDCS significantly enhanced, cathodal stimulation diminished the amplitude of the N70 component. Cathodal tDCS could slightly (but not significantly) increase the amplitude of P100. They concluded that cathodal stimulation was more effective than anodal stimulation in this paradigm. This is in agreement with the findings from previous animal and human studies (4,17,26).

Antal and coworkers used TMS elicited phosphenes to determine whether anodal or cathodal DC can modulate phosphene thresholds (PTs) (28). They elicited phosphenes by applying short trains of 5 Hz rTMS delivered over the V1. They found that cathodal stimulation significantly increased PT, probably due to diminished cortical excitability. Anodal stimulation resulted in the opposite effect, probably via enhanced cortical excitability. The results provide furthermore evidence that external modulation of visual neural excitability using tDCS goes beyond V1 and could influence complex, visual adaptation related processes. Over medio-temporal area (MT+/V5) in that neural cells are particularly sensitive to motion, tDCS affected the strength of perceived motion after-effect (MAE) and supported the involvement of MT+/V5 in motion adaptation processes (29). Interestingly, both cathodal and anodal stimulation over MT+/V5 resulted in a significant reduction of the perceived MAE duration, but had no effect on performance in a luminance-change-detection task used to determine attentional load during adaptation.

In comparison to the M1, the after-effects in the V1 are relatively short. This suggests that V1 might be less prone to plastic alterations as compared to M1. Furthermore, the shorter duration of the after-effects may be due to the differences in anatomical structure of visual and motor cortices, leading to different effects in the stimulated cortical layers. Besides this, for M1 stimulation, cathodal tDCS was more effective in women, whereas anodal tDCS was more effective in the V1 in women as compared to men (30,31).

Although the motor and visual cortices are the most common targets with regards to tDCS, the effect of stimulation is not restricted concerning these brain areas. tDCS was effective over the prefrontal (32) and somatosensory (33,34), cortices, however, the direction and length of the aftereffects was highly dependent on the paradigm used.

Pharmacological studies

Efforts have been made to characterize the neuronal populations affected by tDCS. The primary effects of tDCS on neuronal excitability during stimulation are due to neuronal membrane polarization shifts, as the respective excitability enhancements are prevented by sodium and calcium channel blockers (18). Blocking these ion channels also abolishes the after-effects of facilitatory tDCS, thus membrane polarization is essential for their induction. However, the after-effects are not due to reverberating excitation of neuronal circuits. Indeed, these effects were demonstrated to be protein synthesis-dependent (35) and were accompanied by modifications of intracellular cAMP- and calcium-levels in animals (36,37). Thus they share some features with the nowadays more commonly known neuroplastic phenomena, namely long-term potentiation (LTP) and long-term depression (LTD). In humans it has been demonstrated that the after-effects of tDCS depend on modifications of NMDA receptor-efficacy as they are blocked by the NMDA receptor antagonist dextrometorphan, but prolonged by the partial NMDA receptor-agonist D-Cycloserine (38,39). NMDA-receptor and intracellular sigma 1 receptor blocker dextromethorphan intake prevented both anodal and cathodal tDCS-induced after-effects, demonstrating that dextromethorphan critically interferes with the functionality of tDCS irrespective of the polarity of DC stimulation (18,38). It is known from animal experiments that long-lasting NMDA-receptor dependent cortical excitability and activity shifts are crucially involved in neuroplastic modifications.

Table 1. This table represents the pharmacological approaches concerning DC stimulation in long- and short-term anodal and cathodal stimulation. -: not examined, ↑: the drug has increased the tDCS-induced effect, ↓: the drug has increased the tDCS-induced effect, Ø: no effect

Drug	Effect	intra - anod	intra - cathod	Long-term anod	Long-term cathod
Carbamazepine	voltage-dependent Na^+-channel-blocker	↓	Ø	↓	Ø
Flunarazine	Ca^{++}-channel blocker	↓	Ø	↓	Ø
Dextrometorphane	NMDA-receptor antagonist	Ø	Ø	↓	↓
D-cycloserine	NMDA agonist	Ø	Ø	↑	Ø
Lorazepam	GABA-A agonist	Ø	Ø	(↑)	Ø
Sulpiride	D2-receptor antagonist	-	-	↓	↓
Pergolide	D1-receptor agonist	-	-	Ø	↑
Rivastigmine	ACh-esterase inhibitor	-	-	↓	↑
Amphetamin	increases catecholamine availability	-	-	↑	Ø

The impact of neuromodulators and transmitters on NMDA receptor-dependent plasticity has been extensively studied in animal experiments. Accordingly, the GABAergic system is able to modulate the tDCS-induced after-effects on excitability, since at least the anodal tDCS-induced intracortical enhancement of facilitation and reduction of inhibition is abolished by lorazepam (40). Furthermore the monoaminergic enhancer amphetamine consolidates the tDCS-driven excitability-enhancement, probably due to ß-adrenergic effects (39). This effect of amphetamine on tDCS-induced neuroplasticity not readily explained by dopaminergic action, since enhancement of D2 – and to a lesser degree – of D1 receptors by pergolide consolidated tDCS-generated excitability diminution up until the morning post stimulation, but did not affect facilitatory plasticity (41). L-dopa had similar effects on inhibitory plasticity, but abolished facilitatory plasticity elicited by tDCS (42). This effect was similar to that of the cholinesterase-inhibitor rivastigmine (43).

Taken together, the results of these studies are in accordance with a primary effect of tDCS on neuronal membrane polarization, which results in neuroplastic modifications of NMDA receptor function. Furthermore the results show a dramatic impact of neuromodulators on tDCS-induced plasticity. Apart from exploring the mechanisms of plasticity induced by tDCS, the results of these studies might be of importance for the application of tDCS in clinical studies with patients under medication. Table 1 gives a brief overview of the pharmacological approaches to DC stimulation and the results on single pulse MEP amplitudes.

Conclusions

According to previous studies and results from our own laboratory, tDCS is a promising method to induce acute as well as prolonged cortical excitability and activity modulations. To make this tool relevant not only for basic research purposes but also for clinical application, additional studies are necessary. However, we can see already that there are exciting prospects for the use of tDCS as tool to promote changes of brain activity paralleled by behavioural improvements.

TDCS differs from other plasticity-inducing interventions, such as rTMS, in some respect, which might be important for clinical application. (i) tDCS differs qualitatively from other brain stimulation techniques such as TES and TMS by not inducing neuronal action potentials since static fields in this range do not yield the rapid depolarization required to produce action potentials in neural membranes. Hence, tDCS might be considered a neuromodulatory intervention. The exposed tissue is polarized and tDCS modifies spontaneous neuronal excitability and activity by a tonic de- or hyperpolarization of resting membrane potential. In contrast, rTMS induces externally triggered changes in the neuronal spiking pattern and interrupts or excites cortical activity in a spatially and temporally restricted fashion. (ii) rTMS produces clicks, that acoustically can be observed, and often induces muscle contractions during the stimulation. Furthermore when longer stimulation durations are used, a coil-holder is needed. The application of tDCS completely silent, and induces only light itching of the skin under the electrode at the beginning of the stimulation. Therefore, it represents a real condition for sham stimulation. (iii) Compared to TMS, tDCS is less focal. Spatially, relatively big electrode size (25 - 35 cm^2) is used and temporally, the resolution of the stimulation is significantly less. (iv) It is easier to administer tDCS than rTMS, even during a task. Furthermore, compared to TMS, it is easier to conduct placebo stimulation-controlled studies with tDCS, because, with the exception of a slight itching sensation and sensory phenomena including retinal phosphenes with current switching, subjects rarely experience sensations related to the treatment. (v) The administration of tDCS is more economical and cost effective.

TDCS, as presented here, should be considered as safe (44,45). Conventional electrical brain stimulation can cause excitotoxic damage to over-driven neurons, however, (i) the effects of tDCS inducing changes in cortical excitability are most probably due to a mild effect on cation channels and not being able to induce firing in cells that are not spontaneously active; and (ii) tDCS has been shown in animals to increase spontaneous neuronal firing rate only to a moderate degree, i.e., within the physiologic range (iii) and is unlikely to reach the threshold for excitotoxicity, even over long periods.

There is no data in the literature reporting epileptic jerks elicited by tDCS. Furthermore the anticonvulsant effect of cathodal DC stimulation in a rat model was published (46). This group also described the histologic analysis of rat brain tissue after tDCS. The samples underwent either light microscopic (haematoxylin and eosin) or immunhistological (expression of activated microglial marker) investigation. No cortical oedema, necrosis, nor any sign of cell death (karyopyknosis, karyolysis and karyohexis) was observed. In a recent study (47) fifty-eight rats received single cathodal stimulations at 1-1000 microA for up to 270 min through an epicranial electrode (3.5 mm^2). Histological evaluation (H&E) was performed 48 hours later. Brain lesions occurred at a current density of 142.9 A/m^2 for durations greater than 10 min. For current densities between 142.9 and 285.7 A/m^2, lesion size increased linearly with charge density; with a calculated zero lesion size intercept of 52,400 C/m^2. Brains stimulated below either this current density or charge density threshold, including stimulations over 5 consecutive days, were morphologically intact.

There is only one publication discussing the increment of intracellular calcium level following repetitive anodal polarization of the rat brain. This phenomenon is thought to be a part of the process underlying the observed neuroplastic changes (37). The measurement of the level of serum neurone-specific enolase (a known marker of neuronal death) did not change during and after DC stimulation. This, combined with the results of MRI studies also indicate that tDCS at current parameters, is relatively safe to use within the human population (16). 102 subjects (who performed altogether 567 DC sessions over different cortical areas) participated in a retrospective post-DC questionnaire study (48). Most of the participants were healthy volunteers (75.5%). 8.8% of the subjects were migraine patients, 5.9% post-stroke patients and 9.8% suffered from tinnitus. Subjects described the following, mainly non-specific adverse events during stimulation: 70.6% tingling sensation, 11.8% fatigue, 2.9% nausea, 0.98% insomnia. Interestingly, the intensity of the perceived tingling sensation was significantly higher in healthy subjects than in patients.

The investigation of tDCS for therapeutic effects is in its at initial stages; but the preliminary data for example with regard to chronic pain and stroke are promising (e.g. 49,50). Nevertheless, several questions still need to be addressed before any firm conclusion about this therapy is made. The parameters of stimulation need to be further explored. The duration of the therapeutic effects is another important issue to be considered, further trials must determine the optimum parameters of stimulation. After that, confirmatory, larger studies are mandatory.

References

[1] Fregni F, Pascual-Leone A. Technology insight: noninvasive brain stimulation in neurology-perspectives on the therapeutic potential of rTMS and tDCS. Nat Clin Pract Neurol 2007;3:383-93.

[2] Nitsche MA, Cohen LG, Wassermann EM, Priori A, Lang N, Antal A, Paulus W, Hummel F, Boggio PS, Fregni F, Pascual-Leone A. Transcranial direct current stimulation: state of the art 2008. Brain Stimulat 2008;1:206-23.

[3] Hellwag CF, Jacobi M. Erfahrungen über die Heilkrafte des Galvanismus. Hamburg, 1802.

[4] Bindman LJ, Lippold OCJ, Redfearn JWT. The action of brief polarizing currents on the cerebral cortex of the rat (1) during current flow and (2) in the production of long-lasting after-effects. J Physiol 1964;172:369-82.

[5] Rush S, Driscoll DA. Current distribution in the brain from surface electrodes. Anaest Analg Curr Res 1968; 47:717-23.

[6] Dymond AM, Coger RW, Serafetinides EA. Intracerebral current levels in man during electrosleep therapy. Biol Psychiatry 1975;10:101-4.

[7] Pfurtscheller G. Spectrum analysis of EEG: before, during and after extracranial stimulation in man. Elektromed Biomed Tech 1970;15:225-30.

[8] Lolas F. Brain polarization: behavioral and therapeutic effects. Biol Psychiatry 1977;12:37-47.

[9] Elbert T, Lutzenberger W, Rockstroh B, Birbaumer N. The influence of low-level transcortical DC-currents on response speed in humans. Int J Neurosci 1981;14:101-14.

[10] Jaeger D, Elbert T, Lutzenberger W, Birbaumer N. The effects of externally applied transcephalic weak direct currents on lateralization in choice reaction tasks. J Psychophysiol 1987;1:127-33.

[11] Nitsche MA, Paulus W. Excitability changes induced in the human motor cortex by weak transcranial direct current stimulation. J Physiol 2000;527:633-9.

[12] Nitsche, MA, Paulus W. Sustained excitability elevations induced by transcranial DC motor cortex stimulation in humans. Neurology 2001;57:1899-1901.

[13] Nitsche, MA, Nitsche, MS, Klein, CC, Tergau F, Rothwell JC, Paulus W. Level of action of cathodal DC polarisation induced inhibition of the human motor cortex. Clin Neurophysiol 2003;114:600-4.

[14] Dundas JE, Thickbroom GW, Mastaglia FL. Perception of comfort during transcranial DC stimulation: effect of NaCl solution concentration applied to sponge electrodes. Clin Neurophysiol 2007; 18:1166-70.

[15] Iyer MB, Mattu U, Grafman J, et al. Safety and cognitive effect of frontal DC brain polarization in healthy individuals. Neurology 2005;64:872-5.

[16] Nitsche MA, Niehaus L, Hoffmann KT, Hengst S, Liebetanz D, Paulus W, Meyer BU. MRI study of human brain exposed to weak direct current stimulation of the frontal cortex. Clin Neurophysiol 2004;115:2419-23.

[17] Creutzfeldt OD, Fromm GH, Kapp H. Influence of transcortical d-c currents on cortical neuronal activity. Exp Neurol 1962;5:436-52.

[18] Nitsche MA, Fricke K, Henschke U, Schlitterlau A, Liebetanz D, Lang N, Henning S, Tergau F, Paulus W. Pharmacological modulation of cortical excitability shifts induced by transcranial direct current stimulation in humans. J Physiol. 2003;553:293-301.

[19] Purpura DP, McMurtry JG. Intracellular activities and evoked potential changes during polarization of motor cortex. J Neurophysiol 1965;28:166-85.

[20] Roth BJ. Mechanisms for electrical stimulation of excitable tissue. Crit Rev Biomed Eng 1994;22:253-305.

[21] Edgley SA, Eyre JA, Lemon RN, Miller S. Comparison of activation of corticospinal neurons and spinal motor neurons by magnetic and electrical transcranial stimulation in the lumbosacral cord of the anaesthetized monkey. Brain 1997;120:839-53.
[22] Ardolino G, Bossi B, Barbieri S, Priori A. Non-synaptic mechanisms underlie the after-effects of cathodal transcutaneous direct current stimulation of the human brain. J Physiol 2005;568:653-63.
[23] Nitsche MA, Seeber A, Frommann K, Klein CC, Rochford C, Nitsche MS, Fricke K, Liebetanz D, Lang N, Antal A, Paulus W, Tergau F. Modulating parameters of excitability during and after transcranial direct current stimulation of the human motor cortex. J Physiol 2005;568:291-303.
[24] Kujirai T, Caramia MD, Rotwell JC, Day BL, Thompson PD, Ferbert A, Wroe S, Asselman P, Marsden CD. Corticocortical inhibition in human motor cortex. J. Physiol 1993;471:501-19.
[25] Ziemann U. TMS and drugs. Clin Neurophysiology, 2004;115:1717-29.
[26] Antal A, Nitsche MA, Paulus W. External modulation of visual perception in humans. Neuroreport. 2001;12:3553-5.
[27] Antal A, Kincses TZ, Nitsche MA, Bartfai O, Paulus W. Excitability changes induced in the human primary visual cortex by transcranial direct current stimulation: direct electrophysiological evidence. Invest Ophthalmol Vis Sci 2004;45:702-7.
[28] Antal A, Kincses TZ, Nitsche MA, Paulus W. Manipulation of phosphene thresholds by transcranial direct current stimulation in man. Exp Brain Res 2003;150:375-8.
[29] Antal A, Varga ET, Nitsche MA, Chadaide Z, Paulus W, Kovács G, Vidnyánszky Z. Direct current stimulation over MT+/V5 modulates motion aftereffect in humans. Neuroreport. 2004; 15:2491-4.
[30] Kuo MF, Paulus W, Nitsche MA. Sex differences of cortical neuroplasticity in humans. Neuroreport 2006;17:1703-7.
[31] Chaieb L, Antal A, Paulus W. Gender-specific modulation of short-term neuroplasticity in the visual cortex induced by transcranial direct current stimulation. Vis Neurosci 2008;25:77-81.
[32] Boros K, Poreisz C, Münchau A, Paulus W, Nitsche MA. Premotor transcranial direct current stimulation (tDCS) affects primary motor excitability in humans. Eur J Neurosci 2008;27:1292-300.
[33] Rogalewski A, Breitenstein C, Nitsche MA, Paulus W, Knecht S. Transcranial direct current stimulation disrupts tactile perception. Eur J Neurosci. 2004;20:313-6.
[34] Matsunaga K, Nitsche MA, Tsuji S, Rothwell J. Effect of trenscranial DC sensorimotor cortex stimulation on somatosensory evoked potentials in humans. Clin Neurophysiol 2004;115:456-60.
[35] Gartside IB. Mechanisms of sustained increases of firing rate of neurones in the rat cerebral cortex after polarization: Role of protein synthesis Nature 1968;220:383-4.
[36] Hattori Y, Moriwaki A, Hori Y. Biphasic effects of polarizing current on adenosine-sensitive generation of cyclic AMP in rat cerebral cortex. Neurosci Lett 1990;116:320-4.
[37] Islam N, Aftabuddin M, Moriwaki A, Hattori Y, Hori Y. Increase in the calcium level following anodal polarization in the rat brain. Brain Res 1995;684:206-8.
[38] Liebetanz D, Nitsche MA, Tergau F, Paulus W. Pharmacological approach to the mechanisms of transcranial DC-stimulation-induced after-effects of human motor cortex excitability. Brain 2002;125:2238-47.
[39] Nitsche MA, Jaussi W, Liebetanz D, Lang N, Tergau F, Paulus W. Consolidation of human motor cortical neuroplasticity by D-cycloserine. Neuropsychopharmacology 2004;29:1573-8.
[40] Nitsche MA, Grundey J, Liebetanz D, Lang N, Tergau F, Paulus W. Catecholaminergic consolidation of motor cortical neuroplasticity in humans. Cereb Cortex 2004;14:1240-5.
[41] Nitsche MA, Lampe C, Antal A, Liebetanz D, Lang N, Tergau F, Paulus W. Dopaminergic modulation of long-lasting direct current-induced cortical excitability changes in the human motor cortex. Eur J Neurosci 2006;23:1651-7.
[42] Kuo MF, Paulus W, Nitsche MA. Boosting Focally-Induced Brain Plasticity by Dopamine. Cereb Cortex, 2008;18:648-51.

[43] Kuo M-F, Grosch J, Fregni F, Paulus W, Nitsche MA. Focusing effect of acetylcholine on neuroplasticity in the human motor cortex. J Neurosci 2007;27:1442-7.
[44] Agnew WF, McCreery DB. Considerations for safety in the use of extracranial stimulation for motor evoked potentials. Neurosurgery 1987;20:143-7.
[45] Gandiga PC, Hummel FC, Cohen LG. Transcranial DC stimulation (tDCS): a tool for double-blind sham-controlled clinical studies in brain stimulation. Clin Neurophysiol 2006;117:845-50.
[46] Liebetanz D, Klinker F, Hering D, Koch R, Nitsche MA, Potschka H, Loscher W, Paulus W, Tergau F. Anticonvulsant effects of transcranial direct-current stimulation (tDCS) in the rat cortical ramp model of focal epilepsy. Epilepsia. 2006;47:1216-24.
[47] Poreisz C, Boros K, Antal A, Paulus W. Safety aspects of transcranial direct current stimulation concerning healthy subjects and patients. Brain Res Bull 2007;72:208-14.
[48] Fregni F, Boggio PS, Lima MC, Ferreira MJ, Wagner T, Rigonatti SP, Castro AW, Souza DR, Riberto M, Freedman SD, Nitsche MA, Pascual-Leone A. A sham-controlled, phase II trial of transcranial direct current stimulation for the treatment of central pain in traumatic spinal cord injury. Pain 2006;122:197-209.
[49] Hummel F, Celnik P, Giraux P, Floel A, Wu WH, Gerloff C, Cohen LG. Effects of non-invasive cortical stimulation on skilled motor function in chronic stroke. Brain 2005;128:490-9.

In: Pain Management Yearbook 2009
Editor: Joav Merrick

ISBN: 978-1-61209-666-7
©2012 Nova Science Publishers, Inc.

Chapter 27

NON-INVASIVE BRAIN STIMULATION APPROACHES TO FIBROMYALGIA PAIN

Baron Short, MD[*,1,2], *Jeffrey J Borckardt, PhD*[1,3], *Mark George, MD*[1,4,5], *Will Beam, BS*[3] *and Scott T Reeves, MD*[3]

[1]Department of Psychiatry, [2]Department of Internal Medicine, [3]Department of Anesthesia, [4]Department of Radiology, [5]Department of Neurosciences, Medical University of South Carolina, Charleston, South Carolina, United States of America

Abstract

Fibromyalgia is a poorly understood disorder that likely involves central nervous system sensory hypersensitivity. There are a host of genetic, neuroendocrine and environmental abnormalities associated with the disease, and recent research findings suggest enhanced sensory processing, and abnormalities in central monoamines and cytokines expression in patients with fibromyalgia. The morbidity and financial costs associated with fibromyalgia are quite high despite conventional treatments with antidepressants, anticonvulsants, low-impact aerobic exercise and psychotherapy. Noninvasive brain stimulation techniques, such as transcranial direct current stimulation, transcranial magnetic stimulation, and electroconvulsive therapy are beginning to be studied as possible treatments for fibromyalgia pain. Early studies appear promising but more work is needed. Future directions in clinical care may include innovative combinations of noninvasive brain stimulation, pharmacological augmentation, and behavior therapies.

Keywords: Fibromyalgia, transcranial magnetic stimulation, transcranial direct current stimulation, noninvasive brain stimulation, chronic pain, electroconvulsive therapy, prefrontal cortex, primary motor cortex.

---

[*] **Correspondence:** E Baron Short, MD, Assistant Professor, Director of Inpatient Adult General Psychiatry for 3 North Unit, Associate Residency Director of Internal Medicine/ Psychiatry Program, Institute of Psychiatry and Behavioral Sciences, Department of Internal Medicine, Medical University of South Carolina, 67 President Street, PO Box 250861, Charleston, SC 29425 United States. Tel: 843-792-0199; Fax: 843-792-7037; E-mail: shorteb@musc.edu

Introduction

The American College of Rheumatology defines fibromyalgia criteria to include pain of at least three months duration above and below the waist bilaterally, axial skeletal pain, and 11 of 18 discrete tender points (1). Historically, fibromyalgia was often termed fibrositis and categorized as an inflammatory musculoskeletal disease. However investigators have not found significant pathology in the muscle or connective tissue regions where fibromyalgia patients complain of pain, thus the focus has shifted to the central nervous system to explain the pain perception abnormalities. Central sensitization or augmentation is one of the more common pain models for fibromyalgia.

Central sensitization likely involves a cascade of events which culminates in the release of excitatory agents, such as glutamate and substance P, at A and C afferent pain fibers at the synapses of dorsal horn neurons and secondarily prolong the excitability of second-order dorsal horn neurons that drive pain states (2). Spinal glial cells may play a role as they can release proinflammatory cytokines, prostaglandins, glutamate, substance P, and calcitonin gene-related peptides, which can precipitate hyperexcitable dorsal horn neurons. As supporting evidence, AV-411, a glial cell modulation drug, decreased pain sensitivity to mechanical pressure in an animal model of neuropathic pain (3). In both animal and human models of central sensitization, the source of sensory input (e.g., nerve injury) is known and pain sensitivity is reduced if the source of sensory input is removed. However, the source of sensory input among patients with fibromyalgia is unknown. Therefore, many fibromyalgia researchers refer to central augmentation of sensory input rather than central sensitization when they discuss the pathophysiology of fibromyalgia (4). In conjunction with the central sensitization or augmentation model of pain, there is a constellation of other biopsychosocial factors that play a role in fibromyalgia.

Biopsychosocial abnormalities

Familial associations: Arnold et al (5) reported that the first-degree relatives of patients with fibromyalgia, compared with those of patients with rheumatoid arthritis (RA), were more likely to meet diagnostic criteria for fibromyalgia or major depressive disorder (MDD) and exhibited a greater number of sensitive tender points. The frequency of fibromyalgia among the first-degree relatives of probands with fibromyalgia and those with RA was 6.4% and 1.1%, respectively. The frequency of lifetime MDD diagnoses within these two groups of relatives was 29.5% and 18.3%.

Bradley et al (6) assessed pain thresholds for mechanical pressure, thermal and ischemic stimulation as well as blood serum serotonin levels among the siblings of fibromyalgia probands and healthy controls. Preliminary data showed that the fibromyalgia probands and their siblings displayed significantly lower pain threshold levels in response to the 3 forms of pain stimulation compared to healthy controls and their siblings, respectively. Interestingly, none of the proband siblings reported persistent or recurrent musculoskeletal pain. These findings, in conjunction with those of Arnold et al (5) suggested that both fibromyalgia probands and their first-degree relatives display enhanced pain sensitivity to multiple nociceptive stimuli.

Genetic associations: The enhanced pain sensitivity in fibromyalgia may be attributed is the serotonin transporter (5-HTT) gene (7). Offenbaecher et al (8) and Cohen et al (9) in independent samples, reported that a single nucleotide polymorphism in the regulatory region of the 5-HTT gene occurs significantly more often in patients with fibromyalgia than in healthy controls. These findings are consistent with Bradley et al (6) wherein both the fibromyalgia probands and their siblings exhibit significantly lower blood serum levels of 5-HT than healthy controls and their siblings, respectively. This particular polymorphism is found more frequently not only in fibromyalgia but patients with MDD (10), and diarrhea-predominant irritable bowel syndrome (11,12) compared with healthy controls. This data lends support to the hypothesis that fibromyalgia may be a part of a group of affective spectrum disorders (ASD) that share 1 or more physiologic abnormalities important to their etiology (13). The ASD grouping contains 10 psychiatric disorders, including major depression, and 4 medical disorders, including migraine and irritable bowel syndrome.

Environmental factors: Environmental triggers including, physical trauma and psychosocial stressors, may be involved in the pathophysiology of fibromyalgia (14,15). Harkness et al (16) reported that both physical and psychosocial stressors predict the development of chronic widespread body pain, and psychosocial factors may, in fact, initiate the development of widespread pain. Davis (17) and Okonkwo et al (18) independently found evidence that inducing negative mood and stress exposure could worsen pain ratings in patients with fibromyalgia.

Stress response dysregulation: Stress response abnormalities are present in fibromyalgia primarily involving the hypothalamic-pituitary-adrenal (HPA) axis and autonomic nervous systems. McCain and Tilbe (19) observed patients with fibromyalgia or RA for 3 days and found that fibromyalgia patients exhibited higher peak and trough levels of plasma cortisol compared with those with RA. Furthermore, fibromyalgia patients displayed significantly higher overall plasma cortisol levels than RA patients. In response to dexamethasone, 35% of patients with fibromyalgia had unsuppressed plasma cortisol levels compared with only 5% of patients with RA. They also found patients with fibromyalgia lost diurnal cortisol response. Crofford (20) revealed a decreased response to corticotropin releasing hormone, which is released to enact a stress response. Hence, there is emerging support that fibromyalgia may involve neuroendocrine abnormalities.

Patients with fibromyalgia also have autonomic nervous system dysfunction that includes hypotension (21-23), variations in heart rate (22), decreased microcirculatory vasoconstriction (24), and sleep disturbance (25, 26). A dysregulated autonomic nervous system may contribute to enhanced pain and other clinical problems associated with fibromyalgia through alterations of physiologic responses required for effective stress management (e.g., blood pressure increases) and pain inhibition (e.g., neurotransmitter availability).

Monoamines: Several lines of evidence suggest that both serotonin and norepinephrine systems are dysfunctional in fibromyalgia patients (27-29). Wolfe et al (7)., found that fibromyalgia subjects had lower serotonin levels even after adjusting for age and sex than those without fibromyalgia p-chlorophenylalanine, a centrally acting serotonin synthesis inhibitor, can induce symptoms similar to those associated with fibromyalgia (30). Tricyclic antidepressants and selective serotonin-norepinephrine reuptake inhibitors may also reduce pain independent of their antidepressant actions as a result of their serotonin- and norepinephrine-mediated effects on the descending pain inhibitory pathways in the brain and spinal cord (31).

While serotonin and norepinephrine have been studied more extensively, there is possibly a role for dopamine in fibromyalgia pathophysiology (32). Wood and Holman (33) using positron emission tomography found reductions in 6-[(18)F]fluoro-L-DOPA uptake on in several brain regions that involve pain perception, suggesting a disruption of presynaptic dopamine activity wherein dopamine plays an important role in endogenous analgesia.

Cytokines: Inflammatory cytokines play a role in diverse clinical processes and phenomena such as fatigue, fever, sleep, pain, depression, stress, and aching (34). Cytokines related to acute or repetitive tissue injuries may be responsible for long-term activation of spinal cord glia and dorsal horn neurons, thus resulting in central sensitization. Cytokines might cause depressive symptoms through modulation of the HPA axis or they may cause downregulation of the synthesis of serotonin; both of these effects might contribute to the development of depression and enhanced pain perception (35-37). Cytokines can directly induce pain sensitization (38) and the inflammatory cytokines IL-1,IL-6, and IL-8 may be dysregulated in FM (39).

Neuroanatomic abnormalities: Multiple brain regions are involved in pain processing. Sensory components include thalamus and sensory cortices, but affective and cognitive components to pain involving other limbic, prefrontal and associative cortices (40). There have been several neuroanatomic abnormalities observed in patients with fibromyalgia. In a single-photon emission computed tomography study, patients with fibromyalgia (compared to healthy controls) showed a decrease in regional cerebral blood flow in the thalamus, caudate nucleus, and pontine tegmentum (41). Gracely et al (42) used functional magnetic resonance imaging (fMRI) to examine the pattern of cerebral activation during the application of painful pressure in patients with fibromyalgia compared with controls. The fMRI results revealed that when moderate levels of pressure were applied to the patients and the controls, no common regions of activation were observed and a greater effect was noticed in patients. When the stimulation was increased to deliver a subjective level of pain in the control group similar to that experienced by fibromyalgia patients, similar activation patterns were seen in patients and controls. Hence, fibromyalgia patients exhibited enhanced sensory processing. This enhanced sensory processing may be nonspecific to fibromyalgia as similar brain regions (contralateral primary [S1] and secondary [S2] somatosensory cortices, inferior parietal lobule, cerebellum, and ipsilateral S2) were activated in idiopathic chronic back pain and fibromyalgia in comparison to healthy controls (43). Additional functional neuroimaging studies have suggested that fibromyalgia is associated with changes in the activity of brain structures involved in pain processing (44-46).

Morbidity and cost burden with conventional treatments: Fibromyalgia has a prevalence range of 0.5 to 5.0% in the general population and up to 15% in medical clinics. Females are 7 times more likely than males to have the disorder (47, 48). Age-adjusted incidence rates were 6.88 cases per 1000 person-years for males and 11.28 cases per 1000 person-years for females in a retrospective cohort study of 62,000 enrollees in nationwide sample (48). Current treatment strategies include treating targeted symptoms of pain and depression with pharmacological and non-pharmacological treatments (49). Pharmaceutical pain management with anti-inflammatory agents, antidepressants and opiates can offer some pain relief but can have significant side effects and adverse reactions (50-52). Despite current treatment, patients with fibromyalgia still incur significant medical utilization, work absence and disability (53). In a prospective cohort study of 34,100 employees, an excess rate of absence due to sickness was 61 episodes/100 person-years among people with fibromyalgia alone (54). In a retrospective cohort including 4,699 persons with fibromyalgia, total annual costs for fibromyalgia claimants were $5,945 versus $2,486 for the typical beneficiary. Six percent of these costs were attributable to fibromyalgia-specific claims but did not include indirect costs. The prevalence of disability was twice as high among employees with fibromyalgia compared to overall employees. For every dollar spent on fibromyalgia-specific claims, the employer spent another $57 to $143 on additional direct and indirect costs (55). Patients with fibromyalgia from 6 rheumatology centers had higher lifetime and current rates of medical service utilization with mean disability rates at 16% (56,57). In the same sample of 538 patients, measures of pain, fatigue, sleep disturbance, depression, and health status did not significantly change over seven years despite treatment (58).

To date, there are limited effective treatment options available to patients with fibromyalgia. Better therapeutic options are needed to reduce fibromyalgia morbidity and costs. Given that fibromyalgia involves abnormal central pain processing, noninvasive brain stimulation techniques are being studied as a means of modulating central nervous system pain processing.

Rationale for non-invasive brain stimulation for fibromyalgia

Noninvasive brain stimulation techniques, such as electroconvulsive therapy (ECT), repetitive transcranial magnetic stimulation (rTMS), have more evidence in psychiatric disorders. ECT and rTMS are both effective for the treatment of depression and rTMS was approved for the treatment of major depressive disorder in 2008. Other noninvasive brain stimulation methods, such as transcranial direct current stimulation (tDCS) have been less well studied in mood disorders but may be useful in both depression (59) and pain disorders (60-62).

The relationship between depression and pain is of significant interest in fibromyalgia and other disorders. When rigorous criteria are applied to diagnose depression, the prevalence of depression and concurrent chronic pain varies from 30-54% (63). The prevalence rate is higher in the general population than for either disorder alone (64). While many believe that depression is secondary to a loss of functioning due to persistent pain, there is some evidence to suggest that depressed individuals are more susceptible to developing pain disorders and they tend to have lower pain thresholds (65-67). Significant research has been done to better understand the biological and psychosocial mechanisms underlying pain and depression. There is significant overlap in the neurochemical processes and neuroanatomical structures thought to be involved in both biological and psychosocial explanations (63,68-72). Since fibromyalgia pain and depression frequently co-exist and there is overlap in terms of neurological substrates between the two conditions, investigators have begun to study noninvasive brain stimulation interventions that have potential to impact affective and sensory dimensions of the pain experience. Currently ECT, rTMS, tDCS have been employed in attempt to modulate fibromyalgia pain.

Electroconvulsive therapy: ECT was introduced in 1938 and remains one of the most effective treatments in psychiatry. ECT has developed into a technically sophisticated procedure with a proven record of safety. The procedure involves passing electrical pulses of approximately 1 ampere into the brain in order to provoke an epileptic seizure. The mechanism is action is not fully known but literature supports ECT may increase Brain

Derived Neurotrophic Factor (BDNF) (73, 74). BDNF likely plays a critical role in the action of antidepressants through neuronal plasticity.

Many studies, dating back to the 1940s, have reported the beneficial effects of ECT upon a variety of pain states. Several studies have demonstrated the clinical effectiveness of ECT treatment for neuropathic pain with low-blood flow in one side of the thalamus (75-77). However, some other reports have not resulted in demonstrable pain relief following ECT (78,79). In addition, there is one report that describes the use of ECT to effectively treat depression associated with fibromyalgia, but had no effect upon pain or other physical symptoms associated with fibromyalgia (80).

Usui and colleagues (81) prospectively designed an ECT study to assess changes in fibromyalgia pain that excluded patients that were diagnosed with concomitant organic disorders or mental disorders as classified by the Diagnostic and Statistical Manual of Mental Disorders. The study group consisted of 15 patients, seven men and eight women, aged 22–76 years (mean age = 42.1, SD = 13.1). The mean duration of fibromyalgia was 4.6 years (SD = 1.2). Fourteen patients had been taking antidepressant medication (milnacipran or paroxetine or amitriptyline) for fibromyalgia. Two patients were on low-dose steroid therapy. The medication was kept constant during the research trial. All patients received bilateral ECT set at 110 volts for 5 seconds. Twelve patients received six sessions, while three patients received only four sessions due to excellent responses. The number of tender points and the pain score (according to Visual analogue scale (VAS)) were significantly improved after ECT. Tender points dropped from a mean of 16.47 ± 0.59 to 6.73 ± 1.04 three days post-ECT. VAS pain scores increased at 3 months and returned to baseline in two patients. Beck Depression Inventory (BDI) scores did not reveal the presence of clinical depression and there were not significant changes in depression ratings post-ECT. The ECT treatment effect on fibromyalgia pain reduction appeared independent of mood changes in the study. Regional cerebral blood flow (rCBF) was also assessed (using single photon emission computed tomography [SPECT]) in each patient before and three days after the course of ECT. For quantitative SPECT analysis, they measured rCBF by using a three-dimensional stereotaxic region of interest template (3DSRT) (82) in addition to regional quantitative analysis. The mean thalamus-to-cerebellum ratio was significantly increased ($P < 0.01$) post-ECT in comparison to before ECT. The SPECT results suggest that improvement of rCBF in the thalamus may correlate with ECT analgesia. It has been shown that improvement in mood following administration of ECT is associated with an increase in rCBF (83). ECT may activate inhibitory pathways via the activation of serotonergic, noradrenergic, and dopaminergic neurotransmission systems in the brain (84). Abnormal sensory processing in fibromyalgia may be modulated by ECT treatment for fibromyalgia. Small sample size, open labeled design, and no other fibromyalgia quality of life instruments limited this study. Further work is needed to understand if ECT can reduce fibromyalgia pain and whether co-morbid depression would be suitable for treatment given a prior study showing no difference in fibromyalgia pain despite reduction in depression. A complicating factor of further ECT research with fibromyalgia is the "invasiveness" (i.e. anesthetic induction, seizure induction, potential cognitive side effects) of this noninvasive brain stimulation technique. Thus less invasive techniques may be more likely to gain ground in fibromyalgia research.

Transcranial direct current stimulation: Transcranial direct current stimulation (tDCS) is the application of weak electrical currents (1-2 mA) to modulate the activity of neurons in the brain. Neuronal firing increases when the positive pole (anode) is located near the cell body or dendrites. Neuronal firing is inhibited when cathode stimulation is applied (85,86). However, when the electrodes are placed on the scalp, the current density produced in the brain is exceedingly small, changing membrane potentials only by a fraction of a millivolt (87). The mechanism of action is unknown but pharmacological studies hint at ionic channel modulation. Sodium and calcium channel blockers eliminate both the immediate and long-term effects of anodal stimulation while blocking NMDA (glutamate) receptors prevents the long-term effects of tDCS, regardless of direction (88). Nitsche et al (89) investigated the short- and long-term effects of anodal and cathodal tDCS on the motor cortex by measuring intracortical inhibition and facilitation as well as indirect-wave (I-wave) interactions. The effects on cortical inhibition suggested that tDCS modulates the excitability of both inhibitory interneurons as well as excitatory neurons. Furthermore, anodal stimulation had a significant positive effect on I-wave facilitation. I-waves are modified by GABAergic drugs and ketamine, an NMDA receptor antagonist, but not by ion channel blockers, thus implicating effects on inhibitory synaptic pathways in the mechanism of action of anodal stimulation (90,91).

There are limited parameters that can be set with tDCS, primarily involving locations of the cathode and anode, voltage intensity, electrode size, and time per session. The typical levels administered are 1 or 2 milliamperes of direct current applied for a maximum of 20 minutes in a given session. In contrast to TMS, this technique does not produce a strongly localized effect; however, increasing the size of the reference electrode and reducing the size of the stimulation electrode allows for more focal treatment effects (92). A feeling of tingling under the electrodes is the most common side effect, although there have been some reports of mild skin burning associated with repeated daily tDCS sessions (93).

Currently tDCS is being studied in a variety of disease processes including stroke recovery (94), depression (59), and pain (60,61). There are two published studies applying tDCS for fibromyalgia pain and sleep disturbance. Fregni et al (95) conducted tests to determine whether active stimulation of the primary motor cortex (M1) or the dorsolateral prefrontal cortex (DLPFC) is associated with a reduction of pain and other symptoms of fibromyalgia as compared with sham stimulation. The primary motor cortex and the DLPFC were chosen as targets, because stimulation of the primary motor cortex induces a significant anti-nociceptive effect using rTMS (62, 96), and stimulation of the DLPFC using tDCS is associated with a significant antidepressant effect (97). Thirty-two female patients participated in this study. Patients were on stable doses of analgesics for at least two months prior to the beginning of the study and were included in the analysis in an attempt to address it as confound. Subjects underwent a two week observation period during which baseline levels of pain were established, followed by a randomization and implementation of double-blinded treatment, during which patients received daily treatment with sham tDCS, tDCS of the primary motor cortex, or tDCS of the DLPFC for five consecutive days, with a 21 day followup. Subjects underwent assessment with clinical visual analogue scale (CVAS), Fibromyalgia Impact Questionnaire (FIQ), Short-Form 36 Health Survey (SF-36), Clinical Global Impression Scale (CGI), Beck Depression Inventory (BDI), and an anxiety visual analog scale. Using the 10/20 system of electrode placement, the anode was placed over C3 for primary motor cortex, F3 for DLPFC with the cathode over contralateral supraorbital area. Electrodes were 35 cm^2. The sham group received thirty seconds of stimulation over M1 so subjects felt the initial itching sensation but received no current for the rest of the session. A constant current of 2-mA intensity was applied for 20 minutes. Eleven enrolled in each treatment arm, ten in the sham group with one drop out in the M1 group due to minor skin irritation at the site of stimulation. Pain VAS revealed that DLFPC was not statistically different from sham regarding pain change over time. M1 had beta coefficient of .31, thus a .31 mean reduction in pain with each evaluation. CGI differences in repeated-measures ANOVA revealed a group effect difference. Post hoc comparisons showed a significant difference between M1 and DLPFC stimulation, M1 and sham stimulation, and DLPFC and sham stimulation. There was no time effect with CGI, suggesting pain improvement was constant throughout the trial. There was a significant difference across the three groups in regards to percent change in the tender point scores after five days of treatment. Post hoc tests revealed a significant difference between the M1 group and the sham group but not between the sham group and the DLPFC group. On day 5, tender point scores decreased by 17.1+/-11.8% in the M1 group, by 11.8+/-8.3% in the DLPFC group, and by 2.3+/-10.9% in the sham group. The 3 groups had a decrease in FIQ scores over the course of the trial. The decrease in the M1 group was significantly different from that seen in the sham group and the DLPFC group. There was no significant difference in Beck Depression Inventory scores across the 3 groups of treatment, but the DLPFC group had absolute mean change of 3 points. There was no cognitive impairment associated with tDCS. In this study, anodal tDCS of the primary motor cortex in fibromyalgia patients induced a significant reduction in pain compared to sham and DLFPC that lasted for several weeks after treatment had ended.

As an extension of the Fregni study, Roizenblatt and colleagues investigated correlations of sleep modulation with decreases in pain with fibromyalgia patients receiving tDCS at M1, DLPFC, or sham. There are sleep disturbances in fibromyalgia and whether alterations of alpha sleep patterns play an etiologic role are unclear (98, 99). Interestingly, slow wave sleep (SWS) fragmentation by alpha rhythm or extrinsic stimuli (100-103) is connected to non-restorative sleep and musculoskeletal pain. Prior work (104) has shown subjects had deeper sleep in the end of active tDCS and during the subsequent 15 minutes after stimulation when compared to placebo conditions. Hence, the work of Roizenblatt (105) is relevant. The methods were essentially the same for all elements other than sleep assessment with polysomnography (PSG). A baseline pretreatment PSG and post-treatment PSG was acquired in addition to the other phases previously described. A minimum of 7 hours of PSG recording was obtained. Total sleep time (TST) was defined as the time elapsed between the first and last recorded sleep period. Sleep efficiency corresponded to the percentage of TST in relation to the total recording time. Sleep latency was considered the time period measured from lights going out to the beginning of sleep and REM sleep latency, as the time interval from sleep onset to the first appearance of REM sleep. There was a statistically significant sleep efficiency modulation. Post-hoc comparisons showed that sleep efficiency was improved by 11.8% after M1 tDCS and significantly worsened by 7.5% after DLPFC stimulation. Additionally, DLPFC stimulation led to a significant worsening in other parameters of sleep such as an increase in sleep latency by 133.4% and REM latency by 47.7%. Conversely, M1 stimulation led to decrease in arousals by 35%. Finally, the alpha/delta index significantly increased after M1 tDCS and decreased after DLPFC tDCS. Thus tDCS at M1 increased sleep efficiency, decreased arousals and increased delta activity in non-REM sleep. DLPFC stimulation was associated with a decrease in sleep efficiency and an increase in REM and sleep latency. Additional, alpha activity increased and delta activity decreased in non-REM sleep after DLPFC stimulation. There was a significant correlation of quality of life improvement as assessed by FIQ changes with a decrease in sleep latency and with an increase in sleep efficiency after M1 stimulation. Finally, patients in whom DLPFC stimulation did not induce a worsening of sleep efficiency were those who obtained the largest pain improvement as indexed by VAS. The authors hypothesized the excitatory effects of anodal tDCS at M1 led to improvement of sleep architecture as a result of a normalization of the dysfunctional neural network activity that is associated with pain and sleep. The alpha/delta index decrease after DLPFC anodal stimulation is in accordance with rTMS and sleep deprivation which lead to an increase in DLPFC activity (106). Interestingly, ECT is associated with an alpha-EEG sleep pattern in depressed patients that is observed at the end of the ECT series (107). In this sense, the sleep alterations observed after DLPFC stimulation in the current study correlate with the Fregni study showing that a 5-day anodal tDCS of the left DLPFC improves mood in major depression (62).

Repetitive transcranial magnetic stimulation: One of the early uses of TMS in the treatment of pain grew out of the surgical implantation of motor cortex stimulation (MCS) (108). With TMS, current is rapidly turned on and off in the electromagnetic coil through the discharge of capacitors. The end result of TMS is thus electrical stimulation of the brain, and some refer to TMS as 'electrodeless electrical stimulation'. The electrical energy stored in a capacitor discharges and creates about 3,000 Amps. Through Maxwell's equations and Faraday's law, this creates a powerful magnetic field, on the order of 2 Tesla. This rapidly changing magnetic field (~30KT/s) then travels across the scalp and skull and induces an electric field within the brain (~30V/m). This induces current to flow in the brain by creating a transmembrane potential (for a thorough discussion see (109)). This localized pulsed magnetic field over the surface of the head depolarizes underlying superficial neurons (110,111), which then induces electrical currents in the brain. TMS therefore differs from techniques where direct electrical or magnetic energy is applied to the brain or body (such as ECT). TMS can induce varying brain effects depending on: 1) the cortical region stimulated, 2) the activity that the brain is engaged in, and 3) the TMS device parameters (particularly frequency, time-interval and intensity). TMS has been shown to produce immediate effects (e.g., thumb movement, phosphenes, temporary aphasia) (112) that are thought to result from direct excitation of inhibitory or excitatory neurons. TMS at different intensities, frequencies and coil angles excites different elements (e.g., cell bodies, axons) of different neuronal groups (e.g., interneurons, neurons projecting into other cortical areas) (113-115). Intermediate effects of TMS (seconds to minutes) likely arise from transient changes in local pharmacology (e.g., gamma-aminobuteric acid, glutamate) (116) and much research has focused on whether different TMS frequencies might have different intermediate biological effects. Repeated low-frequency stimulation of a single neuron in culture produces long-lasting inhibition of cell-cell communication (117,118) while high frequency stimulation can improve communication (119).

It has been hypothesized that TMS can produce sustained inhibitory or excitatory effects in a way analogous to single-cell electrical stimulation (120). Several studies have shown that chronic stimulation of the motor cortex can produce inhibitory or excitatory intermediate effects (lasting several minutes) following stimulation (121,122). Investigations of the intermediate effects of TMS have been used to develop a better understanding of brain functioning with respect to movement, vision, memory, attention, speech, neuroendocrine hormones and mood (123-129). Longer term effects of TMS (days to weeks) are not well understood at a neurobiological level, but there is evidence to support longer-term effects on mood, seizure activity and pain (96, 130-134). With respect to mood, it is hypothesized that chronic repetitive stimulation of the prefrontal cortex initiates a cascade of events in the prefrontal cortex and in connected limbic regions (135). TMS/fMRI interleaved studies as well as PET studies by Paus and others provide evidence to support this hypothesis. Prefrontal TMS sends information to important mood-regulating regions including the cingulate gyrus, orbitofrontal cortex, insula and hippocampus, and there is PET evidence that prefrontal TMS causes dopamine release in the caudate nucleus (and reciprocal activity with the anterior cingulate gyrus) (132,133,135). rTMS is currently been studied for a variety of pain conditions including laboratory induced, neuropathic pain, postoperative pain, and fibromyalgia.

Neuroimaging studies (136,137) have shown that hemodynamic changes induced in the brain by epidural electrical stimulation are not confined to the motor system, but instead involve a set of cortical (e.g. cingulate, orbitofrontal and prefrontal cortices, thalamus and striatum) and subcortical (e.g. periaqueductal gray matter) areas, involved in pain processing and modulation (138-140). Similar changes in brain activity have been demonstrated after the application of rTMS to the motor cortex (141-143), suggesting that rTMS can also modulate the activity of brain structures involved in pain perception. In particular, the analgesic effects of rTMS may involve the pain modulation systems of the diencephalon and/or descending from the brainstem to the spinal cord (144) although other mechanisms such as changes in intracortical inhibitory mechanisms have also been suggested (145). Consistent with these hypotheses, rTMS of the motor cortex, has been shown to reduce experimental pain both in healthy volunteers and in patients with chronic pain (96, 30,146-151).

To date there have been three published studies involving rTMS and fibromyalgia (152,153). (See References on additional text attached for subsequent citation numbering) Sampson (152) examined the effect of slow-frequency (1 Hz) rTMS in subjects with treatment-resistant depression and borderline personality disorder (BPD). Four subjects in this study also had a previous diagnosis of fibromyalgia. Low-frequency rTMS (1 Hz) applied to the right DLPFC was shown to increase bilateral pain tolerance in healthy volunteers (154) and has reduced depressive symptoms (155). The design was sham-controlled, double-blinded. rTMS was produced using a Magstim Super Rapid repetitive stimulator and a 70-mm figure-of-eight coil. Single transcranial magnetic stimuli were used to identify motor threshold (MT). One-hertz rTMS was applied 5 cm anterior to the optimal motor cortex stimulation site to approximate localization of the R-DLPFC. rTMS was applied using a frequency of 1 Hz, intensity of 110% MT, and two 800 second trains with an intertrain interval of 60 seconds, for a total of 1,600 stimuli per session. One of the four subjects with FM received 10 sham rTMS treatments using a 90-degree coil rotation before receiving active rTMS. Subjects received active rTMS over 4 weeks, and one subject received an additional 12 treatments over 6 weeks as part of a taper protocol for those who had remission of depression (> 50% decline and <10 on the Hamilton Rating Scale for Depression (HRSD)). Although improvement on HRSD and ratings were statistically significant, only one subject had a remission of depression. All subjects noted an improvement in fibromyalgia pain, with two subjects reporting complete resolution of pain. One subject received sham rTMS for 2 weeks with no pain improvement during that time. One subject noted improvement in pain during the first week of treatment, and two noted improvement during week 3 of treatment. Two subjects provided pain ratings during treatment and two described changes in pain retrospectively when contacted after it was noted that rTMS might be altering pain. The subjects were contacted repeatedly after finishing the acute series of treatment to assess the recurrence of pain. The subjects were defined as having recurrence of pain when reported ratings increased by at least 1.5 points. The duration of pain improvement ranged from 15 to 27 weeks. Given the limited reduction in depression ratings, the reduction in fibromyalgia pain cannot be explained by the treatment of depression alone. Notably, the subjects' pain improvement was sustained for a number of weeks after rTMS, and suggests the possibility that rTMS applied to the R-DLPFC may be clinically useful in reducing fibromyalgia pain. This study was not prospectively designed or powered to assess changes in fibromyalgia pain and hence there is only 4 subjects reported. Half the subject data was retrospectively gathered. Furthermore it is unclear what sham system was implemented. Nonetheless this is the first rTMS publication detailing prefrontal cortical stimulation in fibromyalgia with rTMS.

Carretero and colleagues (154) recently published a replication study using similar parameters as Sampson but in a larger sample with randomization and a placebo controlled arm. There were 14 subjects that underwent real TMS and 12 that received sham TMS. The real rTMS was employed with DANTEC TMS equipment at the same R-DLPFC location as with Sampson's work. Subjects received 1 Hz 60 seconds on and 45 seconds off at 110% MT for approximately 30 minutes for a total of 1200 pulses per session. Subjects received 20 daily sessions in total. Both groups improved in fatigue and CGI but there was no improvement in pain and depression. Furthermore there was no significant difference between real and sham TMS in this sample. However, the sham system was suboptimal with simply a shift in the TMS coil to 45 degrees so that sound is heard but no cutaneous sensation was experienced. More importantly subjects received 400 fewer pulses per session for a total of 8000 fewer pulses than the Sampson group. Thus subjects may have been relatively "underdosed" in comparison.

Passard and colleagues (153), hypothesized that rTMS of the motor cortex might reduce chronic widespread pain in patients with fibromyalgia. They employed a randomized, double blind, sham-controlled parallel group study analyzing the analgesic effects of repeated daily sessions of unilateral rTMS in patients with widespread pain, quality of life, mood, and anxiety due to fibromyalgia. Tender point pain threshold was a secondary outcome. A Super-Rapid Magstim Stimulator (Magstim Co., Whitland, UK) with a figure-of-eight-shaped coil was employed. Each treatment session consisted of 25 series of 8-second pulse trains, with 52 seconds interval between series, at a stimulation frequency of 10 Hz and 80% resting motor threshold intensity, giving a total of 2000 pulses per session. The resting motor threshold (MT) was determined before each session, using a single-pulse stimulation over the left primary motor cortex. The primary outcome measure was self-reported average pain intensity over the last 24 hours using the 11-point numerical scale of the BPI. Average pain intensity was reported for 1 week as a baseline, during treatment (days 1-14) and until the first followup visit to make it possible to determine the onset of treatment effects, then was assessed at each follow-up visit on days 15, 30, and 60. Changes between the baseline and the endpoint after treatment in the BPI average pain severity score and all secondary efficacy variables (BPI-Interference scores, number of tender points, scores for the FIQ, HAD, BDI and HDRS, pressure pain thresholds) were compared between the active and sham stimulation groups. A repeated measures analysis of variance (ANOVA) was carried out in which the dependent variable was one of the outcome measures and the factors were treatment group (active or sham rTMS) and time (baseline, day 15, day 30 and day 60). Four patients (two per treatment group) withdrew from the trial between days 30 and 60. Pain intensity was similar in the two groups at baseline and rTMS had a significant effect on average pain intensity score between baseline and day 15 in comparison with sham stimulation. This effect was not maintained on days 30 and 60. Average pain intensity was significantly lower in the active rTMS group than in the sham stimulation from day 5 to day 14. On day 15, McGill Pain Questionnaire total score and the sensory and affective subscores were significantly lower in the active rTMS group than in the sham-stimulation group. The difference in affective subscore persisted until day 30, whereas the sensory subscore did not. Subjective global pain relief over the last week, as reported by the patients, was significantly greater in the active than in the sham-stimulation group up to day 30. Mean depression and anxiety scores were similar in the two treatment groups at baseline and were not significantly changed by active or sham stimulation. rTMS had no significant effect on the number of tender points. This study showed that rTMS of the primary motor cortex induced a long-lasting decrease in pain and improved quality of life in patients with fibromyalgia, without affecting mood or anxiety levels. The analgesic effects of rTMS differed for the sensory and affective dimensions of pain with the affective dimension change lasting 15 days longer. One critique of this study is the design of the sham system. Per description, it makes similar sounds as active rTMS, however there is no form of superficial stimulation to the scalp, which can be problematic as otherwise the active and sham are easily discerned when compared.

Our laboratory is currently investigating the effects of rTMS in left DLPFC with the following TMS parameters: 10 Hertz - pulse train duration (on time) 5 seconds, power (intensity) level 120% of motor threshold, and inter-train interval (off time) 10 seconds (15 second cycle time). The rationale for high frequency left prefrontal is related to current work with similar parameters for the treatment of depression and findings from implanted motor cortex stimulator research, and laboratory and clinical studies conducted in our laboratory. Much of the variance in clinical response to implanted motor cortex stimulation seems to be explained by limbic activity (136,156). If one of the mechanisms by which cortical stimulation alleviates pain is by modulating the processing of the affective dimension of pain experience, the prefrontal cortex might be a more efficient cortical target for pain management (135). Consistent with this notion, a few studies have demonstrated acute and transient anti-nociceptive effects with prefrontal cortex TMS (154,157).

We are employing a double blind (rater blinded to condition) sham-controlled design. In order to maintain study blind, the length of treatment and the number of pulses on the head is the same for all subjects. What differs is whether they receive active or sham. The sham group only receives sham at all treatments. Our sham system incorporates a transcutaneous electrical nerve stimulator (TENS) that does not appreciably penetrate through the skull, yet does elicit uncomfortable stimuli similar to the cutaneous sensation from rTMS. Additionally the TENS unit is triggered in concert with rTMS pulses. Subjects receive 4000 pulses per session, 10 sessions over 2 weeks for a total of 40,000 pulses. Early interim analysis, using Hierarchical Linear Modeling and a 0-10 Likert pain scale, (3 active TMS participants, 1 placebo TMS participant) suggested main effects of treatment versus placebo by time (P=.0479), a decrease of 0.16 points in average pain-per-day in the treatment arm (P=.0006), and an average pain reduction of 1.79 at the end of treatment (P<.0001). The treatment arm maintained a reduction in average pain of 1.12 at the end of the last assessment in week 4 (P = .0164). Statistical significance of change per day from baseline began at day 8 and ended at day-20. The baseline HRSD mean score was 18.75 and there was an insignificant decrease in depression from baseline to end of treatment (week 2). There was a decrease in depression from baseline to last followup (P = .0307) of 4.3 points. These interim analyses are tentative at best and more confident statements can be made upon completing enrollment and full analysis. If the interim results are maintained, then fast rTMS stimulation to the LDLPFC may significant lower fibromyalgia pain and be observed before any improvement in mood.

Future directions

Noninvasive brain stimulation is in its infancy, particularly related to chronic pain disorders such as fibromyalgia. Although there are few studies to date, there are potentially promising results of at least three noninvasive techniques (ECT, tDCS, rTMS) in the treatment of fibromyalgia. More work is needed on the site of stimulation and optimal stimulation parameters. Neurophysiological markers may be useful to discern optimal parameters. Applying TMS and tDCS with event-related potentials (ERPs) may assist in describing the underlying neurophysiologic mechanisms of normal and abnormal pain responses. The laser-evoked potential is the ERP response secondary to a mild laser stimulus. Depending on the manner in which this stimulation is performed, it is possible to stimulate A delta fibers or C fibers, and TMS can be applied to modulate these evoked potentials (158). LEP changes and subjective relief on VAS were also observed after tDCS treatments (61,159).

These brain stimulation techniques do not necessarily have to occur separately. tDCS has been used for rTMS "priming" (86). Noninvasive brain stimulation techniques might be used to locate the optimum sites for pain relief and possibly to aid in the implantation process of permanent devices for more constant stimulation. Additionally, pharmacological agents have the potential to act synergistically with brain stimulation techniques (160). Specific medications eventually might be given before or after stimulation to enhance neuroplasticity changes associated with stimulation. Mental activities during stimulation may also enhance neuroplasticity changes. Gracely (161) found that catastrophizing influences pain perception through altering attention and anticipation, and heightening emotional responses to pain. Potentially, other techniques of altering attention and cognitive processing, such as hypnosis, mindfulness, or cognitive therapy in conjunction with brain stimulation may be fruitful. The wide range of techniques and parameters of brain stimulation in conjunction with pharmacological and behavioral methods makes this area of research quite innovative. All three noninvasive brain stimulation techniques are readily available, thus more clinical trial work is needed to confer evidence for employing them for the treatment of fibromyalgia.

Acknowledgments

Dr. Short's work is funded in part by NIAMS. Dr. Borckardt's work is funded in part by the following NINDS: 5K23NS050485-03, NINR: 1R21NR010635-01, NIDA: 1R21DA026085-01, The Robert Wood Johnson Foundation, Neuropace Inc and Cyberonics Inc.

References

[1] Wolfe F, Smythe HA, Yunus MB, Bennett RM, Bombardier C, Goldenberg DL, et al. The American College of Rheumatology 1990 Criteria for the Classification of Fibromyalgia. Report of the Multicenter Criteria Committee. Arthritis Rheum 1990;33(2):160-72.

[2] Bradley LA. Pathophysiologic mechanisms of fibromyalgia and its related disorders. J Clin Psychiatry 2008;69 Suppl 2:6-13.

[3] Ledeboer A, Hutchinson MR, Watkins LR, Johnson KW. Ibudilast (AV-411). A new class therapeutic candidate for neuropathic pain and opioid withdrawal syndromes. Expert Opin Investig Drugs 2007;16(7):935-50.

[4] Watkins LR, Milligan ED, Maier SF. Glial proinflammatory cytokines mediate exaggerated pain states: implications for clinical pain. Adv Exp Med Biol 2003;521:1-21.

[5] Arnold LM, Hudson JI, Hess EV, Ware AE, Fritz DA, Auchenbach MB, et al. Family study of fibromyalgia. Arthritis Rheum 2004; 50(3):944-52.

[6] Bradley L FR, Sotolongo A, et al. Family aggregation of pain sensitivity in fibromyalgia. J Pain 2006;7(4):S1.

[7] Wolfe F, Russell IJ, Vipraio G, Ross K, Anderson J. Serotonin levels, pain threshold, and fibromyalgia symptoms in the general population. J Rheumatol 1997;24(3):555-9.

[8] Offenbaecher M, Bondy B, de Jonge S, Glatzeder K, Kruger M, Schoeps P, et al. Possible association of fibromyalgia with a polymorphism in the serotonin transporter gene regulatory region. Arthritis Rheum 1999;42(11):2482-8.

[9] Cohen H, Buskila D, Neumann L, Ebstein RP. Confirmation of an association between fibromyalgia and serotonin transporter promoter region (5- HTTLPR) polymorphism, and relationship to anxiety-related personality traits. Arthritis Rheum 2002;46(3):845-7.

[10] Hoefgen B, Schulze TG, Ohlraun S, von Widdern O, Hofels S, Gross M, et al. The power of sample size and homogenous sampling: association between the 5-HTTLPR serotonin transporter polymorphism and major depressive disorder. Biol Psychiatry 2005; 57(3):247-51.

[11] Yeo A, Boyd P, Lumsden S, Saunders T, Handley A, Stubbins M, et al. Association between a functional polymorphism in the serotonin transporter gene and diarrhoea predominant irritable bowel syndrome in women. Gut 2004; 53(10):1452-8.

[12] Park JM, Choi MG, Park JA, Oh JH, Cho YK, Lee IS, et al. Serotonin transporter gene polymorphism and irritable bowel syndrome. Neurogastroenterol Motil 2006;18(11):995-1000.

[13] Aaron LA, Buchwald D. Chronic diffuse musculoskeletal pain, fibromyalgia and co-morbid unexplained clinical conditions. Best Pract Res Clin Rheumatol 2003;17(4):563-74.

[14] Al-Allaf AW, Dunbar KL, Hallum NS, Nosratzadeh B, Templeton KD, Pullar T. A case-control study examining the role of physical trauma in the onset of fibromyalgia syndrome. Rheumatology (Oxford) 2002;41(4):450-3.

[15] Demitrack MA, Crofford LJ. Evidence for and pathophysiologic implications of hypothalamic-pituitary-adrenal axis dysregulation in fibromyalgia and chronic fatigue syndrome. Ann N Y Acad Sci 1998; 840:684-97.

[16] Harkness EF, Macfarlane GJ, Nahit E, Silman AJ, McBeth J. Mechanical injury and psychosocial factors in the work place predict the onset of widespread body pain: a two-year prospective study among cohorts of newly employed workers. Arthritis Rheum 2004; 50(5):1655-64.

[17] Davis MC, Zautra AJ, Reich JW. Vulnerability to stress among women in chronic pain from fibromyalgia and osteoarthritis. Ann Behav Med 2001;23(3):215-26.

[18] Okonkwo R BL, Sotolongo A, et al. Effect of stressful imagery on thermal pain ratings of patients with fibromyalgia: what mediates this relationship? J Pain 2007;8(4):S25.

[19] McCain GA, Tilbe KS. Diurnal hormone variation in fibromyalgia syndrome: a comparison with rheumatoid arthritis. J Rheumatol Suppl 1989;19:154-7.

[20] Crofford LJ, Pillemer SR, Kalogeras KT, Cash JM, Michelson D, Kling MA, et al. Hypothalamic-pituitary-adrenal axis perturbations in patients with fibromyalgia. Arthritis Rheum 1994;37(11):1583-92.

[21] Bou-Holaigah I, Calkins H, Flynn JA, Tunin C, Chang HC, Kan JS, et al. Provocation of hypotension and pain during upright tilt table testing in adults with fibromyalgia. Clin Exp Rheumatol 1997; 15(3):239-46.

[22] Martínez-Lavín M HA, Rosas M, et al. Circadian studies of autonomic nervous balance in patients with fibromyalgia: a heart rate variability analysis. Arthritis Rheum 1998;41:1966–71.

[23] Martinez-Lavin M, Hermosillo AG, Mendoza C, Ortiz R, Cajigas JC, Pineda C, et al. Orthostatic sympathetic derangement in subjects with fibromyalgia. J Rheumatol 1997;24(4):714-8.

[24] Vaeroy H, Qiao ZG, Morkrid L, Forre O. Altered sympathetic nervous system response in patients with fibromyalgia (fibrositis syndrome). J Rheumatol 1989;16(11):1460-5.

[25] Roizenblatt S, Moldofsky H, Benedito-Silva AA, Tufik S. Alpha sleep characteristics in fibromyalgia. Arthritis Rheum 2001; 44(1):222-30.

[26] Harding SM. Sleep in fibromyalgia patients: subjective and objective findings. Am J Med Sci 1998;315(6):367-76.

[27] Russell IJ, Vaeroy H, Javors M, Nyberg F. Cerebrospinal fluid biogenic amine metabolites in fibromyalgia/fibrositis syndrome and rheumatoid arthritis. Arthritis Rheum 1992;35(5):550-6.

[28] Yunus MB, Dailey JW, Aldag JC, Masi AT, Jobe PC. Plasma tryptophan and other amino acids in primary fibromyalgia: a controlled study. J Rheumatol 1992;19(1):90-4.

[29] Schwarz MJ, Spath M, Muller-Bardorff H, Pongratz DE, Bondy B, Ackenheil M. Relationship of substance P, 5-hydroxyindole acetic acid and tryptophan in serum of fibromyalgia patients. Neurosci Lett 1999;259(3):196-8.

[30] Sicuteri F. Headache as possible expression of deficiency of brain 5-hydroxytryptamine (central denervation supersensitivity). Headache 1972;12(2):69-72.

[31] Fishbain D. Evidence-based data on pain relief with antidepressants. Ann Med 2000;32(5):305-16.

[32] Wood PB, Patterson JC, 2nd, Sunderland JJ, Tainter KH, Glabus MF, Lilien DL. Reduced presynaptic dopamine activity in fibromyalgia syndrome demonstrated with positron emission tomography: a pilot study. J Pain 2007;8(1):51-8.

[33] Wood PB, Holman AJ. An elephant among us: the role of dopamine in the pathophysiology of fibromyalgia. J Rheumatol 2009; 36(2):221-4.

[34] Gur A, Oktayoglu P. Status of immune mediators in fibromyalgia. Curr Pain Headache Rep 2008;12(3):175-81.

[35] Maier SF. Bi-directional immune-brain communication: Implications for understanding stress, pain, and cognition. Brain Behav Immun 2003;17(2):69-85.

[36] Watkins LR, Maier SF. The pain of being sick: implications of immune-to-brain communication for understanding pain. Annu Rev Psychol 2000;51:29-57.

[37] Anisman H, Merali Z. Cytokines, stress and depressive illness: brain-immune interactions. Ann Med 2003;35(1):2-11.

[38] Schaible HG, Ebersberger A, Von Banchet GS. Mechanisms of pain in arthritis. Ann N Y Acad Sci 2002;966:343-54.

[39] Wallace DJ. Is there a role for cytokine based therapies in fibromyalgia. Curr Pharm Des 2006;12(1):17-22.

[40] Roberts K, Papadaki A, Goncalves C, Tighe M, Atherton D, Shenoy R, et al. Contact heat evoked potentials using simultaneous EEG and fMRI and their correlation with evoked pain. BMC Anesthesiol 2008; 8(8):8.

[41] Kwiatek R, Barnden L, Tedman R, Jarrett R, Chew J, Rowe C, et al. Regional cerebral blood flow in fibromyalgia: single-photon-emission computed tomography evidence of reduction in the pontine tegmentum and thalami. Arthritis Rheum 2000; 43(12):2823-33.

[42] Gracely RH, Petzke F, Wolf JM, Clauw DJ. Functional magnetic resonance imaging evidence of augmented pain processing in fibromyalgia. Arthritis Rheum 2002;46(5):1333-43.
[43] Giesecke T, Gracely RH, Grant MA, Nachemson A, Petzke F, Williams DA, et al. Evidence of augmented central pain processing in idiopathic chronic low back pain. Arthritis Rheum 2004; 50(2):613-23.
[44] Mountz JM, Bradley LA, Modell JG, Alexander RW, Triana-Alexander M, Aaron LA, et al. Fibromyalgia in women. Abnormalities of regional cerebral blood flow in the thalamus and the caudate nucleus are associated with low pain threshold levels. Arthritis Rheum 1995;38(7):926-38.
[45] Gracely E. The role of quasi-experimental designs in pain research. Pain Med 2004;5(2):146-7.
[46] Giesecke T, Gracely RH, Williams DA, Geisser ME, Petzke FW, Clauw DJ. The relationship between depression, clinical pain, and experimental pain in a chronic pain cohort. Arthritis Rheum 2005; 52(5):1577-84.
[47] Neumann L, Buskila D. Epidemiology of fibromyalgia. Curr Pain Headache Rep 2003;7(5):362-8.
[48] Weir PT, Harlan GA, Nkoy FL, Jones SS, Hegmann KT, Gren LH, et al. The incidence of fibromyalgia and its associated comorbidities: a population-based retrospective cohort study based on International Classification of Diseases, 9th Revision codes. J Clin Rheumatol 2006;12(3):124-8.
[49] Crofford LJ. Pharmaceutical treatment options for fibromyalgia. Curr Rheumatol Rep 2004;6(4):274-80.
[50] Hajjar ER, Hanlon JT, Artz MB, Lindblad CI, Pieper CF, Sloane RJ, et al. Adverse drug reaction risk factors in older outpatients. Am J Geriatr Pharmacother 2003;1(2):82-9.
[51] Arnold LM, Rosen A, Pritchett YL, D'Souza DN, Goldstein DJ, Iyengar S, et al. A randomized, double-blind, placebo-controlled trial of duloxetine in the treatment of women with fibromyalgia with or without major depressive disorder. Pain 2005;119(1-3):5-15.
[52] Duloxetine: new indication. Depression and diabetic neuropathy: too many adverse effects. Prescrire Int 2006;15(85):168-72.
[53] Penrod JR, Bernatsky S, Adam V, Baron M, Dayan N, Dobkin PL. Health services costs and their determinants in women with fibromyalgia. J Rheumatol 2004;31(7):1391-8.
[54] Kivimaki M, Leino-Arjas P, Kaila-Kangas L, Virtanen M, Elovainio M, Puttonen S, et al. Increased absence due to sickness among employees with fibromyalgia. Ann Rheum Dis 2007;66(1):65-9.
[55] Robinson RL, Birnbaum HG, Morley MA, Sisitsky T, Greenberg PE, Claxton AJ. Economic cost and epidemiological characteristics of patients with fibromyalgia claims. J Rheumatol 2003;30(6):1318-25.
[56] Wolfe F, Anderson J, Harkness D, Bennett RM, Caro XJ, Goldenberg DL, et al. A prospective, longitudinal, multicenter study of service utilization and costs in fibromyalgia. Arthritis Rheum 1997; 40(9):1560-70.
[57] Wolfe F, Anderson J, Harkness D, Bennett RM, Caro XJ, Goldenberg DL, et al. Work and disability status of persons with fibromyalgia. J Rheumatol 1997;24(6):1171-8.
[58] Wolfe F, Anderson J, Harkness D, Bennett RM, Caro XJ, Goldenberg DL, et al. Health status and disease severity in fibromyalgia: results of a six-center longitudinal study. Arthritis Rheum 1997;40(9):1571-9.
[59] Boggio PS, Rigonatti SP, Ribeiro RB, Myczkowski ML, Nitsche MA, Pascual-Leone A, et al. A randomized, double-blind clinical trial on the efficacy of cortical direct current stimulation for the treatment of major depression. Int J Neuropsychopharmacol 2008;11(2):249-54.
[60] Boggio PS, Zaghi S, Lopes M, Fregni F. Modulatory effects of anodal transcranial direct current stimulation on perception and pain thresholds in healthy volunteers. Eur J Neurol 2008;15(10):1124-30.

[61] Antal A, Brepohl N, Poreisz C, Boros K, Csifcsak G, Paulus W. Transcranial direct current stimulation over somatosensory cortex decreases experimentally induced acute pain perception. Clin J Pain 2008;24(1):56-63.

[62] Fregni F, Boggio PS, Lima MC, Ferreira MJ, Wagner T, Rigonatti SP, et al. A sham-controlled, phase II trial of transcranial direct current stimulation for the treatment of central pain in traumatic spinal cord injury. Pain 2006;122(1-2):197-209.

[63] Banks S, and Kerns, R. Explaining high rates of depression in chronic pain. A diathesis-stress framework. Psychol Bull 1996;(119):95-110.

[64] Magni G, Marchetti, M., Roreschi, C., Merskey, H., Rigatti-Luchini, S. Chronic musculoskeletal pain and depressive symptoms in the National Health and Nutritional Examination I: Epidemiologic follow-up study. Pain 1993;53:163-8.

[65] Campbell LC, Clauw DJ, Keefe FJ. Persistent pain and depression: a biopsychosocial perspective. Biol Psychiatry 2003;54(3):399-409.

[66] Dohrenwend BP, Raphael KG, Marbach JJ, Gallagher RM. Why is depression comorbid with chronic myofascial face pain? A family study test of alternative hypotheses. Pain 1999;83(2):183-92.

[67] McWilliams LA, Cox BJ, Enns MW. Mood and anxiety disorders associated with chronic pain: an examination in a nationally representative sample. Pain 2003;106(1-2):127-33.

[68] Bornhovd K, Quante M, Glauche V, Bromm B, Weiller C, Buchel C. Painful stimuli evoke different stimulus-response functions in the amygdala, prefrontal, insula and somatosensory cortex: a single-trial fMRI study. Brain 2002;125(Pt 6):1326-36.

[69] Brooks JC, Nurmikko TJ, Bimson WE, Singh KD, Roberts N. fMRI of thermal pain: effects of stimulus laterality and attention. Neuroimage 2002;15(2):293-301.

[70] Davis KD. The neural circuitry of pain as explored with functional MRI. Neurol Res 2000;22(3):313-7.

[71] Petrovic P, Ingvar M. Imaging cognitive modulation of pain processing. Pain 2002;95(1-2):1-5.

[72] Sheline YI. Neuroimaging studies of mood disorder effects on the brain. Biol Psychiatry 2003;54(3):338-52.

[73] Piccinni A, Del Debbio A, Medda P, Bianchi C, Roncaglia I, Veltri A, et al. Plasma Brain-Derived Neurotrophic Factor in treatment-resistant depressed patients receiving electroconvulsive therapy. Eur Neuropsychopharmacol 2009;13:13.

[74] Okamoto T, Yoshimura R, Ikenouchi-Sugita A, Hori H, Umene-Nakano W, Inoue Y, et al. Efficacy of electroconvulsive therapy is associated with changing blood levels of homovanillic acid and brain-derived neurotrophic factor (BDNF) in refractory depressed patients: a pilot study. Prog Neuropsychopharmacol Biol Psychiatry 2008;32(5):1185-90.

[75] Hsieh JC, Belfrage M, Stone-Elander S, Hansson P, Ingvar M. Central representation of chronic ongoing neuropathic pain studied by positron emission tomography. Pain 1995;63(2):225-36.

[76] Fukui S, Shigemori S, Nosaka S. Central pain associated with low thalamic blood flow treated by electroconvulsive therapy. J Anesth 2002;16(3):255-7.

[77] Fukui S, Shigemori S, Yoshimura A, Nosaka S. Chronic pain with beneficial response to electroconvulsive therapy and regional cerebral blood flow changes assessed by single photon emission computed tomography. Reg Anesth Pain Med 2002;27(2):211-3.

[78] Salmon JB, Hanna MH, Williams M, Toone B, Wheeler M. Thalamic pain--the effect of electroconvulsive therapy (ECT). Pain 1988; 33(1):67-71.

[79] McCance S, Hawton K, Brighouse D, Glynn C. Does electroconvulsive therapy (ECT) have any role in the management of intractable thalamic pain? Pain 1996;68(1):129-31.

[80] Huuhka MJ, Haanpaa ML, Leinonen EV. Electroconvulsive therapy in patients with depression and fibromyalgia. Eur J Pain 2004; 8(4):371-6.

[81] Usui C, Doi N, Nishioka M, Komatsu H, Yamamoto R, Ohkubo T, et al. Electroconvulsive therapy improves severe pain associated with fibromyalgia. Pain 2006;121(3):276-80.

[82] Takeuchi R, Yonekura Y, Matsuda H, Konishi J. Usefulness of a three-dimensional stereotaxic ROI template on anatomically standardised 99mTc-ECD SPET. Eur J Nucl Med Mol Imaging 2002; 29(3):331-41.
[83] Vangu MD, Esser JD, Boyd IH, Berk M. Effects of electroconvulsive therapy on regional cerebral blood flow measured by 99mtechnetium HMPAO SPECT. Prog Neuropsychopharmacol Biol Psychiatry 2003; 27(1):15-9.
[84] Newman ME, Gur E, Shapira B, Lerer B. Neurochemical mechanisms of action of ECS: evidence from in vivo studies. J Ect 1998; 14(3):153-71.
[85] Wasserman EA EC, Ziemann U, et al. The Oxford handbook of transcranial stimulation. New York: Oxford Univ Press, 2008.
[86] Been G, Ngo TT, Miller SM, Fitzgerald PB. The use of tDCS and CVS as methods of non-invasive brain stimulation. Brain Res Rev 2007;56(2):346-61.
[87] Nitsche M A PW. Excitability changes induced in the human motor cortex by weak transcranial direct current stimulation. J Physiol 2000; 527(3):633-9.
[88] Nitsche MA, Fricke K, Henschke U, Schlitterlau A, Liebetanz D, Lang N, et al. Pharmacological modulation of cortical excitability shifts induced by transcranial direct current stimulation in humans. J Physiol 2003;553(Pt 1):293-301.
[89] Nitsche MA, Seeber A, Frommann K, Klein CC, Rochford C, Nitsche MS, et al. Modulating parameters of excitability during and after transcranial direct current stimulation of the human motor cortex. J Physiol 2005;568(Pt 1):291-303.
[90] Ghaly RF, Ham JH, Lee JJ. High-dose ketamine hydrochloride maintains somatosensory and magnetic motor evoked potentials in primates. Neurol Res 2001;23(8):881-6.
[91] Ziemann U, Tergau F, Wischer S, Hildebrandt J, Paulus W. Pharmacological control of facilitatory I-wave interaction in the human motor cortex. A paired transcranial magnetic stimulation study. Electroencephalogr Clin Neurophysiol 1998;109(4):321-30.
[92] Nitsche MA, Doemkes S, Karakose T, Antal A, Liebetanz D, Lang N, et al. Shaping the effects of transcranial direct current stimulation of the human motor cortex. J Neurophysiol 2007;97(4):3109-17.
[93] Poreisz C, Boros K, Antal A, Paulus W. Safety aspects of transcranial direct current stimulation concerning healthy subjects and patients. Brain Res Bull 2007;72(4-6):208-14.
[94] Schlaug G, Renga V, Nair D. Transcranial direct current stimulation in stroke recovery. Arch Neurol 2008;65(12):1571-6.
[95] Fregni F, Gimenes R, Valle AC, Ferreira MJ, Rocha RR, Natalle L, et al. A randomized, sham-controlled, proof of principle study of transcranial direct current stimulation for the treatment of pain in fibromyalgia. Arthritis Rheum 2006;54(12):3988-98.
[96] Lefaucheur JP, Drouot X, Keravel Y, Nguyen JP. Pain relief induced by repetitive transcranial magnetic stimulation of precentral cortex. Neuroreport 2001;12(13):2963-5.
[97] Fregni F, Boggio PS, Nitsche MA, Marcolin MA, Rigonatti SP, Pascual-Leone A. Treatment of major depression with transcranial direct current stimulation. Bipolar Disord 2006;8(2):203-4.
[98] Doherty M, Smith J. Elusive 'alpha-delta' sleep in fibromyalgia and osteoarthritis. Ann Rheum Dis 1993;52(3):245.
[99] Schneider-Helmert D, Whitehouse I, Kumar A, Lijzenga C. Insomnia and alpha sleep in chronic non-organic pain as compared to primary insomnia. Neuropsychobiology 2001;43(1):54-8.
[100] Hauri P, Hawkins DR. Alpha-delta sleep. Electroencephalogr Clin Neurophysiol 1973;34(3):233-7.
[101] Moldofsky H, Scarisbrick P. Induction of neurasthenic musculoskeletal pain syndrome by selective sleep stage deprivation. Psychosom Med 1976;38(1):35-44.
[102] Older SA, Battafarano DF, Danning CL, Ward JA, Grady EP, Derman S, et al. The effects of delta wave sleep interruption on pain thresholds and fibromyalgia-like symptoms in healthy subjects; correlations with insulin-like growth factor I. J Rheumatol 1998;25(6):1180-6.

[103] Lentz MJ, Landis CA, Rothermel J, Shaver JL. Effects of selective slow wave sleep disruption on musculoskeletal pain and fatigue in middle aged women. J Rheumatol 1999;26(7):1586-92.
[104] Marshall L, Molle M, Hallschmid M, Born J. Transcranial direct current stimulation during sleep improves declarative memory. J Neurosci 2004;24(44):9985-92.
[105] Roizenblatt S, Fregni F, Gimenez R, Wetzel T, Rigonatti SP, Tufik S, et al. Site-specific effects of transcranial direct current stimulation on sleep and pain in fibromyalgia: a randomized, sham-controlled study. Pain Pract 2007;7(4):297-306.
[106] Eichhammer P, Kharraz A, Wiegand R, Langguth B, Frick U, Aigner JM, et al. Sleep deprivation in depression stabilizing antidepressant effects by repetitive transcranial magnetic stimulation. Life Sci 2002; 70(15):1741-9.
[107] Hauri P, Chernik D, Hawkins D, Mendels J. Sleep of depressed patients in remission. Arch Gen Psychiatry 1974;31(3):386-91.
[108] Tsubokawa T KY, Yamamoto T, et al.: (Wien). Chronic motor cortex stimulation for the treatment of central pain. Acta Neurochir Suppl 1991;52:137-9.
[109] Bohning DE. Introduction and overview of TMS psyics. In: George MS, Belmaker RH, eds. Transcranial magnetic stimulation in neuropsychiatry. Washington, DC: Am Psychiatr Press, 2000:13-44.
[110] George MS, Belmaker RH. Transcranial magnetic stimulation In: Meorge MS, Belmaker RH, eds. Neuropsychiatry, 1 ed. Washington, DC: Am Psychiatr Press, 2000.
[111] George MS, Lisanby SH, Sackeim HA. Transcranial magnetic stimulation: applications in neuropsychiatry. Arch Gen Psychiatry 1999;56(4):300-11.
[112] Epstein CM, Meador KJ, Loring DW, Wright RJ, Weissman JD, Sheppard S, et al. Localization and characterization of speech arrest during transcranial magnetic stimulation. Clin Neurophysiol 1999; 110(6):1073-9.
[113] Amassian VE, Eberle L, Maccabee PJ, Cracco RQ. Modelling magnetic coil excitation of human cerebral cortex with a peripheral nerve immersed in a brain-shaped volume conductor: the significance of fiber bending in excitation. Electroencephalogr Clin Neurophysiol 1992;85(5):291-301.
[114] Davey KR, Cheng CH, Epstein CM. Prediction of magnetically induced electric fields in biological tissue. IEEE Trans Biomed Eng 1991;38(5):418-22.
[115] Nagarajan SS, Durand DM, Roth BJ, Wijesinghe RS. Magnetic stimulation of axons in a nerve bundle: effects of current redistribution in the bundle. Ann Biomed Eng 1995;23(2):116-26.
[116] George MS, Nahas Z, Kozol FA, Li X, Yamanaka K, Mishory A, et al. Mechanisms and the current state of transcranial magnetic stimulation. CNS Spectr 2003;8(7):496-514.
[117] Bear MF. Homosynaptic long-term depression: a mechanism for memory? Proc Natl Acad Sci U S A 1999;96(17):9457-8.
[118] Stanton PK, Sejnowski TJ. Associative long-term depression in the hippocampus induced by hebbian covariance. Nature 1989; 339(6221):215-8.
[119] Malenka RC, Nicoll RA. Long-term potentiation--a decade of progress? Science 1999;285(5435):1870-4.
[120] Wang H, Wang X, Scheich H. LTD and LTP induced by transcranial magnetic stimulation in auditory cortex. Neuroreport 1996; 7(2):521-5.
[121] Chen R, Classen J, Gerloff C, Celnik P, Wassermann EM, Hallett M, et al. Depression of motor cortex excitability by low-frequency transcranial magnetic stimulation. Neurology 1997;48(5):1398-403.
[122] Wu T, Sommer M, Tergau F, Paulus W. Lasting influence of repetitive transcranial magnetic stimulation on intracortical excitability in human subjects. Neurosci Lett 2000;287(1):37-40.
[123] Cohrs S, Tergau F, Korn J, Becker W, Hajak G. Suprathreshold repetitive transcranial magnetic stimulation elevates thyroid-stimulating hormone in healthy male subjects. J Nerv Ment Dis 2001;189(6):393-7.

[124] Desmurget M, Epstein CM, Turner RS, Prablanc C, Alexander GE, Grafton ST. Role of the posterior parietal cortex in updating reaching movements to a visual target. Nat Neurosci 1999;2(6):563-7.
[125] Epstein CM, Verson R, Zangaladze A. Magnetic coil suppression of visual perception at an extracalcarine site. J Clin Neurophysiol 1996;13(3):247-52.
[126] Flitman SS, Grafman J, Wassermann EM, Cooper V, O'Grady J, Pascual-Leone A, et al. Linguistic processing during repetitive transcranial magnetic stimulation. Neurology 1998;50(1):175-81.
[127] George MS, Wassermann EM, Williams WA, Steppel J, Pascual-Leone A, Basser P, et al. Changes in mood and hormone levels after rapid-rate transcranial magnetic stimulation (rTMS) of the prefrontal cortex. J Neuropsychiatry Clin Neurosci 1996; 8(2):172-80.
[128] Grafman J, Wassermann E. Transcranial magnetic stimulation can measure and modulate learning and memory. Neuropsychologia 1999;37(2):159-67.
[129] Szuba MP, O'Reardon JP, Rai AS, Snyder-Kastenberg J, Amsterdam JD, Gettes DR, et al. Acute mood and thyroid stimulating hormone effects of transcranial magnetic stimulation in major depression. Biol Psychiatry 2001;50(1):22-7.
[130] Lefaucheur JP, Drouot X, Menard-Lefaucheur I, Nguyen JP. Neuropathic pain controlled for more than a year by monthly sessions of repetitive transcranial magnetic stimulation of the motor cortex. Neurophysiol Clin 2004; 34(2):91-5.
[131] Li X, Teneback CC, Nahas Z, Kozel FA, Large C, Cohn J, et al. Interleaved transcranial magnetic stimulation/functional MRI confirms that lamotrigine inhibits cortical excitability in healthy young men. Neuropsychopharmacology 2004;29(7):1395-407.
[132] Paus T, Castro-Alamancos MA, Petrides M. Cortico-cortical connectivity of the human mid-dorsolateral frontal cortex and its modulation by repetitive transcranial magnetic stimulation. Eur J Neurosci 2001;14(8):1405-11.
[133] Strafella AP, Paus T, Barrett J, Dagher A. Repetitive transcranial magnetic stimulation of the human prefrontal cortex induces dopamine release in the caudate nucleus. J Neurosci 2001; 21(15):RC157.
[134] Teneback CC, Nahas Z, Speer AM, Molloy M, Stallings LE, Spicer KM, et al. Changes in prefrontal cortex and paralimbic activity in depression following two weeks of daily left prefrontal TMS. J Neuropsychiatry Clin Neurosci 1999;11(4):426-35.
[135] George MS, Wassermann EM. Rapid-rate transcranial magnetic stimulation and ECT. Convuls Ther 1994;10(4):251-4,255-8.
[136] Garcia-Larrea L, Peyron R, Mertens P, Gregoire MC, Lavenne F, Le Bars D, et al. Electrical stimulation of motor cortex for pain control: a combined PET-scan and electrophysiological study. Pain 1999; 83(2):259-73.
[137] Peyron R, Kupers R, Jehl JL, Garcia-Larrea L, Convers P, Barral FG, et al. Central representation of the RIII flexion reflex associated with overt motor reaction: an fMRI study. Neurophysiol Clin 2007; 37(4):249-59.
[138] Peyron R, Laurent B, Garcia-Larrea L. Functional imaging of brain responses to pain. A review and meta-analysis (2000). Neurophysiol Clin 2000;30(5):263-88.
[139] Apkarian AV, Bushnell MC, Treede RD, Zubieta JK. Human brain mechanisms of pain perception and regulation in health and disease. Eur J Pain 2005;9(4):463-84.
[140] Tracey I. Nociceptive processing in the human brain. Curr Opin Neurobiol 2005;15(4):478-87.
[141] Bohning DE, Shastri A, McGavin L, McConnell KA, Nahas Z, Lorberbaum JP, et al. Motor cortex brain activity induced by 1-Hz transcranial magnetic stimulation is similar in location and level to that for volitional movement. Invest Radiol 2000;35(11):676-83.
[142] Bestmann S, Baudewig J, Siebner HR, Rothwell JC, Frahm J. Functional MRI of the immediate impact of transcranial magnetic stimulation on cortical and subcortical motor circuits. Eur J Neurosci 2004;19(7):1950-62.

[143] Bestmann S, Baudewig J, Siebner HR, Rothwell JC, Frahm J. BOLD MRI responses to repetitive TMS over human dorsal premotor cortex. Neuroimage 2005;28(1):22-9.
[144] Lefaucheur JP. New insights into the therapeutic potential of non-invasive transcranial cortical stimulation in chronic neuropathic pain. Pain 2006;122(1-2):11-3.
[145] Lefaucheur JP, Drouot X, Menard-Lefaucheur I, Keravel Y, Nguyen JP. Motor cortex rTMS restores defective intracortical inhibition in chronic neuropathic pain. Neurology 2006;67(9):1568-74.
[146] Kanda M, Mima T, Oga T, Matsuhashi M, Toma K, Hara H, et al. Transcranial magnetic stimulation (TMS) of the sensorimotor cortex and medial frontal cortex modifies human pain perception. Clin Neurophysiol 2003; 114(5):860-6.
[147] Summers J, Johnson S, Pridmore S, Oberoi G. Changes to cold detection and pain thresholds following low and high frequency transcranial magnetic stimulation of the motor cortex. Neurosci Lett 2004;368(2):197-200.
[148] Tamura Y, Okabe S, Ohnishi T, D NS, Arai N, Mochio S, et al. Effects of 1-Hz repetitive transcranial magnetic stimulation on acute pain induced by capsaicin. Pain 2004;107(1-2):107-15.
[149] Johnson S, Summers J, Pridmore S. Changes to somatosensory detection and pain thresholds following high frequency repetitive TMS of the motor cortex in individuals suffering from chronic pain. Pain 2006;123(1-2):187-92.
[150] Migita K, Uozumi T, Arita K, Monden S. Transcranial magnetic coil stimulation of motor cortex in patients with central pain. Neurosurgery 1995;36(5):1037-40.
[151] Khedr EM, Kotb H, Kamel NF, Ahmed MA, Sadek R, Rothwell JC. Longlasting antalgic effects of daily sessions of repetitive transcranial magnetic stimulation in central and peripheral neuropathic pain. J Neurol Neurosurg Psychiatry 2005;76(6):833-8.
[152] Sampson SM, Rome JD, Rummans TA. Slow-frequency rTMS reduces fibromyalgia pain. Pain Med 2006;7(2):115-8.
[153] Passard AF, Attal N, Attal NF, Benadhira R, Benadhira RF, et al. Effects of unilateral repetitive transcranial magnetic stimulation of the motor cortex on chronic widespread pain in fibromyalgia. Personal communication.
[154] Graff-Guerrero A, Gonzalez-Olvera J, Fresan A, Gomez-Martin D, Mendez-Nunez JC, Pellicer F. Repetitive transcranial magnetic stimulation of dorsolateral prefrontal cortex increases tolerance to human experimental pain. Brain Res Cogn Brain Res 2005; 25(1):153-60.
[155] Kauffmann CD, Cheema MA, Miller BE. Slow right prefrontal transcranial magnetic stimulation as a treatment for medication-resistant depression: a double-blind, placebo-controlled study. Depress Anxiety 2004;19(1):59-62.
[156] Peyron R, Garcia-Larrea L, Gregoire MC, Convers P, Richard A, Lavenne F, et al. Parietal and cingulate processes in central pain. A combined positron emission tomography (PET) and functional magnetic resonance imaging (fMRI) study of an unusual case. Pain 2000;84(1):77-87.
[157] Pridmore S, Oberoi G, Marcolin M, George M. Transcranial magnetic stimulation and chronic pain: current status. Australas Psychiatry. 2005;13(3):258-65.
[158] Kakigi R, Inui K, Tamura Y. Electrophysiological studies on human pain perception. Clin Neurophysiol 2005;116(4):743-63.
[159] Csifcsak G, Antal A, Hillers F, Levold M, Bachmann CG, Happe S, et al. Modulatory effects of transcranial direct current stimulation on laser-evoked potentials. Pain Med 2009;10(1):122-32.
[160] Rigonatti SP, Boggio PS, Myczkowski ML, Otta E, Fiquer JT, Ribeiro RB, et al. Transcranial direct stimulation and fluoxetine for the treatment of depression. Eur Psychiatry 2008;23(1):74-6.
[161] Gracely RH, Geisser ME, Giesecke T, Grant MA, Petzke F, Williams DA, et al. Pain catastrophizing and neural responses to pain among persons with fibromyalgia. Brain 2004;127(Pt 4):835-43.

Chapter 28

NON-INVASIVE BRAIN STIMULATION THERAPY FOR THE MANAGEMENT OF COMPLEX REGIONAL PAIN SYNDROME (CRPS)

Ricardo A Cruciani, MD, PhD[*,1,2], *Santiago Esteban, MD*[1], *Una Sibirceva, MD*[1] *and Helena Knotkova, PhD*[1,2]

[1]Institute for Noninvasive Brain Stimulation of New York, Research Division, Department of Pain Medicine and Palliative Care, Beth Israel Medical Center, New York, United States of America
[2]Department of Neurology and Anesthesiology, Albert Einstein College of Medicine, Bronx, New York, United States of America

Abstract

Neuropathic pain is an abnormal response to painful stimuli that can be caused by a variety of insults that may or may not involve direct nerve injury, and ranges from very common conditions like lumbar radiculopathy, to unusual causes like HTLV-1 myelopathy. Neuropathic pain syndromes that in addition to pain present with allodynia, hyperalgesia, changes in coloration of the skin and edema, are classified under the umbrella known as Complex Regional pain Syndrome (CRPS). Although full blown CRPS is easily recognizable, when the associated symptoms are subtle, then it can become a diagnostic challenge. The underlying mechanism responsible for CRPS is not well understood but due to the variability in its presentation and to the different nature of the symptoms, it is believed to be multifactorial. Sensitization of nociceptors, increase release of neurotransmitters and changes in the phenotype of certain receptors in the posterior horn of the spinal cord, and modifications in the excitability and topographical cortical representation of the sensorimotor and motor cortices that receive projections from the affected body part, have been identified and recognized as important contributors. Indeed, recent findings suggest that pain in CRPS is positively associated with a functional reorganization of the somatosensory and motor cortex. Cortical reorganization is the result of

---

[*] **Correspondence:** Ricardo Cruciani, MD, PhD, Department of Pain Medicine and Palliative Care, 350 East 17th Street, Baird Hall, 12th floor, Beth Israel Medical Center, New York, NY 10003 United States. Tel: 212-420-2432; E-mail: rcrucian@bethisraelny.org

changes in somatotopic organization, and changes in excitability of the somatosensory and motor cortices. Preliminary data suggests that both rTMS and tDCS under certain conditions can alleviate pain in patients with CRPS and that may be related to reversal of excitability and topographical changes.

Keywords: Transcranial direct current stimulation (tDCS), Pain management, Repetitive transcranial magnetic stimulation (rTMS), Complex regional pain syndrome (CRPS), brain plasticity, neuronal excitability.

Introduction

Complex Regional Pain Syndrome (CRPS) can have a dramatic impact on the patient's quality of life. It is clinically characterized by pain, allodynia, edema, abnormal regulation of blood flow of the affected area, movement disorders and changes in the skin trophism that affects more frequently the upper limbs. CRPS includes CRPS I (formerly known as Reflex Sympathetic Distrophy), that typically follows trauma, and CRPS II (formerly called Causalgia), which develops after nerve damage, and may or may not have a sympathetic component. Managing CRPS, represents a challenge to pain specialists because it may progress into a chronic pain state that can be refractory to pharmacological therapy and interventions. Although its underlying mechanism is not clearly understood, the current theory implicates both central and peripheral generators, and recognizes a role for the neocortex in the pathogenesis and chronicity of the syndrome (1). Recent findings suggest that the somatosensory, motor and autonomic signs and symptoms that can be present in patients with CRPS are associated with a functional reorganization and hyperexitability of the somatosensory and motor cortex, as well as subcortical structures and that reversal of this cortical reorganization correlates with pain relief (2). Hence, there has been a great deal of effort in developing novel strategies that may modulate cortical excitability to alleviate pain. Recently, non-invasive brain stimulation techniques such as repetitive transcranial magnetic stimulation (rTMS) and transcranial direct current stimulation (tDCS) have been proposed as suitable methods for modulation of cortical excitability in patients with pain. Both techniques (rTMS and tDCS) have been used in a variety of pain syndromes (3-7). Preliminary data on the management of CRPS related pain with both techniques opens up the possibility of new strategies to treat this challenging syndrome.

Molecular mechanisms for pain and other symptoms associated to CRPS

CRPS is a very complex syndrome and the mechanisms involved in its development and sustainability are multiple and diverse. It has been suggested that the changes that occur in patients with CRPS are not only molecular in nature but that also affect anatomical structures and the electrical properties of neurons at several levels of the nervous system.

The products of the inflammatory response and tissue damage, including prostanoids, bradykinin, cytokines, protons, free radicals, proteinases (e.g. tryptase), growth factors, and adenosine-5'-triphosphate (ATP), may activate nociceptors through direct or indirect mechanisms (8-11). In addition these agents can sensitize the nociceptors to further stimuli, increasing the response to a range of mechanical, thermal, and chemical stimuli at the site of injury. Also, there is increased migration of autologous leukocytes and nonspecific immunoglobulins towards the CRPS affected location indicating a participation of these systems (12). Neuroimmune changes occur not only at the site of the affected area, but are also detected in the neuronal pathways that convey the information to the central nervous system (CNS). Indeed, neuropeptides are released within the dorsal horn of the spinal cord by depolarization provoked by afferent impulses, as part of a very complex mechanism, for the central sensitization that can be observed in these patients (12). Clinically, central sensitization translates into allodynia, hyperalgesia, and spontaneous pain. There are some studies utilizing immunomodulators in patients with CRPS that suggest a role for this type of therapy, but more detailed studies are needed before making any strong recommendation regarding their use (12).

The electrical impulse generated at the level of the site of injury, that can be abnormal due to changes in the milieu at the level of the nociceptor, may encounter also abnormal changes in the posterior horn of the spinal cord where the primary neuron that carries the impulse from the periphery, synapses with the projection neuron that carries the information to the thalamus and through a third neuron, to the somatosensory cortex. The abnormal changes observed in that region include receptors that mediate pain signals and the neuromodulators and neurotransmitters that transmit the pain signals between neurons. Over time, this increase in stimulation and response to the pain stimuli, results in sensitization of the dorsal horn pain-transmitting neurons (PTNs), and produces a state of central sensitization responsible for the development of mechanical hyperalgesisa and allodynia (13). Glutamate plays an important role in this process because it is one of the key excitatory amino acids and is the main neurotransmitter, along with substance P, at the level of the lamina I-II and IV. Other EAAs that are involved in the process of central sensitization is aspartate that, as glutamate, is also released from small afferent fibers (14). The EAAs exert their action trough the activation of ionotropic metabotropic receptors (13). The iontropic include the N-methyl-D-aspartate (NMDA), alpha-amino-3-hydroxy-5-methyl-4-isoxazole-propionic acid (AMPA), and kainate receptors. The neuropeptides that participate in the process of central sensitization include substance P, CGRP, cholecystokinin and bradikinin. In addition to an increase in signal mediators small-fibers (15,16) can undergo axonal neurodegeneration in patients with CRPS, as an epiphenomenon of a pathological change of the nociceptors, but also as part of pathological neuroplastic changes. The current line of thinking suggests that aggressive pain interventions and disengagement of gene expression to prevent neurodegeneration might result in uncoupling of the phenotypic shift and reversal of the syndrome into a pain condition more easily manageable.

In addition to the changes at the neuronal level described above, recent evidence suggests that the spinal cord microglia may play a relevant role in the hyperexcitability of pain transmitting neurons in the dorsal horn (PTNs) that can be seen in neuropathic pain syndromes (17-22). When microglia cells are activated, they undergo hypertrophy, hyperplasia, and begin to release factors including nerve growth factors, TNF-alpha, IL-1 beta, IL-6, prostaglandins, and nitric oxide that vastly amplify dorsal horn PTNs excitability (17). Preclinical studies in sciatic nerve lesions show that the changes are not limited to the damaged nerve fibers but that also extend to the neighboring intact axons. A great deal of attention has been placed on sodium channels that increase in number and also change their phenotype. Del Valle et al (23) described significant microglial and astrocytic cell activation in spinal cord tissues obtained from the autopsies of 1 patient with longstanding pain related to CRPS, but not in 4 matching controls. Although the number of the sample is small, these results are in agreement with prior observations done in tissues of autopsies performed in cadavers of patients with history of neuropathic pain.

At the macroscopic level Geha et al (24) reported changes in the white and grey matter of patients with CRPS that included anterior portion of the right insula (AI), the right ventromedial prefrontal cortex (VMPFC), and the right nucleous accumbens (NAc). These changes were independent of the side of the lesion and proportional to the intensity and duration of the symptoms. Interestingly they also suggested that the location of the atrophy could correlate with a particular symptom and proposed that atrophy of the AI would be responsible, at least in part, for autonomic symptoms and the constant negative emotional state frequently observed in patients with CRPS. They also observed an association between atrophy of the VMPFC, possibly involving autonomic changes through projections to the hypothalamus and the brainstem, with the poor performance in emotional decision making tasks that can be seen in patients with CRPS. Partial atrophy of the VMPFC and the periaqueductal grey area has been speculated to result in a reduced inhibition of the ascending nociceptive pathways that result in increased pain. In addition they also proposed an association between the decrease in white matter branching between the VMPFC, NAc and the AI and high anxiety levels also seen in this patient population. These results suggest that the brain anatomical changes may be the cause for pain, some of the autonomic and cognitive symptoms that can be observed in patients with CRPS.

Although sympathetically maintained pain (SMP), (pain sustained by the activity of sympathetic flow), has been observed in some patients with CRPS, its prevalence in this patient population has not been established with certainty, and its presence is not a requirement for its diagnosis. The mechanism of SMP is unclear but it has been proposed that it may be related to an increase in sympathetic outflow or to "de novo" expression of adrenergic receptors in nociceptive fibers. The presence of an increase out flow of the sympathetic system in this syndrome is based upon the observation that central sympathetic stimulation arouses pain, that abnormal vasoconstriction can be seen in patients with CRPS, and to the presence of increased sympathetic skin reflexes in these patients. The theory that support that the "de novo" expression of alpha-adrenergic receptors in nociceptive fibers (25) activated by noradrenaline, a circumstance that does not occur under normal physiological conditions, is supported by the fact that a reversal of this phenotypic shift is associated with the reduction of neuropathic pain (26), observation that is supported by several clinical studies (27-29).

Pain adaptation seems to be affected in CRPS patient as described in a case-control trial, where patients with CRPS depicted decreased adaptation to repetitive high current density electrical stimuli (rHCDES), on both the affected and the unaffected limb. Furthermore, in the CRPS group hyperalgesic areas, resulting from the rHCDES, were significantly enhanced on the affected side. The changes did not correlate to individual disease symptoms. In addition, the authors hypothesized that differential activity in endogenous pain modulation systems would not only be the result of CRPS but could also a predisposing factor to its development (30).

Cortical reorganization in CRPS

Recent results in patients with neuropathic pain suggest that there is a close relationship between the degree of cortical reorganization and the magnitude of pain (31-35). In patients with CRPS I, Pleger and colleagues (36) reported shrinkage of the cortical representation of the CRPS-affected hand and an enlargement/expansion of the cortical map of the non-affected as compared with healthy controls and that the changes correlated with mean sustained pain level and that the intensity correlated with the magnitude of the difference between the two sides. Similarly, Maihöfner and colleagues (35) observed a significant shrinkage of the size of the cortical representation of the affected hand in patients with CRPS with a shift toward the lip that is neighboring representation. The degree of cortical reorganization correlated with the extent of mechanical hyperalgesia, and with the magnitude of CRPS-related pain and that the changes in the primary somatosensory cortex (SI) reversed after a year or more with various therapies paralleling reduction of CRPS-related pain (37) consistent with observation by Pleger and colleagues (33,34) made a similar observation in patients with CRPS that received behavioral treatment over several months. Somatotopic reorganization in CRPS, as detected in the primary and secondary somatosensory cortex, has also been observed in the motor cortex by Krause and colleagues (38) that observed a significant increase of the motor cortical representation of the unaffected limb as compared to healthy controls. The expansion of the motor representation in the unaffected hemisphere could be explained by the interhemisphere callosal connection as suggested by Maihöfner and colleagues (39), who observed that in patients with CRPS somatotopic reorganization within the motor cortex is strikingly different from somatotopic changes in the somatosensory cortex possibly due to incongruence that lead to an abnormal self–perception and disrupted body scheme. The data from somatosensory and cortical representation taken as a whole, suggest that in CRPS patients there are deficient inhibitory mechanisms in response to sensory stimuli while the integrity of the sensorimotor pathways is preserved. It has been hypothesized that these changes are the result of persistent nociceptive input that might interfere with cortical relays of sensory perception, progressively decreasing representational area of the pain-affected limb. And also that suppression of SI activity might "per se" sustain the experience of pain (36) possible through a "gating effect" in which two somatosensory modalities of different quality (pain and non-painful tactile stimuli) (40) compete for common pathways.

There is significant evidence suggesting an changes in excitability of the motor and somatosensory cortices in patients with in patient with neuropathic pain including CRPS (39,41-43), and that its regulation can result in pain relief (4,36,44). Patient with CRPS present with decreased cortical inhibition that is possibly the consequence of decreased activity of GABA-ergic inhibitory neurons (46). These early findings have been confirmed with quantitative sensory testing and transcranial magnetic stimulation that showed significant differences in cold, heat and mechanical pain thresholds between the affected and contralateral limb in patient with CRPS reflecting a reduction of intracortical inhibition of the affected site rather than an increase intracortical facilitation (42). Schwenkreis and colleagues (43) compared intracortical facilitation, intracortical inhibition and motor thresholds in CRPS patients vs. healthy subjects and did not find significant differences in intracortical facilitation and motor thresholds between the two groups, whereas intracortical inhibition was markedly reduced (i.e. disinhibition occurred) in the two hemispheres of patients with CRPS only.

Interestingly Valeriani and colleagues (45) showed that painful noxious heat stimulation induced inhibition of the primary motor area that lead Pleger and others to use TMS and later to apply tDCS to regulate the motor cortex excitability and thereby achieve pain relief (4,36).

rTMS for the treatment of CRPS

Pleger et al (36) used rTMS in ten right-handed patients with CRPS of one upper limb. All central acting drugs were stopped at least 48 hs before the study started. Patients were randomly assigned either to the sham rTMS (n=5) or to the verum rTMS (n=5) group. The next day, the groups were reversed. On the verum rTMS group, an eight-shaped coil was applied on the motor cortex contralateral to the affected limb. After determining motor threshold (MT) for the first dorsal interosseum muscle, rTMS applications started. The trial consisted of a series of 10 applications, at a pulse intensity of 110% of MT, a frequency of 10 Hz and during a lapse of 1,2 s. Between each series there was a 10 s interruption. Patients were instructed to determine pain intensity using a visual analog scale (VAS). For the sham rTMS the coil was applied to the same position over the motor cortex, but it was angled at 45 degrees, with only the edge of the coil resting on the scalp. Out of the ten patients, seven responded to verum rTMS and showed significant decreased in pain level starting 30s after stimulation and reaching maximum analgesic effect 15 min later, but it re-intensified 45 min later. Sham rTSM caused no changes in individual pain intensity (see figure 1).

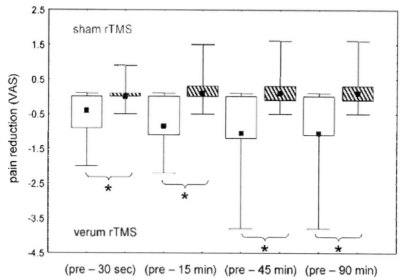

The box-whisker-plot shows the benefit of verum rTMS when compared to sham rTMS. Pain levels (VAS) differences between pre-rTMS and the four successive evaluations over 90 min post-rTMS (the black point within the box gives the median of data. The top and bottom of the box gives the 25 and 75 percentiles respectively. The top and bottom of the wishker gives the maximum and the minimum, respectively). To elucidate the difference between the two conditions a Student's paired t-test was utilized ($p<0.005$).

Figure 1. Pain scores in verum rTMS vs. sham in patient with CRPS type I. (from Pleger et al., 2004, with permission).

tDCS for the treatment of CRPS

Although the are no controlled studies published on tDCS in CRPS/RSD population, there is an empirical evidence from clinical settings (47) indicating that tDCS can relieve CRPS/RSD-related pain that does not respond to conventional pharmacological treatment. At our site at the Institute for Non-invasive Brain Stimulation, Department of Pain Medicine and Palliative Care, Beth Israel Medical Center, New York, we utilize tDCS for research purposes, and also in clinical settings to relieve chronic pain in patients, whose pain did not respond to conventional therapies. We have conducted more than 500 tDCS sessions, i.e. more than 100 blocks of tDCS (each block consists of 5 tDCS treatments on 5 consecutive days), in patients with chronic pain of various origin. Figure 2 shows a decrease in pain intensity during one block of tDCS in 19 CRPS/RSD patients (47). Patients received anodal tDCS over the motor cortex at the intensity of 2 mA for 20 min, on 5 consecutive days, using two saline-soaked sponge electrodes of size of 25 cm2 placed over the motor cortex contralateral to the painful site, and over ipsilateral supraorbital region.

Pain intensity was measured using the 11 points numerical rating scale (NRS, 0-10) before and immediately after tDCS. All patients were then treated in an open label fashion, and all of them received tDCS utilizing the same parameters. Pain relief was significant from day 2: p<0.01 on Day 2; p<0.001 on Day 3, 4, 5 (see figure 2).

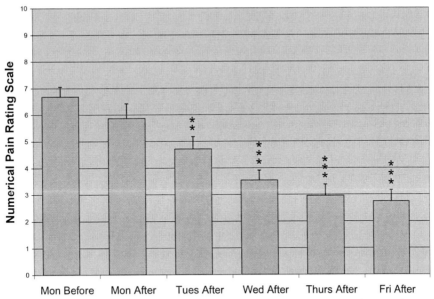

Mean pain scores in 19 patients treated with 20 min duration, 5 consecutive sessions of anodal tDCS applied over the contralateral motor cortex of the affected limb. Significant pain relief was observed from the end of the second application (Day 2, p<0.01; Days 3-5 p<0.001).

Figure 2. Pain scores obtained from patients with CRPS/RSD treated with tDCS.

Further, there is a case report (48) of CRPS/RSD patient with intractable CRPS/RSD-related pain in lower limb who received a total of 5 blocks of anodal tDCS (2 mA for 20 min, saline-soaked sponge electrodes 25cm^2) applied over the primary motor cortex over the course of 42 weeks in "as needed" regime. Each block of tDCS resulted in significant pain relief, which substantially over-lasted the stimulation (by up to 11 weeks). Furthermore, the patient gained secondary benefits from tDCS (for example improvement in sleep, mood and activity) that over-lasted the stimulation by weeks. The repeated stimulation (5 blocks) did not cause any serious adverse effects, and did not show the effect of "desensitization" to the tDCS treatment (48).

Conclusions

CRPS is characterized for a myriad of signs and symptoms where pain plays a pivotal role (49). Pain can be very intense, constant, refractory to treatment and can impose severe limitations to the patient's activities of daily living. In search for more effective therapies to manage the pain and associated symptoms, several investigators have studied a possible role for tDCS, TMS and behavioral therapies, on the reversal of the changes in plasticity and neuronal excitability documented in this patient population. Although there is evidence that supports the use of both TMS and tDCS to induce pain relief in patients with CRPS, there are only a few studies and more controlled trials need to be conducted.

References

[1] Karin Swart CM, Stins JF, Beek PJ. Cortical changes in complex regional pain syndrome. Eur J Pain 2008 Dec 18. {Epub ahead of print}

[2] Maihöfner C, Handwerker HO, Neundorfer B, Birklen F. Patterns of cortical reorganization in complex regional pain syndrome. Neurology 2003;61(12):1707-15.

[3] Pleger B, Janssen F, Schwenkreis P, Volker B, Maier C, Tegenthoff M. Repetitive transcranial magnetic stimulation of the motor cortex attenuates pain perception in complex regional pain syndrome type I. Neurosci Lett 2004;356:87-90.

[4] Andre-Obadia N, Peyron R, Mertens P, Mauguiere F, Laurent B, Garcia-Larea L. Transcranial magnetic stimulation for pain control. Double-blind study of different frequencies against placebo, and correlation with motor cortex stimulation efficacy. Clin Neurophysiol 2006;117:1536-44.

[5] Khedr EM, Kotb H, Kamel NF, Ahmed MA, Sadek R, Rothwell JC. Longlasting antalgic effects of daily sessions of repetitive transcranial magnetic stimulation in central and peripheral neuropathic pain. J Neurol Neurosurg Psychiatry 2005;76:833-838.

[6] Rollnik JD et al. Repetitive transcranial magnetic stimulation for the treatment of chronic pain- a pilot study. Eur Neurol 2002;48:6-10.

[7] Lefaucheur JP, Drouot X, Nguyen JP. Interventional neurophysiology for pain control: duration of pain relief following repetitive transcranial magnetic stimulation of the motor cortex. Neurophysiol Clin 2001;31:247-52.

[8] Maihöfner C, Handwerker HO, Neundorfer B, Birklein F. Mechanical hyperalgesia in complex regional pain syndrome: a role for TNF-alpha? Neurology 2005;65:311-3.

[9] Huygen FJ, De Bruijn AG, De Bruin MT, Groeneweg JG, Klein J, Zijistra FJ. Evidence for local inflammation in complex regional pain syndrome type 1. Mediators Inflamm 2002;11:47-51.

[10] Alexander GM, van Rijn MA, van Hilten JJ, Perreault MJ, Schwartzman RJ. Changes in cerebrospinal fluid levels of pro-inflammatory cytokines in CRPS. Pain 2005;116:213-9.

[11] Allan SM, Tyrrell PJ, Rothwell NJ. Interleukin-1 and neuronal injury. Nat Rev Immunol 2005;5:629-40.
[12] de Mos M, Sturkenboom MC, Huygen FJ. Current Understandings on Complex Regional Pain Syndrome. Pain Pract 2009 Feb 9. [Epub ahead of print]
[13] Woolf CJ, Costigan M. Transcriptional and posttranslational plasticity and the generation of inflammatory pain. Proc Natl Acad Sci USA 1999;96:7723-30.
[14] Pappagallo M, Knotkova H, DeNardis L. Multifaceted CRPS/RSD: Emerging mechanisms and pharmacotherapy. Crit Rev in Phys Rehab Med 2006;18(3):257-82.
[15] Oaklander AL, Rissmiller JG, Gelman LB, Zheng L, Chang Y, Gott R. Evidence of focal small - fiber axonal degeneration in complex regional pain syndrome-1 (Reflex Sympathetic Dystrophy). Pain 2006;120(3)235-43.
[16] Albrecht PJ, Hines S, Eisenberg PE, Pud D, Finlay DR, Connolly MK, Pare M, Davar G, Rice FL. Pathologic alterations of cutaneous innervation and vasculature in affected limbs from patients with complex regional pain syndrome. Pain 2006;120(3):244-66.
[17] Watkins LR, Maier SF. Beyond neurons: evidence that immune and glial cells contribute to pathological pain states. Physiol Rev 2002;82:981-1011.
[18] Ledeboer A, Sloane EM, Milligan ED. Minocycline attenuates mechanical allodynia and proinflammatory cytokine expression in rat models of pain facilitation. Pain 2005;115:71-83.
[19] Hashizume H, Rutkowski MD, Weinstein JN. Central administration of methotrexate reduces mechanical allodynia in an animal model of radiculopathy/sciatica. Pain 2000;87:159-69.
[20] Sweitzer SM, Schubert P, DeLeo JA. Propentofylline, a glial modulating agent, exhibits antiallodynic properties in a rat model of neuropatinc pain. J Pharmacol Exp Ther 2001;297:1210-7.
[21] Jin SX, Zhuang ZY, Wolf CJ. P38 mitogen-activated protein kinase is activated after a spinal nerve ligation in spinal cord microglia and dorsal root ganglinon neurons and contributes to the generation of neuropathic pain. J Neurosci 2003;23:4017-22.
[22] Raghavendra V, Tanga F, Deleo JA. Inhibition of microglial activation attenuates the development but not existing hypersensitivity in a rat model of neuropathy. J Pharmacol Exp Ther 2003;306:624-30.
[23] Del Valle L, Schwartzman RJ, Alexander G. Spinal cord histopathological alterations in a patient with longstanding complex regional pain syndrome. Brain Behav Immun 2009;23(1):85-91.
[24] Geha PY, Baliki MN, Harden RN, Bauer WR, Parrish TB, Apkarian AV. The brain in chronic CRPS pain: abnormal gray-white matter interactions in emotional and autonomic regions. Neuron 2008;60(4):570-81.
[25] Baron R, Levine JD , Fields HL. Causalgia and reflex sympathetic dystrophy: does the sympathetic nervous system contribute to the generation of pain? Muscle Nerve 1999;22:678-695.
[26] Scholz J, Woolf CJ. Mechanism of neuropathic pain. In: Pappagallo M, ed. The neurological basis of pain. New York: McGraw Hill 2005:71-94.
[27] Drummond PD, Skipworth S, Finch PM. 1- Adrenoceptors in normal and hyperalgesic human skin. Clin Sci 1996;91:73-77.
[28] Wasner G, Schattschneider J, Heckmann K. Vascular abnormalities in reflex sympathetic dystrophy (CRPS I): Mechanisms and diagnostic value. Brain 2001;124:587-99.
[29] Ali Z, Raja SN, Wesselmann U. Intradermal injection of norepinephrine evokes pain in patients with sympathetically maintained pain. Pain 2000;88:161-8.
[30] Seifert F, Kiefer G, Decol R, Schmelz M, Maihöfner C. Differential endogenous pain modulation in complex-regional pain syndrome. Brain 2009 Jan 19. [EPub ahead of print]
[31] Flor H, Elbert T, Knecht S, Wienbruch C, Pantev C, Birbaumer N, Larbig W, Taub E. Phantom limb pain as a perceptual correlate of cortical reorganization. Nature 1995;357:482-4.

[32] Birbaumer N, Lutzenberger W, Montoya P, Larbig W, Unertl K, Topfner S, Grodd W, Taub E, Flor H. Effects of regional anesthesia on phantom limb pain are mirrored in changes in cortical reorganization. J Neurosci 1997;17(14):5503-8.
[33] Pleger B et al. Sensorimotor returning in complex regional pain syndrome parallels pain reduction. Ann Neurol 2005;57(3):425-9.
[34] Pleger B et al. Patterns of cortical reorganization parallel impaired tactile discrimination and pain intensity in complex regional pain syndrome. Neuroimage 2006;32(2):503-10.
[35] Maihöfner C, Handwerker HO, Neundorfer B, Birklen F. Patterns of cortical reorganization in complex regional pain syndrome. Neurology 2003;61(12):1707-15.
[36] Pleger B, Janssen F, Schwenkreis P, Völker B, Maier C, Tegenthoff M. Repetitive transcranial magnetic stimulation of the motor cortex attenuates pain perception in complex regional pain syndrome type I. Neurosci Lett 2004;356(2):87-90.
[37] Maihöfner C, Handwerker HO, Neundorfer B, Birklein F. Cortical reorganization during recovery from complex regional pain syndrome. Neurology 2004;63(4):693-701.
[38] Krause P, Forderreuther S, Straube A. TMS motor cortical brain mapping in patients with Complex Regional Pain Syndrome type I. Clinical Neurophysiol 2006;117(1):169-176.
[39] Maihöfner C et al. The motor system shows adaptive changes in complex regional pain syndrome. Brain 2007;130(Pt 10):2671-87.
[40] Larbig W, Montoya P, Braun C, Birbaumer N. Abnormal reactivity of the primary somatosensory cortex during the experience of pain in complex regional pain syndrome: a magnetoencephalograhic case study. Neurocase 2006;12(5):280-5.
[41] Juottonen K, Gockel M, Silen T, Hurri H, Hari R, Forss N. Altered central sensorimotor processing in patients with complex regional pain syndrome. Pain 2002;98(3):315-23.
[42] Eisenberg E, Chistyakov AV, Yudashkin M, Kaplan B, Hafner H, Feinsod M. Evidence for cortical hyperexcitability of the affected limb representation area in CRPS: a psychophysical and transcranial magnetic stimulation study. Pain 2005;113(1-2):99-105.
[43] Schwenkreis P et al. Bilateral motor cortex disinhibition in complex regional pain syndrome(CRPS)type I of the hand. Neurology 2003;61(4):515-9.
[44] Khedr EM, Kotb H, Kamel NF, Ahmed MA, Sadek R, Rothwell JC. Longlasting antalgic effects of daily sessions of repetitive transcranial magnetic stimulation in central and peripheral neuropathic pain. J Neurol Neurosurg Psychiatry 2005;76:833-8.
[45] Valeriani M et al. Inhibition of the human primary motor area by painful heat stimulation of the skin. Clin Neurophysiol 1999;110(8):1475-80.
[46] Jacobs KM, Donoghue JP. Reshaping the cortical motor map by unmasking latent intracortical connections. Science 1991;22:251(4996):944-7.
[47] Cruciani RA, Knotkova H. Clinical potential of tDCS in the treatment of neuropathic pain. Ground Rounds, oral presentation. New York: Beth Israel Med Center, Oct 2008.
[48] Knotkova H, Sibirceva U, Factor A, Feldman D, Ragert P, Flor H, Cohen LG: Repeated transcranial direct current stimulation (tDCS) for the treatment of neuropathic pain due to CRPS. Poster Presentation, Book of Abstracts, World Congress on Pain, Glasgow, UK. IASP Press, 2008:156.
[49] Knotkova H, Dmochowska J, Sibirceva U, Flor H, Cruciani RA. Cortical reorganization in the complex regional pain syndrome. J Pain Manage 2008;1:207-14.

Chapter 29

SAFETY OF TRANSCRANIAL DIRECT CURRENT STIMULATION (TDCS) IN PROTOCOLS INVOLVING HUMAN SUBJECTS

Arun Sundaram[1], Veronika Stock, MD[1], Ricardo A Cruciani, MD, PhD[1,2,3] and Helena Knotkova, PhD[*1,2]

[1]Institute for Noninvasive Brain Stimulation of New York, Research Division, Department of Pain Medicine and Palliative Care, Beth Israel Medical Center, New York, [2]Department of Neurology, Albert Einstein College of Medicine, Bronx, New York and [3]Department of Anesthesiology, Albert Einstein College of Medicine, Bronx, New York, United States of America

Abstract

The purpose of this review was to evaluate safety of Transcranial Direct Current Stimulation (tDCS) in humans. We have performed a focused search in two major medical databases, Medline and PubMed, for original articles on tDCS in humans (healthy subjects and patients with various diagnoses) published in English. A primary search yielded 141 articles. Fifty-two articles were excluded for the following reasons: 17 articles were review papers, 26 articles were deemed not related to tDCS, and nine articles did not provide a complete list of the stimulation-parameters. A total of 89 articles involving tDCS protocols in human subjects were analyzed in the scope of safety parameters, with the main focus on the Current Density and Total Charge. The findings of the review further support the existing evidence on tDCS safety.

Keywords: Transcranial direct current stimulation (tDCS), human subjects, safety, non-invasive brain stimulation.

---

[*] **Correspondence:** Helena Knotkova, PhD, Institute for Noninvasive Brain Stimulation of New York, Research Division, Dept of Pain Medicine and Palliative Care, 350 East 17th Street, Baird Hall, 12th floor, Beth Israel Medical Center, New York, NY 10003 United States. Tel: 212-844-8541; E-mail: HKnotkov@chpnet.org

Introduction

TDCS (Transcranial Direct Current Stimulation) has been developed as a noninvasive technique for modulation of cortical excitability (1). The principle of tDCS is based on influencing neuronal excitability and modulating the firing rates of individual neurons by a low amplitude direct current, which is delivered non-invasively and painlessly through the scalp to the selected brain structures (2,3). The nature of tDCS-induced changes on cortical excitability depends on the polarity of the current. It is well accepted that the anodal tDCS increases cortical excitability, while the cathodal tDCS decreases it (2-6). Some of tDCS induced changes occur immediately during the stimulation (so called intra-tDCS effects), while others occur later as short-lasting and long-lasting after-effects (2). The intra-tDCS effects which elicit no after-effects can be induced by a short (seconds) single application of tDCS. The intra-tDCS effect of cathodal tDCS is the reduction of intracortical facilitation, while anodal tDCS has no intra-effect on intracortical facilitation or inhibition. All effects of anodal stimulation occur later as after-effects. The short-lasting after-effects outlast the end of stimulation by 5-10 min and can be induced by application of seven min of 1 mA tDCS, while to obtain long-lasting effects (about one hr), 13 min of 1 mA tDCS is needed. Both, anodal and cathodal tDCS can produce short-lasting and long-lasting effects (7). After-effects of anodal tDCS involve reduction of intracortical inhibition and enhancement of intracortical facilitation, while cathodal tDCS after-effect represent enhancement of intracortical inhibition.

TDCS is not only a useful tool of neurophysiological research, but it also shows a promising clinical potential in alleviation of symptoms related to diseases and pathological conditions that have shown to involve changes in cortical excitability, for example post-stroke syndrome, complex regional pain syndrome, fibromyalgia, major depression, Parkinson's disease, and others. As the principle of this technique is based on delivering direct current through the skull to the brain tissue, evidence of the safety of tDCS needs to be regularly evaluated and updated to protect subjects receiving tDCS in both research and clinical settings.

General considerations of tDCS safety

Generally, there are several mechanisms of potential current-induced tissue damage (8) that need to be considered in protocols using current-delivering procedures:

- Electrochemically produced toxic brain products and metallic electrode dissolution products caused by the electrode-tissue interface.
- Heat development under the electrodes.
- Current-induced neuronal hyper-excitability and brain tissue heating.

TDCS technique has not been shown to conflict with any of the general mechanisms associated with potential current-induced tissue damage mentioned above (1,3,9). Importantly:

- In tDCS, electrodes and brain tissue do not come into direct contact. Further, to minimize chemical processes at the electrode-skin interface, sponge electrodes, instead of metallic ones, have been utilized in tDCS protocols.
- Heating under the electrodes has been shown not to occur during the tDCS protocol (1). Damage from the heating of neuronal tissue can be also ruled out as a potential safety concern, since excessive heating directly on the skin under the electrodes was not experienced (1).
- Potential damaging effects due to neuronal hyperactivity refer to high frequency of supra-threshold stimulation lasting for hours (10). As pointed out by Nitsche et al. (9), the effects of tDCS are sub-threshold in the means of eliciting action potentials in neurons at resting membrane potentials. Furthermore, tDCS induced only moderate changes in cortical excitability (1,3,4,7).

Thus, tDCS as a technique of noninvasive modulation of cortical excitability has been shown to comply with safety considerations in the means of above described current-induced tissue damage mechanisms.

However, besides the general safety parameters of the tDCS technique, safety parameters of stimulation within each particular tDCS protocol need to be strongly considered and exercised to ensure safety of subjects receiving tDCS stimulation.

Major safety parameters of stimulation as tested in studies using a high frequency supra-threshold stimuli (a train of high frequency pulses) are Current Density, Total Charge, Charge per Phase, and Charge Density (8,11,12). Not all of these parameters apply for tDCS, as tDCS delivers direct current, i.e. one continuous stimulus per session. Thus, the appropriate parameter for deriving safety limits of tDCS (9) is Current Density [A/cm2] (=stimulation strength [A]/electrode size [cm2]), together with Total Charge [C/cm2] (=stimulation strength [A]/electrode size [cm2] x total stimulation duration[s]), since duration of stimulation is an important factor contributing to potential tissue damage (9).

In this review, we evaluate existing tDCS protocols published on human subjects from the point of the aforementioned safety parameters, Current Density and Total Charge, and discuss them in the context of reported side effects and other safety related issues.

Methods

We searched in two major medical databases, PubMed and Medline, for tDCS-related articles published in English between January 1999 and January 2009 precluding other than human subjects. The search words used were: "transcranial direct current stimulation" and "tDCS". Inclusion criteria were: complete information about parameters of stimulation (including electrode size) must be given, and the article must be primary source regarding the use of tDCS performed on human subjects.

Using the search words, 141 articles were found. Fifty-two articles did not meet the Inclusion criteria: 26 articles were not relevant, 17 articles were reviews, and 9 studies did not completely list parameters of stimulation. Thus, the application of the Inclusion criteria yielded the final pool of 89 articles (1-7,9,13-93), which were evaluated in this review.

Discussion

Parameters of stimulation are dictated to a high degree by the purpose of stimulation. While not all studies in healthy subjects aim to induce the tDCS after-effects (see Introduction) and thus the duration of stimulation can be short, the desired result of tDCS in patients with various diagnoses is usually a relief of symptoms that outlast the stimulation as long as possible. To induce long-lasting after-effects, the tDCS stimulation needs to be applied for about 13 min or more (1,4,7,9). Thus, it may translate to higher Total Charge in studies involving patients as compared to protocols designed for healthy subjects. For that reason, we analyzed separately protocols on healthy subjects and protocols involving patients with various diagnoses. As tDCS effects have been shown to be cumulative (74,76,80-83,89,93), some tDCS protocols delivered a block of treatments consisting of tDCS sessions on several consecutive days, rather than a single session. Thus, when evaluating parameters of existing protocols, we commented on not only Total Charge per Session, but (when applicable) on Total Charge per Complete Block of Treatments as well. Ranges of evaluated parameters, i.e. Current Density, Total Charge per Session, and Total Charge per Complete Block of Treatments, separately for anodal and cathodal stimulation, in patients and healthy subjects, appear in table 1.

Table 1. Range of parameters "Current Density" and "Total Charge" in tDCS protocols involving human subjects

	Current Density (mA/cm2)	Total Charge per Session (C/cm2)	Total Charge per Complete Block of Treatments (C/cm2)
Healthy subjects – anodal tDCS	0.025-0.0667	0.0045-0.08	N/A
Healthy subjects – cathodal tDCS	0.0204-0.08	0.00245-0.096	N/A
Patients – anodal tDCS	0.0286-0.0571	0.00514-0.0686	0.0206-0.686
Patients – cathodal tDCS	0.0286-0.0571	0.00514-0.0686	0.0206-0.172

Current Density (mA/cm2) = stimulation strength (mA)/electrode size (cm2)

Total Charge per Session(C/cm2) = stimulation strength (A)/electrode size (cm2) x total tDCS stimulation duration (s).

Total Charge per Complete Block of Treatments (C/cm2) = stimulation strength (A)/electrode size (cm2) x total tDCS stimulation duration (s) x number of sessions.

tDCS protocols in healthy subjects

Sixty-eight (1-7,9,13-72) of the total pool of 89 analyzed studies involved anodal or cathodal tDCS stimulation in healthy subjects (total n=1208). For anodal stimulation the Current Density ranged between 0.025 (13) and 0.0667(69) mA/cm2, and the Total Charge per Session was between 0.0045 (13) – 0.08 (69) C/cm2. The highest Total Charge per Session was delivered in the study aiming to determine contralateral and ipsilateral motor effects after tDCS (71). Seven healthy subjects received the anodal stimulation at intensity of 1mA with 15cm2 electrodes placed over the right supraorbital region and the left motor cortex, with a Current Density of 0.0667mA/cm2, for 20 min, resulting in the Total Charge of 0.08 C/cm2 (71). No adverse effects were reported in this study.

As shown by McCreery (11) and noted by Nitsche (9), Current Densities below 25mA/cm2 do not induce brain tissue damage even when applying high-frequency stimulation over several hours. Thus, the Current Density of 0.0667mA/cm2, as reported above, is well within the safety limit. As for Total Charge per Session, tissue damage has been detected at a minimum charge of 216 C/cm2 (12). Thus, the Total Charge per Session in the analyzed anodal tDCS protocols, with the highest value of 0.08 C/cm2, is clearly within safety limits.

For cathodal stimulation, the Current Density ranged between 0.0204 (34) and 0.08mA/cm2 (72), and the Total Charge per Session was between 0.00245 (34) and 0.096C/cm2 (72). In the study employing the cathodal stimulation of the highest Current Density of 0.08mA/cm2 and highest Total Charge per Session of 0.096 C/cm2 (72), 12 healthy subjects received 20 min of cathodal stimulation at intensity of 1.2mA, using two sponge electrodes 15cm2, placed over the left Brodman's area and contralateral supraorbital area to study a potential enhancement of working memory. The study monitored possible side effects, but none were reported. Again, both Current Density and Total Charge per Session in protocols using cathodal stimulation were well within the safety limits (11,12).

tDCS protocols in patients with various diagnoses

In the pool of analyzed articles, 21 studies (73-93) involved patients (total n=278) with various diagnoses including e.g. major depression, Parkinson's disease, stroke, uncontrollable food cravings, alcohol dependence, and chronic pain syndromes. Safety parameters of anodal tDCS were drawn from 20 studies (73-85,86,88-93), while 12 studies yielded safety data on cathodal stimulation (73,76-80,83,84,87,90-92).

For anodal stimulation, the Current Density ranged between 0.0286 (73,75,77,81,83-84,91) and 0.0571 (74,76,79-80,82,86,90,93)mA/cm2, the Total Charge per Session was between 0.00514 (83) and 0.0686 (74,76,80,82,86,93)C/cm2, while the Total Charge per Block of Treatments ranged from 0.0206 (83) to 0.686 (74)C/cm2. The highest Total Charge per Session (0.0686C/cm2), the Total Charge per Block of Treatment (0.686C/cm2), and also the highest values for the Current Density (0.0571mA/cm2) of anodal stimulation were delivered in the study on the efficacy of cortical DCS for the treatment of major depression (74). Forty patients with major depression took part in the study, with 35cm2 electrodes placed over the dorsolateral prefrontal cortex or occipital cortex, and the contralateral supraorbital area. A 2mA current was delivered for 20 minutes for 10 days. The side effects that were reported by some patients were minor and transient, and included itching, redness of the skin under the electrode, and transient headache.

As for parameters of anodal tDCS specifically in population of patients with chronic pain, the highest parameters for anodal stimulation (82) were as follows: The Current Density 0.0571mA/cm2, Total Charge per Session 0.0686C/cm2, and Total Charge per Complete Block of Treatments (one block = 5 session on 5 consecutive days) was 0.343C/cm2.

Seventeen patients with spinal cord injury participated in the study (82), and the stimulation was delivered at current intensity of 2mA, for 20 minutes, on 5 consecutive days, with sponge-electrodes of size 35cm2 placed over the primary motor cortex and the contralateral supraorbital area (82). Only minor side effects like itching were reported.

For cathodal stimulation in the patients with various diagnosis, the Current Density in analyzed studies varied between 0.0286 (73,77,83-84,91) and 0.0571mA/cm2 (76,80,90), the Total Charge per Session was between 0.00514 (83) and 0.0686 (76,80) C/cm2, while the Total Charge per Block of Treatments was from 0.0206 (83) to 0.172 (77) C/cm2.

The cathodal stimulation of the highest Total Charge per Block of Treatments, as mentioned above, was utilized in the study of Boggio and his colleagues (77). Nine stroke patients received 5 sessions of the cathodal tDCS at the intensity of 1mA, for 20 min with sponge-electrodes of size 35cm2 placed over primary motor cortex. All reported side effects were transient, tolerable, and not serious. The side effects included tingling, burning, and itching sensations under the area of the electrode.

As for cathodal stimulation in the treatment of chronic pain, there are no published controlled studies using cathodal stimulation to elicit relief of chronic pain. However, our experience from a case of CRPS/RSD patient receiving cathodal tDCS over the somatosensory cortex to relieve intractable chronic pain associated with CRPS/RSD (94), suggests that cathodal stimulation applied at the current intensity of 2mA for 20 min in 5 sessions on 5 consecutive days, with sponge electrodes of 25cm2, can be safely delivered without occurrence any substantial side effects. These parameters translated into the Current Density of 0.08mA/cm2, the Total Charge per Session of 0.096C/cm, and the Total Charge per Block of Treatment of 0.480C/cm2.

Conclusions

1. Highest parameters applied in the analyzed studies in humans were for anodal and cathodal tDCS as follows: Anodal stimulation Current Density 0.0667mA/cm2, Total Charge per Session 0.08C/cm2, and Total Charge per Block of Treatments 0.686 C/cm2. Cathodal tDCS: Current Density of 0.08mA/cm2, Total Charge per Session 0.096C/cm, and the Total Charge per Block of Treatments 0.172C/cm2.

    As indicated by McCreery et al (11) and noted by Nitsche et al (9), Current Densities below 25 mA/cm2 do not induce brain tissue damage even applied at high-frequency stimulation over several hours. For Total Charge per Session, tissue damage has been detected at a minimum charge of 216 C/cm2 (12). Thus, Current Density, and Total Charge in tDCS protocols as they were described in 89 analyzed tDCS studies in humans are within aforementioned safety limits.
2. TDCS stimulation when delivered even at the highest parameters reported above, did not elicit any serious side effects.
3. The findings of the review further support the existing evidence on tDCS safety.

References

[1] Nitsche MA, Paulus W. Excitability changes induced in the human motor cortex by weak transcranial direct current stimulation. J Physiol 2000;527:633-9.
[2] Nitsche MA, Seeber A, Frommann K, Klein CC, Rochford C, et al. Modulating parameters of excitability during and after transcranial direct current stimulation of the human motor cortex. J Physiol 2005; 568:291-303.
[3] Nitsche MA, Paulus W. Sustained excitability elevations induced by transcranial DC motor cortex stimulation in humans. Neurology 2001;57:1899-1901.
[4] Nitsche MA, Nitsche MS, Klein CC, Tergau F, Rothwell JC, Paulus W. Level of action of cathodal DC polarization induced inhibition of the human motor cortex. Clin Neurophysiol 2003;114:600-4.
[5] Liebetanz D, Nitsche MA, Tergau F, Paulus W. Pharmacological approach to the mechanisms of transcranial DC stimulation induced after effects of human motor cortex excitability. Brain 2002;125: 2238-47.
[6] Nitsche MA, Liebetanz D, Schlitterlau A, Henschke U, Fricke K, et al. GABAergic modulation of DC stimulation induced motor cortex excitability shifts in humans. Eur J Neurosci 2004;19:2720-6.
[7] Nitsche MA, Fricke K, Henschke U, Schlitterlau A, Liebetanz D, et al. Pharmacological modulation of cortical excitability shifts induced by transcranial direct current stimulation in humans. J Physiol 2003; 553:293-301.
[8] Agnew WF, McCreery DB. Considerations for safety in the use of extracranial stimulation for motor evoked potentials. Neurosurgery 1987;20:143-7.
[9] Nitsche MA, Liebetanz D, Lang N, Antal A, Tergau F, Paulus W. Safety criteria for transcranial direct durrent stimulation (tDCS) in humans. Clin Neurophysiol 2003;114:2220-2.
[10] Agnew WF, Yuen TG, McCreery DB. Morphologic changes after prolonged electrical stimulation of the cat's cortex at defined charge densities. Exp Neurol 1983;79:379-411.
[11] McCreery DB, Agnew WF, Yuen TG, Bullara LA. Charge density and charge per phase as cofactors in neural injury induced by electrical stimulation. IEEE Trans Biomed Eng 1990;37:996-1001.
[12] Yuen TGH, Agnew WF, Bullara LA, Skip Jaques BS, McCreery DB. Histological evaluation of neural damage from electrical stimulation: considerations for the selection of parameters for clinical application. Neurosurgery 1981;9:292-9.
[13] Accornero N, Li Voti P, La Riccia M, Gregori B. Visual evoked potentials modulation during direct current polarization. Exp Brain Res 2007;178:261-6.
[14] Antal A, Begemeier S, Nitsche MA, Paulus W. Prior state of cortical activity influences subsequent practicing of a visuomotor coordination task. Neuropsychologia, 2008;46:3157-61.
[15] Antal A, Terney D, Poreisz C, Paulus W. Towards unraveling task-related modulations of neuroplastic changes induced in the human motor cortex. Eur J Neurosci 2007;26:2687-91.
[16] Antal A, Kincses T, Nitsche MA, Paulus W. Manipulation of phosphene thresholds by transcranial direct current stimulation in man. Exp Brain Res 2003;150:375-8.
[17] Antal A, Nitsche MA, Kinces TZ, Kruse W, Hoffmann KP, Paulus W. Facilitation of visuomotor learning by transcranial direct current stimulation of the motor and extrastriate visual areas in humans. Eur J Neurosci 2004;19:2888-92.
[18] Antal A, Nitsche MA, Paulus W. External modulation of visual perception in humans. NeuroReport 2001;12:3553-5.
[19] Antal A, Kincses TZ, Nitsche MA, Bartfai O, Paulus W. Excitability changes induced in the human primary visual cortex by transcranial direct current stimulation: Direct electrophysiological evidence. IOVS 2004;45:702-7.

[20] Antal A, Varga ET, Nitsche MA, Chadaide Z, Paulus W, Kovacs G, Vidnyanszky Z. Direct current stimulation over MT+/V5 modulates motion aftereffect in humans. NeuroReport 2004;15:2491-4.

[21] Antal A, Varga ET, Kincses TZ, Nitsche MA, Paulus W. Oscillatory brain activity and transcranial direct current stimulation in humans. NeuroReport 2004;15:1307-10.

[22] Antal A, Brepohl N, Poreisz C, Boros K, Csifcsak G, Paulus W. Transcranial Direct Current Stimulation over somatosensory cortex decreases experimentally induced acute pain perception. Clin J Pain 2008;24:56-63.

[23] Antal A, Kincses TZ, Nitsche MA, Paulus W. Modulation of moving phosphene thresholds by transcranial direct current stimulation of V1 in human. Neuropsychol 2003;41:1802-7.

[24] Ardolino G, Bossi B, Barbieri S, Priori A. Non-synaptic mechanisms underlie the after-effects of cathodal transcutaneous direct current stimulation of the human brain. J Physiol 2005;568:653-63.

[25] Baudewig J, Nitsche MA, Paulus W, Frahm J. Regional Modulation of BOLD MRI Responses to Human Sensorimotor Activation by Transcranial Direct Current Stimulation. Magn Reson Med 2001;45: 196-201.

[26] Beeli G, Casutt G, Baumgartner T, Jäncke L. Modulating presence and impulsiveness by external stimulation of the brain. Behav Brain Funct 2008;4:33.

[27] Beeli G, Koeneke S, Gasser K, Jancke L. Brain stimulation modulates driving behavior. Behav Brain Funct 2008;4:34.

[28] Boggio PS, Zaghi S, Lopes M, Fregni F. Modulatory effects of anodal transcranial direct current stimulation on perception and pain thresholds in healthy volunteers. Eur J Neurol 2008;15:1124-30.

[29] Boggio PS, Castro LO, Savagim EA, Braite R, Cruz VC, Rocha RR, Rigonatti SP, Silva MTA, Fregni F. Enhancement of non-dominant hand motor function by anodal transcranial direct current stimulation. Neurosci Lett 2006;404:232-6.

[30] Boggio PS, Rocha RR, da Silva MT, Fregni F. Differential modulatory effects of transcranial direct current stimulation on a facial expression go-no-go task in males and females. Neurosci Lett 2008;447(2-3):101-5.

[31] Boros K, Poreisz C, Munchau A, Paulus W, Mitsche MA. Premotor transcranial direct current stimulation (tDCS) affects primary motor excitability in humans. Eur J Neurosci 2008;27:1292-1300.

[32] Cogiamanian F, Marceglia S, Ardolino G, Barbieri S, Priori A. Improved isometric force endurance after transcranial direct current stimulation over the human motor cortical areas. Eur J Neurosci 2007;26:242-9.

[33] Dieckhofer A, Waberski TD, Nitsche M, Paulus W, Buchner H, Gobbele R. Transcranial direct current stimulation applied over the somatosensory cortex – differential effect on low and high frequency SEPs. Clin Neurophysiol 2006;117:2221-7.

[34] Dundas JE, Thickbroom GW, Mastaglia FL. Perception of comfort during transcranial DC stimulation: Effect of NaCl solution concentration applied to sponge electrodes. Clin Neurophysiol 2007; 118:1166-70.

[35] Fecteau S, Pascual-Leone A, Zald DH, Liguori P, Theoret H, Boggio PS, Fregni F. Activation of prefrontal cortex by transcranial direct current stimulation reduces appetite for risk during ambiguous decision making. J Neurosci 2007;27(23):6212-8.

[36] Fecteau S, Knock D, Fregni F, Sultani N, Boggio P, Pascual-Leone A. Diminishing risk taking behavior by modulating activity in the prefrontal cortex: a direct current stimulation study. J Neurosci 2007; 27(46):12500-5.

[37] Fregni F, Boggio PS, Nitsche M, Bermpohl F, Antal A, et al. Anodal transcranial direct current stimulation of prefrontal cortex enhances working memory. Exp Brain Res 2005;166:23-30.

[38] Fregni F, Liguori P, Fecteau S, Nitsche MA, Pascual-Leone A, Boggio PS. Cortical stimulation of the prefrontal cortex with transcranial direct current stimulation reduces cue-provoked smoking craving: a randomized, sham-controlled study. J Clin Psychiatry 2008;69(1):32-40.

[39] Jeffrey DT, Norton JA, Roy FD, Gorassini MA. Effects of transcranial direct current stimulation on the excitability of the leg motor cortex. Exp Brain Res 2007;182:281-7.

[40] Kincses TZ, Antal A, Nitsche MA, Bartfai O, Paulus W. Facilitation of probabilistic classification learning by transcranial direct current stimulation of the prefrontal cortex in the human. Neuropsychol 2003;42:113-7.

[41] Knoch D, Nitsche MA, Fischbacher U, Eisenegger C, Pascual-Leone A, Fehr E. Studying the neurobiology of social interaction with transcranial direct current stimulation – The example of punishing unfairness. Cerebral Cortex 2008;18:1987-90.

[42] Kuo MF, Paulus W, Nitsche MA. Boosting focally induced brain plasticity by dopamine. Cerebral Cortex 2008;18:648-51.

[43] Kuo MF, Paulus W, Nitsche MA. Sex differences in cortical neuroplasticity in humans. NeuroReport 2006;17:1703-7.

[44] Kuo MF, Grosch J, Fregni F, Paulus W, Nitsche MA. Focusing effect of acetylcholine on neuroplasticity in the human motor cortex. J Neurosci 2007;27(52):14442-7.

[45] Kuo MF, Unger M, Liebetanz D, Lang N, Tergau F, Paulus W, Nitsche MA. Limited impact of homeostatic plasticity on motor learning in humans. Neuropsychol 2008;46:2122-8.

[46] Kwon YH, Ko MH, Ahn SH, Kim YH, Song JC, Lee CH, Chang MC, Jang SH. Primary motor cortex activation by transcranial direct current stimulation in the human brain. Neurosci Lett 2008;435:56-9.

[47] Lang N, Siebner HR, Ward NS, Lee L, Nitsche MA, Paulus W, Rothwell JC, Lemon RN, Frackowiak RS. How does transcranial DC stimulation of the primary motor cortex alter regional neuronal activity in the human brain? Eur J Neurosci 2005;22:495-504.

[48] Lang N, Nitsche MA, Paulus W, Rothwell JC, Lemon RN. Effects of transcranial direct current stimulation over the human motor cortex on corticospinal and transcallosal excitability. Exp Brain Res 2004;156: 439-43.

[49] Lang N, Siebner HR, Chadaide Z, Boros K, Nitsche MA, Rothwell JC, Paulus W, Antal A. Bidirectional modulation of primary visual cortex excitability: a combined tDCS and rTMS study. IVOS 2007; 48:5782-7.

[50] Lang N, Siebner HR, Ernst D, Nitsche MA, Paulus W, Lemon RN, Rothwell JC. Preconditioning with transcranial direct current stimulation sensitizes the motor cortex to rapid rate transcranial magnetic stimulation and controls the direction of after effects. Biol Psychiatry 2004;56:634-9.

[51] Marshall L, Molle M, Siebner H, Born J. Bifrontal transcranial direct current stimulation slows reaction time in a working memory task. BMC Neurosci 2005;6:23.

[52] Marshall L, Molle M, Hallschmid M, Born J. Transcranial direct current stimulation during sleep improves declarative memory. J Neurosci 2004;24(44): 9985-92.

[53] Matsunaga K, Nitsche MA, Tsuji S, Rothwell JC. Effect of transcranial DC sensorimotor cortex stimulation on somatosensory evoked potentials in humans. Clin Neurophysiol 2004;115:456-60.

[54] Miranda PC, Lomarev M, Hallett M. Modeling the current distribution during transcranial direct current stimulation. Clin Neurophysiol 2006;117:1623-9.

[55] Nitsche MA, Lampe C, Antal A, Liebetanz D, Lang N, Tergau F, Paulus W. Dopaminergic modulation of long lasting direct current induced cortical excitability changes in the human motor cortex. Eur J Neurosci 2006;23:1651-7.

[56] Nitsche MA, Grundey J, Liebetanz D, Lang N, Tergau F, Paulus W. Catecholaminergic consolidation of motor cortical neuroplasticity in humans. Cerebral Cortex 2004;14:1240-5.

[57] Nitsche MA, Doemkes S, Karakose T, Antal A, Liebetanz D, et al. Shaping the effects of transcranial direct current stimulation of the human motor cortex. J Neurophysiol 2007;97:3109-17.

[58] Nitsche MA, Roth A, Kuo MF, Fischer AK, Liebetanz D, et al. Timing dependent modulation of associative plasticity by general network excitability in the human motor cortex. J Neurosci 2007; 27(14):3807-12.

[59] Nitsche MA, Niehaus L, Hoffman KT, Hengst S, Liebetanz D, et al. MRI study of human brain exposed to weak direct current stimulation of the frontal cortex. Clin Neurophysiol 2004; 115:2419-23.

[60] Ohn SH, Park C, Yoo WK, Ko MH, Choi KP, et al. Time dependent effect of transcranial direct current stimulation on the enhancement of working memory. NeuroReport 2008;19:43-7.

[61] Poreisz C, Boros K, Antal A, Paulus W. Safety aspects of transcranial direct current stimulation concerning healthy subjects and patients. Brain Res Bull 2007;72:208-14.

[62] Power H, Norton J, Porter C, Doyle Z, Hui I, Chan KM. Transcranial direct current stimulation of the primary motor cortex affects cortical drive to human musculature as assessed by intermuscular coherence. J Physiol. 2006; 577: 795-803

[63] Priori A, Mameli F, Cogiamanian F, Marceglia S, Tiriticco M, et al. Lie specific involvement of dorsolateral prefrontal cortex in deception. Cerebral Cortex 2008;18:451-5.

[64] Quartarone A, Morgante F, Bagnato S, Rizzo V, Sant'Angelo A, et al. Long lasting effects on transcranial direct current stimulation on motor imagery. NeuroReport 2004;15:1287-91.

[65] Ragert P, Vandermeeren Y, Camus M, Cohen LG. Improvement of spatial acuity by transcranial direct current stimulation. Clin Neurophysiol 2008;119:805-11.

[66] Rogalewski A, Breitenstein C, Nitsche MA, Paulus W, Knecht S. Transcranial direct current stimulation disrupts tactile perception. Eur J Neurosci 2004;20:313-6.

[67] Siebner HR, Lang N, Rizzo V, Nitsche MA, Paulus W, Lemon RN, Rothwell JC. Preconditioning of low-frequency repetitive transcranial magnetic stimulation with transcranial direct current stimulation: evidence for homeostatic plasticity in the human motor cortex. J Neurosci 2004;24(13):3379-85.

[68] Sparing R, Dafotakis M, Meister IG, Thirugnanasambandam N, Fink GR. Enhancing language performance with non-invasive brain stimulation – A transcranial direct current stimulation study in healthy humans. Neuropsychol 2008;46:261-8.

[69] Terney D, Bergmann I, Poreisz C, Chaieb L, Boros K, et al. Pergolide increases the efficacy of cathodal direct current stimulation to reduce the amplitude of laser evoked potentials in humans. J Pain Symptom Manage 2008;36:79-91.

[70] Vines BW, Cerruti C, Schlaug G. Dual-hemisphere tDCS facilitates greater improvements for healthy subjects' non-dominant hand compared to uni-hemisphere stimulation. BMC Neurosci 2008;9:103.

[71] Vines BW, Nair DG, Schlaug G. Contralateral and ipsilateral motor effects after transcranial direct current stimulation. NeuroReport 2006;17:671-4.

[72] Vines BW, Schnider NM, Schlaug G. Testing for causality with transcranial direct current stimulation: pitch memory and the left supramarginal gyrus. NeuroReport 2006;17:1047-50.

[73] Antal A, Lang N, Boros K, Nitsche M, Siebner HR, Paulus W. Homeostatic metaplasticity of the motor cortex is altered during headache free intervals in migraine with aura. Cerebral Cortex 2008; 18:2701-5.

[74] Boggio PS, Rigonatti SP, Riberio RB, Myczkowski ML, Nitsche MA, Pascual-Leone A, Fregni F. A randomized, double blind clinical trial on the efficacy of cortical direct current stimulation for the treatment of major depression. Int J Neuropsychopharmacol 2008;11:249-54.

[75] Boggio PS, Ferrucci R, Rigonatti SP, Covre P, Nitsche M, Pascual-Leone A, Fregni F. Effects of transcranial direct current stimulation on working memory in patients with Parkinson's disease. J Neurol Sci 2006;249:31-8.

[76] Boggio PS, Sultani N, Fectau S, Merabet L, Mecca T, Pascual-Leone A, Basaglia A, Fregni F. Prefrontal cortex modulation using transcranial DC stimulation reduces alcohol craving: A double blind, sham controlled study. Drug Alcohol Depend 2008;92:55-60.

[77] Boggio PS, Nunes A, Rigonatti SP, Nitsche MA, Pascual-Leone A, Fregni F. Repeated sessions of noninvasive brain DC stimulation is associated with motor function improvement in stroke patients. Restor Neurol Neurosci 2007;25(2):123-9.
[78] Chadaide Z, Arlt S, Antal A, Nitsche MA, Lang N, Paulus W. Transcranial direct current stimulation reveals inhibitory deficiency in migraine. Cephalalgia 2007;27:833-9.
[79] Ferrucci R, Mameli F, Guidi I, Mrakic-Sposta S, Vergari M, et al. Transcranial direct current stimulation improves recognition memory in Alzheimer disease. Neurology 2008;71:493-8.
[80] Fregni F, Orsati F, Pedrosa W, Fecteau S, Tome FAM, et al. Transcranial direct current stimulation of the prefrontal cortex modulates the desire for specific foods. Appetite 2008;51:34-41.
[81] Fregni F, Boggio PS, Nitsche MA, Marcolin MA, Rigonatti SP, Pascual-Leone A. Treatment of major depression with transcranial direct current stimulation. Bipolar Disord 2006;8:203-5.
[82] Fregni F, Boggio PS, Lima MC, Ferreira MJL, Wagner T, et al. A sham-controlled, phase II trial of transcranial direct current stimulation for the treatment of central pain in traumatic spinal cord injury. Pain 2006;122:197-209.
[83] Fregni F, Marcondes R, Boggio PS, Marcolin MA, Rigonatti SP, et al. Transient tinnitus suppression induced by repetitive transcranial magnetic stimulation and transcranial direct current stimulation. Eur J Neurol 2006;13:996-1001.
[84] Fregni F, Boggio PS, Mansur CG, Wagner T, Ferreira MJL, et al. Transcranial direct current stimulation of the unaffected hemisphere in stroke patients. NeuroReport 2005;16:1551-5.
[85] Fregni F, Boggio PS, Santos MC, Lima M, Vieira AL, et al. Noninvasive cortical stimulation with transcranial direct current stimulation in Parkinson's Disease. Movement Disord 2006;21:1693-1702.
[86] Fregni F, Gimenes R, Valle AC, Ferreira MJ, Rocha RR, et al. A randomized, sham-controlled, proof of principle study of transcranial direct current stimulation for the treatment of pain in fibromyalgia. Arthritis Rheum 2006;54(12):3988-98.
[87] Gandiga PC, Hummel FC, Cohen LG. Transcranial DC stimulation (tDCS): A tool for double blind sham controlled clinical studies in brain stimulation. Clin Neurophysiol 2006;117:845-50.
[88] Hummel FC, Voller B, Celnik P, Floel A, Giraux P, et al. Effects of brain polarization on reaction times and pinch force in chronic stroke. BMC Neurosci 2006;7:73.
[89] Hummel F, Celnik P, Giraux P, Floel A, Wu WH, et al. Effects of non-invasive cortical stimulation on skilled motor function in chronic stroke. Brain 2005;128:490-9.
[90] Monti A, Cogiamanian F, Marceglia S, Ferrucci R, Mameli F, et al. Improving naming after transcranial direct current stimulation in aphasia. J Neurol Neurosurg Psychiatry 2008;79:451-3.
[91] Quartarone A, Rizzo V, Bagnato S, Morgante F, Sant'Angelo A, et al. Homeostatic-like plasticity of the primary motor hand area is impaired in focal hand dystonia. Brain 2005;128:1943-50.
[92] Quartarone A, Lang N, Rizzo V, Bagnato S, Morgante F, et al. Motor cortex abnormalities in amyotrophic lateral sclerosis with transcranial direct current stimulation. Muscle Nerve 2007;35:620-4.
[93] Roizenblatt S, Fregni F, Gimenes R, Wetzel T, Rigonatti SP, et al. Site specific effects of transcranial direct current stimulation on sleep and pain in fibromyalgia: A randomized sham controlled study. Pain Pract 2007;7:297-306.
[94] Knotkova H, Homel P, Cruciani R. Cathodal tDCS over the somatosensory cortex relieved chronic neuropathic pain in a patient with complex regional pain syndrome (CRPS/RSD). J Pain Manage 2009, in press.

In: Pain Management Yearbook 2009
Editor: Joav Merrick

ISBN: 978-1-61209-666-7
©2012 Nova Science Publishers, Inc.

Chapter 30

THE POTENTIAL ROLE OF BRAIN STIMULATION IN THE MANAGEMENT OF POSTOPERATIVE PAIN

Jeffrey J Borckardt[*]*, PhD, Scott Reeves, MD and Mark S George, MD*

Department of Psychiatry and Behavioral Sciences, Department of Anesthesiology and Perioperative Medicine, Medical University of South Carolina, Charleston, South Carolina, United States of America

Abstract

There is limited evidence to date of the effectiveness of minimally-invasive brain stimulation in controlling post-operative pain. Two studies have provided preliminary evidence that transcranial magnetic stimulation (TMS) can significantly reduce post-operative pain, and no studies have been published on the effects of transcranial direct current stimulation (tDCS) on postoperative pain. The evidence supporting the role of brain stimulation in producing general anesthetic effects is also limited but there is a possibility that appropriately targeted electrical stimulation might have a role in the future if the technology permits such stimulation in a non-invasive manner. The present article provides a brief overview of the available evidence supporting the role of minimally invasive brain stimulation technology in perioperative medicine. More studies and well-controlled trials are needed to establish a clear role for minimally-invasive brain stimulation technologies in the perioperative arena.

Keywords: Transcranial magnetic stimulation, pain, direct current stimulation, postoperative, perioperative.

---

[*] **Correspondence:** Jeffrey J. Borckardt, PhD, Assistant Professor, Department of Psychiatry and Behavioral Sciences, 4 South, Institute of Psychiatry, 67 President Street, POBox 250861, Charlesston, SC 29425, United States. E-mail: borckard@ musc.edu

Introduction

To date, little is known about the potential role of brain stimulation in perioperative pain management. However, based on some very preliminary research, it is becoming possible to imagine some possibilities for the application of technologies such as transcranial magnetic stimulation (TMS) and/or transcranial direct current stimulation (tDCS) to manage acute post-operative pain, and perhaps even to produce general anesthesia in patients. This paper provides a brief review of the available evidence to date on the potential effectiveness of minimally invasive brain stimulation technologies on perioperative pain. First, we discuss the potential role of TMS and tDCS in post-operative pain management, and then we consider the possibility of brain stimulation in general anesthesia applications.

Brain stimulation and postoperative pain management

There is accumulating evidence that TMS can provide significant analgesic effects in patients with neuropathic pain of various etiologies (1-3), some non-neuropathic pain syndromes (4) and in healthy adults (5-8) using laboratory evocative pain procedures. Despite some theoretical speculation that TMS might be capable of engendering more permanent cortical (and perhaps subcortical) reorganization in patients with chronic central pain, most of the evidence to date suggests short-lived analgesic effects (9). Thus, in order to provide clinically useful and meaningful results in patients with chronic pain, TMS may have to be delivered repeatedly over days or weeks, and it may be that regular "booster" sessions are necessary to produce long-term analgesic effects in this population.

Several surgical procedures result in postoperative pain that can last hours to days, but then remits and never returns. After surgery, management of this acute pain becomes a focus of good post-operative clinical care and is typically accomplished via the use of opioid analgesic medications. While the use of systemic opioid analgesics is largely an appropriate pain-management strategy given the current analgesic options available to clinicians, there are some limitations associated with their ubiquitous use. Because opioid analgesics are usually delivered intravenously or orally in the postoperative environment (and therefore the effects are systemic instead of localized to the painful area), patients are subject to some undesirable side-effects including nausea, constipation, drowsiness, lightheadedness, dysphoria, confusion, urinary retention, respiratory depression, and pruritus (10). Some of these effects can be more or less problematic depending upon the nature of the surgical procedure. For example, patients undergoing gastric-bypass surgery for weight loss have substantially increased likelihood of apnea and cardiac problems that can be exacerbated by high doses of opioid medication (11). While the risks of addiction following opioid use for postoperative pain management are quite low, this remains a concern for many patients and physicians.

Given the findings that a single-session (or a few sessions) of TMS appears capable of producing somewhat reliable short-term analgesic effects, and given some of the limitations associated with current post-operative pain management techniques, TMS may be well-suited for clinical situations in which acute pain is the primary target.

In 2006, Borckardt and colleagues conducted the first pilot study investigating the effects of a single 20-minute session of prefrontal TMS on postoperative pain (11). Twenty patients undergoing gastric-bypass surgery for weight loss received 20-minutes of either real or sham TMS (randomly determined) immediately following surgery in this single-blind trial. Patient-controlled analgesia (PCA; morphine or equivalent) use was tracked over the remainder of each patient's inpatient hospital stay as well as visual-analogue scale (VAS) mood and pain ratings. Patients that received real TMS used 40% less PCA morphine than patients that received sham TMS at the time of discharge from the hospital. Further, no differences were observed between groups with respect to mood ratings at any point during the study suggesting that the observed effects were not due to effects of TMS on mood alone.

In 2008, Borckardt and colleagues published a replication trial in which another 20 patients were studied using the same methods as the pilot (12). In this replication trial, a 35% reduction in PCA morphine was observed in the real TMS group compared to sham. When the data from both preliminary trials were combined, a 36% reduction in PCA morphine was found to be associated with real TMS compared to sham. Additionally, VAS pain ratings were found to be significantly lower among patients receiving real TMS compared to sham. Specifically, patients that received real TMS had significantly lower VAS ratings for "pain on average" and "pain at its worst" than those receiving sham, and better "mood at its worst" ratings as well.

An interesting observation regarding this finding is that this difference in pain ratings was found despite patients in the real-TMS group using substantially less morphine. It might be expected to find a difference in either morphine use or VAS ratings as these two factors should be inter-related. The fact that patients receiving real TMS used less morphine and had lower VAS ratings raises interesting questions about possible mechanisms of TMS action. For example, these findings support the possibility that prefrontal TMS increases the efficiency of both endogenous and exogenous opioids thereby resulting in a lower morphine requirement to produce analgesic effects. Additionally, when one considers the improved "mood at its worst" ratings among patients receiving real TMS, it seems possible that prefrontal TMS may be associated with inhibition of cortical processes associated with pain catastrophizing thereby reducing pain experience and the perceived need for morphine to provide pain control. However, more work is needed to further establish the analgesic effects of TMS in the postoperative setting and to clarify mechanisms.

These studies are the only published post-operative TMS trials to date and the preliminary findings are promising. Unfortunately, these trials were single-blind so it is impossible to rule-out potential confounding influences of the investigators on patient responses. Additionally, the sham TMS procedures, while consistent with the standard methodology employed in the field, have limits too. Real TMS is capable of producing scalp discomfort in patients, whereas sham TMS does not. More rigorous studies are needed that employ double-blind methodology and more sophisticated TMS sham procedures before the field can start to feel confident that there is a place for TMS in post-operative pain management.

While there is some preliminary evidence supporting the effectiveness of TMS in managing postoperative pain, little attention has been paid to the potential role of transcranial direct current stimulation (tDCS) in perioperative medicine. There is accumulating evidence that tDCS can produce short-term analgesic effects in laboratory as well as clinical studies (13-15). However, there are no published studies investigating the effects of tDCS on postoperative pain. This is unfortunate given that there are some advantages to using tDCS compared to TMS in the postoperative setting. First, tDCS delivery does not require that a motor threshold assessment be conducted (as is necessary for TMS delivery) before starting treatment. Motor threshold assessment can be challenging in the postoperative settings as the patients are sometimes disoriented, drowsy, in a lot of pain, and have little tolerance for the complicated methods involved in motor threshold assessment. Second, tDCS appears to be less painful and more tolerable to patients. Third, tDCS does not produce magnetic fields that can interfere with physiology measurement equipment like TMS, and fourth tDCS is silent whereas TMS makes noise that can be heard by most other patients in the post-anesthesia care unit. However, studies of the effects of tDCS in the management postoperative pain are needed to determine whether it may have a place in the perioperative setting.

General anesthesia and brain stimulation

The discovery of general anesthesia, over 150 years ago revolutionized medicine. The ability to render a patient unconscious made modern surgery possible and general anesthetics have become both indispensable as well as one of the most widely used class of drugs (16). The mechanisms through which general anesthetics cause reversible loss of consciousness are unclear, however a small number of important molecular targets have emerged, and drug action at the molecular level is becoming clearer. Recent work suggests that the thalamus and the neuronal networks that regulate its activity are the key to understanding how anaesthetics cause loss of consciousness (16).

Little attention has been paid to the potential role of electrical stimulation of the brain to produce general anesthetic effects, although it may be possible to use focused electrical stimulation to produce controlled, reversible unconsciousness. Reynolds (17) first reported producing general anesthetic effects in rats using only brain stimulation in 1969. Chronic monopolar electrodes were implanted in the region of the midbrain central gray in eight rats. Continuous 60Hz sine-wave stimulation resulted in an electrical analgesia defined by the elimination of responses to aversive stimulation while general motor responsiveness was retained. Exploratory laparotomy was carried-out during continuous brain stimulation without the use of chemical anesthetics. Following surgery, brain stimulation was terminated, and responses to aversive stimuli returned. Electrodes effective in inducing electrical analgesia at the lowest currents were located at the dorsolateral perimeter of the midbrain. It was concluded that focal brain stimulation in this region can induce analgesia.

TMS over the motor cortex has been shown to decrease cortical excitability and even reduce thalamic activity (18), however it is unclear whether this technology will ever be capable of causing continuous, reversible loss of consciousness like general anesthetics. As technologies like TMS and tDCS continue to develop, it is conceivable that the key cortical and/or sub-cortical targets could be identified and stimulated in a manner that replicates the effects of chemically-induced general anesthesia. This notion is likely far from realization, but as the field of minimally-invasive brain stimulation continues to explode, realization of this possibility is probably closer than ever before.

Conclusions

To date, there is limited evidence of the effectiveness of minimally-invasive brain stimulation in controlling post-operative pain. Two studies found that TMS over the prefrontal cortex significantly reduce post-operative pain, and no studies have been published on the effects of tDCS on postoperative pain. The evidence supporting the role of brain stimulation in general anesthesia is also limited but there is a possibility that appropriately targeted electrical stimulation could produce general anesthetic effects if the technology permits such stimulation in a non-invasive manner. More pilot studies and well-controlled trials are needed to investigate and perhaps establish a clear role for minimally-invasive brain stimulation technologies in the perioperative arena.

Acknowledgments

Dr. Borckardt's work is funded in part by the following NINDS: 5K23NS050485-03, NINR: 1R21NR010635-01, NIDA: 1R21DA026085-01, The Robert Wood Johnson Foundation, Neuropace Inc, and Cyberonics Inc. Dr. George receives research funding from the National Institute for Mental Health at NIH, Jazz Pharmaceuticals, GlaxoSmithKline, and Cyberonics Inc. He is a consultant for Argolyn Pharmaceuticals, Abbott, Neuropace, Dantec, and Philips, however he has no equity ownership in any device or pharmaceutical company.

References

[1] Canavero S, Bonicalzi V, Dotta M, et al. Transcranial magnetic cortical stimulation relieves central pain. Stereo Funct Neurosurg 2002;78(3-4):192-6.
[2] Khedr EM, Kotb H, Kamel NF, Ahmed MA, Sadek R, Rothwell JC. Longlasting antalgic effects of daily sessions of repetitive transcranial magnetic stimulation in central and peripheral neuropathic pain. J Neurol Neurosurg Psychiatry 2005;76:833-8.
[3] Pleger B, Janssen F, Schwenkreis P et al. Repetitive transcranial magnetic stimulation of the motor cortex attenuates pain perception in complex regional pain syndrome type I. Neurosci Letters 2004;356: 87-90.
[4] Sampson SM, et al. (2006) Slow-frequency rTMS reduces fibromyalgia pain. Pain Med 2006;7:115-8.
[5] Kanda M, Tatsuya M, Oga T, et al. Transcranial magnetic stimulation of the sensorimotor and medial frontal cortex modifies human pain perception. Clin Neurophysiol 2003;114:860-6.
[6] Tamura Y, Okabe S, Ohnishi T, et al. Effects of 1-Hz repetitive transcranial magnetic stimulation on acute pain induced by capsaicin. Pain 2004;107:107-15.
[7] Borckardt JJ, Smith AR, Reeves ST, Weinstein M, Kozel FA, et al. Fifteen Minutes of Left Prefrontal Repetitive Transcranial Magnetic Stimulation Acutely Increases Thermal Pain Thresholds in Healthy Adults. Pain Res Manage 2007;12(4):287-90.
[8] Summers J, Johnson S, Pridemore S, Oberoi G. Changes to cold detection and pain thresholds following low and high frequency transcranial magnetic stimulation of the motor cortex. Neurosci Letters 2004;368:197-200.
[9] Lefaucheur JP. Transcranial magnetic stimulation in the management of pain. Suppl Clin Neurophysiol 2004;57:737-48.

[10] Meylan N, Elia N, Lysakowski C, Tramèr MR. Benefit and risk of intrathecal morphine without local anaesthetic in patients undergoing major surgery: meta-analysis of randomized trials. Br J Anaesth 2009; 102(2):156-67.

[11] Borckardt JJ, Weinstein M, Reeves ST, Kozel FA, Nahas Z, et al. Post-operative left prefrontal repetitive transcranial magnetic stimulation reduces patient-controlled analgesia use. Anesthesiology 2006;105(3):1-6.

[12] Borckardt JJ, Reeves ST, Weinstein M, Smith AR, Shelley N, et al. Significant analgesic effects of one session of postoperative left prefrontal cortex repetitive transcranial magnetic stimulation: A replication study. Brain Stimulat 2008;1(2):122-7.

[13] Been G, Ngo TT, Miller SM, Fitzgerald PB. The use of tDCS and CVS as methods of non-invasive brain stimulation. Brain Res Rev 2007;56(2):346-61.

[14] Fregni F, Pascual-Leone A. Technology insight: noninvasive brain stimulation in neurology-perspectives on the therapeutic potential of rTMS and tDCS. Nat Clin Pract Neurol 2007;3(7):383-93.

[15] Fregni F, Freedman S, Pascual-Leone A. Recent advances in the treatment of chronic pain with non-invasive brain stimulation techniques. Lancet Neurol 2007;6(2):188-91.

[16] Franks NP. General anaesthesia: from molecular targets to neuronal pathways of sleep and arousal. Nat Rev Neurosci 2008; 9(5):370-86.

[17] Reynolds DV. Surgery in the rat during electrical analgesia induced by focal brain stimulation. Science 1969;164(878):444-5.

[18] Huang YZ, Rothwell JC, Lu CS, Wang J, Weng YH, et al. The effect of continuous theta burst stimulation over premotor cortex on circuits in primary motor cortex and spinal cord. Clin Neurophysiol 2009, in press.

Chapter 31

DEEP BRAIN STIMULATION FOR CHRONIC PAIN

Morten L Kringelbach, DPhil[*,1,2,3], *Erlick AC Pereira, MBChB*[4], *Alexander L Green, FRCS (SN)*[4], *Sarah LF Owen, DPhil*[2] *and Tipu Z Aziz, D Med Sci*[2,3,4]

[1]University of Oxford, Department of Psychiatry, Warneford Hospital, Oxford, United Kingdom, [2]University of Oxford, Department of Physiology, Anatomy and Genetics, Oxford, United Kingdom, [3]University of Aarhus, Centre for Functionally Integrative Neuroscience (CFIN), Aarhus, Denmark and [4]Nuffield Department of Surgery, John Radcliffe Hospital, Oxford, United Kingdom

Abstract

As a clinical intervention, deep brain stimulation (DBS) has provided remarkable therapeutic benefits for otherwise treatment-resistant movement and affective disorders including chronic pain. In this review, we concentrate on the experience of using DBS to treat chronic pain in Oxford. We provide a brief historical background as well as details of our methods for patient selection, surgical techniques and assessment. While the precise mechanisms of action for DBS remain uncertain, we describe how DBS can help for treatment-resistant chronic pain and have great potential to advance our general understanding of the human brain. In particular, we show how DBS can be used in conjunction with methods such as local field potentials and magnetoencephalography to map the underlying mechanisms of normal and abnormal oscillatory synchronization in the brain related to the pleasure of pain relief.

Keywords: Chronic pain, neuroimaging, magnetoencephalography, local field potentials, obsessive compulsive disorder, functional neurosurgery, amputation, neuropathic pain, thalamus, cingulate, periaqueductal gray, pleasure.

---

[*] **Correspondence:** Professor Morten L Kringelbach, University of Oxford, Department of Psychiatry, Warneford Hospital, Oxford OX3 7JX, United Kingdom. E-mail: Morten.Kringelbach@psych.ox.ac.uk

Introduction

Deep brain stimulation (DBS) has become the basis of important successful therapies for treating otherwise treatment-resistant movement and affective disorders such as Parkinson's disease, tremor, dystonia and chronic pain (1). Despite the long history of DBS, its underlying principles and mechanisms are still not clear but what is clear is that DBS directly changes brain activity in a controlled manner, the effects are reversible (unlike those of lesioning techniques) and that DBS is one of only a few neurosurgical methods that allows blinded studies (2).

Modulation of brain activity by way of direct electrical stimulation of the brain has been in use at least since 1870, when Fritsch and Hirtzig showed that stimulation of the motor cortex of the dog can elicit limb movement (3). Direct neuromodulation and recordings have since proved to be very useful for improving human neurosurgical procedures as first shown in 1884 by Horsley (4).

It is over fifty years since the initial studies used DBS in the hypothalamus to treat chronic pain (5). Around the same time ablative surgery of thalamic nuclei (ventral posterior lateral and medial, VPL/VPM) and adjacent structures was used for the alleviation of pain (6-9). This evidence led Hosobuchi to try stimulation of the VPM for treating anaesthesia dolorosa (10). Similarly, other groups were successfully experimenting with DBS of the thalamus (11-14). Some groups also reported some success with using DBS in the internal capsule (15-17).

Other DBS targets for chronic pain were identified over time, which included the periventricular and periaqueductal gray (PVG/PAG) regions. Reynolds and colleagues discovered that they could use PAG stimulation to induce analgesia during surgery in awake rodents (18,19). This was then translated into using DBS of the PVG/PAG in human patients (20-23).

Other targets such as the more medial thalamic nuclei including the centromedian-parafascicular complex came from investigations into inadvertent localisation errors and current spread from existing targets (24-27).

This rapid progress in electrical stimulation treatments for chronic pain and for movement disorders such as Parkinson's Disease led the United States Food and Drug Administration (FDA) to try to evaluate their merits. A symposium was organised (28), which found that DBS treatments for pain were both safe and effective (29, 30). The United States Medical Device Amendments of 1976 and an additional ruling in 1989 meant that DBS manufacturers were subsequently required to conduct clinical trials to demonstrate safety and efficacy.

Two multi-centre trials for DBS of chronic pain were conducted by Medtronic. The first trial in 1976 had 196 patients (using the Medtronic Model 3380 electrode) and a second trial in 1990 had 50 patients (using Model 3387) (31). The two trials were far from ideal as they consisted of prospective case series from various neurosurgical centres, which were not randomised or case controlled, and in addition had poor enrolment and high attrition. There were inconsistencies across centres in the selection of number of DBS targets, numbers of electrodes used per patient and stimulation parameters chosen. Heterogeneous case mixes with underspecified patient selection criteria, and subjective and unblinded assessment of patient outcomes added to the confusion.

The second trial tried to improve the data by limiting deep brain sites stimulated to two per patient and using visual analogue scores (VAS) to rate pain intensity for outcome assessment, but was on a much smaller scale with a mean of five and median of three patients treated per centre.

The study criteria for efficacy was that at least half of patients should report at least 50% pain relief one year after surgery. This was not met by either trial and FDA approval for analgesic DBS was therefore not sought by the device manufacturer (31).

As a consequence, during the last decade most of the research in DBS for chronic pain has gone on outside the US with only five centres outside the US having produced case series of more than six patients: (32-40).

These studies have in general been much better controlled and shown significant improvements for patients with primarily pain after amputation and stroke, and head pain including anaesthesia dolorosa, as documented below.

In addition to chronic pain states, there are other affective disorders with pain components that have been successfully treated with DBS. Patients with cluster headache have been successfully treated with DBS in the hypothalamus (41-43). Depression is another condition, where the targets have included thalamus (44, 45) and the subgenual cingulate cortex (46). Another recent study of DBS in the nucleus accumbens found a significant reduction in anhedonia in three patients with treatment-resistant depression (47). DBS for obsessive compulsive disorder have targeted the anterior internal capsule (48). DBS of the thalamus (49) and GPi (50) have been reported effective in treating Tourette syndrome.

It should, however, be noted that owing to the lack of good animal models of depression, obsessive compulsive disorder and Tourette syndrome, the mechanisms underlying these interventions are much more speculative than for example the targets used in Parkinson's disease. We have previously argued that the MPTP model may also be useful (1), since many of the involved brain structures are also implicated in affective disorders as e.g. demonstrated by how severe depression can be reversibly induced by DBS for Parkinson's disease (51, 52). The ethical implications of DBS for the treatment of affective disorders should be carefully considered to avoid comparisons to the psychosurgery of last century – but it should be remembered that DBS is, in principle, reversible.

Mechanics of DBS surgery

The specific methods used for DBS vary between neurosurgical teams. Here we present the methods adopted in Professor Tipu Aziz' neurosurgical centre in Oxford and focus specifically on the selection and surgical procedures used for DBS for pain relief (see figure 1).

Patient selection

There are two main challenges to chronic pain patient selection for DBS, which is to determine that 1) the patient's pain is neuropathic and neither factitious nor psychogenic, and 2) this neuropathic pain is likely to be successfully treatable with DBS.

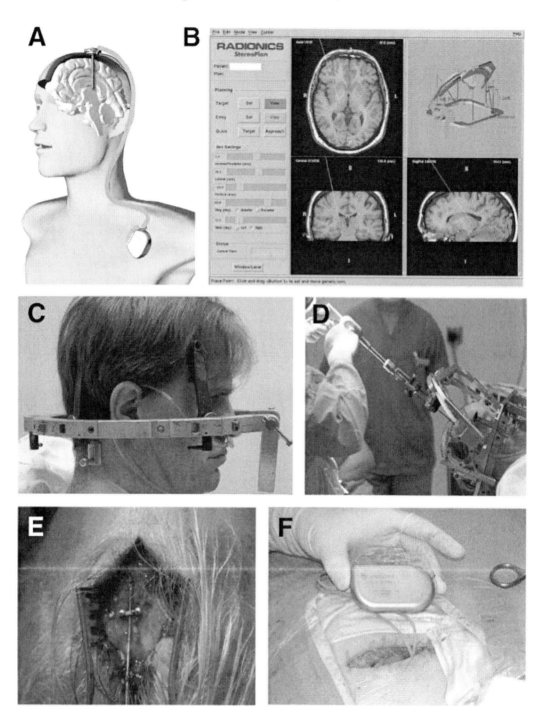

Figure 1. The neurosurgical procedures involved in DBS. A) Schematic of the principles of DBS. B) Illustration of the process of the neurosurgical pre-planning. C) Application of the Cosman-Roberts-Wells stereotactic head frame on the patient. Note that the base ring is parallel to the orbitomeatal line. D) The precise positioning of the electrode through perforating the calvarium with a twist drill. E) Securing the electrode to the skull with a titanium miniplate and screws. F) Placement of the implantable pulse generator in a subcutaneous pectoral pouch.

Assessment by a multi-disciplinary team consisting as a minimum of a pain specialist, neuropsychologist and neurosurgeon is essential to the patient selection process. Comprehensive neuropsychological evaluation forms best practice in patient selection for DBS to exclude psychoses, addiction and medically refractory psychiatric disorders and ensure minimal cognitive impairment (53-56).

Quantitative assessment of the pain and health related quality of life should be a requirement of the pre-operative patient selection process. Our preference is to use both VAS (scale 1-10) to rate pain intensity and the McGill pain questionnaire (MPQ) for pain evaluation (57, 58), the latter giving additional qualitative information. Quality of life is assessed using the Short Form 36 (SF-36) and VAS part of the Euroqol five-dimensional assessment tool (EQ-5D), (59-61). The patient records their VAS twice daily in a pain diary over a period of 12 days. The 24 VAS scores are reviewed to ensure consistency. The EQ-5D, SF-36 and MPQ are administered by the pain specialist pre-operatively. The MPQ is repeated on a separate occasion independently by the neuropsychologist and scored using the ranked pain rating index. Our experience is that certain items of the MPQ can predict a good response to DBS. In particular, over 80% of our patients who describe 'burning' pain have found benefit from DBS, regardless of whether VPL/VPM, PVG/PAG or both are stimulated.

The specific aetiology of the chronic pain is less important than its symptom history which may involve hyperalgesia, allodynia and hyperpathia. The pain must have a definable organic origin with the patient refractory to or poorly tolerant of pharmacological treatments. Surgical treatments may have been attempted, for example peripheral neuroablative or decompressive procedures for trigeminal neuralgia, however we do not consider failure of other neurostimulatory therapies a prerequisite for DBS.

Our preference is to trial DBS rather than SCS or MCS in carefully selected patients wherever the aetiologies of chronic pain are consistent with neuronal reorganisation at multiple levels of the central neuromatrix. Our experience of DBS for pain after limb or plexar injury includes ten successfully implanted patients to date (38, 40) has led us to consider DBS rather than SCS as first-line treatment for complex regional pain syndromes, in other words for plexar injuries and stump pain after amputation as well as phantom limb pain.

Overall, optimal patient selection includes expert opinion after multi-disciplinary assessment demonstrating quantitatively severe pain refractory to medication for at least one year with significantly impaired quality of life and likely neuropathic aetiology without predominantly spinal involvement. We do not advocate opiate or naloxone administration to determine suitability for DBS. Medical contraindications to DBS include uncorrectable coagulopathy obviating neurosurgery and ventriculomegaly sufficient to preclude direct electrode passage to the surgical target.

Surgical procedures

A T1-weighted MRI scan of each patient's brain is performed several weeks before surgery. For surgery, a Cosman-Roberts-Wells base ring is applied to the patients' head under local anesthesia. A stereotactic computed tomography (CT) scan is then performed and using the Radionics Image Fusion® and Stereoplan® (Integra Radionics, Burlington, Mass) program the coordinates for the PVG and ventro-posterior lateral thalamus (VPL) are calculated. A double oblique trajectory is used with an entry point just anterior to the coronal suture and laterality of approach dictated by ventricular width. The PVG/PAG is proximally located 2–3 mm lateral to the wall of the third ventricle and 2 mm anterior to the level of the posterior commissure and distally the deepest electrode lay in the superior colliculus. The VPL is located 8-14 mm lateral and 5–8 mm posterior to the mid-commissural point, at the depth of the anterior/posterior commissure plane. After washing the patient's scalp with alcoholic chlorhexidine, a parasaggital posterior frontal scalp incision 3.0 cm from the midline is made contralateral to the side of pain.

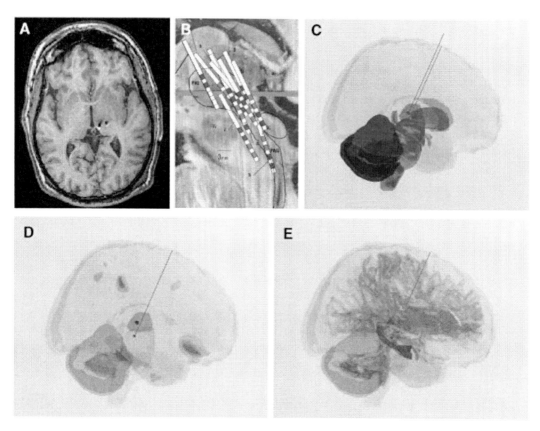

Figure 2. DBS for chronic pain. A) Axial MRI slice showing the implantation of electrodes in PVG/PAG and thalamus in a patient. B) Schematic illustration of the vertical placement of electrodes in the PVG/PAG in a series of chronic pain patients. C) Three-dimensional rendering of human brain showing the placement of the two electrodes in the PVG/PAG and thalamus, as well as some of the important subcortical structures. D) Three-dimensional rendering showing the whole-brain DBS induced activity from stimulation in the PVG/PAG. E) The connectivity of the PVG/PAG measured with diffusion tensor imaging.

The VPL is usually implanted with a Medtronic 3387 (Medtronic, Minneapolis, Minn) electrode with stimulation induced parasthesia in the area of pain. The PVG is also implanted with a Medtronic 3387 electrode with stimulation induced relief of pain or a sensation of warmth in the area of pain. The deepest electrode is noted to be in a satisfactory position if eye bobbing was induced at intensity of stimulation at least twice that required for sensory effects. The electrodes are fixed to the skull with a miniplate prior to externalization. In most patients the electrodes are externalized for a week of trial stimulation.

Pain is assessed before surgery and during stimulation by a self-rated visual analog scale. If the patients are satisfied with the degree of pain relief, full implantation of a pulse generator is performed in the following week under general anesthesia.

Other surgical centres around the world use slightly different procedures with one of the main differences being the use of microelectrode recordings to improve the accuracy of targeting in stereotactic placement. Some of the benefits of this procedure include the potential for differentiation of gray and white matter locations, localization of white matter tracts with particular responses to stimulation, and real-time correction for intraoperative shifts in implantation sites. This procedure is, however, somewhat controversial and perhaps superfluous since studies have shown a good correspondence between the MRI-defined target and the proposed electrophysiology-derived map (62). Furthermore, a review comparing modern techniques with the older unguided lesioning procedures of the 1960s argued that the modern technique of multiple microelectrode passes for localization results in no significant difference in outcome and more intracranial haemorrhages (63).

Safety and complications

The safety of DBS and the procedure involved has been demonstrated in many world-wide trials and in the long-term follow-up in DBS for the treatment of chronic pain (64). The long-term efficacy of DBS depends on the generators where most will last around 3-5 years depending on the current demands of the pulse protocol; although in the case of dystonia this can be less than one year. Rechargeable pulse generators are available for spinal cord generators and are being trialled for DBS.

Stereotactic neurosurgical procedures always carry a significant risk and can lead to intracranial bleeding, usually in around 2.0-2.5% of DBS implants (65, 66). Other potential complications include hardware-related complications such as dislocation, lead fracture, and infection (6%). The infection rate is equal to that of other surgical procedures but may necessitate explantation of the stimulator (67). Stimulation-induced side effects (3%) are also quite common effects, such as paresthesia, dyskinesia, tonic muscle contractions and gait ataxia, as well as the less common effects like aggression (68), mirthful laughter (69), penile erection (70), depression (51) and mania (71). These side-effects are closely related to the location of lead/contact used for stimulation.

The principles of DBS

The similar therapeutic outcomes of DBS and neurosurgical lesions have been used for trying to understand the mechanisms of DBS. This in turn raises the deceptively simple general question of whether DBS inhibits or excites neurons, which we will address in the following.

Fundamentally, DBS of the normal and diseased brain must fundamentally depend on the stimulation parameters, the properties of the neural tissue and their interaction. In other words, these parameters include 1) the stimulation parameters including amplitude and temporal characteristics, 2) the physiological properties of the brain tissue which may change with disease state, and 3) the interactions between the electrode and the surrounding tissue arising from the specific geometric configurations.

The stimulation parameters of DBS of therapeutic value have been derived primarily by trial and error by using the near immediate effects on e.g. tremor, rigidity, paresthesia, bradykinesia, and chronic pain in patients on the operating table (72). The exact DBS parameters vary with treatment and targeted brain region but are usually between 1-9 volts stimulus amplitude; 60-240 μseconds stimulus pulse duration; monopolar cathodic; and either low (5-50 Hz) or high (130-180Hz) stimulus frequencies (73). Currently a charge-density limit of 30 μC/cm2 is used as a safety factor based on post-mortem studies of tissue damage (73). Most commercially available stimulators will allow for these parameters to be changed and fine-tuned over time but based solely on the patient's behavioural state. The technology is open-loop continuous stimulation which can not be adjusted real-time to the continuous changes in brain state of the individual patient. In some ways, the current technology is like that of cardiac pacing technologies of twenty years ago, and the field is wide open for further innovation.

The physiological properties of normal and diseased brain tissue have variable electrical properties depending on the types of neurons and supporting glial cells which utilize different types of ion channels with variable voltage-sensitive properties. The most excitable neural elements are the myelinated axons (74, 75). The effect of DBS on the various neural elements depends on the nonlinear relationship between stimulus duration (pulse width) and amplitude (voltage or current) necessary to stimulate the neural element (74). The minimal current necessary to stimulate a neural element with a long stimulus duration is called rheobase, which is the amplitude threshold. The chronaxie time measurement is the minimum interval of time required to excite a neural element using half the intensity that elicits a threshold response. The chronaxie of myelinated axons is around 30-200 μsecs, while the chronaxies of cell bodies and dendrites are substantially larger at around 1-10 msec (76). This means that with usual DBS parameters, the postsynaptic responses are the result of activity from efferent axons rather than from cell bodies (77).

The geometrical configuration of neural elements in relation to the electrode is important for determining the effects of stimulation on local and global elements. For example, the orientation of the axons and the cell body is an important determinant of neural responsiveness (74). The distance of the neural elements from the electrode is also an important factor with both the rheobase and chronaxie rising in proportion to distance, such that the responsiveness of more distal elements is increasingly unlikely (76). The stimulation volume is not a fixed cylinder around the stimulation electrode but varies with electrode position and surrounding neural tissue. Usual clinical parameters lead to the stimulation of a large volume of neural tissue (75, 78). For example, modelling the excitability effects for STN stimulation using realistic white-matter pathways has shown that at 3V the stimulation spreads outside the STN proper and the pattern of excitation is consistent with known stimulation side-effects (78). Finally, currents from monopolar cathodes of more than eight times threshold may block action potentials in axons. This leads to the intriguing possibility that the effective stimulation from an electrode blocks activity in nearby elements and give rise to sub-threshold activity in distal elements, leaving the intermediate neural elements to be the most likely to receive the effects of stimulation and pass on to mono- and poly-synaptic connected brain structures.

The relative contribution of these parameters in determining the underlying mechanisms of DBS on local and whole-brain activity can be assessed experimentally in humans and other animals through direct neural recordings (79-83), neurochemistry (84, 85) and functional neuroimaging methods (86-88). In addition, computational modelling can be used to test and predict the effects of DBS on simulated neural elements (75, 78).

Functional neuroimaging

Unlike neurophysiological studies, functional neuroimaging methods allow for the study of the whole-brain activity elicited by DBS. The most widespread of these neuroimaging methods are positron emission tomography (PET) and functional magnetic resonance (fMRI), which can measure indirect changes of neural activity such as blood flow, blood oxygenation and glucose consumption. Presently it is not entirely clear how well these indirect measurements correlate with various aspects of neural activity but some progress has been made under normal physiological conditions (89, 90). This means that these methods entail a number of assumptions which may or may not prove to be important for interpreting the subsequent results.

In addition, fMRI studies clearly pose a large degree of risk to DBS patients since the large magnitude of the magnetic fields will interfere with active pulse generators and DBS electrodes. One study showed that extreme caution must be exercised when studying DBS with fMRI since strong heating, high induced voltage, and even sparking at defects in the connecting cable have been observed (91). It has also been shown that fMRI using the blood-oxygen level dependent (BOLD) signal as a measurement may be problematic, since near-infrared spectroscopy showed considerable variations in blood oxygenation in frontal cortex following GPi and thalamic stimulation (92). Despite these important caveats, a case report has been published using fMRI to study STN stimulation in a patient with Parkinson's disease. The results showed increases in the BOLD signal in primary motor areas and decreases in supplementary motor areas during STN stimulation (93). It should be noted that safety guidelines and procedures have since been issued by DBS manufacturers.

Similarly, PET is not without health risks due to the ionized radiation, but has been used for measuring the effects of DBS. It should be noted, however, that the long acquisition times (on the scale of minutes) make the ensuing brain changes difficult to interpret, and investigators have to carefully address the potential movement artefacts when studying movement disorders.

Using PET to study DBS for affective disorders is less challenging in terms of potential movement artefacts. One PET study investigated the effects of hypothalamic stimulation for cluster headache in ten patients (94) and found that hypothalamic stimulation modulated the pain processing network. Another PET study used stimulation of subgenual cingulate cortex for treatment-resistant depression in seven patients showed marked reduction in mood symptoms in four patients (46). The results are harder to interpret given the small numbers of patients and the paucity of knowledge about the brain structures involved in depression, but suggest that the mode of functioning of DBS would appear one of modulating an existing network of interacting brain regions.

Single-photon emission computed tomography (SPECT) is another invasive neuroimaging technique which has been used to measure regional cerebral blood flow changes following DBS for chronic pain. In one study DBS for intractable neuropathic pain were assessed in three patients using SPECT (95). Pain relief was achieved in all patients with one patient had having electrodes in the VPL, another with electrode in the PVG, and one patient had electrodes in both targets. DBS consistently increased perfusion in the posterior subcortical region between VPL and PVG, regardless of the site of stimulation. Furthermore, thalamic and dual target DBS increased thalamic perfusion, yet PVG DBS decreased perfusion in the PVG-containing midbrain region and thalamus. Dual target stimulation decreased perfusion in the anterior cingulate and insular cortices.

In contrast to PET, SPECT and fMRI, magnetoencephalography (MEG) is non-invasive and almost without risks for use in patients, and can provide novel spatiotemporal information on the underlying whole-brain activity with the current density of MEG sensors affording sensitivity such that the spatial resolution is comparable to fMRI (typically around 5 mm3) but with much better temporal resolution (in milliseconds) (96).

The first MEG study of DBS was carried out in a patient with low-frequency PVG/PAG stimulation for severe phantom limb pain (88, 97). When the stimulator was turned off the patient reported significant increases in subjective pain. Corresponding significant changes in the elicited power of neural activity were found in a wide-spread network including the mid-anterior orbitofrontal and subgenual cingulate cortices; these areas are known to be involved in pain relief (98). Similarly, MEG of high-frequency hypothalamic stimulation for cluster headache showed a similar pattern of changes in neural activity in a wide-spread cortical and sub-cortical network including the orbitofrontal cortex (99). Due to its non-invasive nature and high spatial and temporal resolution MEG holds great promise in elucidating the underlying whole-brain neural mechanisms of DBS by for example measuring oscillatory communication between brain regions (100).

Synthesis of mechanisms

The experimental evidence collected so far allows for some conclusions to be drawn about the neural and systems level mechanisms of action of DBS. The effects of DBS do vary with the stimulation parameters (including frequency, amplitude, pulse width and duration); with the intrinsic physiological properties; and with the interactions between the electrode and the geometric configuration of the surrounding neural tissue and specific anatomy of the targeted region. DBS affects multiple neural elements including foremost myelinated axons and to a lesser degree cell bodies.

Overall, the weight of the evidence so far suggests that the most likely mode of action for DBS is through stimulation-induced modulation of brain activity (1, 2, 101-103), rather than competing hypotheses such as synaptic inhibition (81), depolarization blockade (104) or synaptic depression (105).

Findings using DBS for chronic pain

To date over 1300 cases of DBS for chronic pain have been reported (33, 35, 38, 106-108). This compares to the nearly 4000 patients who have been implanted with spinal cord stimulators (SCS) (109, 110) and the nearly 400 patients with motor cortex stimulators (MCS) (111, 112).

Over the last decade, over 65 patients (70% men, mean age 51 years old) have been treated with DBS for chronic pain in Oxford with DBS of thalamus and/or PVG/PAG. We have published detailed results for the majority of implanted patients amenable to follow-up elsewhere (37-40, 113, 114). Approximately 70% of our patients gained pain relief during the week post-procedure and proceeded to full implantation. DBS remained effective for pain relief in over 60% of patients one year after surgery.

The Oxford data shows that DBS is superior to MCS for selected refractory pain syndromes (115), and that DBS is more appropriate than SCS for certain pain aetiologies. In particular, our results suggests that DBS is most effective in patients with pain after amputation, either phantom or stump, cranial and facial pain including anaesthesia dolorosa.

We also found very good efficacy of DBS for stroke patients complaining of burning hyperaesthesia (37) but overall less efficacy in patients with stroke, demonstrating the importance of patient selection.

We have also obtained good outcomes using DBS for facial and head pain including post-herpetic trigeminal neuralgia and anaesthesia dolorosa (39, 116), multiple sclerosis (107), genital pain, brachial plexus injuries and malignancy (38).

We are currently looking for new ways to improve to improve patient selection and thus outcomes. One intriguing possibility is the future use of autonomic measures as a potential objective markers (117), such as shown by the subjective preference for PVG/PAG stimulation over VPL/VPM in stroke together with the correlations revealed between cardiovascular effects, analgesic efficacy of DBS and burning hyperaesthesia.

It should, however, be noted that the complexity of chronic pain is such that the relief of one component of the chronic pain, for example burning hyperaesthesia, may unmask other pain components and thus may not overall lead to an quantitative reduction in pain scores. The large variability of results in case series to date reflects not just limitations in pain assessment tools and study design and execution, but also individual differences between patients as to what constitutes success. It is therefore important to include quality of life measures in outcome assessment to overcome the limitations of using VAS scores and pain questionnaires.

Conclusions

Deep brain stimulation is an important tool both for alleviating human suffering and for obtaining novel insights into the nature of fundamental brain function. Due to the existence of the robust MPTP translational model, DBS has so far proven most useful for controlling movement disorders as well as for controlling chronic pain. It is, however, imperative to find novel ways to treat affective disorders such as depression, which are far more prevalent than movement disorders in the general population (98).

Possible future innovations such as closed-loop demand-driven stimulators have great potential for transforming the therapeutic potential of DBS. Through the use of MEG and DBS we will come to understand the normal oscillatory activity of specific brain regions better (83), and such 'neural signatures' may come to help drive specific DBS interventions.

We now also have potential evidence of such a neural signature of pain in DBS patients who showed characteristically enhanced low frequency (8-12 Hz) power spectra of both PVG/PAG and VPL/VPM LFPs when in pain (118). Further research is required to elucidate if such neural signatures could aid patient selection, in particular if combined with technical advances in MEG to characterise whole-brain functional neuronal connectivity (88).

In general, such research on feedback-driven neural protheses may open up for more advanced brain-computer interfaces, which can in time come to help patients in a number of pathological states, such as helping patients with spinal cord injuries or even come to help to drive brain activity to help individuals in vegetative and minimally conscious states (119).

In this review we have tried to share our experience of what chronic pain patients to offer DBS and which targets to select. In our experience, successful indications include amputation, stroke, anaesthesia dolorosa, brachial plexus injuries and post-operative wound pain. We have shown how improving patient selection is essential to improving outcomes. In our view, DBS should only be performed in experienced, specialist centres willing to carefully study the patients and publish the results. The intensive experimental study of small groups of patients can help generate hypotheses creating opportunity for larger randomized, case-controlled, clinical trials.

Overall, DBS is a remarkable therapeutic tool which has great future potential both in terms of improving its clinical efficacy and in terms of understanding the fundamental mechanisms of normal human brain function.

Acknowledgments

The authors were funded by the UK Medical Research Council, TrygFonden Charitable Foundation, Norman Collisson Foundation, Oxford Biomedical Research Centre and Charles Wolfson Charitable Trust.

References

[1] Kringelbach ML, Jenkinson N, Owen SLF, Aziz TZ. Translational principles of deep brain stimulation. Nature Rev Neurosci 2007;8:623-35.
[2] Kringelbach ML, Owen SLF, Aziz TZ. Deep brain stimulation. Future Neurol 2007;2(6):633-46.
[3] Fritsch G, Hitzig E. Über die elektrische Erregbarkeit des Grosshirns. Arch Anat Physiol 1870;37:300-32. [German]
[4] Gildenberg PL. Evolution of neuromodulation. Stereotactic Funct Neurosurgery 2005;83(2-3):71-9.
[5] Pool JL, Clark WD, Hudson P, Lombardo M. Steroid hormonal response to stimulation of electrodes implanted in the subfrontal parts of the brain. In: Fields WS, Guillemin R, Carton CA, eds. Hypothalamic-Hypophysial Interrelationships. Springfield, IL: Charles C Thomas, 1956:114-24.
[6] White JC, Sweet WH. Pain and the Neurosurgeon. Springfield, IL: Charles C Thomas, 1969.
[7] Ervin FR, Brown CE, Mark VH. Striatal influence on facial pain. Confin Neurol 1966;27(1):75-90.
[8] Mark VH, Ervin FR. Role of Thalamotomy in Treatment of Chronic Severe Pain. Postgrad Med 1965;37:563-71.

[9] Mark VH, Ervin FR, Hackett TP. Clinical aspects of stereotactic thalamotomy in the human. Part I. The treatment of chronic severe pain. Arch Neurol 1960;3:351-67.
[10] Hosobuchi Y, Adams JE, Rutkin B. Chronic thalamic stimulation for the control of facial anesthesia dolorosa. Arch Neurol 1973;29(3):158-61.
[11] Mazars G, Merienne L, Cioloca C. [Treatment of certain types of pain with implantable thalamic stimulators]. Neurochirurgie 1974;20(2):117-24.
[12] Mazars G, Merienne L, Ciolocca C. [Intermittent analgesic thalamic stimulation. Preliminary note]. Rev Neurol (Paris) 1973;128(4):273-9.
[13] Mazars GJ. Intermittent stimulation of nucleus ventralis posterolateralis for intractable pain. Surg Neurol 1975;4(1):93-5.
[14] Mazars G, Roge R, Mazars Y. (Results of the stimulation of the spinothalamic fasciculus and their bearing on the physiopathology of pain.). Rev Prat 1960;103:136-8.
[15] Adams JE, Hosobuchi Y, Fields HL. Stimulation of internal capsule for relief of chronic pain. J Neurosurgery 1974;41(6):740-4.
[16] Fields HL, Adams JE. Pain after cortical injury relieved by electrical stimulation of the internal capsule. Brain 1974;97(1):169-78.
[17] Hosobuchi Y, Adams JE, Rutkin B. Chronic thalamic and internal capsule stimulation for the control of central pain. Surg Neurol 1975;4(1):91-2.
[18] Mayer DJ, Wolfle TL, Akil H, Carder B, Liebeskind JC. Analgesia from electrical stimulation in the brainstem of the rat. Science 1971;174(16):1351-4.
[19] Reynolds DV. Surgery in the rat during electrical analgesia induced by focal brain stimulation. Science 1969;164(878):444-5.
[20] Richardson DE, Akil H. Long term results of periventricular gray self-stimulation. Neurosurgery 1977;1(2):199-202.
[21] Richardson DE, Akil H. Pain reduction by electrical brain stimulation in man. Part 1: Acute administration in periaqueductal and periventricular sites. J Neurosurgery 1977;47(2):178-83.
[22] Richardson DE, Akil H. Pain reduction by electrical brain stimulation in man. Part 2: Chronic self-administration in the periventricular gray matter. J Neurosurgery 1977;47(2):184-94.
[23] Hosobuchi Y, Adams JE, Linchitz R. Pain relief by electrical stimulation of the central gray matter in humans and its reversal by naloxone. Science 1977;197(4299):183-6.
[24] Ray CD, Burton CV. Deep brain stimulation for severe, chronic pain. Acta Neurochir Suppl (Wien) 1980;30:289-93.
[25] Thoden U, Doerr M, Dieckmann G, Krainick JU. Medial thalamic permanent electrodes for pain control in man: an electrophysiological and clinical study. Electroencephalogr Clin Neurophysiol 1979;47(5):582-91.
[26] Boivie J, Meyerson BA. A correlative anatomical and clinical study of pain suppression by deep brain stimulation. Pain 1982;13(2):113-26.
[27] Andy OJ. Parafascicular-center median nuclei stimulation for intractable pain and dyskinesia (painful-dyskinesia). Appl Neurophysiol 1980;43(3-5):133-44.
[28] Gildenberg PL. Symposium on the safety and clinical efficacy of implanted neuroaugmentive devices. Appl Neurophysiol 1977;40:69-240.
[29] Gildenberg PL. Neurosurgical statement on neuroaugmentive devices. Appl Neurophysiol 1977;40:69-71.
[30] Gildenberg PL. History of electrical neuromodulation for chronic pain. Pain Med 2006;7(Suppl 1):S7-S13.
[31] Coffey RJ. Deep brain stimulation for chronic pain: results of two multicenter trials and a structured review. Pain Med 2001;2(3):183-92.
[32] Hamani C, Schwalb JM, Rezai AR, Dostrovsky JO, Davis KD, Lozano AM. Deep brain stimulation for chronic neuropathic pain: Long-term outcome and the incidence of insertional effect. Pain 2006;125(1-2):188-96.

[33] Krauss JK, Pohle T, Weigel R, Burgunder JM. Deep brain stimulation of the centre median-parafascicular complex in patients with movement disorders. J Neurol Neurosurg Psychiatry 2002;72(4):546-8.
[34] Marchand S, Kupers RC, Bushnell MC, Duncan GH. Analgesic and placebo effects of thalamic stimulation. Pain 2003;105(3):481-8.
[35] Tronnier VM. Deep brain stimulation. Amsterdam: Elsevier, 2003.
[36] Nandi D, Aziz T, Carter H, Stein J. Thalamic field potentials in chronic central pain treated by periventricular gray stimulation -- a series of eight cases. Pain 2003;101(1-2):97-107.
[37] Owen SL, Green AL, Stein JF, Aziz TZ. Deep brain stimulation for the alleviation of post-stroke neuropathic pain. Pain 2006;120(1-2):202-6.
[38] Owen SLF, Green AL, Nandi D, Bittar RG, Wang S, Aziz TZ. Deep brain stimulation for neuropathic pain. Neuromodulation 2006;9(2):100-6.
[39] Green AL, Owen SL, Davies P, Moir L, Aziz TZ. Deep brain stimulation for neuropathic cephalalgia. Cephalalgia 2006;26(5):561-7.
[40] Bittar RG, Otero S, Carter H, Aziz TZ. Deep brain stimulation for phantom limb pain. J Clin Neurosci 2005;12(4):399-404.
[41] Franzini A, Ferroli P, Leone M, Broggi G. Stimulation of the posterior hypothalamus for treatment of chronic intractable cluster headaches: first reported series. Neurosurgery 2003;52(5):1095-1101.
[42] Leone M, Franzini A, Broggi G, May A, Bussone G. Long-term follow-up of bilateral hypothalamic stimulation for intractable cluster headache. Brain 2004;127(Pt 10):2259-64.
[43] Owen SL, Green AL, Davies P, Stein JF, Aziz TZ, Behrens T, et al. Connectivity of an effective hypothalamic surgical target for cluster headache. J Clin Neurosci 2007;14(10):955-60.
[44] Andy OJ, Jurko F. Thalamic stimulation effects on reactive depression. Appl Neurophysiol 1987;50(1-6):324-9.
[45] Jimenez F, Velasco F, Salin-Pascual R, Hernandez JA, Velasco M, Criales JL, et al. A patient with a resistant major depression disorder treated with deep brain stimulation in the inferior thalamic peduncle. Neurosurgery. 2005;57(3):585-93.
[46] Mayberg HS, Lozano AM, Voon V, McNeely HE, Seminowicz D, Hamani C, et al. Deep brain stimulation for treatment-resistant depression. Neuron 2005;45(5):651-60.
[47] Schlaepfer TE, Cohen MX, Frick C, Kosel M, Brodesser D, Axmacher N, et al. Deep brain stimulation to reward circuitry alleviates anhedonia in refractory major depression. Neuropsychopharmacology 2007;33(2):368-77.
[48] Nuttin BJ, Gabriels LA, Cosyns PR, Meyerson BA, Andreewitch S, Sunaert SG, et al. Long-term electrical capsular stimulation in patients with obsessive-compulsive disorder. Neurosurgery 2003;52(6):1263-72.
[49] Visser-Vandewalle V, Temel Y, Boon P, Vreeling F, Colle H, Hoogland G, et al. Chronic bilateral thalamic stimulation: a new therapeutic approach in intractable Tourette syndrome. Report of three cases. J Neurosurgery 2003;99(6):1094-100.
[50] Ackermans L, Temel Y, Cath D, van der Linden C, Bruggeman R, Kleijer M, et al. Deep brain stimulation in Tourette's syndrome: two targets? Mov Disord 2006;21(5):709-13.
[51] Bejjani BP, Damier P, Arnulf I, Thivard L, Bonnet AM, Dormont D, et al. Transient acute depression induced by high-frequency deep-brain stimulation. N Engl J Med 1999;340(19):1476-80.
[52] Temel Y, Kessels A, Tan S, Topdag A, Boon P, Visser-Vandewalle V. Behavioural changes after bilateral subthalamic stimulation in advanced Parkinson disease: a systematic review. Parkinsonism Relat Disord 2006;12(5):265-72.
[53] Saint-Cyr JA, Trepanier LL. Neuropsychologic assessment of patients for movement disorder surgery. Mov Disord 2000;15(5):771-83.
[54] Voon V, Kubu C, Krack P, Houeto JL, Troster AI. Deep brain stimulation: neuropsychological and neuropsychiatric issues. Mov Disord 2006;21(Suppl 14):S305-27.

[55] Lang AE, Houeto JL, Krack P, Kubu C, Lyons KE, Moro E, et al. Deep brain stimulation: preoperative issues. Mov Disord 2006;21(Suppl 14):S171-96.
[56] Shulman R, Turnbull IM, Diewold P. Psychiatric aspects of thalamic stimulation for neuropathic pain. Pain 1982;13(2):127-35.
[57] Carlsson AM. Assessment of chronic pain. I. Aspects of the reliability and validity of the visual analogue scale. Pain 1983;16(1):87-101.
[58] Melzack R. The McGill Pain Questionnaire: major properties and scoring methods. Pain 1975;1(3):277-99.
[59] Ware JE, Snow KK, Kosinski M, Gandek B. SF-36 Health Survey Manual and Interpretation Guide. Boston, MA.: New Engl Med Center, Health Institute, 1993.
[60] Euroqol. EuroQol--a new facility for the measurement of health-related quality of life. The EuroQol Group. Health Policy 1990;16(3):199-208.
[61] Medical Outcomes T. How to Score the SF-36 Health Survey. Boston, MA: Med Outcomes Trust, 1991.
[62] Hamani C, Richter EO, Andrade-Souza Y, Hutchison W, Saint-Cyr JA, Lozano AM. Correspondence of microelectrode mapping with magnetic resonance imaging for subthalamic nucleus procedures. Surg Neurol 2005;63(3):249-53.
[63] Hariz MI. Safety and risk of microelectrode recording in surgery for movement disorders. Stereotactic Functl Neurosurg 2002;78(3-4):146-57.
[64] Hosobuchi Y. Subcortical electrical stimulation for control of intractable pain in humans. Report of 122 cases (1970-1984). J Neurosurgery 1986;64(4):543-53.
[65] Benabid AL, Pollak P, Gao D, Hoffmann D, Limousin P, Gay E, et al. Chronic electrical stimulation of the ventralis intermedius nucleus of the thalamus as a treatment of movement disorders. J Neurosurg 1996;84(2):203-14.
[66] Beric A, Kelly PJ, Rezai A, Sterio D, Mogilner A, Zonenshayn M, et al. Complications of deep brain stimulation surgery. Stereotactic Funct Neurosurg 2001;77(1-4):73-8.
[67] Hariz MI. Complications of deep brain stimulation surgery. Mov Disord 2002;17:S162-6.
[68] Bejjani BP, Houeto JL, Hariz M, Yelnik J, Mesnage V, Bonnet AM, et al. Aggressive behavior induced by intraoperative stimulation in the triangle of Sano. Neurology 2002;59(9):1425-7.
[69] Krack P, Kumar R, Ardouin C, Dowsey PL, McVicker JM, Benabid AL, et al. Mirthful laughter induced by subthalamic nucleus stimulation. Mov Disord 2001;16(5):867-75.
[70] Temel Y, van Lankveld JJ, Boon P, Spincemaille GH, van der Linden C, Visser-Vandewalle V. Deep brain stimulation of the thalamus can influence penile erection. Int J Impot Res 2004;16(1):91-4.
[71] Kulisevsky J, Berthier ML, Gironell A, Pascual-Sedano B, Molet J, Pares P. Mania following deep brain stimulation for Parkinson's disease. Neurology 2002;59(9):1421-4.
[72] Volkmann J, Herzog J, Kopper F, Deuschl G. Introduction to the programming of deep brain stimulators. Mov Disord 2002;17:S181-7.
[73] Kuncel AM, Grill WM. Selection of stimulus parameters for deep brain stimulation. Clin Neurophysiol 2004;115(11):2431-41.
[74] Ranck JB, Jr. Which elements are excited in electrical stimulation of mammalian central nervous system: a review. Brain Res 1975;98(3):417-40.
[75] McIntyre CC, Grill WM, Sherman DL, Thakor NV. Cellular effects of deep brain stimulation: model-based analysis of activation and inhibition. J Neurophysiol 2004;91(4):1457-69.
[76] Holsheimer J, Demeulemeester H, Nuttin B, de Sutter P. Identification of the target neuronal elements in electrical deep brain stimulation. Eur J Neurosci 2000;12(12):4573-7.
[77] Nowak LG, Bullier J. Axons, but not cell bodies, are activated by electrical stimulation in cortical gray matter. II. Evidence from selective inactivation of cell bodies and axon initial segments. Exp Brain Res 1998;118(4):489-500.
[78] Durand DM. Electric field effects in hyperexcitable neural tissue: a review. Radiat Prot Dosimetry 2003;106(4):325-31.

[79] Hashimoto T, Elder CM, Okun MS, Patrick SK, Vitek JL. Stimulation of the subthalamic nucleus changes the firing pattern of pallidal neurons. J Neurosci 2003;23(5):1916-23.

[80] Anderson ME, Postupna N, Ruffo M. Effects of high-frequency stimulation in the internal globus pallidus on the activity of thalamic neurons in the awake monkey. J Neurophysiol 2003;89(2):1150-60.

[81] Dostrovsky JO, Levy R, Wu JP, Hutchison WD, Tasker RR, Lozano AM. Microstimulation-induced inhibition of neuronal firing in human globus pallidus. J Neurophysiol 2000;84(1):570-4.

[82] Pralong E, Debatisse D, Maeder M, Vingerhoets F, Ghika J, Villemure JG. Effect of deep brain stimulation of GPI on neuronal activity of the thalamic nucleus ventralis oralis in a dystonic patient. Neurophysiol Clin 2003;33(4):169-73.

[83] Brown P, Mazzone P, Oliviero A, Altibrandi MG, Pilato F, Tonali PA, et al. Effects of stimulation of the subthalamic area on oscillatory pallidal activity in Parkinson's disease. Exp Neurol 2004;188(2):480-90.

[84] Windels F, Bruet N, Poupard A, Urbain N, Chouvet G, Feuerstein C, et al. Effects of high frequency stimulation of subthalamic nucleus on extracellular glutamate and GABA in substantia nigra and globus pallidus in the normal rat. Eur J Neurosci 2000;12(11):4141-6.

[85] Boulet S, Lacombe E, Carcenac C, Feuerstein C, Sgambato-Faure V, Poupard A, et al. Subthalamic stimulation-induced forelimb dyskinesias are linked to an increase in glutamate levels in the substantia nigra pars reticulata. J Neurosci 2006;26(42):10768-76.

[86] Perlmutter JS, Mink JW, Bastian AJ, Zackowski K, Hershey T, Miyawaki E, et al. Blood flow responses to deep brain stimulation of thalamus. Neurology 2002;58(9):1388-94.

[87] Hershey T, Revilla FJ, Wernle AR, McGee-Minnich L, Antenor JV, Videen TO, et al. Cortical and subcortical blood flow effects of subthalamic nucleus stimulation in PD. Neurology 2003;61(6):816-21.

[88] Kringelbach ML, Jenkinson N, Green AL, Owen SLF, Hansen PC, Cornelissen PL, et al. Deep brain stimulation for chronic pain investigated with magnetoencephalography. Neuroreport 2007;18(3):223-8.

[89] Lauritzen M. Reading vascular changes in brain imaging: is dendritic calcium the key? Nat Rev Neurosci 2005;6(1):77-85.

[90] Logothetis NK, Wandell BA. Interpreting the BOLD signal. Annu Rev Physiol 2004;66:735-69.

[91] Georgi JC, Stippich C, Tronnier VM, Heiland S. Active deep brain stimulation during MRI: a feasibility study. Magn Reson Med 2004;51(2):380-8.

[92] Sakatani K, Katayama Y, Yamamoto T, Suzuki S. Changes in cerebral blood oxygenation of the frontal lobe induced by direct electrical stimulation of thalamus and globus pallidus: a near infrared spectroscopy study. J Neurol Neurosurg Psychiatry 1999;67(6):769-73.

[93] Stefurak T, Mikulis D, Mayberg H, Lang AE, Hevenor S, Pahapill P, et al. Deep brain stimulation for Parkinson's disease dissociates mood and motor circuits: a functional MRI case study. Mov Disord 2003;18(12):1508-16.

[94] May A, Leone M, Boecker H, Sprenger T, Juergens T, Bussone G, et al. Hypothalamic deep brain stimulation in positron emission tomography. J Neurosci 2006;26(13):3589-93.

[95] Pereira EA, Green AL, Bradley KM, Soper N, Moir L, Stein JF, et al. Regional cerebral perfusion differences between periventricular grey, thalamic and dual target deep brain stimulation for chronic neuropathic pain. Stereotactic Funct Neurosurg 2007;85(4):175-83.

[96] Hillebrand A, Barnes GR. A quantitative assessment of the sensitivity of whole-head MEG to activity in the adult human cortex. Neuroimage 2002;16(3 Pt 1):638-50.

[97] Kringelbach ML, Jenkinson N, Green A, Hansen PC, Cornelissen PL, Holliday IE, et al. Deep brain stimulation and chronic pain mapped with MEG. Society Neurosci 2006;782.1.

[98] Kringelbach ML. The human orbitofrontal cortex: linking reward to hedonic experience. Nature Rev Neurosci 2005;6(9):691-702.

[99] Ray NJ, Kringelbach ML, Jenkinson N, Owen SLF, Davies P, Wang S, et al. Using magnetoencephalography to investigate deep brain stimulation for cluster headache. Biomed Imaging Intervent J 2007;3:e25.
[100] Schnitzler A, Gross J. Normal and pathological oscillatory communication in the brain. Nat Rev Neurosci 2005;6(4):285-96.
[101] Montgomery EB, Jr., Baker KB. Mechanisms of deep brain stimulation and future technical developments. Neurol Res 2000;22(3):259-66.
[102] McIntyre CC, Savasta M, Kerkerian-Le Goff L, Vitek JL. Uncovering the mechanism(s) of action of deep brain stimulation: activation, inhibition, or both. Clin Neurophysiol 2004;115(6):1239-48.
[103] Vitek JL. Mechanisms of deep brain stimulation: excitation or inhibition. Mov Disord 2002;17:S69-72.
[104] Beurrier C, Bioulac B, Audin J, Hammond C. High-frequency stimulation produces a transient blockade of voltage-gated currents in subthalamic neurons. J Neurophysiol 2001;85(4):1351-6.
[105] Urbano FJ, Leznik E, Llinas RR. Cortical activation patterns evoked by afferent axons stimuli at different frequencies: an in vitro voltage sensitive dye imaging study. Thalamus Rel Syst. 2002;1:371-8.
[106] Gybels J. Brain stimulation in the management of persistent pain, 4th ed. Philadelphia, PA: Saunders, 2000.
[107] Hamani C, Schwalb JM, Rezai AR, Dostrovsky JO, Davis KD, Lozano AM. Deep brain stimulation for chronic neuropathic pain: Long-term outcome and the incidence of insertional effect. Pain 2006;125(1-2):188-96..
[108] Levy RM. Deep brain stimulation for the treatment of intractable pain. Neurosurg Clin North Am 2003;14(3):389-99, vi.
[109] Cameron T. Safety and efficacy of spinal cord stimulation for the treatment of chronic pain: a 20-year literature review. J Neurosurg 2004;100(3 Suppl Spine):254-67.
[110] Taylor RS, Van Buyten JP, Buchser E. Spinal cord stimulation for chronic back and leg pain and failed back surgery syndrome: a systematic review and analysis of prognostic factors. Spine 2005;30(1):152-60.
[111] Brown JA, Barbaro NM. Motor cortex stimulation for central and neuropathic pain: current status. Pain 2003;104(3):431-5.
[112] Smith H, Joint C, Schlugman D, Nandi D, Stein JF, Aziz TZ. Motor cortex stimulation for neuropathic pain. Neurosurg Focus 2001;11(3).
[113] Green AL, Shad A, Watson R, Nandi D, Yianni J, Aziz TZ. N-of-1 trials for assessing the efficacy of deep brain stimulation in neuropathic pain. Neuromodulation 2004;7(2):76-81.
[114] Nandi D, Aziz TZ. Deep brain stimulation in the management of neuropathic pain and multiple sclerosis tremor. J Clin Neurophysiol 2004;21(1):31-9.
[115] Nandi D, Smith H, Owen S, Joint C, Stein J, Aziz T. Peri-ventricular grey stimulation versus motor cortex stimulation for post stroke neuropathic pain. J Clin Neurosci 2002;9(5):557-61.
[116] Green AL, Nandi D, Armstrong G, Carter H, Aziz T. Post-herpetic trigeminal neuralgia treated with deep brain stimulation. J Clin Neurosci 2003;10(4):512-4.
[117] Green AL, Wang S, Owen SL, Xie K, Bittar RG, Stein JF, et al. Stimulating the human midbrain to reveal the link between pain and blood pressure. Pain 2006;124(3):349-59.
[118] Green AL, Wang S, Stein JF, Pereira EA, Kringelbach ML, Liu X, et al. Neural signatures in patients with neuropathic pain. Neurology 2009;72(6):569-71.
[119] Tsubokawa T, Yamamoto T, Katayama Y, Hirayama T, Maejima S, Moriya T. Deep-brain stimulation in a persistent vegetative state: Follow-up results and criteria for selection of candidates. Brain Inj 1990;4:315-27.

In: Pain Management Yearbook 2009
Editor: Joav Merrick

ISBN: 978-1-61209-666-7
©2012 Nova Science Publishers, Inc.

Chapter 32

INVASIVE TREATMENT OF CHRONIC NEUROPATHIC PAIN SYNDROMES: EPIDURAL STIMULATION OF THE MOTOR CORTEX

Dirk Rasche[*], *MD and Volker M Tronnier, MD, PhD*

Department of Neurosurgery, University of Lübeck, Lübeck, Germany

Abstract

The aim of this paper is to demonstrate the current status of motor cortex stimulation (MCS) as an invasive treatment option in chronic neuropathic pain patients. Epidural lead placement and MCS is performed in selected patients suffering from pain syndromes of central or peripheral neuropathic origin. To date a total number of about 500 cases and more than 30 prospective or retrospective clinical studies, patients samples or reviews have been published. The clinical experience of the authors, the perioperative management and a recent review of the relevant literature are presented.

Keywords: Motor cortex stimulation, central neuropathic pain, trigeminal neuropathic pain, post-stroke pain, neuromodulation.

---

[*] **Correspondence:** Dirk Rasche, MD, Department of Neurosurgery, University of Lübeck, Ratzeburger Allee 160, 23538 Lübeck, Germany. Tel: +49-451 5002075; Fax: +49-451 5006191; E-mail: dirk.rasche@uk-sh.de

Introduction

Over more than 20 years extradural electrical stimulation of cortical areas (motor cortex stimulation = MCS) surrounding the central sulcus is performed for various chronic pain conditions (see table 1).

Table 1. Overview listing all relevant publications regarding neuropathic pain and MCS

Author	Year	Patient#	Diagnosis	Follow-Up	Responder
Tsubokawa et al.	1993	11	PSP	24	8 (5)
Meyerson et al.	1993	5	TNP	28	5
Katayama et al.	1994	3	central pain	12	2
Migita et al.	1995	15	PSP, spinal cord lesion pain	>24	11
Ebel et al.	1996	6	TNP	24	3
Katayama et al.	1998	31	PSP	>24	15
Garcia-Larrea et al.	1999	10	PSP, Plexus avulsion	6	5
Nguyen et al.	1999	31	PSP, TNP, SCI, PHP	>24	7
Mertens et al.	1999	23	central neuropathic pain, SCI, BPA	74	11
Carroll et al.	2000	10	PSP, phantom limb pain, traumatic neuralgia, brachyalgia	>24	5
Saitoh et al.	2000	8	PSP, peripheral deafferentation pain	26	6
Drouot et al.	2002	31	peripheral neuropathy and central lesions	18	21
Rainov et al.	2003	2	TNP	18	2
Tirakotai et al.	2004	5	central pain	24	5
Brown et al.	2005	10	central and neuropathic facial pain	24	8
Nuti et al.	2005	31	PSP, SCI	48	16
Cioni et Meglio	2007	14	PSP, TNP, SCI	n.s.	3 (2)
Hosomi et al.	2008	34	PSP, TNP, BPA, SCI, PLP	112	12
Velasco et al.	2008	11	central and peripheral neuropathic pain	12	8
Rasche et al.*	2009	35	TNP, PSP, BPA, SCI, PHP	180	17

* = unpublished patient sample including Rasche et al. 2006. (n.s. = not specified; Follow-Up: months).

Chronic pain is defined as persistent and constant pain over at least six months. Neuropathic pain is defined, according to the International Association for the Study of Pain (IASP), as pain initiated or caused by a lesion (or dysfunction) of the central or peripheral nervous system. The cause of this lesion or dysfunction can be trauma, inflammation, metabolic diseases, tumour and iatrogenic.

Undoubtedly the pioneering work of Penfield and colleagues (1) with mapping of the cortical surface, in detail the motor strip and central region, was the groundwork for many functional procedures. To date the cortical representation of the motor "homunculus" is the background for targeting the somatotopic correlate of the affected part of the body.

According to this information leads are placed interhemispherically to treat pain syndromes of the lower extremities, over the convexity for the upper extremities or, moving more laterally, for facial pain.

In the 1950s many invasive procedures with destruction of somatosensory or spinothalamic pathways were performed to treat chronic pain patients. Nowadays most of these procedures are obsolete; others are very rarely performed so that they do not play a specific role in pain therapy anymore. This is due to the ongoing development of pharmacological agents for the treatment of pain (e.g. opioids, anticonvulsants...) on the one side, on the other side these operations can not be learned by younger neurosurgeons and therefore will not be performed in the future anymore.

Beginning in the 1980's the first leads were implanted sub- or epidurally over the motor or somatosensory cortex. The stimulation mode may be cyclic or continuous, but is always subthreshold of motor evoked responses. This invasive neurosurgical treatment is used in patients who do not respond to any pharmacological or conservative treatment, usually at the end of the patients treatment course as a "last resort", comparable with e. g. deep brain stimulation in chronic pain. Therefore the indication for cortical stimulation is limited to a small patient collective with intractable chronic pain conditions. Until now Medline search reveals about 500 cases and more than 30 studies, trials or reviews dealing with MCS in different chronic pain syndromes, movement disorders, stroke rehabilitation and chronic tinnitus (2-7). These include on the one hand pain of central origin involving pain pathways in the central nervous system (brain, spinal cord) and on the other hand neuropathic pain following peripheral nerve injury (cranial nerves, brachial plexus, nerve roots). The first results were published by Tsubokawa in patients with post-stroke pain (PSP) in the early 1990s (8,9). A few years later Meyerson et al. reported the first treated patients with chronic facial pain syndromes (10). The indication list was expanded by Nguyen et al. in the late 1990s, which treated patients with Parkinson's disease to improve the movement disorder (7). Until today several review articles regarding MCS and neuropathic pain are published by different experts in the field (see table 2).

Methods and results

Summarizing our clinical experience from 1994 until 2009 we have treated 35 patients with central pain or post-stroke-pain (PSP; n=12), trigeminal neuropathic pain (TNP; n=17), brachial plexus avulsion (BPA; n=4) and one patient each with spinal cord injury (SCI) and post herpetic neuropathic pain (PHP). The cause of the central pain was mainly due to ischemic or post hemorrhagic lesion of the central pain pathway itself. In detail this was the posterior thalamus (eight patients), pons (three patients) or the parietal lobe (one patient). In all patients a unilateral neuropathic pain, contralateral to the affected brain area was obvious and hemisensory deficits including different kinds of A-beta, A-delta and C-fibres function were found. Pain affected mainly the upper limb or face in eight cases and in four patients additional pain was described in the lateral trunk or lower limb. Patients with pain located only in the lower limb or with paralysis or severe motor deficit of the affected pain area, e.g. upper limb, were not considered for MCS.

Table 2. List of reviews and meta-analysis of different experts in the field

Authors	Year
Brown et Barbaro (43)	2003
Henderson et Lad (57)	2006
Osenbach (58)	2006
Canavero et Bonicalzi (38)	2007
Cioni et Meglio (22)	2007
Lazorthes et al (51)	2007
Saitoh et Yoshimine (59)	2007
Arle et Shils (3)	2008
Lima et Fregni (6)	2008

17 patients suffered from chronic neuropathic facial pain after partial destruction or lesion of the trigeminal nerve itself or peripheral branches. This was mainly following operative procedures for trigeminal neuralgia, tumours surrounding the cranial pathway of the trigeminal nerve or dental manipulations. TNP was diagnosed according to the criteria of the 2nd edition of the International Classification of Headache Disorders (11).

Four male patients suffered from posttraumatic unilateral BPA and chronic neuropathic pain of the upper limb. In two of these patients operative procedures like dorsal root entry zone lesions of the cervical spinal cord were performed several years before. Despite initial positive effect pain syndrome and allodynia recurred over time. In one patient spinal cord stimulation was tested ineffectively.

In one patient each spinal cord injury at the thoracic level and postherpetic neuropathic pain in the dermatoma Th 6-8 was ineffectively treated by various conservative methods before selection for MCS was performed.

In all of these cases a specific sensory nerve deficit, e.g. tactile hypo- or hyperaesthesia, was found in the pain area. In 16 cases this was quantified using a standardized quantitative sensory testing.

All patients were selected from a patient population of the outpatient clinic of a special neurosurgical pain unit. MRI scans of the brain were performed to rule out other symptomatic causes of pain and to visualize the precentral gyrus, the size and area of infarction in PSP patients, brain atrophy etc. Neuropsychological assessment and testing was performed by an independent neuropsychologist and implemented in the preoperative evaluation to rule out major depression, psychosis etc. Over time more than 10 patients were excluded from this treatment option due to psychiatric disorders including severe depression and drug abuse.

Among the patients are 26 women and nine men. The mean age was 58.1 years (SD= 14.3; range 26-82 years) and mean pain duration was 6 years (SD= 2.7; range 2-12 years).

During follow-up one patient died at the age of 90 years, independently and not related to the MCS. The mean postoperative follow-up was 3.5 years (SD = 4.0; range 0.5-15 years) for patients with active MCS. Multiple prior treatments and pharmacological therapies were ineffective or the patient claimed major intolerable side effects. Four weeks before and also during the test trial the current medication was not changed. After information about the procedure, test-trial, double-blind testing and procedure-related complications all patient signed written consent.

Intravenously testing of barbiturate, propofol and morphine was performed in 5 cases but a predictive effect was not derived. Also repetitive transcranial magnetic stimulation (rTMS) of the motor cortex was performed in 10 patients. A predictive value was not evaluated and negative or no response to rTMS was no contraindication for MCS (12).

Preoperative imaging/fMRI

A standardized MRI data set with 3-D-volume reconstruction of the brain and cortical surface was achieved and transferred to the neuronavigation system. Because of an implanted cardia pacemaker or other MRI contraindications a 3-D neuronavigation data set was performed using computed tomography (CT) in 3 patients. In 27 of the 35 cases preoperative motor-function MRI using standardized paradigms (13-20) was performed. These data were also transferred to the neuronavigation system and coregistered with the 3-D-volume MRI data sets in 20 cases. Due to motion artifacts matching was not possible or incorrect in 5 cases. In 8 cases a postoperative CT-scan was performed as a 3-D-volume data set and matching with preoperative MRI was achieved. The position of the lead was defined by using the midpoint of the induced artefacts in the CT-scan and this position was matched on the MRI data set (see also figure 1).

Further development of imaging modalities, e.g. MRI diffusion tensor imaging (DTI), may be helpful to visualize if corticothalamic or other fibre connections are intact or what cortical or even subcortical localisation are the best targets for neuromodulation.

Operative procedure

The intraoperative details were described in an earlier publication in 2006 (21). Fixation of the head was performed with application of local anaesthetics and a 3 point pin holder. Standard neuronavigation system and also electrophysiological monitoring system were prepared and installed. Positioning of one or more leads via the burr-hole technique was performed in 30 patients (see also figure 2).

In three patients with TNP a craniotomy was performed. In these cases an octapolar lead was used and sutured to the dura. In all patients somatosensory evoked potentials (SEP) of the median and/or tibial nerve, especially in the patients with BPA, were recorded in a bipolar mode using two electrodes of the quadripolar lead. With the help of the phase reversal of the N20 (median SEP) or P40 (tibial SEP) component the pre- and postcentral gyrus was identified (22-27).

Additionally suprathreshold stimulation via the lead was performed and focal muscle contractions of the face, upper or lower limb were evoked with a frequency of 5 or 100 Hertz and an intensity varying from 4-10 milliampere. In case of phase reversal of the SEP or a short focal seizure the lead was left in place on the convexity over the precentral gyrus. Somatosensory phenomena induced by MCS were not reported by the patients. In one case the lead was placed subdurally because of brain atrophy. The lead extension was fixed to prevent dislocation and the extension cable was tunnelled subcutaneously to the frontotemporal region.

Postoperative clinical test trial

After insertion of the lead a test trial of up to 14 days was conducted in all patients. On the first postoperative day a plane x-ray and a CT-scan of the head were performed to document the position of the lead and to rule out any complications like epidural bleeding. A test trial of minimum 6 days up to 14 days using a standardized protocol with different stimulation settings and an external stimulation device (DualScreen, Model 3628, Medtronic Inc., Minneapolis, MN, USA) was conducted. As long as the connection cables were externalized a prophylactic oral antibiotic was administered.

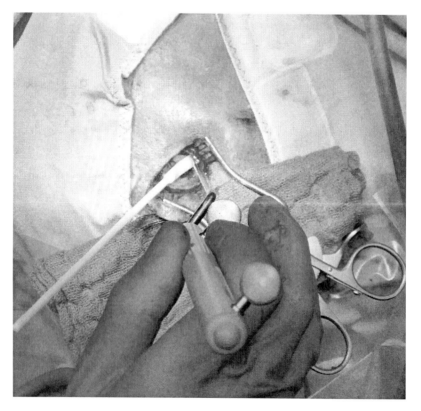

Figure 1. Intraoperative photograph demonstrating the burr-hole technique and neuronavigation guidance of epidural spacing and lead positioning.

Invasive treatment of chronic neuropathic pain syndromes

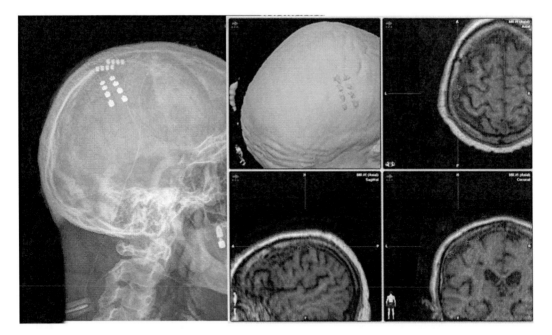

Figure 2. Postoperative x-ray (left) and image fusion of the postoperatice CT-scan and the preoperative MRI-data set with reconstruction of the lead position.

Stimulation intensity was adjusted between 50 and 75% of the intraoperatively evoked motor threshold. Therefore stimulation intensities varied from 0.5 up to 7.0 milliampere. Pain intensity was measured using a visual analogue scale (VAS) and the patient was asked to complete a pain diary. The external stimulation device was programmed by an independent physician according a standardized protocol.

Positive effect of MCS was defined as pain reduction of more than 30% on the VAS, subjective impression of improvement and reduction of daily medication intake. If the patient was detected as responder to MCS a permanent neurostimulator (Itrel 2 or 3, Model 7425; Synergy, Model 7427, Medtronic Inc., Minneapolis, MN, USA) was implanted. After permanent implantation of the stimulation device parameters varied from 2.0 up to 7.0 milliampere, a frequency of 30 to 85 Hertz and stimulus duration of 210 to 450 μsec.

In the patients with PSP only 4 out of 12 (33%) were positive responders to MCS and pain reduction of > 30% was achieved. Interestingly, in 2 of the 4 patients pain was due to lesion of the pons and the thalamic area was unaffected.

In the TNP patient group 10 out of 17 patients were screened as responders to MCS and a permanent neurostimulator was implanted. Looking at the four male patients with posttraumatic BPA and chronic pain of the affected upper limb we found in all patients motor weakness or paralysis of the forearm. Also a sensory deficit with tactile hypoesthesia, beginning at the upper arm, was detectable. In one case a tactile hyperesthesia and in three cases an allodynia was present. Phase reversal of tibial nerve evoked somatosensory potentials was performed to identify the precentral gyrus and the lead was placed over the motor strip of the forearm and hand. All three patients mentioned improvement of the allodynia and tension pain in the affected limb using subthreshold stimulation. In all patients a > 50% pain reduction was achieved while no effect was documented during double-blind or placebo stimulation.

Considering the long-term follow-up a positive effect of MCS with lasting improvement of pain was observed in 11/17 patients. Only minor changes of the stimulation parameters were necessary. Only 4 of 12 patients with PSP were permanently implanted and during follow-up a slowly diminishing effect was observed in two patients with pain reduction of about 30%. In all patients additional pain medication was necessary, but in the remaining two patients daily dosage was significantly reduced.

More than 50% pain reduction was achieved in 10 of the 17 patients with TNP. Of the remaining seven patients one patient had only minor pain relief of about 30%, in one case the generator was inactivated because of seizures and one patient died of other reasons. Three patients with BPA and long-term response to MCS reported more than 50% pain reduction and a stable effect over more than 3 years. In the forth patient a slowly diminishing effect of the MCS was detected after 18 months. Dislocation of the lead and technical failure of the implanted devices was ruled out. Even with reprogramming the stimulation parameters no positive clinical effect was stated by the patient.

No positive effect was observed during the test phase regarding the patient with PHP. No pain reduction could be achieved with any stimulation settings or placebo testing. During the double-blinded stimulation phase of the patient with SCI pain reduction was mentioned during placebo stimulation and also active MCS. Therefore the patient was considered as false positive responder and the lead was explanted.

All responders reported improvement of pain immediately or within 30-60 minutes after activation of MCS. After deactivation the positive effect lasted for up to several hours. Active MCS lead to improvement of sensory phenomena like allodynia or dysesthesia in 17 patients, including the three patients with BPA.

In all patients initially a cyclic stimulation mode varying from stimulating 3 x 0.5 hours/day up to stimulating 1 hour followed by 0.5 hours off-stimulation was adjusted. In 10 patients it was necessary to change the stimulation mode to continuous stimulation due to diminishing effect of the MCS in the cycling mode. 8 patients perform a stimulation pause during the night to spare battery capacity. In 7 patients one or more exchanges of the stimulation device were necessary due to low battery capacity.

In long term use stimulation parameters were as follows: stimulus intensity varying from 2.5 to 6.0 milliampere, frequency from 30 to 85 Hertz and stimulus duration from 210 to 450 μsec.

Double blinded testing

Subthreshold stimulation intensities without induction of clinical sensible effects as compared to spinal cord stimulation allow a blinded or even double blinded testing of MCS. Therefore it is necessary to blind the patient, physician and the nurse staff on the ward. An independent physician is needed to program and control the stimulation device, which is covered and shielded for the setting of the lead combinations. Evaluation of the test protocol allows detection of false positive responders with pain reduction during the placebo settings. Using this method we were able to identify three patients with PSP, four patients with TNP and 1 patient with SCI as false-positive responders and the stimulation lead was explanted.

Complications

Reported complications regarding this treatment method were mostly related to local wound infections and postoperative seizures (see also table 3).

Table 3. List of complications and conditional propability as reported by different trials

Complications	%
wound infection	≤12
seizures	≤4
hardware failure	≤5
haematoma	≤9,5
neurological worsening	≤8

In some cases local headache or tenderness at the implanted devices were mentioned. Fracture of the lead or connection cable is rare. Intraoperative seizures due to suprathreshold stimulation were seen in 15 patients and in 12 cases phenytoine was administered iv by the anaesthesiologist. It has to be mentioned that in 30/33 patients a pharmacological pain therapy with pregabalin, gabapentin and/or carbamazepine was performed as long-term prescription. Therefore also a seizure protection effect can be assumed. Nevertheless, in one case, a patient with TNP, MCS had to be deactivated because of persisting postoperative focal seizures. Pain reduction was achieved by intrathecal application of ziconotide and an infusion pump was permanently implanted.

In all operated cases a postoperative cranial CT-scan was performed after lead insertion to exclude intracranial complications. No epidural haematomas were observed. In one patient local wound infection was followed by removal of the connection cable and stimulation device. Contralateral reimplantation of the stimulation device and connection cable after several months was possible and positive effect regained.

Discussion

Central pain syndromes like PSP are the most difficult to treat and success rates are lower than in other neuropathic pain syndromes. This can be due to the fact that the pain origin is located in the central pain transmission network. The mode of action of MCS is unclear and only theories exist based on morphological anatomical examinations and imaging techniques like functional MRI or positron emission tomography (PET). Using positron emission tomography (PET) studies in nine patients with MCS Garcia-Larrea et al (28-30) were able to demonstrate regional changes in cerebral blood flow (rCBF) effects of active MCS in the region of the ipsilateral lateral thalamus, anterior cingulate gyrus, left insula and upper brainstem. Until today no standardized protocol or guidelines exist for this procedure. When looking at the published data no clear indications for surgery, site of stimulation and stimulation parameters exist (12,15,22,31-36). The rating of efficacy is different and has a wide spectrum (6,14,26,37-39). It was shown by Carroll et al (39) and Yamamoto et al (40) that severe motor weakness or paralysis in the area of pain with injury of the corticospinal tract is of negative predictive value for pain relief by MCS. In the presented collective two out of seven patients with PSP showed a spastic hemiparesis (Grade 3-4/5 according to BMC). Only in one case of the TNP group a facial palsy (Grade 2-3 according to House and Brackmann) was detected.

An overview concerning selected publications regarding MCS is given in table 1. The first operated patients with PSP were reported by Tsubokawa et al in 1990, respectively 1991 (8). In 1993 Tsubokawa et al (9) reported an initial success-rate in 8 of 11 patients (73%) with PSP. Two years after implantation only five patients were still positive responders (45%).

Meyerson et al (10) reported the first patients with TNP and MCS. Initial positive effect of MCS is demonstrated in all cases with a follow-up of 4-28 months. Reporting positive MCS effect in 50% (three of six) of the patients with TNP and a follow-up of 5-24 months was performed by Ebel et al (41). Pain relief by MCS in seven out of 12 (58%) patients with TNP was reported by Nguyen et al in 1999 (24). Reporting a series of 20 patients with central neuropathic pain and a follow-up of more than one year, Mertens et al (42) reported an excellent pain relief in 5 (25%), good in 7 (35%) and fair in 3 (15%) patients. Five patients (25%) were negative responders. The success-rates reported for TNP and PSP are higher than in the present collective. A literature review is reported by Canavero in 2002 and 2007 (37,38). Recently Brown et Pilitsis (43) reported the results of a prospective series of 10 patients with central and neuropathic facial pain. In eight of ten cases (80%), all patients with trigeminal neuropathic pain, implantation of the stimulation device after successful trial was performed. Of the two patients without positive effect there was one case of central pain after lateral medullary infarction and one with pain of unknown origin. Positive effect of the MCS was also evaluated in three patients with improvement of facial weakness and sensory impairment and in one case dysarthria improved. All patients with implanted devices were able to reduce daily pain medication by more than 50%.

In 2005 Nuti et al (44) published the results of their patient sample with 31 patients and PSP or SCI. A positive effect and pain relief was evaluated in 16 patients and it was stated that efficacy of MCS may be predicted in the first month of therapy. Less impressive were the results reported by Cioni et Meglio (4). Only 2/14 patients experienced pain relief by chronic MCS. In contrast to these findings, Velasco reported positive effects of MCS in 8/11 patients with unilateral neuropathic pain of different origin in a randomized double-blind trial with postoperative follow-up of 12 months (26).

Direct stimulation of the cortical surface by implantation of the lead within the central sulcus and on the precentral gyrus was performed by Hosomi et al. (45). Out of a collective of 34 patients 12 responded well to MCS. In detail, 10/12 patients experienced pain relief by direct stimulation within the central sulcus and in 4/10 patients positive effects maintained at follow-ups. The efficacy of direct lead positioning and electrical stimulation within the central sulcus needs to be evaluated and compared with MCS in a prospective randomized trial (31,45).

When looking at the relevant publications regarding MCS and peripheral neuropathic pain different peripheral pain syndromes, including cases of mixed neuropathic and nociceptive pain, are reported. The most experiences are reported for patients with TNP, followed by pain syndromes from plexus or nerve root avulsion. Trigeminal neuropathic pain (TNP) is one of the main indications for MCS. Totally about 60 patients are reported in retrospective studies and three prospective trials. More than 50% of these patients are positive responders to MCS and constant pain reduction of more than 50% of the VAS is achieved, even in long term follow-up. This may be due to the very good representation of the facial area on the motor strip. In 1993 Meyerson et al (10) reported the first results of MCS in nine patients with TNP. A positive effect and implantation of the neurostimulator was described in 8/9 patients with a follow-up of 8-40 months. Ebel et al. (41) were able to show that in 6/7 patients with TNP an initial positive effect was achieved, but long term follow-up up to 24 months revealed that 3/6 patients documented pain relief of >50%. Nguyen et al. (24) published a series with 12 patients and pain relief by MCS in 7 cases (58%). The results of a prospective series of 6 patients with neuropathic facial pain were reported by Brown et Pilitsis (46). In four patients with TNP and two patients with postherpetic neuralgia, implantation of the stimulation device after a successful trial was performed.

Concerning BPA only about 20 patients are reported. The first published patients by Mertens et al. (42) suffered from chronic posttraumatic pain following brachial plexus avulsion. In 4 cases a subdural or epidural lead was placed over the motor area of the upper limb and 2 patients were screened to achieve pain reduction by stimulation during a follow-up of about two years. The largest collective was reported by Hosomi et al (45) with seven patients suffering from chronic pain following brachial plexus avulsion. In 6/7 patients a permanent neurostimulator was implanted. Pain reduction of the remaining patients varied from 10 to 90%. After a follow-up from 9-112 months the lead was removed in 2 cases and one patient died after 36 months due to a cerebral haemorrhage. Only in one case the pain reduction achieved by subdural stimulation of the precentral gyrus was stable with 50% over a follow-up of 50 months. In all other cases the effect diminished over time.

Until now about 14 patients with phantom limb pain and MCS are reported. Two out of three patients published by Carroll et al. (39) showed a benefit by MCS in phantom limb pain. Saitoh et al (47,48) reported two patients with phantom limb pain and lasting positive effect over 6-20 months. In 2001 Katayama et al (49) published five cases, but only one patient improved by this therapy with a follow-up of more than 24 months. Four patients are reported in the patient series of Hosomi et al (45). Only in one patient a stable pain reduction of 90% was achieved for 54 months. In the remaining three patients the system was removed during the first six postoperative months.

Only a small number of cases with chronic postherpetic pain are published. Recently Velasco et al (26) reported five patients with postherpetic neuralgia in a prospective randomized double-blind trial. The pain distribution involved was cervical in two patients, the thoracic spine in two patients and only in one patient the first branch of the trigeminal nerve was affected. Two patients with postherpetic neuralgia of the spine and one with trigeminal pain improved by MCS and pain reduction of 56-80% were achieved. The positive effect was stable over the follow-up period of one year.

In contrast to other centres the burr hole technique with epidural spacing for positioning of one or two leads was used in 30/33 patients in our series. Only in three cases a craniotomy was performed to place the paddle shaped octapolar lead. A small craniotomy over the central sulcus is the preferred technique in other centres. In our series no intra- or postoperative bleeding could be observed in routine cranial CT-scan on the first postoperative day.

In all patients the lead was placed over the convexity of the precentral gyrus running with the motor area from medially to laterally. This is in contrast to other centres and different possibilities to position one or more sub- or epidural leads in various orientations (24,26,31,42,45,50,51). FMRI-studies revealed that the localisation of the cortical motor area can vary (52-54) and the correct or ideal place of stimulation is still a matter of debate (22,31,33,35).

Most of the published series represent a very inhomogeneous and mixed collective of pain patients. Also some cases of rare pain syndromes including both neuropathic and nociceptive pain were reported (e. g. stumb pain, neuroma, scleroder etc.) with different results (34,55). From these individual case reports no general conclusions can be drawn.

Additionally, in most of the clinical trials no information is given if placebo or double blind testing was conducted. Therefore it can be assumed that in many studies no double blind testing phase was performed.

The scientific and clinical evidence of MCS in chronic pain treatment is insufficient. Only three prospective studies were found. In 2005 Brown et Pilitsis (46) reported 10 patients with neuropathic pain treated by MCS. In eight patients a permanent neurostimulator was implanted after a successful test-trial. Another prospective study was reported by Velasco et al (26). Again 10 patients with different chronic pain syndromes were treated with MCS. In eight of the ten patients pain reduction was achieved. Randomization procedure to "ON" or "OFF" stimulation was performed at day 60 or 90 after permanent implantation in a double-blinded fashion. It was demonstrated that randomization to "OFF" stimulation lead to significant increase of pain ($p<.05$) and that significant improvement of pain was induced by MCS ($p<.01$).

In synopsis the evidence classification, according to the guidelines of the EFNS, of the published studies and case-reports for cortical stimulation in chronic pain syndromes is only level IV and no level of recommendation can be performed (56).

Conclusions

MCS is an alternative invasive procedure for a selected patient group with chronic peripheral neuropathic pain. Well located neuropathic pain syndromes after nerve injury, like in cases with TNP, seem to respond more favourable than pain syndromes after lesion of the central pain pathways itself, like in patients with PSP. The authors patient sample showed that in PSP an initial success rate of 33% (4/12), TNP of 59% (10/17) and in BPA 100% (4/4) was achieved. Long-term follow-up with pain reduction of at least 30% or more was achieved in 2/4, 8/10, respectively 3/4 patients.

Indications for MCS, site of stimulation and standard protocols with defined stimulation parameters should be evaluated for routine clinical use. MCS should be performed in an experienced centre of neurosurgical pain therapy following a standardized protocol including double blinded or placebo testing. Undoubtedly, there is a urgent need for a prospective randomized controlled trials of the experienced centres to gain a level of evidence and recommendations for the significance of MCS as an invasive pain therapy.

Acknowledgments

This study was in part sponsored by the German Research Network on Neuropathic Pain (GNNP), granted by the German Ministry of Education and Research (BMBF), C 2.1.1; 01 EM 01 05 to VT.

References

[1] Penfield W, Rasmussen T. The cerebral cortex of man. New York: Macmillan 1950.
[2] Arle JE, Apetauerova D, Zani J, Vedran Deletis D, Penney DL, Hoit D, Gould C, Shils JL. Motor cortex stimulation in patients with Parkinson disease: 12-months follow-up in 4 patients. J Neurosurg 2008;109:133-9.
[3] Arle JE, Shils JL. Motor cortex stimulation for pain and movement disorders. Neurotherapeutics 2008;5(1):37-49.
[4] Cioni B, Megglio M. Motor cortex stimulation for chronic non-malignant pain: current state and future prospects. Acta Neurochir Suppl 2007;97(2):45-9.
[5] Friedland DR, Gaggl W, Runge-Samuelson C, Ulmer JL, Kopell BH. Feasibility of auditory cortical stimulation for the treatment of tinnitus. Otol Neurotol 2007;28:1005-12.
[6] Lima MC, Fregni F. Motor cortex stimulation for chronic pain: systematic review and meta-analysis of the literature. Neurology 2008;70:2329-37.
[7] Nguyen JP, Pollin B, Feve A, Geny C, Cesaro P. Improvement of action tremor by chronic cortical stimulation. Mov Disord 1998;13:84-8.
[8] Tsubokawa T, Katayama Y, Yamamoto T, Hirayama T, Koyama S. Chronic motor cortex stimulation for the treatment of central pain. Acta Neurochirur (Wien) Suppl 1991;52:137-9.
[9] Tsubokawa T, Katayama Y, Yamamoto T, Hirayama T, Koyama S. Chronic motor cortex stimulation in patients with thalamic pain. J Neurosurg 1993;78:393-401.
[10] Meyerson BA, Lindblom U, Linderoth B, Lind G, Herregodts P. Motor cortex stimulation as treatment of trigeminal neuropathic pain. Acta Neurochir (Wien) Suppl 1993;58:150-3.
[11] Olesen J, Bousser MG, Diener HC, Dodick D, First M, el al. Headache classification committee of the international headache society. The international classification of headache disorders, 2nd ed. Cephalalgia 2004;24(s1):126-35.
[12] Starafella AP, Vanderwerf Y, Sadikot AF. Transcranial magnetic stimulation of the human motor cortex influences the neuronal activity of subthalamic nucleus. Eur J Neurosci 2004;20:2245-9.
[13] Nguyen JP, Lefaucheur JP, Le Guerinel C, Fontanine D, Nakano N, et al. Treatment of central and neuropathic facial pain by chronic stimulation of the motor cortex: value of neuronavigation guidance for the localization of the motor cortex. Neurochirurgie 2000;46:483-91.
[14] Peyron R, Laurent B, Garcia-Larrea L. Functional imaging of brain responses to pain. A review and analysis. Neurophysiol Clin 2000;30:263-88.
[15] Pirotte B, Voordecker P, Neugroschl C, Baleriaux D, Wikler D, et al. Combination of functional magnetic resonance imaging-guided neuronavigation and intraoperative cortical brain mapping improves targeting of motor cortex stimulation in neuropathic pain. Neurosurgery 2005;56(ONS Suppl 2):344-59.
[16] Rao SM, Binder JR, Hammeke TA, Bandettini PA, Bobholz JA, et al. Somatotopic mapping of the human primary motor cortex with functional magnetic resonance imaging. Neurology 1995;45:919-24.
[17] Sol JC, Casaux J, Roux FE, Lotterie JA, Bousquet P, et al. Chronic motor cortex stimulation for phantom limb pain: correlations between pain relief and functional imaging studies. Stereotact Funct Neurosurg 2001;77:172-6.
[18] Stippich C, Ochmann H, Sartor K. Somatotopic mapping of the human primary sensorimotor cortex during motor imagery and motor execution by functional magnetic resonance imaging. Neurosci Lett 2002;331:50-4.
[19] Stippich C, Romanowski A, Nennig E, Kress B, Hähnel S, Sartor K. Fully automated localization of the human primary somatosensory cortex in one minute by functional magnetic resonance imaging. Neurosci Lett 2004;364:90-3.
[20] Tirakotai W, Riegel T, Sure U, Rohlfs J, Gharabaghi A, Bertalanffy H, Hellwig D. Image-guided motor cortex stimulation in patients with central pain. Minim Invas Neurosurg 2004;47:273-7.

[21] Rasche D, Ruppolt M, Stippich C, Unterberg A, Tronnier VM. Motor cortex stimulation for long-term relief of chronic neuropathic pain: a 10-year experience. Pain 2006;121:43-52.
[22] Cioni B, Meglio M, Perotti V, De Bonis P, Montano N. Neurophysiological aspects of chronic motor cortex stimulation. Neurophysiol Clin 2007;37(6):441-7.
[23] King RB, Schnell GR. Cortical localisation and monitoring during cerebral operations. J Neurosurg 1987;67:210-9.
[24] Nguyen JP, Lefaucheur JP, Decp P, Uchiyama T, Carpentier A, et al. Chronic motor cortex stimulation in the treatment of central and neuropathic pain. Correlations between clinical, electrophysiological and anatomical data. Pain 1999;82:245-51.
[25] Velasco M, Velasco F, Brito F, Velasco AL, Nguyen JP, et al. Motor cortex stimulation in the treatment of deafferentation pain. I. Localisation of the motor cortex. Stereotact Funct Neurosurg 2002;79:146-67.
[26] Velasco F, Argüelles C, Carillo-Ruiz JD, Castro G, Velasco AL, Jiménez F, Velasco M: Efficacy of motor cortex stimulation in the treatment of neuropathic pain: a randomized double-blind trial. J Neurosurg 2008;108:698-706.
[27] Wood CC, Spencer DD, Allison T, McCarthy G, Williamson PD, Goff WR. Localization of human sensorimotor cortex during surgery by cortical surface recording of somatosensory evoked potentials. J Neurosurg 1998;68:99-111.
[28] Garcia-Larrea L, Peyron R, Mertens P, Gregoire MC, Lavenne F, et al. Positron emission tomography during motor cortex stimulation for pain control. Stereotact Funct Neurosurg 1997;68:141-8.
[29] Garcia-Larrea L, Peyron R, Mertens P, Gregoire MC, Lavenne F, et al. Electrical stimulation of motor cortex for pain control: a combined PET-scan and electrophysiological study. Pain 1999;83:259-73.
[30] Garcia-Larrea L, Peyron R, Mertens P, Laurent B, Mauguiere F, Sindou M. Functional imaging and neurophysiological assessment of spinal and brain therapeutic modulation in humans. Arch Med Res 2000;31:248-57.
[31] Delavallée M, Abu-Serieh B, de Touchaninoff M, Raftopoulos C. Subdural motor cortex stimulation for central and peripheral neuropathic pain: a long-term follow-up study in a series of eight patients. Neurosurgery 2008;63:101-8.
[32] Fukaya C, Katayama Y, Yamamoto T, Kobayashi K, Kasai M, Oshima. Motor cortex stimulation in patients with post-stroke pain: conscious somatosensory response and pain control. Neurol Res 2003;25(2):153-6.
[33] Holsheimer J, Nguyen JP, Lefaucheur JP, Manola L. Cathodal, anodal or bifocal stimulation of the motor cortex in the management of chronic pain? Acta Neurochir Suppl 2007;97(2):57-66.
[34] Kuroda R, Yamada Y, Kondo S. Electrical stimulation of the second somatosensory cortex for intractable pain: a case report and experimental study. Stereotact Funct Neurosurg 2000;74:226.
[35] Pirotte B, Voordecker P, Brotchi J, Levivier M. Anatomical and physiological basis, clinical and surgical considerations, mechanisms underlying efficacy and future prospects of cortical stimulation for pain. Acta Neurochir Suppl 2007;97(2):81-9.
[36] Rainov NG, Heidecke V. Motor cortex stimulation for neuropathic facial pain. Neurol Res 2003;25:157-61.
[37] Canavero S, Bonicalzi V. Therapeutic extradural cortical stimulation for central and neuropathic pain: a review. Clin Journal Pain 2002;18:48-55.
[38] Canavero S, Bonicalzi V. Extradural cortical stimulation for central pain. Acta Neurochir Suppl 2007;97(2):27-36.
[39] Carroll D, Joint C, Maartens N, Shlugman D, Stein J, Aziz TZ. Motor cortex stimulation for chronic neuropathic pain: a preliminary study of 10 cases. Pain 2000;84:431-7.
[40] Yamamoto T, Katayama Y, Hirayama T, Tsubokawa T. Pharmacological classification of central post-stroke pain: comparison with the results of chronic motor cortex stimulation therapy. Pain 1997;72:5-12.

[41] Ebel H, Rust D, Tronnier V, Spies EH, Böker D, Kunze S. Chronic precentral stimulation in trigeminal neuropathic pain. Acta Neurochir 1996;138:1300-6.
[42] Mertens P, Nuti C, Sindou M, Guenot M, Peyron R, Garcia-Larrea L, Laurent B. Precentral cortex stimulation for the treatment of central neuropathic pain: results of a prospective study in a 20-patients series. Stereotact Funct Neurosurg 1999;73:122-5.
[43] Brown JA, Barbaro NM. Motor cortex stimulation for central and neuropathic pain: current status. Pain 2003;104:431-5.
[44] Nuti C, Peyron R, Garcia-Larrea L, Brunon J, Laurent B, Sindou M, Mertens P. Motor cortex stimulation for refractory neuropathic pain: four year outcome and predictors of efficacy. Pain 2005;118:43-52.
[45] Hosomi K, Saitoh Y, Kishima H, Oshino S, Hirata M, Tani N, Shimokawa T, Yoshimine T. Electrical stimulation of primary motor cortex within central sulcus for intractable neuropathic pain. Clin Neurophysiol 2008;119:993-1001.
[46] Brown JA, Pilitsis JG. Motor cortex stimulation for central and neuropathic facial pain: a prospective study of 10 patients and observations of enhanced sensory and motor function during stimulation. Neurosurgery 2005;56:290-7.
[47] Saitoh Y, Shibata M, Hirano SI, Hirata M, Moshimo T, Yoshimine T. Motor cortex stimulation for central and peripheral deafferentation pain. J Neurosurg 2000;92:150-5.
[48] Saitoh Y, Shibata M, Hirano SI, Kato A, Kishima H, Hirata M, Yamamoto K, Yoshimine T. Motor cortex stimulation for deafferentation pain. Neurosurg Focus 2001;11:1-5.
[49] Katayama Y, Yamamoto T, Kobayashi K, Kasai M, Oshima H, Fukaya C. Motor cortex stimulation for phantom limb pain: a comprehensive therapy with spinal cord and thalamic stimulation. Sterotact Funct Neurosurg 2001;77:159-61.
[50] Gharabaghi A, Hellwig D, Rosahl SK, Shahidi R, Schrader C, Freund HJ, Samii M. Volumetric image guidance for motor cortex stimulation: integration of three-dimensional cortical anatomy and functional imaging. Neurosurgery 2005;57(ONS Suppl 1):114-20.
[51] Lazorthes Y, Sol JC, Fowo S, Roux FE, Verdié JC. Motor cortex stimulation for neuropathic pain. Acta Neurochir Suppl 2007;97(2):37-44.
[52] Flor H, Elbert T, Mühlnickel W, Pantev C, Wienbruch C, Taub E. Cortical reorganization and phantom phenomena in congenital and traumatic upper-extremity amputees. Exp Brain Res 1998;119:205-12.
[53] Karl A, Birbaumer N, Lutzenberger W, Cohen LG, Flor H. Reorganization of motor and somatosensory cortex in upper extremity amputees with phantom limb pain. J Neurosci 2001;21:3609-18.
[54] Tinazzi M, Valeriani M, Moretto G, Rosso T, Nicolato A, Fiaschi A, Aglioti SM. Plastic interactions between hand and face cortical representation in patients with trigeminal neuralgia: a somatosensory-evoked potentials study. Neuroscience 2004;127:769-76.
[55] Lefaucheur JP, Drouot X, Menard-Lefaucheur I, Keravel Y, Nguyen JP. Motor cortex rTMS in chronic neuropathic pain: pain relief is associated with thermal sensory perception improvement. J Neurol Neurosurg Psychiatry 2008;79(9):1044-9.
[56] Brainin M, Barnes M, Baron JC, Gilhus NE, Hughes R, Selmaj K, Waldemar G. Guidance for the preparation of neurological management guidelines by EFNS scientific task forces – revised recommendations 2004. Eur J Neurol 2004;11:577-81.
[57] Henderson JM, Lad SP. Motor cortex stimulation and neuropathic facial pain. Neurosurg Focus 2006;21:E6.
[58] Osenbach RK. Motor cortex stimulation for intractable pain. Neurosurg Focus 2006;21:E7.
[59] Saitoh Y, Yoshimine T. Stimulation of primary motor cortex for intractable deafferentation pain. Acta Neurochir Suppl 2007;97(2):51-6.

In: Pain Management Yearbook 2009
Editor: Joav Merrick

ISBN: 978-1-61209-666-7
©2012 Nova Science Publishers, Inc.

Chapter 33

ELECTRICAL STIMULATION OF PRIMARY MOTOR CORTEX FOR INTRACTABLE NEUROPATHIC DEAFFERENTATION PAIN

*Youichi Saitoh, MD, PhD**

Department of Neurosurgery, Osaka University Graduate School of Medicine, Osaka, Japan

Abstract

The electrical stimulation of the primary motor cortex (M1) has proved to be an effective treatment for intractable neuropathic pain. This treatment started in 1990, and around thirty studies have been reported. The patients who have been operated were suffering from central post-stroke pain (59%), trigeminal neuropathic pain (17%), brachial plexus injury, spinal cord injury, peripheral nerve injury and phantom-limb pain. The method of stimulation was a) epidural, b) subdural and c) within the central sulcus. The mostly reported cases showed epidural implantation of the electrode, a few reports subdural. There has been only one report of the electrode implant within the central sulcus. Overall, considering the difficulty in treating central neuropathic pain, trigeminal neuropathic pain and certain types of refractory peripheral pain, the electrical stimulation of M1 is a promising technique, but still the success rate has not been satisfactory. It is very interesting that the electrode implant within the central sulcus remarkably reduced intractable pain temporally. The mechanism of pain relief has been under investigation. Recently, repetitive transcranial magnetic stimulation (rTMS) of M1 has been reported to be effective on neuropathic pain. In the future, rTMS may compete with the electrical stimulation in the treatment of intractable neuropathic pain.

Keywords: Motor cortex stimulation, primary motor cortex, repetitive transcranial magnetic stimulation (rTMS), deafferentation pain, neuropathic pain.

Introduction

Neuropathic pains including deafferentation pains are one of the most difficult types of pain to treat and are usually medically refractory. In 1990, Tsubokawa et al (1) found the pain reduction by motor cortex stimulation (MCS) in the patients with central post-stroke pain (CPSP). In 1993, pain due to the trigeminal peripheral legion was successfully treated with MCS (2). Phantom limb pain and brachial plexus injuries also responded to MCS well. MCS can provide pain relief in 50-75% of patients with neuropathic pains (2-6).

Around thirty studies have been reported from Japan (7-9), France (4,10-12), Belgium (13,14), USA (15,16), Sweden (2), United Kingdom (17), Germany (18-21), Italy (22,23) and Mexico (24). All but one trial followed an open methodology and no controlled double blind study had been performed. In 2008, Velasco et al (24) performed randomized double-blind trial in 11 cases with various neuropathic pains and evaluated the efficacy of MCS. Several indications have been studied covering most neuropathic pains, but one is clearly far ahead from all others: CPSP (59% of all published cases) followed by trigeminal neuropathic pain (17%). All other indications represent less than 10% each (25).There are several surgical procedures for MCS. Most neurosurgeons implant an electrode (Resume, Medtronic Inc., Minneapolis. MN, USA, Lamitrode, ANS, Plano TX, USA) in the epidural space, but some implant it in the subdural or interhemispheric or within the central sulcus. The location and direction of the implanted Resume remains controversial. In this report, MCS, especially surgical procedures will be summarized.

Pharmacological tests

To clarify pathophysiological mechanisms and for patient choice, pharmacological tests, or drug challenge tests (DCT) have been done in two institutes. One study employed 39 CPSP patients who had intractable hemibody pain with dysesthesias. The correlation between the pharmacological characteristics and the effects of MCS therapy was examined. Yamamoto et al (26) reported that thiopental- and ketamine-responsive and morphine-resistant patients displayed long-lasting pain reduction with long-term use of MCS. Their DCT showed that definite pain reduction occurred in 20% by the morphine test, 56% by thiopental test, and 48% by the ketamine test. Based on these DCT's assessments, there was no obvious difference between thalamic (n=25) and suprathalamic pain (n=14) (26).

Saitoh et al (27) performed DCT including thiopental, ketamine, phentolamine, lidocaine, morphine, and placebo in 18 cases. Of the 18 cases in the DCT, eight cases scoring with "excellent" or "good" pain relief using the MCS were found to have sensitivities to morphine (n=¬5), ketamine (n=4), thiopental (n=4) or lidocaine (n=3). The other 10 cases scoring "fair" or "poor" pain relief had morphine (n=4) or thiopental (n=2) sensitivities. No relationship was found between morphine sensitivity and pain relief with the MCS, and none of the patients was found to be sensitive to phentolamine. Some of the excellent MCS responder did not respond to any drug. They concluded that ketamine might be an useful drug for patient selection (27).

Patients

The most common disease is CPSP, which is the most difficult to treat in general. The other reported cases included brachial plexus injury, spinal cord injury, trigeminal neuropathic pain, peripheral nerve injury, phantom limb pain. All reported cases had a severe neuropathic pain history, two thirds central and one third peripheral neuropathic pain (25).

Surgical methods

All the implanted quadripolar electrodes used in reported studies have been Resumes made by Medtronics or Lamitrode by ANS. Eight electrodes with a Synergy neurostimulator were used in a clinical trial in Europe (NCT00122915). However, this trial has been suspended. The electric current delivered by Synergy to eight electrodes has been used for spinal cord stimulation. Tsubokawa (1) was the first to implant the electrode in the epidural space, and since then most neurosurgeons have used the epidural method. Saitoh et al (9) and Nuti et al (28) used subdural implantation of the electrode. If the painful area is large, two electrodes are used. Finally, some neurosurgeons have used grid electrodes to measure SEP and perform test stimulations. The anatomical landmarks and neurophysiological methods of MCS were summarized previously (29,30).

While both epidural and subdural methods are in use, the former is more popular (6,30). A small craniotomy or burr-hole was made around the central sulcus (1,7). The four-plate electrodes (5 mm in diameter; center of each electrode is 1 cm in distance) is usually placed in the epidural space. The best location and orientation of the electrode array are, therefore generally determined in such a way that bipolar stimulation with an appropriate pair of electrodes can be attained. Nguyen et al's report (31) deals with navigational craniotomy and implantation of the electrode in the epidural space, which they placed perpendicular to the central sulcus in a parietal-to-frontal direction. Tsubokawa (1) and Katayama (7) reported that there were no polarity-related differences in pain relief for most patients with the epidural implantation of the electrode.

Saitoh et al (9) used a subdural implant (cerebral surface and interhemispheric surface) or implantation of the Resume within the central sulcus. The latter seems to be more effective than the former because this method makes it possible to stimulate the primary motor cortex more directly (32,33) (see figure 1). Nuti et al (28) reported using the electrode implantation on the interhemispheric surface for some cases with leg pain. In some patients with brain atrophy, however, the cortical surface and dura mater are few cm apart, so that such cases may fail to respond to stimulation.

After the implantation of test electrodes, most institutes usually perform test stimulation for a few days to two weeks. A second surgery is then performed under general anesthesia. The electrode is implanted after identification of the best location for pain relief, and an implantable pulse generator is placed subcutaneously in the chest or abdomen. At a few institutes, a single surgical procedure is used (34).

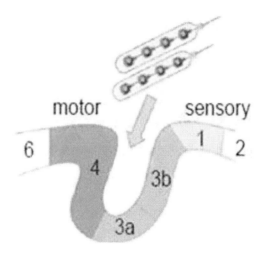

Figure 1. Structure of the central sulcus. M1 (primary motor cortex) locates within the central sulcus mainly.

Representative surgical techniques (see table 1)

Epidural single burr-hole

Tsubokawa et al (1) initiated MCS using a single burr-hole made under local anesthesia. Meyerson's procedure (2), which is very similar, involves making a burr-hole on the central sulcus, usually under local anesthesia. Some neurosurgeons make a small linear skin incision and a burr-hole by using a classical anatomical landmark, such as the Taylor-Haughton line, while others use navigation with fMRI (21). After insertion of one or two Resumes, some practitioners measure SEP by stimulating the contralateral median or tibial nerves, others have tried using MEP measurement for some patients. The Resumes are sometimes implanted perpendicular to the central sulcus above precentral and postcentral gyri (4), and sometimes parallel to the central sulcus (21,34). Tsubokawa et al (1) reported that there was no correlation between pain reduction and the directions of the Resume placement. For leg pain, they placed the Resume at the medial edge of the hemisphere, which is less invasive, but involves some risk of developing epidural hematoma. This technique may require relocations before an optimal position is found, and thus increase the risk of epidural bleeding due to dural detachment. However, this was not a problem in recent navigated procedures (21).

Two epidural burr-holes

Canavero (34) reports making an oblique linear skin incision (6-10cm) parallel to and 1 cm ahead of or behind the projection of the central sulcus and then drilling two burr holes at a distance of 2-4 cm. A Resume is inserted from the edge of one burr hole into the epidural space overlying the precentral gyrus or post central gyrus contralateral to the painful area. The bony bridge between the two holes will then hold the plate in place. Some authors prefer to place the Resume perpendicular to the central sulcus for because of the supposed improved selectivity of this approach, but there appears to be no difference between the results of these two approaches. For facial or leg pain, targeting of the hand area and an approach to the motor area of the face or the foot may be used by moving the electrode caudally by 20mm or rostrally by 20mm along the central sulcus.

Table 1. Representative surgical procedures of motor cortex stimulation

	Electrode placement	targeting	anesthesia	craniotomy	device
Tsubokawa et al (1)	epidural two staged	bone landmark SEP test stimulation	local	paramedian incision burr hole	Resume
Meyerson et al (2)	epidural two staged	bone landmark Scalp SEP test stimulation	local	paramedian incision burr hole	Resume
Canavero et al (34)	epidural single or two staged	bone landmark	local (without head fix)	incision parallel to CS two burr holes	Resume parallel to CS
Nguyen et al (31)	epidural two staged	navigation oblique CT/MRI SEP Muscle twitch	general	flap craniotomy 4-5 cm	Resume vertical to CS
Nuti et al (28)	epidural subdural	navigation SEP single staged	general	flap craniotomy 4-5 cm	Resume, Symix parallel to CS
Rasche et al (21)	epidural two staged	navigation bone landmark	local (head pin) SEP	incision parallel to CS burr hole	Resume parallel to CS
Saitoh et al (9)	subdural within CS two staged	surface MRI SEP	general	flap craniotomy 5 cm vertical to CS within CS	Resume

CS: central sulcus, SEP: somatosensory evoked potential, Resume: 4 array electrode made by Medtronic.

Epidural bone flap

To overcome some problems of burr holes techniques, Nguyen et al (31) made a small craniotomy (4-5 cm) on the central sulcus by using a 3D image-guided navigation system. The center of the craniotomy should correspond to the target as determined by imaging. SEP is then recorded from 16 contacts of a grid-electrodes placed on the dura mater. Test stimulation is also used as previously (mentioned under "electrophysiological localization"). The Resume is then placed perpendicular to the central sulcus and is fixed to the dura mater with two stitches.

Subdural method

In some patients with brain atrophy, the cortical surface and dura mater are a few cm apart, so that such cases may fail to respond to epidural stimulation. The subdural cortical surface and interhemispheric surfaces may be suitable candidates for more direct stimulation of the primary motor cortex. However, large bridging veins sometimes interfere with implantation on the interhemispheric surface and adhesion may occurred by subarachnoid hemorrhage. Nuti et al (28) tried implantation of the Resume on the interhemispheric surface in some painful leg cases. Saitoh et al (9) reported that the implant of an electrode within the central sulcus seemed to be more effective than the epidural implant because their approach makes it possible to stimulate the primary motor cortex more directly (32,33). For upper limb and/or face pain, the arachnoid membrane of the central sulcus was carefully dissected and the vessels within the central sulcus were freed with a microsurgical procedure to expose the hidden lateral walls of the precentral and postcentral gyri. Since the Resume is too stiff to be placed within the central sulcus, it was trimmed off to reduce stiffness (see figure 2). Saitoh et al (9) limited most of the implantations within the central sulcus to the patients with severe motor weakness or lack of function. In their series, test stimulation of the primary motor cortex within the central sulcus was more effective in most cases than was subdural stimulation on the cerebral surface. Interestingly, the patients who received the Resume implantation within the central sulcus gained only temporary pain reduction at longest six months. The dissection of the central sulcus may constitute a key factor in the development of chronic refractory pains. Of course, dissection of the central sulcus may also involve the risk of developing new neurological deficits due to brain damage or vein obstruction. Their results indicate that long-term pain reduction was not significantly superior to other reports. Pain reduction resulting from MCS and Resume implantation within the central sulcus will therefore have to be either considered as a truly important technique or not omitted from consideration because of its dubious advantages and major risks.

Results of motor cortex stimulation

Globally, considering the difficulty to treat central neuropathic pain, trigeminal neuropathic pain and some refractory peripheral pain, MCS is a very promising technique with nearly 60% of the patients treated improved (>50% pain relief) after several months follow up (sometimes a few years) in most reports. Considering the numbers of cases published and outcomes, CPSP and trigeminal neuropathic pain are the only indications with significant results to be considered as validated for MCS (25).

This important number of patients with CPSP can be explained by two factors: CPSP is the biggest number of the patients with neuropathic pain and therapeutic possibilities are very limited. The numbers are more limited for trigeminal neuropathic pain but the results are excellent and very consistent for most teams with more than 70% of responders (2,13,18,31). Other central pains and traumatic spinal cord injury have promising outcomes but more cases are needed to assess more precisely the efficacy of MCS.

Brachial plexus avulsion does not seem to respond very well (less than 50% of responders) (12,15,27,31), results for phantom pain (9,17,27,37) are better but vary from one report to another, too few cases to draw any conclusions. For peripheral nerve injury (SCS failure), results are excellent (2,17). If those excellent results were confirmed the therapeutic strategy between SCS and MCS should be discussed.

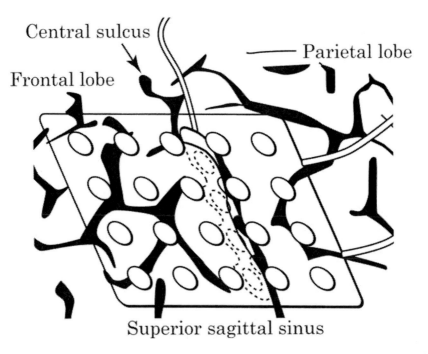

Figure 2A. The Resume was trimmed off to reduce its stiffness and implanted within the central sulcus. Grid electrodes cover the precentral and postcentral gyri. This figure has been copied from Clin Neurophysiol (9).

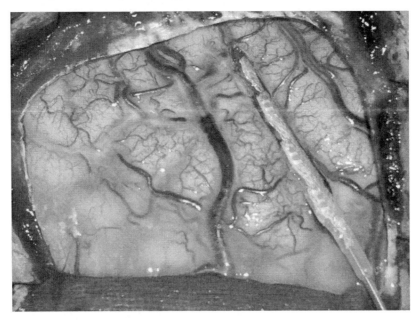

Figure 2B. This photograph indicates the implanted Resume within the central sulcus. The Resume is trimmed off.

More studies with more rigorous methodology are needed to validate some of the indications. rTMS trial have potential anticipating the effectiveness of the MCS in the treatment of neuropathic pain (9,37,38). Hosomi et al reported that there is good correlation between MCS efficacy and that of rTMS (see figure3).

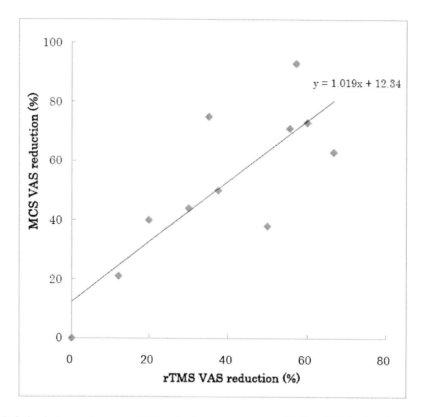

Figure 3. Relation between short-term VAS reduction in response to rTMS and MCS. Simple linea regression indicated that the pain reduction in response to rTMS contributed to that in response to MCS on test stimulation or discgarge (p=0.0021).

Usually intermittent MCS stimulations were performed mainly because of seizure risk. The pain relief with MCS was temporally. The longest MCS effect was 24 hours with 30 minutes' stimulation. Some patients showed pain relief for only about one hour after stimulation. In general, the obtained pain relief with MCS was 3-5 hours (5). A report showed continuous MCS but there was no convulsion (21). Some cases showed decrease of the MCS effectiveness after implantation, however, the reason of decrease has been unknown.

Stimulation parameters were usually relatively low frequency (25-50Hz). The impedance was between 900 and 1500 ohm. The amplitude was subthreshold of inducing muscle twitch.

Complications

Occurrence of epileptic seizures, probably due to differences in testing conditions, has been reported during test stimulation (25). Paresthesia, dysesthesia and chronic contraction during test stimulation are more common than epileptic seizures. Speech disorders, although rare, have also been observed. The low rate of epileptic seizures during chronic stimulation (0.7%) means that stimulation of the primary motor cortex within an appropriate range of parameters is reasonably safe. Paresthesia and dysesthesia have been documented in a small percentage (2.2%) of published cases, while overall, 11.4% was associated with one or more adverse effects. The most serious reported complications are epidural or subdural hematoma, epileptic seizures, and aphasia or dysphasia, which altogether represent 3.6% of the reported cases. A larger craniotomy should reduce the risk of epidural or subdural hematoma and its consequences because it allows for better visual control of the electrode, makes the accidental removal of the grid or four electrode array less likely, and reduces the risk of inadvertent opening of the dura (5,9,28). The risk of peri-operative hemorrhage is also lower compared to deep brain stimulation.

Some wound infections have been reported by most institutes (6). If the infection occurs, all devices including the electrode, extension leads, and pulse generators must be removed temporally. Patients with CPSP frequently have diabetes mellitus, and thus easily develop wound infection.

Some cases of headache reportedly associated with stimulation of the face area may actually be due to contraction of the temporalis muscle (34).

In one study (9), major adverse effects occurred during a long follow-up of the two patients who developed cerebral hemorrhage: one died and the other remained in a vegetative state. However, neither of these complications can be linked to the MCS procedure itself or to chronic stimulation, but are more closely related to the medical history of the patients. This is especially true for patients with CPSP. It has already been demonstrated that stroke patients are likely to develop a second stroke in the years following the first stroke. In another study, one patient developed a speech arrest for three months postoperatively but made a complete recovery (18).

The MCS implanted patients cannot receive MRI because MRI wracks stimulators. Probably some patients with MCS system complained of the contraindication of MRI.

Pain relief mechanism with MCS

Tsubokawa et al suggested that activation of hypothetical sensory neurons by means of MCS might inhibit deafferentation nociceptive neurons within the cortex in patients with central deafferentation pain (1). The mechanism of peripheral deafferentation pain such as phantom-limb pain is unknown, however, both hyperactivity of peripheral nerves and sensitization of spinal neurons may play a part (39,40).

So far, some PET studies using O15-labeled water have been published about MCS. There was no significant change in rCBF in the right primary sensory cortex and the primary motor cortex close to the stimulation position (41-43). Therefore, it was speculated that MCS does not stimulate either of these cortices directly and reduce pain. Tsubokawa's hypothesis is that MCS activates non-nociceptive fourth-order sensory neurons, which in turn inhibit hyperactive nociceptive neurons in sensory cortex. However, no significant changes were induced in the parietal cortex, thus indicating that the sensory cortex is probably not the key structure in MCS-induced pain reduction. A model of MCS action is proposed by Garcia-Larrea et al (44), whereby activation of thalamic nuclei directly connected with motor and premotor cortices would entail a cascade of synaptic events in pain-related structures receiving afferents from these nuclei, including the medial thalamus, anterior cingulate and upper brainstem. MCS could influence the affective-emotional component of chronic pain by way of cingulate/orbitofrontal activation (41,43,44), and lead to descending inhibition of pain impulses by activation of the brainstem, also suggested by attenuation of spinal flexion reflexes (44).

Ipsilateral thalamic hypometabolism has been reported in cases of central pain. Increased rCBF demonstrated on PET scanning indicates increased synaptic activity, which can subserve either excitatory or inhibitory mechanisms. Thalamic CBF changes may reflect the activation of inhibitory processes, which is in line with animal studies showing that pathologically hyperactive thalamic neurons are inhibited by MCS (45).

The mechanism of deafferentation pain and that of MCS have been still under investigation, and will be solved in the near future.

rTMS (repetitive transcranial magnetic stimulation)

Recently rTMS has been applied as a treatment method for psychiatric and neuro-degenerative diseases such as depression (46), dystonia (47), schizophrenia, Parkinson's disease, seizures and so on (48). Based on experiences with MCS, rTMS is now beginning to be applied to cases of intractable deafferentation pain (36,49,50).

Hirayama et al (50) applied rTMS precisely to primary motor cortex with using navigation-guided figure-of-eight coil. Effective treatment was defined as a VAS improvement of more than 30%. Ten of 20 patients (50%) showed significant reductions in pain on the VAS with the stimulation of primary motor cortex. Five Hz stimulation of M1 was able to reduce intractable deafferentation pain in approximately one out of two patients. The pain reduction continued significantly for three hours. Saitoh et al (51) reported that the neuropathic pain caused by spinal cord and peripheral nerve injuries showed more response to rTMS than that caused by CPSP. They also reported that 5 or 10 Hz stimulation of M1 reduced neuropathic pain but 1 Hz failed. Lefaucheur et al (36) reported that 10 Hz rTMS of motor cortex was found to result in a significant but transient relief of chronic pain, influenced by pain origin and pain site. The factors most favorable for rTMS treatment are a trigeminal nerve lesion and the presence of sensation in the painful zone. The factors least favorable are brain stem stroke, limb pain, and severe sensory loss. And some other reports supported the effectiveness of rTMS on pain (52).

Today, rTMS may be a good predictor of MCS efficacy, and thus, Saitoh et al consider that MCS can be recommended to the patients with good results of rTMS (9). Goto et al reported that tractography by MRI diffusion tensor image may predict the responsibility of CPSP to rTMS therapy (53). Preservation of motor and sensory fibers predicts the efficacy of rTMS of M1 for neuropathic pain. Probably the patients with well preserved motor and sensory fibers in MRI tractography also respond to MCS therapy.

Conclusions

MCS is effective therapy of intractable neuropathic pain, but the effective rate is still not satisfactory. It is very interesting evidence that the dissection of the central sulcus remarkably reduced the intractable pain temporally. We have to clarify its mechanism. In the near future, MCS may compete with rTMS as the pole-position of the stimulation therapy for intractable pains. I wish that new technologies will offer the innovative methods.

References

[1] Tsubokawa T, Katayama Y, Yamamoto T, Hirayama T, Koyama S. Chronic motor cortex stimulation in patients with thalamic pain. J Neurosurg 1993;78:393-401.
[2] Meyerson BA, Lindblom U, Linderoth B, Lind G, Herregodts P. Motor cortex stimulation as treatment of trigeminal neuropathic pain. Acta Neurochir (S) 1993;58:150-3.
[3] Katayama Y, Yamamoto T, Kobayashi K, Oshima H, Fukaya C. Deep brain and motor cortex stimulation for post-stroke movement disorders and post-stroke pain. Acta Neurochir (S) 2003;87:121-3.
[4] Nguyen JP, Keravel Y, Feve A, Uchiyama T, Cesaro P, Le Guerinel C, et al. Treatment of deafferentation pain by chronic stimulation of the motor cortex: report of a series of 20 cases. Acta Neurochir(S) 1997;68:54-60.
[5] Saitoh Y, Shibata M, Hirano S, Hirata M, Mashimo T, Kato A, et al. Motor cortex stimulation for central and peripheral deafferentation pain. J Neurosurg 2000;92:150-5.
[6] Canavero S, Bonicalzi V. Therapeutic extradural cortical stimulation for central and neuropathic pain: A review. Clin J Pain 2002; 18:48-55.
[7] Katayama Y, Fukaya C, Yamamoto T. Poststroke pain control by chronic motor cortex stimulation: neurological characteristics predicting a favorable response. J Neurosurg 1998;89:585-91.
[8] Katayama Y, Yamamoto T, Kobayashi K, Kasai M, Oshima H, Fukaya C. Motor cortex stimulation for post-stroke pain: comparison of spinal cord and thalamic stimulation. Stereotact Funct Neurosurg 2001;77:183-6.
[9] Hosomi K, Saitoh Y, Kishima H, Oshino S, Hirata M, Tani N, et al. Electrical stimulation of primary motor cortex within the central sulcus for intractable neuropathic pain. Clin Neurophysiol 2008; 119:993-1001.
[10] Mertens P, Nuti C, Sindou M, Guenot M, Peyron R, Garcia-Larrea L, et al. Precentral cortex stimulation for the treatment of central neuropathic pain: results of a prospective study in a 20-patient series. Stereotact Funct Neurosurg 1999;73:122-5.
[11] Peyron R, Laurent B, Garcia-Larrea L. Functional imaging of brain responses to pain. A review and meta-analysis. Neurophysiol Clin 2000;30:263-88.
[12] Sol JC, Casaux J, Roux FE, Lotterie JA, Bousquet P, Verdie JC, et al. Chronic motor cortex stimulation for phantom limb pain: correlations between pain relief and functional imaging studies. Stereotact Funct Neurosurg. 2001;77:172-6.
[13] Herregodts P, Stadnik T, De Ridder F, D'Haens J. Cortical stimulation for central neuropathic pain: 3-D surface MRI for easy determination of the motor cortex. Acta Neurochir (S) 1995;64:132-5.
[14] Pirotte B, Voordecker P, Neugroschl C, Baleriaux D, Wikler D, Metens T, et al. Combination of functional magnetic resonance imaging-guided neuronavigation and intraoperative cortical brain mapping improves targeting of motor cortex stimulation in neuropathic pain. Neurosurg 2005;56(2S):344-59.

[15] Henderson JM, Boongird A, Rosenow JM, LaPresto E, Rezai AR. Recovery of pain control by intensive reprogramming after loss of benefit from motor cortex stimulation for neuropathic pain. Stereotact Funct Neurosurg 2004;82:207-13.
[16] Hosobuchi Y. Motor cortex stimulation for control of central deafferentation pain. Electrical and magnetic stimulation of the brain and spinal cord. New York: Raven Press, 1993
[17] Carroll D, Joint C, Maartens N, Shlugman D, Stein J, Aziz TZ. Motor cortex stimulation for chronic neuropathic pain: a preliminary study of 10 cases. Pain 2000;84:431-7.
[18] Ebel H, Rust D, Tronnier V, Boker D, Kunze S. Chronic precentral stimulation in trigeminal neuropathic pain. Acta Neurochir (Wien) 1996;138:1300-6.
[19] Rainov NG, Fels C, Heidecke V, Burkert W. Epidural electrical stimulation of the motor cortex in patients with facial neuralgia. Clin Neurol Neurosurg 1997;99:205-9.
[20] Rainov NG, Heidecke V. Motor cortex stimulation for neuropathic facial pain. Neurol Res 2003;25:157-61.
[21] Rasche D, Ruppolt M, Strippich C, Unterberg A, Tronnier VM. Motor cortex stimulation for long-term relief of chronic neuropathic pain: A 10 year experience. Pain 2006;121:43-52
[22] Canavero S, Bonicalzi V. Cortical stimulation for central pain. J Neurosurg 1995;83:1117.
[23] Franzini A, Ferroli P, Servello D, Broggi G. Reversal of thalamic hand syndrome by long-term motor cortex stimulation. J Neurosurg 2000;93:873-5.
[24] Velasco F, Arguelles C, Carrillo-Ruiz JD, Castro G, Velasco AL, Jimenez F, Velasco M. Efficacy of motor cortex stimulation in the treatment of neuropathic pain: a randomized double-blind trial. J Neurosurg 2008;108:698-706.
[25] Saitoh Y, Yoshimine T. Stimulation of primary motor cortex for intractable deafferentation pain. In: DE Sakas, BA Simpson, eds. Operative neuromodulation, Vol. 2. Berlin: Springer, 2007:51-6.
[26] Yamamoto T, Katayama Y, Hirayama T, Tsubokawa T. Pharmacological classification of central post-stroke pain: comparison with the results of chronic motor cortex stimulation therapy. Pain 1997;72:5-12.
[27] Saitoh Y, Kato A, Ninomiya H, Baba T, Shibata M, Mashimo T, et al. Primary motor cortex stimulation within the central sulcus for treating deafferentation pain. Acta Neurochir (S) 2003;87:149-52.
[28] Nuti C, Peyron R, Garcia-Larrea L, Brunon J, Laurent B, Sindou M, et al. Motor cortex stimulation for refractory neuropathic pain: Four year outcome and predictors of efficacy. Pain 2005;118:43-52.
[29] Tirakotai W, Hellwig D, Bertalanffy H, Riegel T. Localization of precentral gyrus in image-guided surgery for motor cortex stimulation. Acta Neurochir (S) 2007;97: 75-9.
[30] Saitoh Y, Hosomi K. From localization to surgical implantation. In: Canavero S, ed. Textbook of therapeutic cortical stimulation. New York: Nova Science, 2009, in press.
[31] Nguyen JP, Lefaucheur JP, Decq P, Uchiyama T, Carpentier A, Fontaine D, et al. Chronic motor cortex stimulation in the treatment of central and neuropathic pain. Correlations between clinical, electrophysiological and anatomical data. Pain 1999;82:245-51.
[32] Takahashi N, Kawamura M, Araki S: Isolation hand palsy due to cortical infarction: localization of the motor hand area. Neurology 2002;58:1412-4.
[33] White LE, Andrewa TJ, Hulette C, Richards A, Groelle M, Paydarfar J, et al. Structure of the human sensorimotor system: I. Morphology and cytoarchitecture of the central sulcus. Cereb Cortex 1997; 7:18-30.
[34] Canavero S, Bonicalzi V. Extradural cortical stimulation for central pain. Acta Neurochir Suppl 2007;97:27-36.
[35] Roux FE, Ibarrola D, Tremoulet M, Lazorthes Y, Henry P, Sol JC, et al. Methodological and technical issues for integrating functional magnetic resonance imaging data in a neuronavigational system. Neurosurg 2001;49:1145-56.

[36] Lefaucheur JP, Drouot X, Menard-Lefaucheur I, Zerah F, Bendib B, Cesaro P, et al. Neurogenic pain relief by repetitive transcranial magnetic cortical stimulation depends on the origin and the site of pain. J Neurol Neurosurg Psychiatry 2004;75:612-6.
[37] Saitoh Y, Shibata M, Sanada M, Mashimo T. Motor cortex stimulation for phantom limb pain. Lancet 1999;353:212.
[38] Migita K, Uozumi T, Arita K, Monden S. Transcranial magnetic stimulation of motor cortex in patients with central pain. Neurosurg 1995;36:1037-40.
[39] Coghill RC, Sang CN, Maisog JM, Iadarola MJ,. Pain intensity processing with in the human brain: a bilateral distributed mechanism. J Neurophysiol 1999;82:1934-43.
[40] Tasker RR. Deafferentation. In: Wall PD, Melzack R, eds. Textbook of pain. Edinburgh: Churchill Livingstone, 1984:119-32.
[41] Peyron R, Garcia-Larrea L, Deiber MP, Cinotti L, Convers P, Sindou M, et al,. Electrical stimulation of precentral cortical area in the treatment of central pain: electrophysiological and PET study. Pain 1995; 62:275-86.
[42] Saitoh Y, Osaki Y, Nishimura H, Hirano S, Kato A, Hashikawa K, et al. Increased regional cerebral blood flow in the contralateral thalamus after successful motor cortex stimulation in a patient with poststroke pain. J Neurosurg 2004;100:935-9.
[43] Kishima H, Saitoh Y, OsakiY, Nishimura H, Kato A, Hatazawa J, Yoshimine T. Motor cortex stimulation activates posterior insula and thalamus in deafferentation pain patients J Neurosurg 2007;107:43-8.
[44] Garcia-Larrea L, Peyron R, Mertens P, Gregoire MC, Lavenne F, Le Bars D, et al. Electrical stimulation of motor cortex for pain control: a combined PET-scan and electrophysiological study. Pain 1999; 83:259-73.
[45] Iadarola MJ, Max MB, Berman KF, Byas-Smith MG, Coghill RC, Gracely RH, et al. Unilateral decrease in thalamic activity observed with positron emission tomography in patients with chronic neuropathic pain. Pain 1995;63:55-64.
[46] Kimbrell TA, Little JT, Dunn RT, Frye MA, Greenberg BD, Wassermann EM, et al. Frequency dependence of antidepressant response to left prefrontal repetitive transcranial magnetic stimulation (rTMS) as a function of baseline cerebral glucose metabolism. Biol Psychiatry 1999;46:1603-13.
[47] Siebner HR, Filipovic SR, Rowe JB, Cordivari C, Gerschlager W, Rothwell JC, et al. Patients with focal arm dystonia have increased sensitivity to slow-frequency repetitive TMS of the dorsal premotor cortex. Brain 2003;126:2710-25.
[48] Wassermann EM, Lisanby SH. Therapeutic application of repetitive transcranial magnetic stimulation: a review. Clin Neurophysiol 2001; 112:1367-77.
[49] Pleger B, Janssen F, Schwenkreis P, Volker B, Maier C, Tegenthoff M. Repetitive transcranial magnetic stimulation of the motor cortex attenuates pain perception in complex regional pain syndrome type I. Neurosci Lett 2004;356:87-90.
[50] Hirayama A, Saitoh Y, Kishima H, Shimokawa T, Oshino S, Hirata M, et al. Reduction of intractable deafferentation pain with navigation-guided repetitive transcranial magnetic stimulation (rTMS) of the primary motor cortex Pain 2006;122:22-7.
[51] Saitoh Y, Hirayama A, Kishima H, Shimokawa T, Oshino S, Hirata M, Tani N, Kato A, Yoshimine T. Reduction of intractable deafferentation pain due to spinal cord or peripheral lesion by high-frequency repetitive transcranial magnetic stimulation of the primary motor cortex J Neurosurg 2007;107:555-9.
[52] Tamura Y, Okabe S, Ohnishi T, Saito D, Arai N, Mochio S, et al. Effects of 1-Hz repetitive transcranial magnetic stimulation on acute pain induced by capsaicin. Pain 2004;107:107-15.
[53] Goto T, Saitoh Y, Hashimoto N, Hirata M, Kishima H, Oshino S, Naoki Tani, Hosomi K, Kakigi R, Yoshimine T. Diffusion tensor fiber tracking in patients with central post-stroke pain; Correlation with efficacy of repetitive transcranial magnetic stimulation. Pain 2008;140:509-18.

In: Pain Management Yearbook 2009
Editor: Joav Merrick

ISBN: 978-1-61209-666-7
©2012 Nova Science Publishers, Inc.

Chapter 34

BRAIN STIMULATION FOR THE TREATMENT OF PAIN: A REVIEW OF COSTS, CLINICAL EFFECTS, AND MECHANISMS OF TREATMENT FOR THREE DIFFERENT CENTRAL NEUROMODULATORY APPROACHES

Soroush Zaghi, BS, Nikolas Heine, BS and Felipe Fregni, MD, PhD[*]

Berenson-Allen Center for Noninvasive Brain Stimulation, Beth Israel Deaconess Medical Center, Harvard Medical School, Boston, United States of America

Abstract

Methods of cortical stimulation including epidural motor cortex stimulation (MCS), repetitive transcranial magnetic stimulation (rTMS), and transcranial direct current stimulation (tDCS) are emerging as alternatives in the management of pain in patients with chronic medically-refractory pain disorders. Here we consider the three methods of brain stimulation that have been investigated for the treatment of central pain: MCS, rTMS, and tDCS. While all three treatment modalities appear to induce significant clinical gains in patients with chronic pain, tDCS is revealed as the most cost-effective approach (compared to rTMS and MCS) when considering a single year of treatment. However, if a 5-year treatment is considered, MCS is revealed as the most cost-effective modality (as compared to rTMS and tDCS) for the neuromodulatory treatment of chronic pain. We discuss the theory behind the application of each modality as well as efficacy, cost, safety, and practical considerations.

Keywords: Chronic pain, brain stimulation, cost-effect analysis, motor cortex stimulation, repetitive transcranial magnetic stimulation, transcranial direct current stimulation, brain polarization.

---

[*] **Correspondence:** Felipe Fregni, MD, PhD, Berenson-Allen Center for Non-invasive Brain Stimulation, 330 Brookline Ave, KS 452, Boston, MA 02215 United States. Tel: 617–667-5272; E-mail: ffregni@bidmc.harvard.edu

"Chronic pain is a thief. It breaks into your body and robs you blind. With lightning fingers, it can take away your livelihood, your marriage, your friends, your favorite pastimes and big chunks of your personality. Left unapprehended, it will steal your days and your nights until the world has collapsed into a cramped cell of suffering." (Claudia Willis, Time Magazine).

Introduction

Central pain syndrome is a prevalent, costly, and disabling neurological disorder that causes unrelenting suffering and disability. The pain ranges in intensity from moderate to severe and is often described as a burning, pressing, lacerating, or aching pain, occasionally accompanied by brief, intolerable bursts of sharp pain (1). Analgesics often provide some relief and treatment with tricyclic antidepressants (e.g. nortriptyline) or anticonvulsants (e.g. gabapentin) may be helpful, but pharmacologic interventions for central pain are nonspecific in focality and at target doses may cause drowsiness, impaired memory, and decreased capacity to carry out activities that require high executive functioning. These side effects result in administration of doses that are often insufficient or ineffective. Other limitations to pharmacologic intervention include concerns of organ toxicity and risk of abuse or addiction (2). Thus, central pain remains inadequately treated, affecting up to 2.6% of women and 1.9% men for an average duration of 9.5 to 11.2 years (3). Indeed, the ensuing chronic pain results in significant loss of function and productivity, and is relatively expensive in terms of health care use. Thus, there remains an unmet clinical need for the development of new therapeutic approaches for the treatment of central pain.

In this setting, cortical stimulation has emerged as an interesting, effective, and promising modality in the investigation of novel approaches for pain relief. Cortical stimulation is based on the delivery of electric current to the motor cortex (among other cortical areas) of the brain; this delivery of current can be accomplished directly via epidural electrodes (as in epidural motor cortex stimulation, MCS) or indirectly and non-invasively via transcranial application of rapidly varying magnetic fields (as in repetitive transcranial magnetic stimulation, rTMS) or weak electrical currents (as in transcranial direct current stimulation, TDCS). A recent meta-analysis has shown that both direct and noninvasive means of motor cortical stimulation can be highly effective in the treatment of chronic pain (4) (5)). Sites of stimulation beyond the motor cortex, such as the dorsal lateral prefrontal cortex, may also be effective. Here we discuss the principles and mechanism in the use of brain stimulation for the treatment of central pain, and we discuss safety and practical considerations, as well as cost, in the application of these modalities.

Mechanisms and components of central pain

Central pain is, by definition, damage to or dysfunction of the central nervous system (brain, brainstem, and spinal cord) that results in long-lasting pain. It can be caused by stroke, multiple sclerosis, tumors, epilepsy, brain or spinal cord trauma, or Parkinson's disease, among other etiologies. However, central pain can also be caused by peripheral nerve injury, as with limb amputation, chemical injury, blunt trauma, or neuropathy that secondarily affects the central nervous system. Central pain often begins shortly after the causative injury or damage, but may be delayed by months or even years, especially if it is related to post-stroke pain (1).

Pain, in general, is mediated by a specific network of peripheral and central neurons that alarm us to the presence of potentially harmful stimuli. Normally, the perception of pain diminishes after resolution of the insult. In chronic pain, however, the nociceptive neural network responsible for pain conduction and processing sustains a hypersensitive state. The result is a hypersensitive network with lowered neural thresholds for sensory stimuli such that noxious stimuli produce an exaggerated and prolonged response to pain and non-noxious stimuli that are normally not painful become more likely to induce pain (6). Indeed, dysfunctional central sensitization is the hallmark of central pain, and a disturbance of pain-related thalamocortical transmission and processing is now acknowledged to be one of the main engines of this dysfunctional state (7).

The sensation commonly referred to as "pain" can be divided into a sensory-discriminative and an affective-motivational component (8). The sensory-discriminative component of pain (i.e. nociception or sensory pain) provides information about the location, modality, and intensity of painful stimuli. Pathways involved in this aspect of pain involve the spinothalamic tract (9) and result in preferential activation of the lateral thalamus and somatosensory cortices (S1 and S2), as well as the posterior insular cortex (10). On the other hand, the affective-motivational component of pain (i.e. the moment-by-moment unpleasantness of pain) refers to the emotional responses elicited by a painful stimulus—that is, painful stimuli invoke feelings of suffering, fear, exhaustion, disgust, sadness, and anxiety, among others, that motivate the individual to escape or reduce the source of pain. Indeed, this emotional pain preferentially activates the anterior cingulate cortex and the anterior insular cortex, which in turn activate other components of the limbic system (i.e. areas of executive processing, such as the medial and dorsolateral prefrontal cortex), (10) which play an integral role in focusing attention to salient stimuli.

Interestingly, this affective dimension of pain relies on neurophysiological systems that are at least partly anatomically distinct from those involved in the sensory perception of pain (11). Even so, the cortico-limbic pathway is known to integrate nociceptive input with information about overall status of the body, in turn regulating (and sometimes amplifying) the affect attributed to pain (12). The cortical perception of pain is then intimately linked with areas of the brain involved in autonomic and neuroendocrine regulation (amygdala, hypothalamus, thalamic reticular nucleus, ventral tegmental area, locus coeruleus, laterodorsal tegmental nucleus), such that the perception of pain manifests physically with changes in blood pressure, heightened reflexes, and skin galvanomic response, among other changes (13). In addition, this integrated system might indicate that pain is not only part of an afferent system in which the final product is a change in behavior, but that the perception of pain itself may be part of a complex two-way afferent-efferent system in which the chronic pain might have profound changes in immune system function and endocrine regulation (14).

Thus, the perception of pain involves a large and complex interconnected network of neural structures, and central pain may result from a dysfunction in any part of this system. That is, lesions or injuries affecting any part of the network that processes sensation, emotion, or attention may all in turn contribute to the genesis of central pain. This is important to consider when discussing focal therapies (as with brain stimulation) because not all types of central pain are caused by a similar etiology, and so not all patients with central pain may benefit from a single, unique parameter of stimulation. Even so, cortical stimulation promises an interesting alternative in the treatment of central pain.

Cortical stimulation for the treatment of central pain

The mechanism of cortical stimulation for the relief of pain is based on the excitability modification of neuronal activity intimately involved in the neural circuits responsible for pain processing and perception. In this way, it is believed that stimulation of the cerebral cortex either inhibits or interrupts and interferes with pain signals that originate from the thalamus and other hyperactive areas in the pain networks of the brain. Thus, stimulation of the cortex may merely be an entry port for the complex pain-related neural network. We discuss two targets for cortical stimulation: motor cortex and prefrontal cortex.

Electrical stimulation of the primary motor cortex has been heralded as an extremely promising technique (15), and indeed the motor cortex has been the primary target for cortical stimulation for pain relief. The role of motor cortex stimulation in the relief of central pain has been best demonstrated for pain of thalamic origin. Animal studies show that transection of the spinal cord results in burst hyperactivity of VPL thalamic neurons that can be decreased by motor, but not sensory, cortex stimulation (7). Furthermore, epidural stimulation of the primary motor cortex has been found to relieve both thalamic hyperactivity and pain in human spinal cord injury pain patients (16). These findings suggest that motor cortex stimulation modulates abnormal thalamic activity via cortico-thalamic fibers to relieve pain in certain chronic pain syndromes (17,18). One possibility is that enhancement of motor cortex activity may result in direct inhibition of thalamic activity through inhibitory cortico-thalamic fibers. The secondary modulation of the thalamic nuclei may perhaps underlie the pain-alleviating attribute of motor cortex stimulation.

The prefrontal cortex is an alternate target of stimulation for the relief of pain, one that may be especially helpful in modulating the emotional, attentional, and affective dimensions of pain. Simulation of the prefrontal cortex has been associated with a modification of a large extensive neural network associated with the limbic system such as the cingulate gyrus and parahippocampal areas (19,20). In fact, stimulation of prefrontal cortex areas is associated with working memory, attentional control, reasoning and decision-making modulation, as well as temporal organization of behavior, and emotional processing (21). Indeed, stimulation of the prefrontal cortex with rTMS has been shown to increase thermal pain thresholds in healthy adults (22) and to reduce of pain in fibromyalgia (23), further suggesting that this area may indeed be a potent target for brain stimulation in the treatment of central pain.

Stimulation of the primary motor cortex (M1) and dorsolateral prefrontal cortex (DLFPC) may both reduce the perception of pain, but recent studies suggest that they likely do so by different mechanisms. Pain and perception thresholds to electrical stimulation were assessed in 20 healthy volunteers before and during anodal TDCS. Four conditions of stimulation were compared: M1, DLPFC, occipital cortex, and sham. Anodal tDCS of M1 increased both perception and pain thresholds, while stimulation of DLPFC increased pain thresholds only. The results suggested that 1) anodal stimulation of M1 but not DLPFC could induce analgesia by modulating sensory discrimination and 2) stimulation of DLPFC could modulate the perception of pain via a mechanism independent of sensory perception (21). An adjunctive study with 22 healthy volunteers showed that anodal tDCS of the DLPFC (but not M1, occipital, or sham) could decrease the perception of unpleasantness and reduces emotional discomfort/pain while subjects viewed emotionally aversive images demonstrating human pain. It is indeed quite interesting that subjects perceived the aversive images as less unpleasant and reported lower levels of emotional discomfort during DLPFC tDCS, as compared to baseline and sham, and that motor cortex stimulation had no effect (22).

Together, these results suggests that while motor cortex stimulation may mediate its analgesic effects by decreasing the somatosensory-discriminative aspect of pain, stimulation of DLPFC may effect the affective-emotional aspect of pain, reducing the unpleasantness of a perceived stimulus. Interestingly, stimulation of DLPFC has also been effective in the treatment of depression and anxiety disorders, as well as the enhancement of attention and memory on cognitive tasks.

Methods of stimulation

Here we consider the three methods of brain stimulation that have been investigated for the treatment of central pain: MCS, rTMS, and tDCS.

Epidural motor cortex stimulation

MCS is a method of introducing electric current to the motor cortex via the surgical implantation of epidural electrodes. Preoperative and intraoperative localization of the motor cortex is achieved through neuronavigation, which includes fMRI and somatosensory evoked potentials, among other neurosurgical mapping techniques. During the neurosurgical procedure, a paddle lead with four electrodes is placed beneath the periosteum of the skull and above the dura mater. The paddle lead is adjusted so that all four contact points cover the precentral gyrus of the brain. Proper positioning is ensured by the application of suprathreshold stimulation to induce contralateral motor response without the induction of parasthesia or other sensory phenomena (24). After the operation, an individualized test trial is performed for each patient to identify the electrode combination and stimulation parameters that generate the greatest pain-relieving effect. The most commonly used settings are 2–3 V (range 0.5–9.5 V) of intensity, 25–50 Hz (range 15–130 Hz) of frequency, and 200 μsec (range 60–450 μsec) for pulse width. In all cases, the stimulation is sub-threshold and bipolar, and the parameters of stimulation (i.e. elevated frequency and intensity) are targeted to cause a disruption in the area of stimulation where the electrodes are placed. Stimulation is provided off-and-on throughout the day according to a cyclic program, where most patients receive about 12 hrs of stimulation daily (25).

According to a recent systematic review the mean weighted responder rate for studies with epidual MCS is 72.6% (95% CI, 67.7-77.4) (4). Another similar review also confirmed the high response rate for this procedure: about 56.7% of patients experience a "good outcome" (= 40–50% improvement) after the implantation of a motor cortex stimulator. In studies where follow-up = 1 year was considered, 45.4% had a "good postoperative outcome." In the 2 studies with the longest follow-up period (49 months in both), 47 and

22.6% of the patients experienced a long-term pain relief of = 50%. Among the subset of patients with less favorable results, for many it has been possible to reduce medication doses and still others are noted to experience substantial yet less significant pain relief and improvements in quality of life. Nevertheless, many neurosurgeons anecdotally suggest that MCS results are not consistent and often disappointing (25).

Repetitive transcranial magnetic stimulation

Transcranial magnetic stimulation (TMS) is a non-invasive technique of brain stimulation based on the principle of electromagnetic induction. A coil of copper wire encased in plastic is rested on the subject's scalp overlying the area of the brain to be stimulated. As current passes through the coil, a magnetic field is generated in a plane perpendicular to the coil. The current passed is strong but extremely brief, thus generating a magnetic field that changes rapidly in time. In fact, the magnetic field reaches 2 Tesla in about 50 µs, but then decays back to 0 in the same amount of time. This very rapidly changing magnetic field penetrates the skin and skull of the subject unimpeded, without causing any discomfort. Due to the rapid change in time, it induces a secondary electrical current in the subject's brain that is strong enough to depolarize neurons. The peak of this induced current is limited to a small volume of brain cortex (1-4 cm3) (26). The stimulation does not penetrate further because the magnetic field decays rapidly in intensity with square of the distance. Even so, depolarization of cortical neurons may result in secondary activation or inhibition of other brain areas, including the contralateral hemisphere and thalamic nuclei, among other cortical and subcortical regions.

If the TMS stimulus is repeated over and over again in trains of stimulation, this is referred to as repetitive transcranial magnetic stimulation (rTMS). A train of rTMS can modulate cortical excitability in manner that lasts beyond the duration of the rTMS itself. This effect may range from suppression to facilitation of activity in an underlying brain area, depending on the stimulation parameters, particularly stimulation frequency. For instance, in the motor cortex, lower rTMS frequencies in the 1 Hz range can usually suppress cortical excitability, while 20 Hz stimulation trains seem to lead to a temporary increase in cortical excitability in most subjects. Although these effects are relatively consistent, other parameters (such as baseline cortical excitability) do play an important role. Indeed, in epileptic patients with chronic valproate use, a study shows that when serum concentration of valproate are low, 1 Hz rTMS has a similar inhibitory effect on corticospinal excitability as in healthy subjects; but, when the serum valproate concentration are high (in the same patients), 1 Hz rTMS paradoxically increases the corticospinal excitability (27). Therefore the therapeutic use of rTMS should take into consideration the interaction between rTMS and drugs that change cortical excitability.

In rTMS, the site of stimulation can be approximated by using brain landmarks and then confirmed by identification of motor or sensory evoked potentials. Motor cortex stimulation is reliable with such an approach, because motor evoked potentials can be appreciated. DLPFC stimulation, on the other hand, is limited, however, because the technician can only approximate and never be entirely sure whether an exact location is being stimulated. Here, it is debatable whether this represents a real limitation as the focality of rTMS is also limited. Alternatively, the use of a frameless stimulation guiding device allows targeting specific areas of the subject's brain by using the subject's own brain MRI to guide placement of the TMS coil on the subject's head (28). Nevertheless, accurate localization and focalization of stimulation area with TMS clearly has greater limitations when compared to direct epidural stimulation.

In patients with chronic neuropathic pain, motor cortex stimulation with rTMS applied at 5-20 Hz for at least 1000 pulses reduces pain scores by about 25-30% (5). In fact a recent meta-analysis, has shown that the mean responders rate is 36.8% (95% C.I., 30. 5– 43. 0 %) (4). Following a single rTMS session, analgesic effects are optimal a few days later and last for less than one week. Repeated daily stimulation sessions appear to increase and prolong the pain-relieving effects, and there may be some role for treatment with maintenance therapy (see Case Report by Zaghi et al. in this journal). Of note, although stimulation of DLPFC has been shown to be effective in depression and anxiety syndromes, including fibromyalgia and PTSD, to our knowledge, the investigation of stimulation of DLPFC stimulation for pain has been limited to healthy volunteers.

Transcranial direct current stimulation

tDCS is based on the application of low-amplitude electric current to the scalp. A battery-powered current generator (capable of delivering up to 2 mA of constant current flow) is attached to two sponge-based electrodes (20-35 cm^2). The sponge electrodes are then soaked, applied to the scalp, and held in place by a non-conducting rubber montage affixed around the head. During tDCS, low amplitude direct currents penetrate the skull to enter the brain. Although there is substantial shunting of current at the scalp, sufficient current penetrates the brain to modify the transmembrane neuronal potential (29,30) and, thus, influence the level of excitability and modulate the firing rate of individual neurons. However, it should be noted that the effects of tDCS are strongly dependent on electrode montage and parameters of stimulation (i.e. intensity and duration of stimulation). Furthermore, DC currents do not induce action potentials; rather, the current appears to modulate the spontaneous neuronal activity in a polarity-dependent fashion: for example, anodal tDCS applied over the motor cortex increases the excitability of the underlying motor cortex, while cathodal tDCS applied over the same area decreases it (31,32). Similarly, anodal tDCS applied over the occipital cortex produces short-lasting increases in visual cortex excitability (33,34). Hence, TDCS is believed to deliver its effects by polarizing brain tissue, and while anodal stimulation generally increases excitability and cathodal stimulation generally reduces excitability, the direction of polarization depends strictly on the orientation of axons and dendrites in the induced electrical field.

It has been demonstrated that the functional effects of tDCS are generally restricted to the area under the electrodes (35,36). However, of significant interest are recent studies that show that TDCS can induce effects beyond the immediate site of stimulation (37,38). This supports the notion that TDCS has a functional effect not only on the underlying cortico-spinal excitability but also on distant neural networks (39). In addition, fMRI studies reveal that tDCS not only has effects on the underlying cortex (40), but that it moreover provokes sustained and widespread changes in regional neuronal activity (41). EEG studies support these findings showing that stimulation induces synchronous changes to oscillatory activity (42,43). Hence, the effects of DC stimulation are likely perpetuated throughout the brain via networks of inter-neuronal circuits (44). But, this raises an interesting question as to whether the observed clinical effects (e.g. pain, depression alleviation) are mediated primarily through the cortex or secondarily via activation or inhibition of other cortical and/or sub-cortical structures (21,45).

tDCS has been valuable in exploring the effect of cortical modulation on various neural networks implicated in decision-making (46), language (47), memory (48), among other high-order cortical processes, including sensory perception and pain (45). Furthermore, preliminary small sample-size studies with TDCS have shown initial positive results in modulating chronic pain (49). For chronic central pain due to traumatic spinal cord injury, 5 daily sessions of TDCS (20 min, 2 mA, motor cortex) resulted in a reduction of pain scores of at least 50% in 6/11 patients receiving active treatment (50). For pain due to fibromyalgia, our studies suggest an approximate improvement of 20-30% with 10 daily sessions among all subjects receiving motor cortex or DLPFC stimulation.

tDCS has some advantages over rTMS because it has longer-lasting modulatory effects on cortical function and is less expensive to administer. The primary limitation is that the sites of stimulation in tDCS are identified based on the cranial landmarks used in 10-20 system for EEG electrode placement. Clearly, because there is great variety in true brain anatomy among subjects, this means that in many cases, the electrode placement may not exactly correspond to the target site of stimulation. Coincidentally, it appears that certain subjects appear more susceptible to the effects of tDCS per the current protocol, and indeed subjects who do respond to treatment with tDCS appear to do quite well when supported with repeated maintenance tDCS sessions (51).

Cost-effectiveness analysis

We performed a preliminary cost-effectiveness analysis involving the three main modalities of brain stimulation (MCS, rTMS and tDCS) for the treatment of chronic pain.

Study population

The target population for this study was patients with chronic pain (see list of conditions in table 1) undergoing cortical stimulation. In carrying out this analysis, we considered the sub-acute effects of the treatments as described in the studies, but we furthermore adopted extrapolative assumptions in the consideration of these modalities for long term-use. In order to obtain estimates of treatment effects, we conducted a systematic investigation throughout MEDLINE and other databases and collected Visual Analogue Scale (VAS) assessments from studies that evaluated the effects of any of these techniques on pain.

Effectiveness measures

For the purpose of evaluation, we decided to use VAS of pain as the primary measure of effectiveness. Quality-Adjusted Life Years (QALYs) were used as a secondary measure of effectiveness and were derived from the VAS of pain using a transformation function to convert VAS values (V) to Standard Gamble (SG) utility scores (U). Several studies found a discrepancy between V and U values due to a well known end-aversion bias of VAS and a slightly concave curve pattern in a direct and systematic relationship of SG and VAS. Despite the fact that this relationship may not be stable at the individual level, comparative group analysis have demonstrated a highly accurate relationship once the VAS values are converted by a transformation function into SG utility scores.

Table 1. Etiology of pain syndrome (number of patients)

Causative Lesion	Number of Patients	Treatment	Causative Lesion	Number of Patients
Deep brain hematoma	5	rTMS	Trigeminal neuralgia	24
Ischemic Stroke	25		Post-stroke pain	24
Arteriovenous malformation	1		Fibromyalgia	8
Avulsion	4		Spinal Cord injury	6
Haemorrhagic stroke	16			
Dental surgery	3			
Trigeminal pain	22	tDCS	Fibromyalgia	11
Thalamic abscess	1		Spinal Cord injury	11
Trauma	8			
Herpetic pain	3			
Nerve injury	6			
No clear cause	2			

Cost measures

We decided to include only costs from the perspective of the health care system. We did not include future or societal costs due to the short time frame of our model. Therefore, we only included direct fixed costs associated with treatment such as: room utilization, equipment maintenance, supplies, technician, neurologist coverage for each session and/or consultation, administrative fees, hospitalization costs, surgeon fee, anesthesiologist fee, surgical fee, electrode costs.

The costs of rTMS and tDCS treatment administration were estimated using data on capital costs (including the treatment suite and machines used during treatment) and cost of professionals' time related to treatment. We searched for these costs in several cities US cities.

For the estimation of costs associated with the treatment suite, we searched for the rental of medical office space with a size of 200 square feet – including utilities. The costs of machinery used in treatment were obtained from suppliers, and the market value of the equipment annuitized at 3.0% over 10 years plus any associated maintenance costs. The annual costs of the treatment suite and machinery were then divided by the number of administrations of treatments for the year – we estimated an average of 400 treatments per year.

To measure staff time, we recorded the profession and grade of the staff involved in the treatment; we estimated the annual salary of the technician over the different US cities and divided by the number of treatments (400 a year). For the neurologist, we estimated his/her annual salary and divided by 8 (estimating that he would dedicate 1/8 of his time to follow-up these patients and then divided by the number of treatments in a year [400]. We then estimated the costs of administrative overhead calculating 10% of the total costs per session for each modality.

To estimate costs of the surgery, we gathered data across the U.S. on hospitalization-related costs, including admission; room and board; operating room; pharmacy; radiology; laboratory; medical and surgical supplies; and other charges (i.e., anesthesia, blood, etc.).

Economic evaluation

A cost-effectiveness analysis summarizes the additional resources consumed for an improvement in the effects (in our study measured as decrease in pain as indexed by VAS) associated with one intervention compared to another. The result can be summarized as an incremental cost-effectiveness ratio (ICER) – a measure of the additional cost per unit of health gain. The underlying calculation for the ICER comparing for instance MCS vs. rTMS in patients with chronic pain was:

$$ICER = \frac{\text{Average Cost}_{MCS} - \text{Average Cost}_{rTMS}}{\text{Average Effect}_{MCS} - \text{Average Effect}_{rTMS}}$$

where costs were measured in US dollars and effects were measured in VAS changes. A cost-effective analysis was conducted by comparing MCS vs. rTMS, MCS vs. tDCS and rTMS vs. tDCS. For each comparison, we calculated the incremental cost per unit of VAS decreased and incremental cost per quality-adjusted life-year (QALY) gained. Incremental cost-effectiveness ratios were not calculated if one treatment strategy dominated the other (i.e., lower costs, better outcomes).

Preliminary results

The demographic and clinical characteristics of the subjects at baseline are shown in table 2. MCS treatment was associated with a mean reduction in VAS of 3.44 and an increase in Standard Gambles Utilities Score of 0.41.

Table 2. Demographic characteristics

	MCS	rTMS	tDCS
Number of patients	96	35	22
Age (mean)	58.14215	56	45.4
Duration of pain (years)	6.433333	4.283333	6.85
Baseline pain (VAS)	8.59	6.666667	7.34

rTMS had the lowest reduction in VAS and lowest increase in Utilities Score, respectively 2.14 and 0.25. On the other hand, tDCS was intermediate in effect with 2.84 for VAS and 0.30 for Utilities Score.

Table 3. Changes in VAS and utilities

	Change in VAS (amount decreased from baseline)	VAS % change	Change in Utilities Scores (amount increased from baseline)
MCS	3.44	41.7%	0.41
TMS	2.14	33.5%	0.25
TDCS	2.84	37.3%	0.30

Costs of treatment

Our analysis showed that the cost per tDCS session is lower than rTMS session (US$167.72 vs. US$207.24). The mean cost of the first treatment (given 10 sessions of non-invasive brain stimulation) is US$ 1677.20 for tDCS, US$ 2072.40 for rTMS and US$ 42,000.00 for MCS (mean cost of neurosurgical procedure including electrodes to implant the cortical stimulation). We then analyzed costs over 1 year and over 5 years. For tDCS and rTMS, we calculated one maintenance session per week – starting 2 weeks after treatment and including two sets of booster treatments of 5 sessions per year – then 70 sessions are needed per year for both treatments, therefore an annual treatment for these two techniques would cost US$ 11,740.40 for tDCS and US$ 14,506.80 for rTMS. For MCS, one monthly visit is necessary to check the parameters of stimulation – therefore, the annual costs of MCS are US$ 3,600.00 (given US$ 300 dollars the cost of one appointment to check parameters of stimulation).

Stipulating a time horizon of 1 year, the costs of treatment are US$45,600.00 for MCS, US$ 11,740.40 for tDCS and US$ 14.506.80 for rTMS treatment. For a time horizon of 5 years, we discounted the costs of years after the first year, adjusting to the beginning of the first year, following a discount rate of 3.0 percent per year. For MCS, with the monthly visit of the second through the fifth year properly discounted and added to the surgery costs, totalized US$ 58591.91. All rTMS discounted costs summed with the first year is US$ 68.311.00. For tDCS the total amount correctly discounted is US$ 55.284.00.

Cost-effectiveness

The main outcome for the cost-effectiveness analysis was the incremental cost per unit of VAS. Because MCS was associated with the best outcome but was also the most expensive treatment, we compared MCS vs. tDCS and MCS vs. rTMS. We performed this analysis for two scenarios: 1 and 5 years of treatment. This comparison was not done for rTMS vs. tDCS as the response to tDCS was larger and less costly than rTMS; therefore, tDCS is always more cost-effective as compared to rTMS.

Scenario 1: 1-year treatment

Initially, we compared rTMS vs. MCS during the first year of treatment. For the first year, rTMS is a less costly procedure but induces less benefit as compared to MCS. The ICER when comparing these two procedures is US$ 23819.84 per unit of VAS. We then performed similar analysis, but used tDCS instead of rTMS. The comparison showed that ICER is US$ 56432.66 per unit of VAS. Therefore, rTMS and tDCS are less costly but also less effective than MCS, and an additional gain of 1.3 or 0.6 units of VAS conferred by MCS would cost US$30,964.70 and US$33,859.60 respectively as compared with rTMS and tDCS.

Scenario 2: 5-year treatment

We then performed similar analysis, but considered the 5-year scenario. The ICER when comparing MCS and rTMS shows a negative value (-9,358.66 dollars); therefore showing that MCS would be a more effective and cost-saving procedure compared to rTMS. However the comparison between MCS and tDCS showed that ICER is US$3,667.95 per unit of VAS, such that the additional gain of 0.6 units of VAS conferred by MCS would cost US$2,200.77.

Summary and future directions

MCS is an invasive technique of brain stimulation that requires neurosurgery and therefore carries significant risk of injury or death. While the procedure is quite expensive, the major benefit is that it allows for a prolonged duration of stimulation (hours a day for years) and in fact might induce the largest benefits as compared to rTMS and tDCS. rTMS, on the other hand, is similarly excellent in targeted brain stimulation and it offers a non-invasive manner of inducing electric current. Even so, the technique is quite challenging requiring a trained technician to be present for the entire duration of stimulation, and so rTMS is relatively more expensive in comparison to tDCS. Furthermore, specific parameters of stimulation must be followed (and certain subjects excluded) to prevent risk of seizure with the application of rTMS. Finally, tDCS offers a less focal method of brain stimulation that is much easier to apply and carries almost no risk of seizure. Indeed, it may be possible to design tDCS devices for home use, so that patients can use the device for extended durations at little or no extra cost. This would make this technique the most cost-effective modality as compared to all the other methods of stimulation. tDCS is limited with respect to the intensity of stimulation that can be applied, such that it generally involves a diffuse spread of electric current.

It is not clear whether the efficacy of these treatments is based on accurate localization of brain targets, intensity of stimulation, and duration. If it is, then it should be expected that MCS would deliver the greatest efficacy followed in turn by tTMS and tDCS. In the future, chronic pain patients who respond beneficially but only transiently to rTMS, may then be offered a trial of tDCS, or as a last resort they may be referred for consideration of epidural motor cortex stimulation.

In addition, in the future, we can hope that more sophisticated regimens and parameters of stimulation will be developed that may be able to dynamically stimulate various brain regions at different frequencies and intensities during a single session. In this way, non-invasive brain stimulation might be physiologically tailored to suit the brain state of each patient in an attempt to maximize efficacy.

References

[1] NINDS. NINDS Central Pain Syndrome Information Page. National Institute of Neurological Disorders and Stroke. 2009; http://www.ninds.nih.gov/disorders/central_pain/central_pain.htm.

[2] Katz NP, Adams EH, Chilcoat H, Colucci RD, Comer SD, Goliber P, et al. Challenges in the development of prescription opioid abuse-deterrent formulations. Clin J Pain 2007;23(8):648-60.

[3] Tunks ER, Crook J, Weir R. Epidemiology of chronic pain with psychological comorbidity: prevalence, risk, course, and prognosis. Can J Psychiatry 2008;53(4):224-34.

[4] Lima MC, Fregni F. Motor cortex stimulation for chronic pain: systematic review and meta-analysis of the literature. Neurology 2008;70(24):2329-37.

[5] Lefaucheur JP. Use of repetitive transcranial magnetic stimulation in pain relief. Expert Rev Neurother 2008;8(5):799-808.

[6] Woolf CJ, Ma Q. Nociceptors--noxious stimulus detectors. Neuron 2007;55(3):353-64.

[7] Canavero S, Bonicalzi V. Central pain syndrome: elucidation of genesis and treatment. Expert Rev Neurother 2007;7(11):1485-97.

[8] Treede RD, Kenshalo DR, Gracely RH, Jones AK. The cortical representation of pain. Pain 1999;79(2-3):105-11.

[9] Ohara PT, Vit JP, Jasmin L. Cortical modulation of pain. Cell Mol Life Sci 2005;62(1):44-52.

[10] Moisset X, Bouhassira D. Brain imaging of neuropathic pain. Neuroimage 2007;37 Suppl 1:S80-8.

[11] Duquette M, Roy M, Lepore F, Peretz I, Rainville P. [Cerebral mechanisms involved in the interaction between pain and emotion]. Rev Neurol (Paris) 2007;163(2):169-79.

[12] Price DD. Central neural mechanisms that interrelate sensory and affective dimensions of pain. Mol Interv 2002;2(6):392-403.

[13] Blackburn-Munro G. Hypothalamo-pituitary-adrenal axis dysfunction as a contributory factor to chronic pain and depression. Curr Pain Headache Rep 2004;8(2):116-24.

[14] Fregni F, Pascual-Leone A, Freedman SD. Pain in chronic pancreatitis: a salutogenic mechanism or a maladaptive brain response? Pancreatology 2007;7(5-6):411-22.

[15] Saitoh Y, Hirayama A, Kishima H, Oshino S, Hirata M, Kato A, et al. Stimulation of primary motor cortex for intractable deafferentation pain. Acta Neurochir Suppl 2006;99:57-9.

[16] Lenz FA, Kwan HC, Dostrovsky JO, Tasker RR. Characteristics of the bursting pattern of action potentials that occurs in the thalamus of patients with central pain. Brain Res 1989;496(1-2):357-60.

[17] Tsubokawa T, Katayama Y, Yamamoto T, Hirayama T, Koyama S. Treatment of thalamic pain by chronic motor cortex stimulation. Pacing Clin Electrophysiol 1991;14(1):131-4.
[18] Tsubokawa T, Katayama Y, Yamamoto T, Hirayama T, Koyama S. Chronic motor cortex stimulation for the treatment of central pain. Acta Neurochir Suppl (Wien) 1991;52:137-9.
[19] Mottaghy FM, Krause BJ, Kemna LJ, Topper R, Tellmann L, Beu M, et al. Modulation of the neuronal circuitry subserving working memory in healthy human subjects by repetitive transcranial magnetic stimulation. Neurosci Lett 2000;280(3):167-70.
[20] Catafau AM, Perez V, Gironell A, Martin JC, Kulisevsky J, Estorch M, et al. SPECT mapping of cerebral activity changes induced by repetitive transcranial magnetic stimulation in depressed patients. A pilot study. Psychiatry Res 2001;106(3):151-60.
[21] Boggio PS, Zaghi S, Fregni F. Modulation of emotions associated with images of human pain using anodal transcranial direct current stimulation (tDCS). Neuropsychologia 2009;47(1):212-7.
[22] Borckardt JJ, Smith AR, Reeves ST, Weinstein M, Kozel FA, Nahas Z, et al. Fifteen minutes of left prefrontal repetitive transcranial magnetic stimulation acutely increases thermal pain thresholds in healthy adults. Pain Res Manag 2007;12(4):287-90.
[23] Sampson SM, Rome JD, Rummans TA. Slow-frequency rTMS reduces fibromyalgia pain. Pain Med 2006;7(2):115-8.
[24] Rasche D, Ruppolt M, Stippich C, Unterberg A, Tronnier VM. Motor cortex stimulation for long-term relief of chronic neuropathic pain: a 10 year experience. Pain 2006;121(1-2):43-52.
[25] Fontaine D, Hamani C, Lozano A. Efficacy and safety of motor cortex stimulation for chronic neuropathic pain: critical review of the literature. J Neurosurg, in press.
[26] Wagner T, Gangitano M, Romero R, Theoret H, Kobayashi M, Anschel D, et al. Intracranial measurement of current densities induced by transcranial magnetic stimulation in the human brain. Neurosci Lett 2004;354(2):91-4.
[27] Fregni F, Boggio PS, Valle AC, Otachi P, Thut G, Rigonatti SP, et al. Homeostatic effects of plasma valproate levels on corticospinal excitability changes induced by 1Hz rTMS in patients with juvenile myoclonic epilepsy. Clin Neurophysiol 2006;117(6):1217-27.
[28] Gugino LD, Romero JR, Aglio L, Titone D, Ramirez M, Pascual-Leone A, et al. Transcranial magnetic stimulation coregistered with MRI: a comparison of a guided versus blind stimulation technique and its effect on evoked compound muscle action potentials. Clin Neurophysiol 2001;112(10):1781-92.
[29] Wagner T, Valero-Cabre A, Pascual-Leone A. Noninvasive human brain stimulation. Annu Rev Biomed Eng 2007;9:527-65.
[30] Miranda PC, Lomarev M, Hallett M. Modeling the current distribution during transcranial direct current stimulation. Clin Neurophysiol 2006;117(7):1623-9.
[31] Wassermann EM, Grafman J. Recharging cognition with DC brain polarization. Trends Cogn Sci 2005;9(11):503-5.
[32] Nitsche MA, Paulus W. Sustained excitability elevations induced by transcranial DC motor cortex stimulation in humans. Neurology 2001;57(10):1899-901.
[33] Antal A, Kincses TZ, Nitsche MA, Paulus W. Manipulation of phosphene thresholds by transcranial direct current stimulation in man. Exp Brain Res 2003;150(3):375-8.
[34] Lang N, Siebner HR, Chadaide Z, Boros K, Nitsche MA, Rothwell JC, et al. Bidirectional modulation of primary visual cortex excitability: a combined tDCS and rTMS study. Invest Ophthalmol Vis Sci 2007;48(12):5782-7.
[35] Nitsche MA, Liebetanz D, Lang N, Antal A, Tergau F, Paulus W. Safety criteria for transcranial direct current stimulation (tDCS) in humans. Clin Neurophysiol 2003;114(11):2220-3.
[36] Nitsche MA, Niehaus L, Hoffmann KT, Hengst S, Liebetanz D, Paulus W, et al. MRI study of human brain exposed to weak direct current stimulation of the frontal cortex. Clin Neurophysiol 2004; 115(10):2419-23.

[37] Boros K, Poreisz C, Munchau A, Paulus W, Nitsche MA. Premotor transcranial direct current stimulation (tDCS) affects primary motor excitability in humans. Eur J Neurosci 2008;27(5):1292-300.
[38] Vines BW, Cerruti C, Schlaug G. Dual-hemisphere tDCS facilitates greater improvements for healthy subjects' non-dominant hand compared to uni-hemisphere stimulation. BMC Neurosci 2008; 9(1):103.
[39] Nitsche MA, Seeber A, Frommann K, Klein CC, Rochford C, Nitsche MS, et al. Modulating parameters of excitability during and after transcranial direct current stimulation of the human motor cortex. J Physiol 2005;568(Pt 1):291-303.
[40] Kwon YH, Ko MH, Ahn SH, Kim YH, Song JC, Lee CH, et al. Primary motor cortex activation by transcranial direct current stimulation in the human brain. Neurosci Lett 2008;435(1):56-9.
[41] Lang N, Siebner HR, Ward NS, Lee L, Nitsche MA, Paulus W, et al. How does transcranial DC stimulation of the primary motor cortex alter regional neuronal activity in the human brain? Eur J Neurosci 2005;22(2):495-504.
[42] Marshall L, Molle M, Hallschmid M, Born J. Transcranial direct current stimulation during sleep improves declarative memory. J Neurosci 2004;24(44):9985-92.
[43] Ardolino G, Bossi B, Barbieri S, Priori A. Non-synaptic mechanisms underlie the after-effects of cathodal transcutaneous direct current stimulation of the human brain. J Physiol 2005;568(Pt 2):653-63.
[44] Lefaucheur JP. Principles of therapeutic use of transcranial and epidural cortical stimulation. Clin Neurophysiol 2008; 119(10):2179-84.
[45] Boggio PS, Zaghi S, Lopes M, Fregni F. Modulatory effects of anodal transcranial direct current stimulation on perception and pain thresholds in healthy volunteers. Eur J Neurol, in press.
[46] Fecteau S, Pascual-Leone A, Zald DH, Liguori P, Theoret H, Boggio PS, et al. Activation of prefrontal cortex by transcranial direct current stimulation reduces appetite for risk during ambiguous decision making. J Neurosci 2007;27(23):6212-8.
[47] Floel A, Rosser N, Michka O, Knecht S, Breitenstein C. Noninvasive brain stimulation improves language learning. J Cogn Neurosci 2008; 20(8):1415-22.
[48] Fregni F, Boggio PS, Nitsche M, Bermpohl F, Antal A, Feredoes E, et al. Anodal transcranial direct current stimulation of prefrontal cortex enhances working memory. Exp Brain Res 2005;166(1):23-30.
[49] Fregni F, Gimenes R, Valle AC, Ferreira MJ, Rocha RR, Natalle L, et al. A randomized, sham-controlled, proof of principle study of transcranial direct current stimulation for the treatment of pain in fibromyalgia. Arthritis Rheum 2006;54(12):3988-98.
[50] Fregni F, Boggio PS, Lima MC, Ferreira MJ, Wagner T, Rigonatti SP, et al. A sham-controlled, phase II trial of transcranial direct current stimulation for the treatment of central pain in traumatic spinal cord injury. Pain 2006;122(1-2):197-209.
[51] Cecilio SB, Zaghi S, Cecilio LB, Correa CF, Fregni F. Exploring a novel therapeutic approach with noninvasive cortical stimulation for vulvodynia. Am J Obstet Gynecol 2008;199(6):e6-7.

In: Pain Management Yearbook 2009
Editor: Joav Merrick

ISBN: 978-1-61209-666-7
©2012 Nova Science Publishers, Inc.

Chapter 35

EFFICACY OF ANODAL TRANSCRANIAL DIRECT CURRENT STIMULATION (tDCS) FOR THE TREATMENT OF FIBROMYALGIA: RESULTS OF A RANDOMIZED, SHAM-CONTROLLED LONGITUDINAL CLINICAL TRIAL

Angela Valle[1], Suely Roizenblatt[2], Sueli Botte[1], Soroush Zaghi, BS[3], Marcelo Riberto[4], Sergio Tufik[2], Paulo S Boggio[5] and Felipe Fregni, MD, PhD[*3]

[1]Pathology Department, Universidade de São Paulo, Brazil, [2]Psychobiology Department, Universidade Federal de São Paulo, UNIFESP, São Paulo, Brazil, [3]Berenson-Allen Center for Noninvasive Brain Stimulation, Beth Israel Deaconess Medical Center, Harvard Medical School, Boston, United States of America, [4]Physical Medicine and Rehabilitation, Universidade de São Paulo, Brazil, [5]Programa de Pós-Graduação em Distúrbios do Desenvolvimento e Núcleo de Neurociências do Comportamento, Centro de Ciências Biológicas e da Saúde, Universidade Presbiteriana Mackenzie, São Paulo, Brazil

Abstract

Fibromyalgia has been recognized as a central pain disorder with evidence of neuroanatomic and neurophysiologic alterations. Previous studies with techniques of noninvasive brain stimulation--transcranial direct current stimulation (tDCS) and repetitive transcranial magnetic stimulation (rTMS)--have shown that these methods are associated with a significant alleviation of fibromyalgia-associated pain and sleep dysfunction. Here we sought to determine whether a longer treatment protocol involving

---

* **Correspondence:** Felipe Fregni, MD, PhD, Berenson-Allen Center for Non-invasive Brain Stimulation, 330 Brookline Ave – KS 452, Boston, MA 02215 United States. Tel: 617–667-5272; E-mail: ffregni@bidmc.harvard.edu

10 sessions of 2 mA, 20 min tDCS of the left primary motor (M1) or dorsolateral prefrontal cortex (DLPFC) could offer additional, more long-lasting clinical benefits in the management of pain from fibromyalgia. *Methods:* Forty-one women with chronic, medically refractory fibromyalgia were randomized to receive 10 daily sessions of M1, DLPFC, or sham tDCS. *Results*: Our results show that M1 and DLPFC stimulation both display improvements in pain scores (VAS) and quality of life (FIQ) at the end of the treatment protocol, but only M1 stimulation resulted in long-lasting clinical benefits as assessed at 30 and 60 days after the end of treatment. *Conclusions:* This study demonstrates the importance of the duration of the treatment period, suggesting that 10 daily sessions of tDCS result in more long lasting outcomes than only five sessions. Furthermore, this study supports the findings of a similarly designed rTMS trial as both induce pain reductions that are equally long-lasting.

Keywords: Transcranial direct current stimulation, brain polarization, healthy subjects, fibromyalgia, pain.

Introduction

Fibromyalgia is a chronic pain syndrome characterized by neuropathic tenderness in all four quadrants of the body in association with sleep alterations, mood dysfunction, musculoskeletal stiffness, and chronic fatigue (1). Recent evidence suggests that patients with fibromyalgia perceive pain differently from healthy individuals (2). Interestingly, although patients with fibromyalgia have similar detection thresholds for electrical, pressure, and thermal stimuli as compared to healthy controls, pain studies reveal that the pain threshold is significantly lower in fibromyalgia (3-5). In fact, converging evidence from neuroimaging (6) and electroencephalography (EEG) (7,8) suggest that fibromyalgia is a condition associated with brain dysfunction, and so fibromyalgia is now recognized as a central pain syndrome (2). Thus, therapeutic approaches should target the central nervous system.

Transcranial direct current stimulation (tDCS) has come to the forefront in the approach to novel treatments for fibromyalgia as this technique of noninvasive brain stimulation has been shown to significantly modulate the perception of sensory tactile, painful, and emotional stimuli (9-11). Furthermore, tDCS as well as other methods of invasive and noninvasive primary motor cortex (M1) stimulation -- including epidural motor cortex stimulation (MCS) and repetitive transcranial magnetic stimulation (rTMS)-- have all been shown to be effective in the alleviation of chronic pain (12). These methods of M1 stimulation are believed to mediate analgesic effects by modulating M1-thalamic inhibitory connections among other cortico-cortical and cortical-subcortical projections involved in pain processing pathways.

Indeed, previous studies by our group have shown that 5 daily sessions of M1 TDCS (2mA, 20 min) can induce significant improvements with respect to pain and sleep parameters in patients with fibromyalgia as compared to sham and dorsolateral prefrontal cortex (DLPFC) stimulation (13,14). Although a regimen of 5 daily sessions of M1 TDCS has already been shown to induce moderately long-lasting effects (up to 3 weeks after the end of stimulation) in our previous study with 32 patients, now we sought to determine the efficacy of a longer treatment protocol. Here we report the results obtained by performing 10 daily sessions of either sham stimulation or M1 or DLPFC tDCS (2 mA, 20 min) in a series of 41 patients with chronic, medically refractory fibromyalgia.

Methods

We conducted a single-center, doubled-blinded, randomized, sham-controlled trial to determine the effect of ten daily sessions of tDCS on pain in women with fibromyalgia. This study conformed to the ethical standards of the Declaration of Helsinki and was approved by the local institutional ethics committee.

Forty-one women (mean age of 54.8 ± 9.6 years, mean ± SD) with chronic, medically refractory fibromyalgia (diagnosed according to the ACR 1990 criteria) were recruited to participate in this study. Patients were selected from a specialized outpatient service. Subjects were regarded as suitable to participate in this study if they fulfilled the following criteria: 1) mean pain score of at least 4 on the visual analog scale (VAS) in the two weeks preceding the clinical trial, 2) sum of tender points score equal to or greater than 11, 3) no clinically significant or unstable medical, neuropsychiatric, or other chronic pain disorder (as assessed by the patient's clinician); 4) not pregnant or lactating; 5) no history of substance abuse or dependence; 6) no use of central nervous system-effective medication in the past 1 month and 7) no history of brain surgery, tumor, or intracranial metal implantation. Patients were carefully evaluated by a licensed rheumatologist before entry into the trial. All study participants provided written, informed consent.

Experimental design

All subjects participated in a baseline observation period of two weeks duration during which baseline parameters were established. The patients were then randomized in a 1:1:1 ratio to receive 10 sessions of either sham tDCS, active tDCS of left M1, or active tDCS of left DLPFC. Randomization was performed using the order of entrance in the study and a previous randomization list generated by a computer using blocks of six (for each six patients, two were randomized to each group) in order to minimize the risk of unbalanced group sizes. The subjects then participated in follow-up assessment at 30 and 60 days after the final tDCS treatment session. Subjects remained blinded to treatment group throughout the study, and blinded raters carried out all assessments.

Transcranial direct current stimulation (tDCS)

tDCS is based on the application of low amplitude direct current to the scalp via two relatively large anode and cathode electrodes (15,16). Although there is substantial shunting at the scalp, a sufficient current penetrates the skull and enters the brain to modify transmembrane neuronal potentials (17,18). In this way, tDCS influence the excitability level of the underlying neurons, such that anodal stimulation generally increases cortical excitability, while cathodal stimulation decreases it (19-21).

In this study, patients received 10 daily sessions (Mon-Fri, 2 weeks) of either sham stimulation or anodal stimulation of left primary motor cortex (M1) or left dorsolateral prefrontal cortex (DLPFC). A pair of thick (.3 cm) rectangular surface sponge electrodes (5cm x 7cm; 35 cm2) were soaked in saline and applied to the scalp at the desired sites of stimulation. Rubber bandages were used to hold the electrodes in place for the duration of stimulation. For anodal stimulation of M1, the anode electrode was placed over C3 according to the 10-20 system for EEG electrode placement (referred in the text as "M1"). The reference cathode electrode was placed over the supraorbital area on the opposite side. Similarly, for anodal stimulation of DLPFC (referred in the text as "DLPFC"), the anode electrode was placed over F3, as confirmed reliable by neuronavigational techniques (22,23), and the cathode electrode was placed over the contralateral supraorbital area. For the active tDCS conditions, a constant current of 2 mA was applied for 20 min; tDCS delivered at a level of 2 mA has been shown to be safe for use in healthy volunteers (24) and patients with varying neurological disorders (25). For SHAM stimulation, the electrodes were placed in the same positions as for anodal M1 stimulation, but the stimulator was turned off after 30 s of stimulation as previously described as being a reliable method of blinding (26), indeed, extensive data from our laboratory suggests that tDCS in healthy subjects is comparable in sensation to sham stimulation regardless of the area stimulated. Finally it should be noted that although M1 is relatively close to DLPFC site given the electrode sizes, this design has shown to be adequate as we have compared cognitive performance (as indexed by working memory tasks) during stimulation of M1 and DLPFC and found differential results, only DLPFC stimulation resulted in a significant effect on working memory performance in healthy subjects (27) and patients with Parkinson's disease (28).

The rationale for the choice of stimulation sites was the following: M1 stimulation via tDCS, rTMS, and epidural stimulation have all been associated with reduced pain in patients with chronic pain syndromes (29,30). DLPFC was chosen as an area of stimulation because the DLFPC is a critical component of the neural circuit involved in processing the cognitive and emotional aspects of pain (31), and because our previous study suggested that anodal stimulation of this area may be able to modulate the emotional processing of pain (11). We chose to stimulate the left M1 and DLPFC regions in keeping with previous studies (13,27,32), yet it should be noted that at least for the DLPFC, non-invasive brain stimulation may result in different modulatory and cognitive-emotional effects depending on the hemisphere used (33,34). Although we did not find significant results for DLPFC stimulation in our previous study (13), the reason might be the number of sessions – i.e., a longer duration of tDCS therapy might be necessary to induce significant effects with stimulation of DLPFC. Although we acknowledge that other studies prefer the use of noncephalic reference electrodes for tDCS to avoid confounding biases (33,36), we placed the reference electrode at the supraorbital cortex under all conditions of stimulation as in our previous tDCS studies with fibromyalgia (13,14).

Clinical assessment

Pain was measured with Visual Analogue Scale for Pain (VAS-pain). Tender point scores were assessed to identify changes in pain quality or location. Quality-of-life and other domains of fibromyalgia were measured using the Fibromyalgia Impact Questionnaire (FIQ) (online at http://www.myalgia.com/FIQ/FIQ.htm) (37). Psychiatric symptoms were assessed with the Beck Depression Inventory (BDI), IDATE state-trait anxiety inventory for anxiety, and Geriatric Depression Scale. Cognition and safety were evaluated by the Mini-Mental State Examination. Finally, we monitored adverse events by asking patients, after each session of stimulation and during the follow-up period, whether they had experienced any adverse event and the relationship of these events to TDCS.

Statistical analysis

Analyses were done with STATA statistical software (version 9.1, Cary, NC, US). In order to compare the effects of stimulation on pain levels, we performed a mixed ANOVA model in which the dependent variable was the level of pain and the independent fixed variables were treatment (baseline, post-treatment, follow-up 1 and follow-up 2), group of stimulation (M1, DLPFC, and sham) and the interaction term group vs. treatment. In addition, we added the random variable subject ID in order to account for the within subjects variability. When appropriate, post-hoc comparisons were carried out using Bonferroni correction for multiple comparisons. We then performed similar models for the other variables. For the main outcome – pain as indexed by VAS – we calculated the mean of the first 3 days for the baseline evaluation and the mean of the last three days for the post-treatment assessment as to give a more reliable assessment as pain has an important variation. Finally, the time points are defined as: baseline, T1 (immediately after the 10 treatment sessions), T2 (30 days after treatment) and T3 (60 days after treatment).

Unless stated otherwise, all results are presented as means and standard deviation, and statistical significance refers to a p value < 0.05.

Results

Fourteen patients were randomized to M1 and sham group and 13 patients to DLPFC group. There were no significant baseline differences in demographics, baseline clinical and pain characteristics (see table 1). There were no dropouts. Patients tolerated the tDCS treatment well. Adverse effects were minor and uncommon – such as skin redness and tingling - and distributed equally across groups of stimulation.

Pain assessment

In order to assess pain (as indexed by VAS), we initially assessed the interaction term time vs. group of stimulation for the main model. This term was statistically significant ($F_{(9,114)}=3.05$, p=0.0026); suggesting, therefore, that pain changed differently according to the group of stimulation. In fact, post-hoc comparisons showed that there were no significant changes in pain scores for the sham group (when comparing baseline vs. T1, T2, and T3). However, for M1 group, there was a significant difference between baseline vs. T1 (p=0.012), baseline vs. T2 (p=0.02) and baseline vs. T3 (p=0.03), indicating a significant pain reduction that lasted up to 2 months after the end of stimulation (see figure 1). Although there was also a significant effect for DLPFC group when comparing baseline vs. T1 (p=0.035), there was no difference between baseline vs. T2 (p=0.17) and baseline vs. T3 (p=0.27). Suggesting that although DLPFC induced a significant pain reduction, this effect was not long lasting. In fact, we then conducted additional models with each condition of stimulation separately to assess time effect and our results were confirmed: only the model for M1 group showed a significant time effect (F(3,52)=4.07, p=0.011). For the DLPFC and sham groups, there was no significant time effect (p>0.19 for both groups).

Table 1. Demographic and baseline clinical characteristics

	DLPFC mean	DLPFC sd	M1 mean	M1 sd	Sham mean	Sham sd	p-value
Age	57.46	6.21	52.79	10.42	54.50	11.37	ns
Duration of disease	7.54	3.93	8.39	7.06	8.69	3.61	ns
BMI	30.67	5.76	26.92	5.82	29.29	7.08	ns
Pain (VAS)	6.99	1.53	6.00	1.52	6.14	2.44	ns
FIQ	92.62	18.29	90.95	23.94	96.28	28.89	ns
BDI	20.17	8.65	15.08	9.14	18.79	6.82	ns
GDS	14.08	5.95	13.17	8.23	19.43	11.60	ns
IDATE	53.85	12.03	48.43	9.44	52.57	14.21	ns
MMSE	25.92	3.40	25.58	3.85	26.36	3.18	ns

age (years), duration of disease (years), BMI- body mass index (kg/m^2), VAS-Pain Score (0= no pain, 10= worst pain), FIQ- Fibromyalgia Impact Questionnaire (0= no impact, 100= worst possible), BDI- Beck Depression Inventory (0= no depression, 29-63=severe depression), GDS- Geriatric Depression Scale (0= no depression, 10-19= mild depression, 20-30= severe depression), IDATE- Anxiety Metric: (0-30= low anxiety, 31-49= medium anxiety, 50-80= high degree of anxiety), MMSE- Mini-Mental Status Exam (scores of 23/30 and lower indicate relative cognitive impairment). ns indicates not significant (one-way ANOVA comparing the three groups).

Analysis of tender point scores was not significant (p>.2 for all the analyses), showing that this outcome was not sensitive to assess the effects of tDCS treatment on pain reduction.

Quality of life

Changes in domains other than pain (e.g. function, fatigue, sleep disturbance, psychological distress) were assessed using the fibromyalgia impact questionnaire (FIQ). However FIQ was assessed at baseline and only immediately after treatment (T1). Repeated measures analysis for the FIQ showed a significant interaction term (time vs. group) effect (F(3,38) =6.54; p=0.001). Although the results showed that the three groups had a decrease in the FIQ scores over the course of the trial, only the decrease in the M1 group (28.3% (±37.1) reduction, p=0.0015) and DLPFC group (27.6% (±26.8) reduction, p=0.02) were significant. The small decrease in the sham group was not significant (13.8 (±39.4) reduction, p=0.15) (see figure 2).

Efficacy of anodal transcranial direct current stimulation ... 419

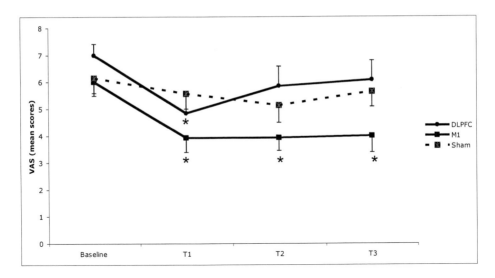

Figure 1. Mean pain scores associated with the three conditions of stimulation: left M1 (primary motor cortex); left DLPFC (dorsolateral prefrontal cortex); and sham tDCS. Pain scores are reported on the Visual Analogue Scale for Pain; 0= no pain, 10= worst pain of life. * Indicates statistically significant (p<0.05) as compared with baseline. Each column represents mean score ± SEM (standard error of mean). T1: end of stimulation, T2: 30 day follow-up, T3: 60 day follow-up.

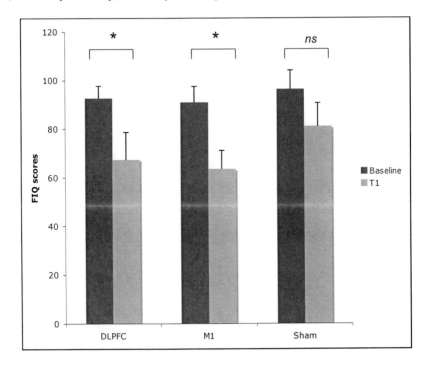

Figure 2. Mean fibromyalgia impact scores associated with the three conditions of stimulation: left M1 (primary motor cortex); left DLPFC (dorsolateral prefrontal cortex); and sham tDCS. The Fibromyalgia Impact Questionnaire (FIQ) quantitates the overall impact of fibromyalgia over many dimensions (e.g. physical functioning, pain level, fatigue, sleep disturbance, psychological distress, etc.) and has been extensively validated; 0= no impact on quality of life, 100= worst impact possible. * Indicates statistically significant (p<0.05). ns – indicates not significant (p>0.05). Each column represents mean FIQ score ± SEM (standard error of mean). T1: end of stimulation, T2: 30 day follow-up, T3: 60 day follow-up.

Psychiatric assessment

For mood assessment, our results showed that there was no significant difference in BDI scores across the three groups of treatment (interaction term group vs. time - $F(3, 38)=0.51$; $p=0.67$), therefore revealing that treatment with tDCS was not associated with mood changes. In fact mean changes in depression scores was less than 10% for three groups of treatment. Similar results were obtained for IDATE state-trait anxiety inventory for anxiety, and Geriatric Depression Scale ($F<1$ for the interaction term for these two analyses).

Correlations

In an exploratory way, we performed correlation tests between pain improvement after M1 and DLPFC stimulation as indexed by VAS score changes (between baseline and after 10 days of treatment) with the following variables: age, duration of pain, sleep (VAS), body mass index (BMI), baseline scores of depression (BDI), pain (VAS) baseline, and fibromyalgia impact questionnaire (FIQ). The results showed no significant correlations.

Discussion

Our results show that 10 daily sessions of 2 mA, 20 min tDCS of left M1 or DLPFC can both induce significant improvements with respect to pain and quality of life in patients with fibromyalgia. These findings are consistent with our previous study of tDCS in patients with fibromyalgia--where 5 daily sessions of M1 tDCS also induced a significant pain reduction. However, in contrast to our previous study where pain scores were noted to take an upward slope at two weeks after treatment completion, here we show that 10 sessions of M1 tDCS can be effective in maintaining the observed diminishment of pain scores for up to 60 days. This difference is in keeping with an rTMS study in patients with fibromyalgia, which shows that 10 daily sessions of 10Hz rTMS applied to the motor cortex can induce similarly long-lasting improvements in pain and measures of quality of life (38). Interestingly, the analgesic effects of the repeated sessions of rTMS were significant only after 5 days of stimulation.

These results are interesting as they underscore the impact of the number of treatment sessions in inducing and maintaining long-lasting clinical effects. Indeed, previous tDCS studies have come to a similar conclusion: Five daily sessions of tDCS in stroke patients yields greater improvements in motor function than a single session alone (39); and, rTMS studies corroborate this session-number dependent efficacy trend: more sessions results in longer-lasting or more significant effects (40-42). In addition, the importance lies not only in the total number of sessions administered, but also in their temporal proximity: 4 weekly sessions of tDCS in stroke patients does not result in changes that are significantly different from single session therapy (39). Therefore, these findings suggest that tDCS induces a cumulative effect that is maximized by consecutive sessions.

tDCS is believed to induce clinical effects through the modulation of synaptic connections (43). Nitsche et al. have shown that anodal stimulation of sufficient duration can enhance cortical excitability beyond the stimulation period (20,21). Further studies have revealed that these changes in post-tDCS cortical excitability are intimately dependent on Na+ channel and NMDA receptor activity (44,45) and that acetylcholine plays an important role in the consolidation of this neuroplasticity (46). These results suggest that long term potentiation of new adaptive synaptic connection is what underlies the improvements in working memory (27), motor function (39), and pain modulation (47) that have been attributed to tDCS. Because LTP underlies the mechanism behind the long-lasting effects of repeated sessions of tDCS, it is therefore not surprising that the changes in cortical excitability and synaptic connections induced by tDCS are prone to extinction and that they can be reinforced with longer and/or additional treatment sessions. Indeed, the difference between our results with 10 sessions of tDCS vs. 5 daily sessions may be attributed to greater synaptic strengthening.

In addition to demonstrating the efficacy of M1 tDCS in relieving pain in fibromyalgia, our study here also demonstrates a potential role for DLPFC stimulation. Whereas our previous study failed to show a significant effect for DLPFC stimulation, here 10 sessions of DLFPC stimulation significantly diminished pain scores compared to sham stimulation. Thus, it is possible that DLPFC is also useful but it is inevitably less effective than M1 for the treatment of fibromyalgia-associated pain. Mechanistically, M1 stimulation produces an analgesic effect by modulating the sensory aspects of pain, while DLPFC stimulation mediates its effects by modulating affective-emotional networks regulating the unpleasantness associated with pain (11). Pain in fibromyalgia has been associated with abnormal information processing characterized by a lack of inhibitory control over somatosensory processing (7,8); thus, it appears appropriate that M1 tDCS would have a more primary analgesic effect in this population.

The treatment protocols resulted in no change to tender points or measures of depression or anxiety as compared to sham stimulation; these parameters may be secondary to central pain in fibromyalgia. In addition we found no significant correlations between baseline characteristics and response to treatment, yet this might be due to low power to perform these correlations.

Here we show that 10 daily sessions of M1 and DLPFC tDCS both generate clinical improvements in patients with fibromyalgia, but that only M1 stimulation results in long-lasting clinical benefits as assessed at 30 and 60 days after the end of treatment. This study demonstrates the importance of the duration of the treatment period, suggesting that protocols with 10 daily sessions of tDCS would result in more long lasting outcomes than protocols with only 5 daily sessions. Furthermore, this study supports the findings of a similarly designed rTMS trial (38), although it should be noted that the magnitude of the effect of 10 sessions of tDCS appears to be greater than the respective rTMS trial— nevertheless, this needs to be compared in a head to head comparison trial of tDCS vs. rTMS using the same study population. Noninvasive forms of brain stimulation hold great promise, yet further studies are indicated to determine the role of maintenance therapy in treatment planning.

References

[1] Wolfe F, Smythe HA, Yunus MB, Bennett RM, Bombardier C, Goldenberg DL, et al. The American College of Rheumatology 1990 Criteria for the Classification of Fibromyalgia. Report of the Multicenter Criteria Committee. Arthritis Rheum 1990;33(2): 160-72.

[2]	Schweinhardt P, Sauro KM, Bushnell MC. Fibromyalgia: A disorder of the brain? Neuroscientist 2008;14(5):415-21.
[3]	Dadabhoy D, Clauw DJ. Therapy Insight: fibromyalgia. A different type of pain needing a different type of treatment. Nat Clin Pract Rheumatol 2006;2(7):364-72.
[4]	Lautenbacher S, Rollman GB. Possible deficiencies of pain modulation in fibromyalgia. Clin J Pain 1997;13(3):189-96.
[5]	Gracely RH, Petzke F, Wolf JM, Clauw DJ. Functional magnetic resonance imaging evidence of augmented pain processing in fibromyalgia. Arthritis Rheum 2002;46(5):1333-43.
[6]	Cook DB, Stegner AJ, McLoughlin MJ. Imaging pain of fibromyalgia. Curr Pain Headache Rep 2007;11(3):190-200.
[7]	Montoya P, Sitges C, Garcia-Herrera M, Rodriguez-Cotes A, Izquierdo R, Truyols M, et al. Reduced brain habituation to somatosensory stimulation in patients with fibromyalgia. Arthritis Rheum 2006;54(6):1995-2003.
[8]	Diers M, Koeppe C, Yilmaz P, Thieme K, Markela-Lerenc J, Schiltenwolf M, et al. Pain ratings and somatosensory evoked responses to repetitive intramuscular and intracutaneous stimulation in fibromyalgia syndrome. J Clin Neurophysiol 2008;25(3):153-60.
[9]	Matsunaga K, Nitsche MA, Tsuji S, Rothwell JC. Effect of transcranial DC sensorimotor cortex stimulation on somatosensory evoked potentials in humans. Clin Neurophysiol 2004;115(2):456-60.
[10]	Rogalewski A, Breitenstein C, Nitsche MA, Paulus W, Knecht S. Transcranial direct current stimulation disrupts tactile perception. Eur J Neurosci 2004;20(1):313-6.
[11]	Boggio PS, Zaghi S, Lopes M, Fregni F. Modulatory effects of anodal transcranial direct current stimulation on perception and pain thresholds in healthy volunteers. Eur J Neurol 2008;15(10):1124-30.
[12]	Lima MC, Fregni F. Motor cortex stimulation for chronic pain: systematic review and meta-analysis of the literature. Neurology 2008;70(24):2329-37.
[13]	Fregni F, Gimenes R, Valle AC, Ferreira MJ, Rocha RR, et al.. A randomized, sham-controlled, proof of principle study of transcranial direct current stimulation for the treatment of pain in fibromyalgia. Arthritis Rheum 2006;54:3988-98.
[14]	Roizenblatt S, Fregni F, Gimenez R, Wetzel T, Rigonatti SP, Tufik S., et al. Site-specific effects of transcranial direct current stimulation on sleep and pain in fibromyalgia: a randomized, sham-controlled study. Pain Pract 2007;7(4):297-306.
[15]	Sparing R, Mottaghy FM. Noninvasive brain stimulation with transcranial magnetic or direct current stimulation (TMS/tDCS)-From insights into human memory to therapy of its dysfunction. Methods 2008;44(4):329-37.
[16]	Priori A. Brain polarization in humans: a reappraisal of an old tool for prolonged non-invasive modulation of brain excitability. Clin Neurophysiol 2003;114(4):589-95.
[17]	Miranda PC, Lomarev M, Hallett M. Modeling the current distribution during transcranial direct current stimulation. Clin Neurophysiol 2006;117(7):1623-9.
[18]	Wagner T, Valero-Cabre A, Pascual-Leone A. Noninvasive human brain stimulation. Annu Rev Biomed Eng 2007;9:527-65.
[19]	Nitsche MA, Paulus W. Excitability changes induced in the human motor cortex by weak transcranial direct current stimulation. J Physiol 2000;527(3):633-9.
[20]	Nitsche MA, Paulus W. Sustained excitability elevations induced by transcranial DC motor cortex stimulation in humans. Neurology 2001;57(10):1899-1901.
[21]	Nitsche MA, Fricke K, Henschke U, Schlitterlau A, Liebetanz D, Lang N, et al. Pharmacological modulation of cortical excitability shifts induced by transcranial direct current stimulation in humans. J Physiol 2003;553(1):293-301.
[22]	Rossi S, Cappa SF, Babiloni C, Pasqualetti P, Miniussi C, Carducci F, et al. Prefrontal [correction of Prefontal] cortex in long-term memory: an "interference" approach using magnetic stimulation. Nat Neurosci 2001;4(9):948-52.

[23] Herwig U, Lampe Y, Juengling FD, Wunderlich A, Walter H, Spitzer M, et al. Add-on rTMS for treatment of depression: a pilot study using stereotaxic coil-navigation according to PET data. J Psychiatr Res 2003;37(4):267-75.
[24] Iyer MB, Mattu U, Grafman J, Lomarev M, Sato S, Wassermann EM. Safety and cognitive effect of frontal DC brain polarization in healthy individuals. Neurology 2005;64(5):872-5.
[25] Poreisz C, Boros K, Antal A, Paulus W. Safety aspects of transcranial direct current stimulation concerning healthy subjects and patients. Brain Res Bull 2007;72(4-6):208-14.
[26] Gandiga PC, Hummel FC, Cohen LG. Transcranial DC stimulation (tDCS): a tool for double-blind sham-controlled clinical studies in brain stimulation. Clin Neurophysiol 2006;117(4):845-50.
[27] Fregni F, Boggio PS, Nitsche M, Bermpohl F, Antal A, et al. Anodal transcranial direct current stimulation of prefrontal cortex enhances working memory. Exp Brain Res 2005;166:23-30.
[28] Boggio PS, Ferrucci R, Rigonatti SP, Covre P, Nitsche M, Pascual-Leone A, et al. Effects of transcranial direct current stimulation on working memory in patients with Parkinson's disease. J Neurol Sci 2006;249(1):31-8.
[29] Fregni F, Pascual-Leone A. Technology insight: noninvasive brain stimulation in neurology-perspectives on the therapeutic potential of rTMS and tDCS. Nat Clin Pract Neurol 2007;3:383-93.
[30] Lefaucheur JP. Use of repetitive transcranial magnetic stimulation in pain relief. Expert Rev Neurother 2008;8(5):799-808.
[31] Duquette M, Roy M, Lepore F, Peretz I, Rainville P. [Cerebral mechanisms involved in the interaction between pain and emotion]. Rev Neurol (Paris) 2007;163(2):169-79. [French]
[32] Boggio PS, Rigonatti SP, Ribeiro RB, Myczkowski ML, Nitsche MA, Pascual-Leone A, et al. A randomized, double-blind clinical trial on the efficacy of cortical direct current stimulation for the treatment of major depression. Int J Neuropsychopharmacol 2008;11(2):249-54.
[33] Fecteau S, Pascual-Leone A, Zald DH, Liguori P, Theoret H, Boggio PS, et al. Activation of prefrontal cortex by transcranial direct current stimulation reduces appetite for risk during ambiguous decision making. J Neurosci 2007;27(23):6212-8.
[34] Avery DH, Holtzheimer PE3rd, Fawaz W, Russo J, Neumaier J, Dunner DL, et al. Transcranial magnetic stimulation reduces pain in patients with major depression: a sham-controlled study. J Nerv Ment Dis 2007;195(5):378-81.
[35] Cogiamanian F, Marceglia S, Ardolino G, Barbieri S, Priori A. Improved isometric force endurance after transcranial direct current stimulation over the human motor cortical areas. Eur J Neurosci 2007:26(1):242-9.
[36] Priori A, Mameli F, Cogiamanian F, Marceglia S, Tiriticco M, Mrakic-Sposta S, et al. Lie-specific involvement of dorsolateral prefrontal cortex in deception. Cereb Cortex 2008;18(2):451-5.
[37] Burckhardt CS, Clark SR, Bennett RM. The fibromyalgia impact questionnaire (FIQ): development and validation. J Rheumatol 1991;18:728-33.
[38] Passard A, Attal N, Benadhira R, Brasseur L, Saba G, Sichere P, et al. Effects of unilateral repetitive transcranial magnetic stimulation of the motor cortex on chronic widespread pain in fibromyalgia. Brain 2007;130(10):2661-70.
[39] Boggio PS, Nunes A, Rigonatti SP, Nitsche MA, Pascual-Leone A, Fregni F. Repeated sessions of noninvasive brain DC stimulation is associated with motor function improvement in stroke patients. Restor Neurol Neurosci 2007;25(2):123-9.
[40] Rumi DO, Gattaz WF, Rigonatti SP, Rosa MA, Fregni F, Rosa MO, et al. Transcranial magnetic stimulation accelerates the antidepressant effect of amitriptyline in severe depression: a double-blind placebo-controlled study. Biol Psychiatry 2005;57(2):162-6.
[41] Avery DH, Holtzheimer PE3rd, Fawaz W, Russo J, Neumaier J, Dunner DL, et al. A controlled study of repetitive transcranial magnetic stimulation in medication-resistant major depression. Biol Psychiatry 2006;59(2):187-94.

[42] Khedr EM, Kotb H, Kamel NF, Ahmed MA, Sadek R, Rothwell JC. Longlasting antalgic effects of daily sessions of repetitive transcranial magnetic stimulation in central and peripheral neuropathic pain. J Neurol Neurosurg Psychiatry 2005;76(6):833-8.

[43] Nitsche MA, Seeber A, Frommann K, Klein CC, Rochford C, Nitsche MS, et al. Modulating parameters of excitability during and after transcranial direct current stimulation of the human motor cortex. J Physiol 2005;568(1):291-303.

[44] Nitsche MA, Jaussi W, Liebetanz D, Lang N, Tergau F, Paulus W. Consolidation of human motor cortical neuroplasticity by D-cycloserine. Neuropsychopharmacology 2004;29(8):1573-8.

[45] Liebetanz D, Nitsche MA, Tergau F, Paulus W. Pharmacological approach to the mechanisms of transcranial DC-stimulation-induced after-effects of human motor cortex excitability. Brain 2002;125(10): 2238-47.

[46] Kuo MF, Grosch J, Fregni F, Paulus W, Nitsche MA. Focusing effect of acetylcholine on neuroplasticity in the human motor cortex. J Neurosci 2007;27(52):14442-7.

[47] Fregni F, Freedman S, Pascual-Leone A. Recent advances in the treatment of chronic pain with non-invasive brain stimulation techniques. Lancet Neurol 2007;6:188-91.

In: Pain Management Yearbook 2009
Editor: Joav Merrick

ISBN: 978-1-61209-666-7
©2012 Nova Science Publishers, Inc.

Chapter 36

CATHODAL tDCS OVER THE SOMATOSENSORY CORTEX RELIEVED CHRONIC NEUROPATHIC PAIN IN A PATIENT WITH COMPLEX REGIONAL PAIN SYNDROME (CRPS/RSD)

Helena Knotkova, PhD[*,1,2], *Peter Homel, PhD*[1]
and Ricardo A Cruciani, MD, PhD[1,2,3]

[1]Institute for Non-invasive Brain Stimulation of New York, Research Division, Department of Pain Medicine and Palliative Care, New York, [2]Department of Neurology, Albert Einstein College of Medicine, Bronx, New York and [3]Department of Anesthesiology, Albert Einstein College of Medicine, Bronx, New York, United States of America

Abstract

Complex Regional Pain Syndrome type I, formerly known as reflex sympathetic dystrophy (CRPS/RSD) is a debilitating neuropathic pain syndrome. Pain in CRPS/RSD is disproportionate to the inciting event, and in many cases CRPS/RSD-related pain does not respond to conventional therapy. The anodal transcranial direct current stimulation (tDCS) has been shown to alleviate intractable pain in CRPS/RSD as well as in some other chronic pain syndromes, while the cathodal tDCS has been shown to reduce experimentally-induced pain in healthy subjects. Up to date, there is no published evidence of the analgesic efficacy of cathodal tDCS over the somatosensory cortex for chronic pain. Here, we report our findings from cathodal stimulation over the somatosensory cortex as compared with "traditional" anodal stimulation over the motor cortex, applied in clinical settings to a patient with intractable CRPS/RSD–related chronic pain in lower limb. The patient received one block of anodal tDCS over the motor cortex and one block of cathodal tDCs over the somatosensory cortex. The period between the two blocks was 6 weeks. Each block consisted of 5 sessions on 5 consecutive days, and the current at intensity of 2 mA was delivered for 20 min. Both cathodal tDCS over the somatosensory cortex and anodal tDCS over the motor cortex resulted in significant pain relief. However, the patient favored the

---

* **Correspondence:** Helena Knotkova, PhD, Department of Pain Medicine and Palliative Care, 350 E 17th Str., Baird Hall, 12th fl, New York, NY, 10003, United States. E-mail: HKnotkov@chpnet.org

cathodal stimulation. Our findings suggest that it is clinically meaningful to further evaluate the analgesic potential of cathodal tDCS by conducting sham-controlled studies in larger samples of patients.

Keywords: Transcranial direct current stimulation (tDCS), non-invasive brain stimulation, Complex Regional Pain Syndrome I (CRPS/RSD), neuropathic pain.

Introduction

Complex Regional Pain Syndrome type I (CRPS I), formerly known as reflex sympathetic dystrophy (RSD), and Complex Regional Pain Syndrome type II, formerly known as causalgia (CRPS II), are debilitating neuropathic pain syndromes. Web-based epidemiological survey of CRPS/RSD conducted in the USA between 2004 and 2005 (www.rsdsa.org) indicates that 93% of CRPS/RSD patients experience neuropathic pain from the time of diagnosis, and that the CRPS-related pain substantially deteriorates quality of life in the majority of the patients (95% of responders), with a disability rate of 60%. Typically, spontaneous pain in CRPS is not limited to the territory of a single peripheral nerve and is disproportionate to the inciting event (1). Moreover, in many CRPS patients, pain does not respond to conventional treatment. A rationale for using modulation of cortical excitability in patients with treatment-resistant chronic pain is based on the evidence that patients with chronic pain may develop pathological changes in the excitability of the somatosensory and motor cortices, and that normalization of the cortical excitability has been paralleled by pain relief (2-4).

Up to date, all published protocols that use tDCS to alleviate chronic pain (5-11) delivered anodal (excitatory) tDCS stimulation over the motor cortex. Cathodal (inhibitory) stimulation over the somatosensory cortex has shown to decrease pain ratings in experimentally-induced acute pain in healthy subjects (12). As there are substantial differences in mechanisms underlying the acute, experimentally induced pain vs. chronic spontaneous pain, it could not be predicted to which extent the findings from cathodal stimulation in healthy subjects with experimentally-induced pain would apply to patients with chronic pain conditions. There is no published evidence of the analgesic efficacy of cathodal tDCS over the somatosensory cortex for chronic pain. Here, we report our findings from cathodal stimulation over the somatosensory cortex as compared with "traditional" anodal stimulation over the motor cortex, applied to a patient with intractable chronic pain of lower limb due to CRPS/RSD.

Case study

The patient is a 55 year old Caucasian male with no prior significant past medical or psychiatric history. The onset of pain was triggered by a surgical procedure done to repair an injury to the knee that he sustained while working as a New York City Police Officer in 1998. During 2003-2007, he underwent multiple drug trials included e.g. lamotrigine, fentanyl patch, hydrocodone/acetaminophen, oxycodone ER, methadone, gabapentine, lidocaine and ketamine infusions. The treatments resulted in either dose-limiting side-effects or sub-optimal pain relief. At the time when the patient opted to receive tDCS to alleviate his CRPS-related neuropathic pain, his pain was severe despite high doses of pain medication taken on daily basis. Here, we report results from one block of anodal tDCS over the motor cortex and a consecutive block of cathodal tDCs over the somatosensory cortex. The period between the two blocks was six weeks. Each block consisted of five sessions on five consecutive days, the current at intensity of 2 mA was delivered for 20 min, with two saline-soaked (9 mg NaCl/liter) sponge electrodes, size 25 cm^2, and the current density was 0.08 mA/cm2 in both conditions (anodal, cathodal). A non-parametric permutation test was used to obtain the p-values for the correlation between level of pain and time.

Results

As shown at figure 1A, the cathodal tDCS over the somatosensory cortex resulted in significant decrease of pain over time (r = -0.92, p= 0.03). The effect was cumulative, with the pattern similar to the analgesic effect of anodal stimulation (figure 1B), r = -.96, p = 0.02. Neither cathodal nor anodal stimulation elicited any substantial side-effects. During both types of stimulation, the patient reported mild tingling and mild burning under the electrodes. The sensation faded immediately after the end of stimulation. Although both modalities (cathodal, anodal) yielded comparable results, i.e. lead to significant pain relief, the patient favored the cathodal stimulation, describing the effect as "more stable", "less flare-ups of pain during hours immediately after the stimulation", and "calming effect on his mood".

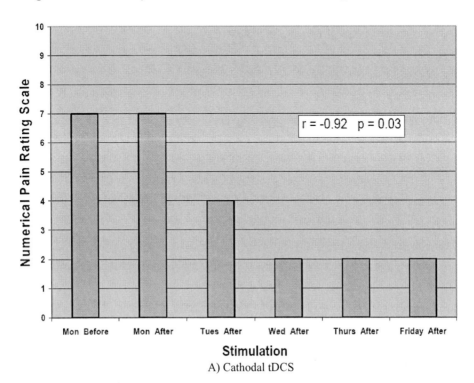

Figure 1. (Continued).

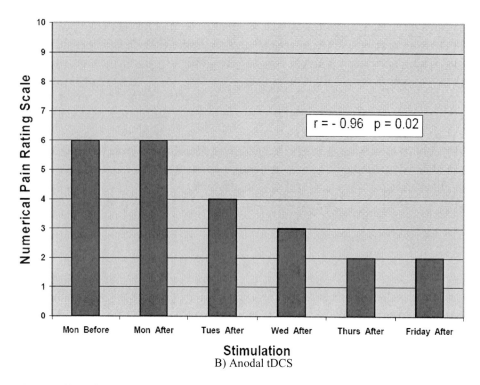

Figure 1 A,B. Effect of anodal tDCS over the motor cortex (A), and cathodal tDCS over the somatosensory cortex (B) in a CRPS/RSD patient. Pain relief was induced by a block (5 tDCS sessions on 5 consecutive days) of either cathodal tDCS over the somatosensory cortex (A), or anodal tDCS over the motor cortex (B) at intensity of 2 mA for 20 min, using saline-soaked sponge electrodes, size 25cm2. The interval between the two blocks of stimulation was 6 weeks. Both modalities (cathodal tDCS over the somatosensory cortex and anodal tDCS over the motor cortex) resulted in significant pain relief.

Conclusions

- Both cathodal stimulation over the somatosensory cortex and anodal stimulation over the motor cortex resulted in significant relief in this patient with CRPS/RSD.
- The procedure was well tolerated by the patient and did not elicit any substantial side effects.
- Although both procedures (anodal and cathodal tDCS) yielded similar results, leading to significant pain relief, the patient favored the cathodal stimulation.
- Our findings suggest that it is clinically meaningful to further evaluate the analgesic potential of cathodal tDCS over the somatosensory cortex, by conducting sham-controlled studies in larger samples of patients with various chronic pain syndromes.

References

[1] Baron R, Binder A. Complex regional pain syndromes. In: Pappagallo M, ed. The neurological basis of pain. New York: McGraw Hill, 2005.

[2] Maihöfner C, Handwerker HO, Neundorfer B, Birklen F. Patterns of cortical reorganization in complex regional pain syndrome. Neurology 2003;61(12):1707-15.
[3] Maihofner CCA, Handwerker HO,Neundorfer B,Birklein F: Cortical reorganization during recovery from complex regional pain syndrome. Neurology 2004;63(4):693-701.
[4] Pleger B, Tegenthoff M, Ragert P, Forster AF, Dinse HR, Schwenkreis P, Nicolas V, Maier C. Sensorimotor returning in complex regional pain syndrome parallels pain reduction. Ann Neurol 2005;57(3):425-9.
[5] Fregni F, Gimenes R, Valle AS, Ferreira MJ, Rocha RR, et al. A randomized,sham-controlled, proof of principle study of transcranial direct current stimulation for the treatment of pain in fibromyalgia. Arthritis Rheum 2006; 54(12):3988-98.
[6] Fregni F, Boggio PS, Lima MC, Ferreira MJ, Wagner T, et al. A sham-controlled, phase II trial of transcranial direct current stimulation for the treatment of central pain in traumatic spinal cord injury. Pain 2006;122(1-2):197-209.
[7] Roizenblatt S, Fregni F, Gimenez R, Werzel T, Rigonatti SP, et al. Site-specific effects of transcranial direct current stimulation on sleep and pain in fibromyalgia: a randomized, sham-controlled study. Pain Pract 2007;7(4):297-306.
[8] Kuhnl S, Terney D, Paulus W, Antal A. The effect of daily sessions of anodal tDCS on chronic pain. Brain Stimulat 2008;1(3):281.
[9] Fenton B, Fanning J, Boggio P, Fregni F. A pilot efficacy trial of tDCS for the treatment of refractory chronic pelvic pain. Brain Stimulat 2008;1(3):260.
[10] Knotkova H, Sibirceva U, Factor A, Feldman D, Ragert P, Flor H, Cohen H, Cruciani R. Repetitive transcranial direct current stimulation (tDCS) for the treatment of neuropathic pain due to complex regional pain syndrome (CRPS). Book of Abstracts, 12th World Congress on Pain, Glasgow, IASP Press 2008:125.
[11] Knotkova H, Feldman D, Factor A, Sibirceva U, Dvorkin E, Cohen L, Ragert P, Cruciani RA. Repeated transcranial direct current stimulation improves hyperalgesia and allodynia in a CRPS patient. Brain Stimulation, 2008;1(3):254.
[12] Antal A, Brepohl N, Poreisz C, Boros K, Csifcsak G. Paulus W. Transcranial direct current stimulation over somatosensory cortex decreases experimentally induced acute pain perception. Clin J Pain 2008;24(1):56-63.

SECTION FOUR - CANCER AND PAIN

Chapter 37

BISPHOSPHONATES IN COMBINATION WITH RADIOTHERAPY FOR THE TREATMENT OF BONE METASTASES: A LITERATURE REVIEW

Shaelyn Culleton, BSc(C), Amanda Hird, BSc(C), Janet Nguyen, BSc(C), Urban Emmenegger, MD, Sunil Verma, MD, Christine Simmons, MD, Elizabeth Barnes, MD, May Tsao, MD, Arjun Sahgal, MD, Cyril Danjoux, MD, Gunita Mitera, MRTT, MBA, Emily Sinclair, MRTT and Edward Chow, MBBS[*]

Rapid Response Radiotherapy Program, Department of Radiation Oncology and Division of Medical Oncology, Odette Cancer Centre, Sunnybrook Health Sciences Centre, University of Toronto, Toronto, Ontario, Canada

Abstract

The purpose was to investigate the clinical benefits of combining radiation and bisphosphonates in bone metastases. Methods: A systematic search on Medline was conducted from 1950 to November 2008. Eligible studies included in-vitro cell studies, animal tumor models, and any human studies combining the use of radiotherapy and bisphosphonates. This search was limited to English publications only. Results: A total of 13 studies involving the combination of bisphosphonates and radiotherapy were identified. Three were in-vitro cell studies, two were animal tumor models, and eight were human studies. Both in-vitro cell studies and animal tumor models demonstrate significant synergistic effects when combining both therapies. There are only two human randomized trials comparing combination therapy to placebo and radiation, which showed greater long term benefits using combination treatment. Conclusion: Preliminary evidence suggests that patients with bone metastases may significantly benefit from concurrent treatment with both radiotherapy and bisphosphonates when compared with either treatment alone.

---

[*] **Correspondence:** Edward Chow, MBBS, PhD, FRCPC, Department of Radiation Oncology, Odette Cancer Centre, Sunnybrook Health Sciences Centre, 2075 Bayview Avenue, Toronto, ON M4N 3M5, Canada. Tel: 416-480-4998; Fax: 416-480-6002; E-mail: Edward.Chow@sunnybrook.ca

Keywords: Bisphosphonates, radiotherapy, bone metastases, combination therapy.

Introduction

Skeletal metastases are a common and often debilitating complication of advanced cancer, with incidences ranging from 23 to 84% (1). Bone metastases can lead to skeletal related events (SREs), which cause significant morbidity, including hypercalcemia, pathological fractures, bone pain and spinal cord compression (1-6). On average, 45-75% of patients with bone metastases experience pain (7). In particular, patients with advanced breast, lung and prostate cancer are among those most commonly impacted by bone metastases (7), accounting for approximately 80% of all cases (8).

With advancements in systemic therapies, patients are now living longer with their diagnosis of bone metastases (8-11). Therefore, this cohort is at an increased risk for experiencing SREs, thereby making the prevention and management of these disease-related events of upmost importance. Two of the most prevalent treatments in managing and preventing adverse events and symptoms associated with bone metastases are radiotherapy (RT) and bisphosphonates (BPs) (12,13).

Radiotherapy is a well-established treatment for the palliation of symptomatic bone metastases (14). Approximately 50-80% of patients receive some pain relief, and approximately 20-30% of patients achieve complete pain relief (13-15). It also has been noted that RT is more effective at reducing incident pain than any analgesic regimen (13).

The most commonly prescribed doses of palliative RT for bone metastases are a single 8Gy fraction, 20Gy in five fractions, and 30Gy in 10 fractions (7,15-17). Palliative doses are considerably less than those used for curative intent, and as such, are usually associated with fewer side effects. Nevertheless, palliative RT not only reduces and often alleviates pain, but it also reduces the tumor burden. For bone metastases treated with RT, the consequence of suppression of progressive osteoclast activity serves to help irradiated bone restore integrity and enables osteoblastic repair. Even though the exact mechanisms of pain relief from RT are not yet fully understood, it is felt that complementary osteoclast inhibition by BPs and RT represents a rationale for the combined use of these two treatment modalities (14).

Since the 1980's, the use of BPs in managing bone metastases has been well established. BPs have a high affinity for bone minerals, allowing these molecules to congregate in areas of active bone destruction. Osteoclasts then take up these BPs and induce apoptosis and inhibit cell differentiation (18). This effect is even more pronounced in newer generation BPs modified with nitrogenous side chains (for example, zoledronic acid) (18). Large meta-analyses of randomized BP trials have shown that they significantly reduce SREs in breast and prostate cancer by 17% and 5.2%, respectively. In addition, both prostate and breast cancer trials have showed significant relief in metastatic bone pain. These effects are associated with an improvement in overall quality of life (6,10,11).

The mechanisms by which BPs suppress osteoclast and osteoblast activity are complex and encompasses various tumor factors, proteins and other molecules. Primarily, BPs act by suppressing both mature and precursor osteoclast cells, and provide physico-chemical protection from hypercalcemia by inhibiting calcium phosphate precipitation (6,14,19). Bisphosphonates have proven to be effective in managing both osteosclerotic and osteolytic lesions since both processes involve the hyperactivity of osteoclast cells (19,20).

Given that RT and BPs are effective in managing bone metastases, particularly with respect to the suppression of osteoclast activity, it is conceivable that combining these two treatments could enhance the overall effect of either treatment in isolation. Data has emerged from the literature within the last 10 years investigating the potential for synergy (21) and the purpose of this review is to summarize relevant studies reporting the potential of this combined approach.

Methods

We conducted a systematic Medline (1950 to November 2008) and Cochrane Central Register of Controlled Trials (4th Quarter 2008) search. Search terms included combinations of "radiotherapy", "irradiation" "bone neoplasm" and "bisphosphonate". Secondary search terms included "zoledronic acid", "zoledronate", "etidronate", "clodronate", "pamidronate", "ibandronate" and "bone metastasis". The search results were manually reviewed, relevant literature was extracted and the references for all these publications were thoroughly examined for additional references.

Inclusion criteria

All studies involving the combination of BPs and palliative RT for the management of bone metastases were included. This criterion also included in-vitro studies.

Exclusion criteria

Studies that were in a language other than English were not considered in our review.

Results

We identified a total of 13 studies that combined both BPs and RT, three of which were in-vitro cell studies, and two of which studied combination therapy in animal tumor models. The remaining eight involved combination BP and RT treatment in humans.

In-vitro cell studies

Three in-vitro studies combining both RT and BPs were identified. The main results of all three studies are summarized in table 1. All studies found a significant synergistic effect when the two treatments were combined, by means of a reduction in cell viability via induction of apoptosis (3,7,18). Only one study evaluated the effect of sequence and fractionation schedules on cell viability. This study found that although all sequences were effective (concurrent, BP before RT, or RT before BP), radiation delivered before BP was most effective, particularly in the ER-positive breast cancer cell line. This study also found no difference in cell response when comparing single or multi-fractionated radiation courses (7).

Table 2 compares the results of cell viability data obtained by all three studies. Each study concluded that in a clinical situation, the combination of both RT and BPs may allow for a reduction in the dose of palliative RT delivered to a patient for their bone metastases. Interestingly, these data also support an advantage for the more potent BP, zoledronic acid, over ibandronate in the ER-positive breast cancer cell line.

Animal tumor models

Two studies were identified that assessed the relationship between BPs and RT in animal tumor models. Primary results of those two studies have been summarized in table 3. In both studies, tumor cells that produced lytic metastases were injected into weight-bearing bones of rodents. Micro-computed tomography analysis was used in both studies to assess the microarchitecture, bone and/or tumor volume, bone density, trabecular number and trabecular separation of both normal and involved bone (1,5). These studies conclude that the combined administration of both BPs and RT may lead to improved mineralization and restabilization when compared with RT alone, and that early administration of BPs before RT was more beneficial than just RT alone (1,5).

Arrington et al (5) also reported on biomechanical testing on both normal and involved bone. In their analysis of the biomechanical properties in treated vs. normal bone, the combined BP and RT approach re-established strength and flexibility of the diseased bone to the equivalent level as that observed in normal bone. The outcome of all treatment schedules to normal bone was also compared, and only treatment with RT and BP was able to improve the microarchitecture of the involved bone to such an extent that it appeared very similar to normal bone under micro-computed tomography analysis. However, statistical analysis was not significant due to the small study population.

Krempien et al (1) also demonstrated that BPs delivered three days prior to RT had a significantly greater impact on bone remodeling and stabilization than concurrent administration of BPs and RT. Of note, both studies showed that RT alone was not able to quickly or completely remineralize and strengthen the involved bone, leaving the subjects at risk for a pathological fracture in the irradiated area.

Human studies

At total of eight human studies involving the combination of BPs and RT were identified and are summarized in table 4. Only two of these studies were randomized, comparing a BP and RT arm with either RT and placebo or placebo alone (22,23). However, the randomized study done by George et al (22), which used a placebo arm, only followed patients for 29 days and the primary outcome only involved pain and analgesic scores.

The majority of the studies are observational and the primary objectives of all studies have a variety of endpoints.

Table 1. Summary of in-vitro studies

Author	Cell lines	Bisphosphonate (BP)	Total Dose of Radiation (RT)	BP + RT	Effect of BP + RT
Journe et al. (7)	MDA-MB-231 (Breast ER-)	Ibandronate (1-1,000 µM)	1-15Gy	significantly reduced clongenic cell survival and increased apoptosis vs. RT, BP and control ($p<0.005$)	Synergistic effects observed irrespective of combined BP + RT dose or sequence
	MCF-7 (Breast ER+)			significantly reduced clongenic cell survival vs. RT, BP and control and increased apoptosis vs. control and BP ($p<0.005$)	Synergistic effects observed in low BP (1-3 µM) irrespective of RT dose or sequence
Algur et al. (18)	C4-2 (Androgen-independent prostate)	Zoledronic Acid (10-200 µM)	1-10Gy	significant reduction in cell viability vs. BP, RT, and control ($p<0.005$)	Synergistic effect of BP + RT is most obvious in lower BP doses (10-100 µM) irrespective of RT dose
	IM-9 (B-lymphoblastic Multiple Myeloma)			significant reduction in cell viability vs. BP, RT, and control ($p<0.005$)	
Ural et al. (3)	MCF-7 (Breast ER +)	Zoledronic Acid (0.1-100 µM)	2-8Gy	significant reduction in cell viability vs. BP, RT, and control ($p<0.005$)	Synergistic effects observed irrespective of combined BP + RT dose

BP = bisphosphonate; RT = radiotherapy.

Table 2. Percent cell viability compared to control

	Journe et al. (7)*		Algur et al. (18)†		Ural et al. (3)‡
	MDA-MB-231 (Breast ER-) (%)	MCF-7 (Breast ER+) (%)	C4-2 (androgen-independent prostate) (%)	IM-9 (B-lymphoblastic Multiple Myeloma) (%)	MCF-7 (Breast ER +) (%)
BP (100 µM)	91	62	35	20	37
RT (4 Gy)	60	62	74	22	64
BP (100 µM) + RT (4 Gy)	51	24	23	13	10

* Analysis was conducted after 160h at 37°C in 5% CO_2 atmosphere.

† Analysis was conducted after 48.5h for the C4-2 cell line and 72.5h for the IM-9 cell line both at 37°C in 5% CO_2 atmosphere.

‡ Analysis was conducted after 72h at 37°C in 5% CO_2 atmosphere.

Table 3. Summary of animal studies

Author	Total Number of Animals	Tumor Cell Variant	Bis-phosphonate (BP)	Radiation (RT)	Groups	Bone Structure	Bone Density	Mechanical testing
Krempien et al. (1)	106	Walker 256B carcinosarcoma (lytic metastases) injected into proximal tibia	Clodronate (20mg/kg)	17 Gy	Group 1: RT treatment only (Day 7 post tumor injection)	Group 2 showed significantly better bone preservation parameters* (p<0.001) vs. groups 1,3. Group 3 only had significantly less trabecular separation vs. Group 1 (P<0.02)	At 6 wks post tumor injection, there was a significant difference in bone density in Groups 1 and 3 vs. normal† (57.6% vs. 100% 56.7% vs. 100% P<0.001). However there was no significant difference in Group 2 vs. normal† (88.1% vs 100%)	None preformed however better weight-bearing 3D trabecular microarchitecture in Group 2 vs. Groups 1 and 3.
					Group 2: Early BP + RT treatment (BP 3-6 days post tumor injection + RT (Day 7)			
					Group 3: Concurrent BP (Days 7-10 post tumor injection) + RT (Day 7)			
Arrington et al. (5)	30	MDAMB-231 Breast cancer (lytic metastases) injected into distal femur	Zoledronic Acid (100µg/kg)	20 Gy	Group 1: No treatment	BV‡ vs. normal for groups 1-3 (70% decrease (P<0.00009), 44% decrease (p<0.0107) and 15% increase (p<0.2602) respectively). Other bone parameters* showed no significant difference in Group 3 vs. Normal.	At 3 wks post tumor injection, Groups 1-3 vs. normal (15% decrease, 4% decrease, 14% increase) in bone density. At 6 wks, Group 2 had lower bone density vs. Group 3 (p< 0.005) and normal (P< 0.035).	No significant difference between groups 1 and 2 in mechanical testing§. Group 3 had no significant difference in mechanical testing§ vs. normal but was significantly better vs. Groups 1 and 2.
					Group 2: RT 3 weeks post tumor injection			
					Group 3: RT 3 wks post tumor injection + BP given once weekly for 6 wks starting 3 days before RT.			

*Histomorphometric bone parameters include: bone area percent (= bone area/ tissue area x 100%), trabecular number and trabecular separation.
† Normal group received no injection of Walker 256B and no treatment.
‡ Bone volume.
§ Biomechanical testing includes: peak torque, energy to failure and initial stiffness of the intact limb through the knee joint.

Table 4. Summary of human studies

Author	Study Type	Population	Bisphosphonate (BP)	Radiation (RT)	Study Group(s)	Pain and analgesics	Skeletal Related Events (SREs)	Bone remodeling (assessed by X-ray or CT comparisons)
Kouloulias et al. (2, 25)	Open-labeled phase I/II Observational study	n=33 Breast cancer with lytic bone metastases	Disodium Pamidronate (180mg every 4 weeks)	30 Gy total dose with patients receiving 3Gy/day	RT and BP given concurrently	Pain scores decreased significantly from baseline to 6 mos*.	One patient had an SRE within 6 mos*. Skeletal complication-free survival was 17 mos*.	Significant bone healing and mineralization at 6 mos*.
Kouloulias et al. (23)	Randomized trial	n=42 Various solid tumors with lytic metastases	Disodium Pamidronate (180mg every 4 weeks)	30 Gy total dose with patients receiving 3Gy/day	Group 1: stepwise 90-180mg BP dose escalation (30mg every 4 wks) + concurrent RT Group 2: 180mg BP + concurrent RT Group 3: RT only	Patients had significantly reduced pain score in all groups at 6 mos* post baseline; most significant improvement noted in Group 2	Patients with BP had significantly delayed new bone metastases (p< 0.011)	Group 2 had greater recalcification vs. Group 1 (p<0.05) while Group 1 and 2 did significantly better than RT alone (P<0.05)
George et al. (22)	Randomized Phase II trial	n=40 Various solid tumors (except prostate or hematological ca) with bone metastases	Pamidronate dose	20Gy/5	Group 1: BP + RT 3 or more days later Group 2: Placebo + RT 3 or more days later	No statistical significance between pamidronate vs. placebo in pain/analgesic scores at day 29 post BP	None reported	None reported

Table 4. (Continued)

Author	Study Type	Population	Bisphosphonate (BP)	Radiation (RT)	Study Group(s)	Pain and analgesics	Skeletal Related Events (SREs)	Bone remodeling (assessed by X-ray or CT comparisons)
Kijima et al. (24)	Retrospective chart review	n=23 Renal cell with cancer with bone metastases	Zoledronic Acid (4mg every 3-4 weeks)	20-45Gy with patients receiving 1.8-2Gy/day	Group 1: RT only / Group 2: RT + BP concurrently	None reported	In Group 1, 10/13 patients had an SRE vs. 1/10 patients in Group 2 (P<0.003) (skeletal event-free survival in Group 2 was 18.7 mos; not reached in Group 2)	6/10 patients in Group 2 had partial recalcification vs. 1/13 in Group 1 (p<0.019)
Micke et al. (28)	Randomized Phase II trial	n=52 Various solid tumors with lytic metastases	Ibandronate	36-40 Gy	Group 1: 4mg BP + RT then 3mg every 28 days for 1 year / Group 2: 1mg BP + RT, 1mg days 8, 15 and 22; 3mg every 28 days for 1 year	No significant difference in pain or analgesic scores in groups 1 vs. 2	None reported	No significant difference in recalcification rates in groups 1 vs. 2
Vassiliou et al. (4)	Phase I observational study	n=45 Various solid tumors with bone metastases	Ibandronate (10 cycles of 6mg monthly)	30-40 Gy	RT + BP concurrently	Opioid use and pain scores decrease significantly at 3, 6, and 10 mos vs. baseline. (P<0.001)	At 10 months, 2 patients had an SRE	Significantly increased bone density at 3 mos*, 6 (45.8%) and 10 (73.2%) vs. baseline. (p<0.001)

Author	Study Type	Population	Bisphosphonate (BP)	Radiation (RT)	Study Group(s)	Pain and analgesics	Skeletal Related Events (SREs)	Bone remodeling (assessed by X-ray or CT comparisons)
Vassiliou et al. (27)	Phase I observational study	n=52 Various solid tumors with bone metastases	Ibandronate (10 cycles of 6mg monthly)	30-40 Gy	Group 1: lytic metastases + concurrent BP + RT Group 2: mixed metastases + concurrent BP + RT Group 3: sclerotic metastases + concurrent BP + RT	In all groups pain and analgesic score significantly decreased at 3, 6, and 10 mos* vs. baseline. Greatest response occurred at 10mos* in Group 1 vs. baseline	None reported	Mean bone density for three groups were significant ($p<0.05$), highest increase in Group 1 at 10 mos*. Recalcification was noted in all groups.

* months- (pls remove period)

The most commonly prescribed doses of RT to treat bone metastases for the majority of these studies were within the range of 30-40Gy. Ibandronate and pamidronate were the BPs of choice in all studies, while a retrospective review by Kijima et al. evaluated zoledronic acid and RT (24). All studies that assessed long term pain and analgesic consumption noted a significant decrease from baseline in patients treated with both BP and RT (2, 4,23,25-27). Additionally, studies that reported bone remodeling found that mean bone density and recalcification rates significantly increased when compared to baseline scores (2,4,23,25,27).

The most compelling study of all those identified was a randomized trial done by Kouloulias et al (23). This study compared two different concurrent BP and RT schedules (high-dose BP versus dose escalated BP) to RT alone. Pain and analgesic scores were shown to significantly decrease in all groups, however high-dose BP and concurrent RT was noted to have the most significant improvement. Patients who received concurrent BP with RT had a significant delay in the development and incidence of new bony lesions when compared to the RT alone group ($p<0.011$).

The high-dose BP and RT group also showed a significantly greater recalcification rate when compared to the RT alone group and dose escalation BP group ($p<0.05$).

This study provided promising evidence regarding the benefits of using combination treatment to manage bone metastases. However, it was limited by its small study population.

Kijima et al (24) comparatively analyzed RT and combination BP treatment in a retrospective study. This report focused on advanced renal cell cancer patients who either received RT alone or concurrent zoledronic acid and RT for painful bone metastases. It was observed that significantly less patients treated with combination BP and RT experienced a SRE compared to those who just received RT ($p<0.003$). In addition, patients treated with combination therapy had achieved a significantly higher recalcification rate than those treated with RT alone ($p<0.019$). They concluded that based on these findings, prospective clinical trials should be established to investigate concurrent therapy in this population.

Human toxicities

No significant toxicities from combined treatments were reported in any of the studies apart from side effects commonly associated with the administration of BPs such as flu-like symptoms, myalgias and arthalgias (2, 4,23,27,28). The combination treatment was reportedly well tolerated among patients in two studies (4,27).

Discussion

Combined modality therapies have recently emerged in the management of the palliative cancer population. As patients with metastatic disease are living longer, quality of life is increasingly recognized as an important outcome. As such, more aggressive therapies for these patients aimed at more rapid and durable palliation of symptoms are emerging, analogous to strategies used in the curative cancer therapeutic approaches (29).

With respect to bone metastases, the combination of BPs and RT is being actively investigated to improve on exiting outcomes with either approach alone. The rationale is to take advantage of the commonalities in both RT and BP pain response pathways with respect to osteoclast suppression and tumor apoptosis (7,14).

In-vitro cell studies that combined both RT and BP have shown a significant synergistic effect (3,7,18). However, the exact mechanism is unknown. Ural et al (30,31) proposed that perhaps BPs have the ability to arrest cells in the M and G2 phase of the cell cycle, thereby increasing the proportion of tumor cells in the more susceptible phases of the cell cycle to RT. The outcome is increased apoptosis.

This is evident when considering data has shown that ibandronate alone had the ability to induce apoptosis in breast tumor cells to a slightly smaller degree than RT alone, however, the combination of both RT and ibandronate had an approximate doubling effect (7). In considering the three in-vitro studies presented in this review, a synergistic relationship between BPs and RT was concluded. Upon further study, this synergistic relationship could one day allow for BP or RT dose-reduction, which would subsequently result in lower treatment toxicities (3,7,18).

Although single or multi-fractionated RT regimens have been shown to be equally efficacious with minimal toxicity, a multi-fraction approach has shown significantly greater effectiveness in inducing remineralization of the bone and reducing re-treatment rates (16,32). Therefore a multi-fractionated course of RT with a BP could provide significantly greater benefits in terms of remineralization and reduced skeletal morbidity. However, human studies exploring BPs and either a single or multi-fractionated course of RT are needed to assess the potential benefits of a multi-fractionated course of RT.

Another factor that has shown to influence the efficacy of combined RT and BP treatment has been the order with which the treatments are scheduled. The one in-vitro cell study that assessed other alternatives to concurrent delivery found that RT given 3-6 days before BP administration had a greater synergistic effect than concurrent administration (7). Further exploration of different treatment schedules was assessed in animal tumor models. Both animal tumor model studies included at least one treatment arm which delivered BPs before RT (1,5). Krempien et al (1) found that BPs delivered 3-6 days before RT was significantly more effective than concurrent BP and RT. This study theorized that early BP administration helped to maintain the microarchitecture of the bone before RT was delivered, reducing the remodeling and chance of fractures in the irradiated area, which subsequently allowed for faster remineralization of the bone following RT (1). Overall, the animal tumor model suggests that early BP administration along with RT has significant benefits in bone remodeling and mechanical restoration within the irradiated area over RT alone. Both the no treatment and RT only groups in both animal tumor studies showed significantly decreased mineralization, bone density and mechanical testing when compared to normal bone (1,5). Though neither study evaluated BPs alone, BPs are not recommended as a first-line therapy for pain relief from bone metastases; RT is a recommended first-line treatment (6). Unfortunately, despite animal tumor model evidence that early BP administration before RT was of significant benefit, all of the published human studies (with one exception) chose to use concurrent (same-day) administration in their study protocols.

To examine how effective combined BP and RT was in human studies, pain scores and analgesic use, SREs, and recalcification rates were all used as determinates. When reviewing pain and analgesic scores of patients receiving combined RT and BPs, only four studies compared baseline and follow-up pain and analgesic scores. All four studies showed that pain scores significantly decreased at six month follow-up (2,4,23,25,27). Analgesic scores, reported only in studies by Vassiliou et al., showed a significant 61% decrease in opioid consumption by 10 month follow-up (4,27). This same study also showed a pain score reduction to zero in 70% of patients at three months and 80% at 10 months (4,27). In comparison, two large separate meta-analyses found that a complete pain reduction from RT alone occurred in only 32-33% of patients, and any response to RT occurred in 60% of patients (16,17,23). This suggests there may be a benefit with regards to pain reduction with combined BP and RT over RT alone, and this could be explored in further large randomized controlled trials. Only two studies were able to directly compare pain and/or analgesic scores of combined RT and BP to RT alone (22,23). Even though these two studies had contradictory findings with respect to pain relief from combination treatment, they both consisted of a small sample population of patients with varying solid tumor types, therefore the significance of these outcomes are somewhat limited.

Of all the eight human studies identified, only three reported SRE data. Two of these studies are observational studies and therefore comparisons are difficult to extrapolate. Nevertheless, one of these studies reported the event-free survival for 33 breast patients receiving 180mg pamidronate and RT was 17 months (2,25). When comparing this statistic to event-free survival of randomized pamidronate trials in breast cancer, the event-free survival was 11.9 months on average (11). However, the dose of pamidronate in the combined pamidronate and RT study was at least double that in pamidronate breast cancer trials (11). The only study that had detailed SRE data was a retrospective review of renal cell patients receiving either zoledronic acid plus RT verses RT alone for bone metastases. This study showed a significant difference in SREs between the two groups, strongly favouring the combination group (24).

With respect to the bone remodeling, five studies reported on recalcification rates following treatment using radiological imaging. All studies reported a significant increase in recalcification or bone density following combination treatment (2,4,23-25,27). Detailed recalcification rates by Vassiliou et al. showed that at 6 months, the average increased bone density was 45.8% from baseline and increased 73.2% at 10 months from baseline (4). In comparison, one of the only studies that evaluated the recalcification rate of lesions from various solid tumors treated with RT alone found that the recalcification rate of multi-fractionated courses at six months was approximately 73% (32). However, this particular study had a higher proportion of breast cancer patients than lung cancer patients when compared to Vassiliou et al (4,32). Patients with breast cancer have a higher response rate with respect to the remineralization to bone (77%) when compared with other primaries such as lung (27%) and renal cell (25%) (33).

Overall, all of the human studies evaluating the effectiveness of BPs and RT had very small patient populations (the largest study contained 52 patients), and the majority of them lacked randomization or a control arm. Though these studies suggest possible benefits from the combined treatment, the variability and subjectivity of all the studies are too great to draw any reasonable conclusions. Suffice to say, both RT and BPs are effective treatments in managing and treating painful bone metastases. This literature review shows that combining the two treatments does not show any added treatment toxicity, nor are either of the two treatments any less effective when combined (3,4,6,7,15,18,27).

Conclusions

We recommend further large randomized trials to evaluate the effectiveness of combining RT and BPs. We also suggest that further randomized studies assess concurrent versus pre-BP administration, as well as assess the potential benefits of using multi-fractionated RT in weight-bearing bones compared with a single fraction. Overall, both animal tumor models and in-vitro cell studies evaluating the use of combined RT and BPs suggest a synergistic effect that may be beneficial for patients with painful bone metastases (1,3,5, 7,18).

Acknowledgments

The studentship was funded by the Michael and Karyn Goldstein Cancer Research Fund. We also thank Stacy Lue, Candi Flynn, Jennifer Wong and Julie Napolskikh for their help. No conflict of interest declared.

References

[1] Krempien R, Huber PE, Harms W, Treiber M, Wannenmacher M, Krempien B. Combination of early bisphosphonate administration and irradiation leads to improved remineralization and restabilization of osteolytic bone metastases in an animal tumor model. Cancer 2003;98(6):1318-24.

[2] Kouloulias V, Matsopoulous G, Kouvaris J, Dardoufas C, Bottomley A, et al. Radiotherapy in conjunction with intravenous infusion of 180 mg of disodium pamidronate in management of osteolytic metastases from breast cancer: Clinical evaluation, biochemical markers, quality of life, and monitoring of recalcification using assessments of grey-level histogram in plain radiographs. Int J Radiation Oncology Biol Phys 2003;57(1):143-57.

[3] Ural AU, Avcu F, Candir M, Guden M, Ozcan MA. In vitro synergistic cytoreductive effects of zoledronic acid and radiation on breast cancer cells. Breast Cancer Res 2006;8(4):R52.

[4] Vassiliou V, Kalogeropoulou C, Christopoulos C, Solomou E, Leotsinides M, Kardamakis D. Combination ibandronate and radiotherapy for the treatment of bone metastases: Clinical evaluation and radiologic assessment. Int J Radiat Oncol Biol Phys 2007;67(1):264-72.

[5] Arrington SA, Damron TA, Mann KA, Allen MJ. Concurrent administration of zoledronic acid and irradiation leads to improved bone density, biomechanical strength, and microarchitecture in a mouse model of tumor-induced osteolysis. J Surg Oncol 2008;97(3):284-90.

[6] Wong R, Wiffen PJ. Bisphosphonates for the relief of pain secondary to bone metastases. Cochrane Database Syst Rev 2002(2):002068.

[7] Journe F, Magne N, Chaboteaux C, Kinnaert E, Bauss F, Body J. Sequence- and concentration-dependent effects of acute and long-term exposure to the bisphosphonate ibandronate in combination with single and multiple fractions of ionising radiation doses in human breast cancer cell lines. Clin Exp Metastasis 2006;23(135):137-47.

[8] Falkmer U, Jarhult J, Wersall P, Cavallin-Stahl E. A systematic overview of radiation therapy effects in skeletal metastases. Acta Oncol 2003;42(5-6):620-33.

[9] Jasmin C, Capanna R, Coleman RE, Coia LR, Saillant G, eds.Textbook of bone metastases. Hoboken, NJ: Wiley, 2005.

[10] Yuen KK, Shelley M, Sze WM, Wilt T, Mason MD. Bisphosphonates for advanced prostate cancer. Cochrane Database Syst Rev 2006(4):006250.

[11] Pavlakis N, Stockler M. Bisphosphonates for breast cancer.update in cochrane database syst rev. Cochrane Database Syst Rev 2002(1):003474 and 2005;(3):CD003474.

[12] Ross J, Saunders Y, Edmonds P, Patel S, Broadley K, Johnston S. Systematic review of bisphosphonates on skeletal morbidity in metastatic cancer. BMJ 2003;327:469.
[13] McQuay HJ, Collins SL, Carroll D, Moore RA. Radiotherapy for the palliation of painful bone metastases. Cochrane Database Syst Rev 2000(2):001793.
[14] Hoskin PJ. Bisphosphonates and radiation therapy for palliation of metastatic bone disease. Cancer Treat Rev 2003;29(4):321-7.
[15] Chow E, Harris K, Fan G, Tsao M, Sze W. Palliative radiotherapy trials for bone metastases: A systematic review. J Clin Oncol 2007;25(11):1423-36.
[16] Sze W, Shelley M, Held I, Mason M. Palliation of metastatic bone pain: Single fraction versus multifraction radiotherapy. Cochrane Database Syst Rev 2004;(2):CD004721.
[17] Wu J, Wong R, Johnston M, Bezjak A, Whelan T. Meta-analysis of dose-fractionation radiotherapy trials for the palliation of painful bone metastases. Int J Radiat Oncol Biol Phys 2003;55(3):594-605.
[18] Algur E, Macklis R, Hafeli U. Synergistic cytotoxic effects of zoledronic acid and radiation in human prostate cancer and myeloma cell line. Int J Radiat Oncol Biol Phys 2005;61(2):535-42.
[19] Fleisch H. The role of bisphosphonates in breast cancer: Development of bisphosphonates. Breast Cancer Res 2002;4:30-4.
[20] Adami S. Bisphosphonates in prostate carcinoma. Cancer 1997;80:1674-9.
[21] Ural AU, Avcu F, Baran Y. Bisphosphonate treatment and radiotherapy in metastatic breast cancer. Med Oncol 2008;25:350-5.
[22] George R, Hephzibah J, John S. Does pamidronate enhance the analgesic effect of radiotherapy? A randomized trial. Palliat Med 2007;21(8):719-20.
[23] Kouloulias EV, Kouvaris RJ, Antypas C, Mystakidou K, Matsopoulos G, Uzunoglu CN, Moulopoulos A, Vlahos JL. An intra-patient dose-escalation study of disodium pamidronate plus radiotherapy versus radiotherapy alone for the treatment of osteolytic metastases. monitoring of recalcification using image-processing techniques. Strahlentherapie Onkologie 2003;179(7):471-9.
[24] Kijima T, Fujii F, Suyama T, Okudo Y, Yamamoto S, Masuda H, Yonese J, Fukui I. Radiotherapy to bone metastases from renal cell carcinoma with or without zoledronate. BJU Int 2009;103(5):620-4.
[25] Kouloulias V, Dardoufas C, Kouvaris J, Antypas C, Sandilos P, Matsopoulos G, Vlahos L. Use of image processing techniques to assess effect of disodium pamidronate in conjunction with radiotherapy in patients with bone metastases. Acta Oncol 2002;41(2):164-9.
[26] Kouloulias V, Kouvaris J, Mystakidou K, Varela M, Kokakis J, Pistevou-Gombaki K, Balafouta M, Gennatas C, Vlahos L. Duration of bisphosphonate treatment: Results of a non-randomised study in patients previously treated with local irradiation for bone metastases from breast cancer. Curr Med Res Opin 2004;20(6):819.
[27] Vassiliou V, Kalogeropoulou C, Giannopoulou E, Leotsinidis M, Tsota I, Kardamakis D. A novel study investigating the therapeutic outcome of patients with lytic, mixed and sclerotic bone metastases treated with combined radiotherapy and ibandronate. Clin Exp Metastasis 2007;24:169-78.
[28] Micke O, Berning D, Schafer F, Bruns F, Willich N. Combination of ibandronate and radiotherapy in metastatic bone disease - final results of a randomized phase II trial. Eur J Cancer Suppl 2003;1(5):S150.
[29] Hillner B, Ingle J, Chlebowski R, Gralow J, Yee G, Janjan N, Cauley J, Blumenstein B, Albain K, Lipton A, Brown S. American society of clinical oncology 2003 update on the role of bisphosphonates and bone health issues in women with breast cancer. J Clin Oncol 2003;21(21):4042-57.
[30] Ural AU, Avcu F. Therapeutic role of bisphosphonate and radiation combination in the management of myeloma bone disease. Clin Cancer Res 2007;13(11):3432.

[31] Ural AU. Zoledronic acid sensitized tumor cells to radiation: In response to algur et al. Int J Radiat Oncol Biol Phys 2005;63(3):970.

[32] Koswig S, Budach V. Remineralization and pain relief in bone metastases after after different radiotherapy fractions (10 times 3 gy vs. 1 time 8 gy). A prospective study. Strahlentherapie Onkologie 1999;175(10):500-8.

[33] Weber W, Rosler HP, Doll G, Dostert M, Kutzner J, Schild H. [The percuaneous irradiation of osteolytic bone metastases—a course assessment]. Strahlentherapie Okologie 1992;168(5):275-80.

In: Pain Management Yearbook 2009
Editor: Joav Merrick

ISBN: 978-1-61209-666-7
©2012 Nova Science Publishers, Inc.

Chapter 38

ARE BASELINE ESAS SYMPTOMS RELATED TO PAIN RESPONSE IN PATIENTS TREATED WITH PALLIATIVE RADIOTHERAPY FOR BONE METASTASES?

*Shaelyn Culleton, BSc (C), Jocelyn Pang, BSc (C), Liying Zhang, PhD, Roseanna Presutti, BSc (C), Janet Nguyen, BSc (C), Gunita Mitera, MRT(T), Emily Sinclair, MRT(T), Elizabeth Barnes, MD, May Tsao, MD, Cyril Danjoux, MD, Arjun Sahgal, MD and Edward Chow, MBBS**

Rapid Response Radiotherapy Program, Department of Radiation Oncology, Odette Cancer Centre, Sunnybrook Health Sciences Centre, University of Toronto, Ontario, Canada

Abstract

The purpose was to assess the relationship between pretreatment symptoms and pain response following palliative radiotherapy for bone metastases. Methods: All patients with bone metastases treated with palliative radiotherapy were followed at baseline, then 1, 2 and 3 months after radiotherapy with the Edmonton Symptom Assessment System (ESAS). This scale includes pain, fatigue, nausea, depression, anxiety, drowsiness, appetite, sense of well being and shortness of breath. Patients were categorized as either a responder or non-responder according to the International Consensus Guidelines for palliative radiotherapy. Statistical analysis included both Wilcoxon rank-sum and one-way ANOVA analysis. Results were considered significant at the 0.5% critical level ($p < 0.005$) applying the Bonferroni statistical correction for multiple comparisons. Results: For the entire cohort of 518 patients, only nausea at baseline was found to significantly correlate with a pain response to radiation at month

---

[*] **Correspondence:** Edward Chow, MBBS, PhD, FRCPC, Department of Radiation Oncology, Odette Cancer Centre, Sunnybrook Health Sciences Centre, 2075 Bayview Avenue, Toronto, ON M4N 3M5, Canada. Tel: 416-480-4998; Fax: 416-480-6002; E-mail: Edward.Chow@sunnybrook.ca

3. No other symptoms at baseline were found to predict a pain response to radiation at months 1, 2 or 3. Conclusion: There are no ESAS symptoms that can accurately predict a patient's pain response to radiation. Patients who are symptomatic from their bone metastases should be treated with palliative radiotherapy irrespective of their baseline ESAS symptoms.

Keywords: Bone metastases, ESAS, palliative radiotherapy.

Introduction

Bone metastases are an unfortunate complication which occurs in approximately 50% of all cancer patients. The most common primary cancer sites which metastasize to bone are breast, prostate and lung carcinomas (1). Symptomatic metastatic bone lesions, which develop in about 50-70% of all patients with bone metastases, can be quite distressing in patients. Most often these patients will experience severe pain and can often have very serious skeletal complications. The most common skeletal related complications include pathological fractures (8-30%), hypercalcemia (10%), and spinal cord compression (5%) (1-4). Palliative radiation has been proven to be an effective treatment for symptomatic bone metastases, with 24% of all patients experiencing complete pain relief and up to 59% reporting some pain relief (2). This treatment is more effective at reducing incident pain than any other analgesic regimen, which is why palliative radiation is considered a first-line therapy for bone metastases (5,6).

Many patients who receive palliative radiotherapy for their painful bone metastases experience other common advanced cancer symptoms as well (7). Though pain from bone metastases may be the most distressing, these other symptoms may also have an effect on a patient's overall quality of life (QOL) and performance status. Some of the most common advanced cancer symptoms apart from pain are fatigue, dypsnea, depression, nausea and lack of appetite (7). It has been suggested that the presence of certain common advanced cancer symptoms prior to radiation may predict a patient's response. In a study by Kovner et al (8), which assessed 42 advanced cancer patients treated with palliative radiotherapy, higher levels of anxiety and depression prior to treatment showed a greater reduction in pain following treatment. Kovner et al (8) also mentioned that this pain reduction had a positive effect on patients' QOL and that this effect was noticed before any medical results were apparent.

The purpose of the present study is to determine if certain advanced cancer symptoms predict a response to radiation treatment by exploring the relationship between pre-RT symptoms and patient response to radiotherapy. To assess changes in symptoms during treatment, the Edmonton Symptom Assessment System (ESAS) was used before radiation (at baseline) and follow-up with advanced cancer patients receiving palliative radiation for bone metastases. This scale has been validated as an effective tool in monitoring common advanced cancer symptoms in the palliative population. This nine item questionnaire includes six symptoms related to physical well-being and three items related to psychological symptoms (9). Comparing ESAS symptoms from baseline to subsequent follow-ups will allow us to determine if the rating of symptoms prior to radiation predicts a patient's response to radiation treatment for bone metastases.

Methods

The Odette Cancer Centre (OCC) is one of two regional cancer centres providing radiotherapy in the Greater Toronto Area. The Rapid Response Radiotherapy Program (RRRP) at the OCC provides timely palliative radiation for symptomatic metastases. On initial consultation, patients with bone metastases were asked to rate the severity of symptoms they were experiencing using the ESAS. This 11-point visual analogue scale asks patients to rate nine of their symptoms from 0 (absence of symptom) to 10 (worst possible feeling of that symptom). Pain, tiredness, nausea, depression, anxiety, drowsiness, appetite, overall sense of well being and shortness of breath are the nine symptoms assessed through ESAS. This tool has been proven to be very indicative of a patient's current status and is noted for its quick and easy administration (9).

Patient demographics such as primary cancer site, age, Karnofsky Performance Status (KPS), analgesic intake and other sites of metastases were also recorded at the time of initial consultation. Radiation dosage and site of radiation were also recorded. The initial baseline assessment was completed before radiation treatment and follow-up interviews were conducted by telephone or in person at months one, two and three after the delivery of radiation treatment.

Statistical analysis

Response to radiation was determined by employing the International Consensus on Palliative Radiotherapy Endpoints. According to these endpoints, a complete response to radiation is defined as a pain score of zero with no concomitant increase in analgesic intake. Partial response is defined as either a pain reduction of two or more at the treated site without an increase in analgesic intake, or a reduction of analgesic intake of 25% or more with no increase in pain score. Patients who responded to radiation treatment are considered to have achieved either a complete or partial response (10).

Results were expressed as mean, standard deviation (SD), and median (range) for continuous variables, and proportion (%) for categorical variables. Mean and median values were calculated for ESAS scales in responders and non-responders at month one, month two and month three. To determine if baseline symptoms predicted response at consecutive months post radiation treatment, two statistical methods were employed. The Wilcoxon rank-sum test (non-parametric) and One-Way ANOVA test (parametric) were both used to search for a relationship between response rate (responders versus non-responders) and baseline ESAS scales. The Bonferroni statistical correction for multiple comparisons, in which the adjusted P-value is found by dividing 0.05 by the number of outcomes, was applied in this study (11). As there are nine items in the ESAS, results were considered significant at the 0.5% critical level ($p < 0.005$). The Statistical Analysis Software (SAS Institute, version 9.1 for Windows) was used for the analysis.

Table 1. Patient demographics

Sex	
Male	280 (54%)
Female	238 (46%)
Karnofsky Performance Status	
Mean	Range
61.2	10-100
Age (Years)	
Mean	Range
68	31-93
Other Metastatic Sites	
Lung	111 (21%)
Liver	90 (17%)
Brain	17 (3%)
Primary Cancer Sites	
Lung	130 (25%)
Breast	127 (25%)
Prostate	117 (23%)
GI	39 (8%)
Unknown Primary	34 (7%)
Others	71 (14%)
Radiation Prescription (cGy/fraction)	
2000/5	219 (42%)
800/1	209 (40%)
3000/10	26 (5%)
1000/1	10 (2%)
Others	54 (11%)
Site of Radiation	
Hip/Pelvis	30%
Spine	29%
Femur	12%
Rib Cage	9%
Humerus	8%
Clavicle	5%
Others	7%

Results

518 patients between January 1999 and January 2002 with bone metastases completed the ESAS at baseline prior to radiation treatment. This population contained approximately an even number of males and females with a median age of 68 years and a mean KPS of 60. The three most prevalent primary cancer sites were lung, breast and prostate, respectively. The majority of patients received either a single dose of 800cGy or 2000cGy in five fractions for their painful bone metastases. The two most common irradiated sites were the pelvis and spine. All other demographic information is included in table 1. The number of responders and non-responders at month one, two and three along with their median and mean scores for all nine symptoms are included in table 2.

Of the 518 patients that completed ESAS at baseline, 256 patients completed the one month follow-up, 223 completed month two follow-up and 189 completed month three follow-up. Table 3 shows the results of the Wilcoxon rank-sum and One-way ANOVA statistical analyses at month one, two and three. These results are however, with the exception of the Wilcoxon rank-sum analysis at month three for nausea, not significant when applying the Bonferroni statistical correction for multiple comparisons (11).

Table 2. ESAS mean and median scores for responders and non-responders

	Responder?	Month 1 N	Month 1 Mean	Month 1 Median	Month 2 N	Month 2 Mean	Month 2 Median	Month 3 N	Month 3 Mean	Month 3 Median
Tired	No	130	4.63	5.00	120	5.01	5.00	92	4.80	5.00
Tired	Yes	130	4.68	5.00	105	4.36	5.00	97	4.13	5.00
Nausea	No	130	1.47	1.00	120	1.72	1.00	92	1.64	1.00
Nausea	Yes	130	1.42	0.00	105	1.10	0.00	97	1.05	0.00
Depressed	No	128	2.41	2.00	116	2.28	2.00	91	2.22	2.00
Depressed	Yes	128	2.42	2.00	103	2.42	2.00	93	2.29	2.00
Anxious	No	129	2.95	3.00	118	3.14	2.00	92	2.83	2.00
Anxious	Yes	129	3.30	3.00	104	3.30	3.00	95	3.35	3.00
Drowsy	No	129	3.38	3.00	120	3.37	3.00	92	3.07	2.00
Drowsy	Yes	129	3.46	3.00	104	3.19	2.50	96	2.97	2.00
Appetite loss	No	130	4.28	5.00	120	4.00	4.00	92	3.84	4.00
Appetite loss	Yes	130	3.68	4.00	105	3.72	4.00	97	3.39	2.00
Sense of Well Being	No	129	4.18	4.00	119	4.13	4.00	88	4.05	4.00
Sense of Well Being	Yes	126	3.94	4.00	102	4.01	4.00	94	3.73	4.00
Short of Breath	No	129	1.93	1.00	119	2.44	1.00	91	2.48	2.00
Short of Breath	Yes	130	2.50	1.00	104	1.99	1.00	97	1.77	1.00

Discussion

There has been very limited research done investigating the relationship between pre-treatment symptoms and response to radiation treatment. A fairly comprehensive analysis done at our centre which analyzed pre-treatment pain scores for 1,053 advanced cancer patients treated with radiotherapy for bone metastases was compared to response following radiation treatment. Patients with mild, moderate or severe pain at the beginning of treatment showed no significant difference in response up to three months post radiation treatment.

Therefore the initial severity of pain was not shown to predict a response to radiation treatment (12). Our study also has yielded similar results when analyzing all other ESAS symptoms (with the exception of pain) in comparison with response. All baseline ESAS symptoms were not significantly related to either responders or non-responders at month one, two and three. Even though Wilcoxon rank-sum test at month three showed that the level of nausea predicted response to radiation, the lack of correlation between other commonly associated symptoms like anxiety and depression make it unlikely that nausea alone could predict for response at month three (13). Also the difference in median and mean nausea levels at baseline is so low between responders and non-responders that this finding would not be of any clinical significance.

Table 3. Wilcoxon rank-sum and One-way ANOVA analysis on ESAS symptoms

	Relationship with response rate (responders vs. non-responders)	
Baseline ESAS	Wilcoxon rank-sum p-value	One-way ANOVA p-value*
Month 1		
Tired	0.8711	0.9106
Nausea	0.1462	0.1833
Depressed	0.9739	0.9744
Anxious	0.5849	0.6720
Drowsy	0.9664	0.5974
Appetite loss	0.1511	0.1118
Well being	0.4407	0.2961
Shortness of breath	0.2789	0.2074
Month 2		
Tired	0.0960	0.0886
Nausea	0.0222	0.0268
Depressed	0.8288	0.6713
Anxious	0.7838	0.7481
Drowsy	0.6618	0.6005
Appetite loss	0.6220	0.5112
Well being	0.7402	0.3567
Shortness of breath	0.4320	0.5672
Month 3		
Tired	0.0988	0.0314
Nausea	0.0038	0.0110
Depressed	0.9864	0.8490
Anxious	0.3159	0.2411
Drowsy	0.7967	0.7444
Appetite loss	0.2891	0.2175
Well being	0.4362	0.2381
Shortness of breath	0.1220	0.1591

*log (baseline ESAS + 1) transformation was used for normalization.
P< 0.005 considered significant.

Kovner et al (8) determined based on their analysis of 42 metastastic cancer patients treated with palliative radiotherapy that had high levels of anxiety and depression prior to treatment had decreased pain and an increase in QOL following radiotherapy. However the analysis done by this study on a significantly greater number of patients refutes the effects of high anxiety and depression on response to radiation. Anxiety and depression are significantly associated with impairment of physical and psychosocial aspects of QOL, even after controlling for pain and illness severity (13). Therefore depression and anxiety have aspects that are independent from pain and levels are not always predictive for reductions in pain and increases in QOL (14).

Overall, a patient's presenting symptomology prior to palliative radiation for bone metastases has no predictive value in determining how a patient will respond. Therefore, it is recommended that patients be referred for palliative radiation to their painful bone metastases irrespective of the level of other ESAS symptoms. It is important that patients presenting even with moderate pain be referred for treatment, in order to avoid symptom progression (12).

Acknowledgments

The studentship was funded by the Michael and Karyn Goldstein Cancer Research Fund. We thank Stacy Lue for secretarial assistance.

References

[1] Falkmer U, Jarhult J, Wersall P, Cavallin-Stahl E. A systematic overview of radiation therapy effects in skeletal metastases. Acta Oncol 2003;42(5-6):620-33.
[2] Chow E, Harris K, Fan G, Tsao M, Sze W. Palliative radiotherapy trials for bone metastases: A systematic review. J Clin Oncol 2007;25(11):1423-36.
[3] Hoegler D. Radiotherapy for palliation of symptoms in incurable cancer. Curr Probl Cancer 1997;21(3):129-83.
[4] Wu J, Wong R, Johnston M, Bezjak A, Whelan T. Meta-analysis of dose-fractionation radiotherapy trials for the palliation of painful bone metastases. Int J Radiat Oncol Biol Phys 2003;55(3):594-605.
[5] Wong R, Wiffen PJ. Bisphosphonates for the relief of pain secondary to bone metastases. Cochrane Database Syst Rev 2002(2):002068.
[6] McQuay HJ, Collins SL, Carroll D, Moore RA. Radiotherapy for the palliation of painful bone metastases. Cochrane Database Syst Rev 2000(2):001793.
[7] Walsh D, Donnelly S, Rybicki L. The symptoms of advanced cancer: Relationship to age, gender, and performance status in 1,000 patients. Support Care Cancer 2000 May;8(3):175-9.
[8] Niv D, Shulamith K. Pain and quality of life. Pain Medicine 2001;1(2):150-61.
[9] Bruera E, Kuehn N, Miller MJ, Selmser P, Macmillan K. The edmonton symptom assessment system (ESAS): A simple method for the assessment of palliative care patients. J Palliat Care 1991;7(2):6-9.
[10] Chow E, Wu JS, Hoskin P, Coia LR, Bentzen SM, Blitzer PH. International consensus on palliative radiotherapy endpoints for future clinical trials in bone metastases. Radiother Oncol 2002;64(3):275-80.
[11] Shaffer JP. Multiple hypothesis testing. Ann Rev Psych 1995;46:561-84.
[12] Kirou-Mauro A, Hird A, Wong J, Sinclair E, Barnes EA, Tsao M, Danjoux C, Chow E. Is response to radiotherapy in patients related to the severity of pretreatment pain? Int J Radiat Oncol Biol Phys 2008;71(4):1208-12.
[13] Smith EM, Gomm SA, Dickens CM. Assessing the independent contribution to quality of life from anxiety and depression in patients with advanced cancer. Palliat Med 2003;17(6):509-13.

[14] Cordova MJ, Andrykowski, MA. Responses to cancer diagnosis and treatment: Posttraumatic stress and posttraumatic growth. Semin Clin Neuropsychiatry 2003;8(4):286-96.

Chapter 39

IMPROVEMENT OF ESAS SYMPTOMS FOLLOWING PALLIATIVE RADIATION FOR BONE METASTASES

*Shaelyn Culleton, BSc(C), Liying Zhang, PhD,
Emily Sinclair, MRT(T), Elizabeth Barnes, MD, May Tsao, MD,
Cyril Danjoux, MD, Sarah Campos, BSc(C), Philiz Goh, BSc
and Edward Chow, MBBS**

Rapid Response Radiotherapy Program, Department of Radiation Oncology, Odette cancer Centre, Sunnybrook Health Sciences Centre, University of Toronto, Toronto, Ontario, Canada

Abstract

The purpose of this paper was to assess pain and other common symptoms using the Edmonton System Assessment scale (ESAS) in patients with bone metastases following palliative radiotherapy. Methods: All patients with bone metastases treated with palliative radiotherapy were followed at baseline, then 1, 2, 4, 8 and 12 weeks after radiotherapy with ESAS. This scale includes pain, tiredness, nausea, depression, anxiety, drowsiness, appetite, sense of well being and shortness of breath. A Chi-squared test was used to search for the association between response effect and ESAS change at different weeks. To evaluate the response effect on the ESAS symptoms over time, a general linear mixed model was performed. Results: For the entire cohort of 518 patients, pain, anxiety, appetite, drowsiness and overall sense of well being significantly improved from baseline to last follow-up. Tiredness was the only symptom which showed worsening following palliative radiation in all patients. When looking at responders and non-responders with respect to pain, the greatest number of symptoms with a significant difference between the two groups occurred at week 12. Also when comparing the significant differences between responder and non-responders from week 1 to 12 inclusive, all ESAS symptoms were significantly better in responders with the exception of shortness of breath. Conclusions: Palliative

---

* **Correspondence:** Edward Chow, MBBS, PhD, FRCPC, Department of Radiation Oncology, Odette Cancer Centre, Sunnybrook Health Sciences Centre, 2075 Bayview Avenue, Toronto, ON M4N 3M5, Canada. Tel: 416-480-4998; Fax: 416-480-6002; E-mail: Edward.Chow@sunnybrook.ca

radiotherapy not only decreased pain at the radiated site in patients with bone metastases, but also improved many other symptoms in ESAS in conjunction with other systemic therapies.

Keywords: ESAS, palliative radiation, advanced cancer symptoms, bone metastases.

Introduction

Skeletal metastases are a common occurrence and are seen in at least 50% of all cancer patients. Breast, prostate and lung cancers are the most frequently reported primaries that metastasize to bone and account for approximately 80% of all cases of bone metastases (1,2). Pain is the most commonly reported distressing symptom in 75% of patients with bone metastases. Palliative radiation has been proven to be an effective treatment for symptomatic bone metastases, with 24% of all patients experiencing complete pain relief and up to 59% reporting some pain relief (3).

Improving pain is the main goal in palliative radiation for bone metastases, however many advanced cancer patients experience other symptoms such as shortness of breath, depression and tiredness. It is therefore important to not only monitor the effects of radiation treatment on pain but to also see how the severities of other associated symptoms respond post-radiotherapy (4).

The Edmonton symptom assessment scale (ESAS) is an effective tool for monitoring pain and other symptoms in patients receiving palliative care. Its nine items include six symptoms related to physical well being (tiredness, drowsiness, appetite, pain, shortness of breath, and nausea) and three relating to psychological symptoms (depression, anxiety and overall well being) (5). Though the effects of radiation on depression and tiredness have been documented, analyzing all ESAS symptoms post radiation as well as comparing the results between responders and non-responders has not been reported (6-8). Therefore it is of interest to assess how response to radiation can affect the most common palliative cancer symptoms as well as a patient's overall sense of well being.

The primary objective of this study was to assess the overall change in ESAS symptoms in all patients following palliative radiation treatment for bone metastases. The secondary objective was to analyze the differences in ESAS symptoms between responders and non-responders to radiation treatment from week 1 to 12.

Methods

The Odette Cancer Centre (OCC) is one of two regional cancer centres providing radiotherapy in the Greater Toronto Area. The Rapid Response Radiotherapy Program (RRRP) at the OCC provides timely palliative radiation for symptomatic metastases. On initial consultation, patients with bone metastases were asked to rate the severity of symptoms they were experiencing using ESAS. This 11-point visual analogue scale asks patients to rate their symptoms from 0 (absence of symptom) to 10 (worst possible feeling of that symptom). The symptoms that ESAS assesses are pain, tiredness, nausea, depression, anxiety, drowsiness, appetite, overall sense of well being and shortness of breath. This tool has been proven to be very indicative of a patient's current status and is noted for its ease of administration as well as its brevity (5).

Patient demographics such as primary cancer site, age, Karnofsky Performance Status (KPS), analgesic intake and other sites of metastases were also recorded at the time of initial consultation. Radiation and site of radiation were also recorded. The initial baseline assessment was completed before radiation treatment and follow-up interviews were conducted by telephone or in person at weeks 1, 2, 4, 8, and 12 after the delivery of radiation treatment. We obtained ethics approval from the hospital for this study.

Statistical analysis

Response to radiation was determined by employing the International Consensus endpoints. A complete response to radiation is defined as a pain score of zero with no analgesic increase. Partial response is defined as a pain reduction of 2 or more without increased analgesic intake or a reduction of analgesic intake of 25% or more with no increase in pain score. Patients who responded to radiation treatment encompassed either one of the definitions for a complete and partial response (9).

To determine the percentage of patients who had an increase, decrease or no change in the severity of their symptoms comparing to the baseline score, an individual linear regression of ESAS symptom was applied for estimation of slope. It was considered as an increase, decrease or no change in the severity of symptom when an individual slope was positive, negative or zero. Chi-squared test was performed to evaluate the relationship between response effect and percentage change of ESAS symptoms at weeks 4, 8, and 12. Mean and median values were calculated for ESAS symptoms from baseline to week 12. General linear mixed model was used to determine the response effect on the ESAS symptoms over time. Results were considered significant at the 5% critical level ($p < 0.05$). All calculations were performed using SAS (version 9.1, SAS institute, Cary, NC) statistical software.

Results

Between January 1999 and January 2002, 518 patients with bone metastases completed baseline ESAS at the time of consultation. Demographic information is included in table 1. There were 280 males (54%) and 238 females (46%) in this study. Median and mean age of the study population was 68 years with an average KPS of 60. The most common primary cancer sites were lung (25%), breast (25%) and prostate (23%). The most frequently prescribed doses of radiation were 2000cGy/5 (42%) and 800cGy/1 (40%). The most common radiated sites were the pelvis (30%) and the spine (29%). Table 2 shows the median and mean scores for all 9 ESAS symptoms from baseline to week 12. At baseline pain, tiredness and lack of appetite were the most distressful symptoms reported by all patients with a median score of 5 for all three symptoms. Nausea and shortness of breath were shown to be the least severe symptoms at baseline with median scores of 0 and 1 respectively.

Of the 518 patients, 349 had at least one completed follow-up and 119 patients had a full five completed follow-ups. Using linear regression to determine percentage change in each patient's score, pain, anxiety, drowsiness, appetite and overall sense of well being all were shown to significantly improve from baseline to last follow-up. Tiredness was the only symptom that significantly worsened from baseline to last follow-up. Nausea, depression and shortness of breath showed no significant correlation from baseline to last follow-up. Table 3 shows all 518 patients' percent changes from baseline to their last follow-up regardless of response to radiation.

When comparing responders and non-responders at weeks 4, 8 and 12 (see table 4), all symptoms which showed a significant difference between the two populations had a greater improvement in the responders. At week 4, pain, anxiety and sense of well being were significantly better in the responders than the non-responders.

Table 1. Patient demographics

Sex	
Male	280 (54%)
Female	238 (46%)
Karnofsky Performance Status	
Median	Range
60	10-100
Age (Years)	
Mean	Range
68	31-93
Other Metastatic Sites	
Lung	111 (21%)
Liver	90 (17%)
Brain	17 (3%)
Primary Cancer Sites	
Lung	130 (25%)
Breast	127 (25%)
Prostate	117 (23%)
GI	39 (8%)
Unknown Primary	34 (7%)
Others	71 (14%)
Radiation Prescription (cGy/fraction)	
2000/5	219 (42%)
800/1	209 (40%)
3000/10	26 (5%)
1000/1	10 (2%)
Others	54 (11%)
Site of Radiation	
Hip/Pelvis	30%
Spine	29%
Femur	12%
Rib Cage	9%
Humerus	8%
Clavicle	5%
Others	7%

Table 2. Mean (M) and Median (P50) of ESAS symptoms in all patients from baseline to week 12

ESAS symptom	Week 0 M	Week 0 P50	Week 1 M	Week 1 P50	Week 2 M	Week 2 P50	Week 4 M	Week 4 P50	Week 8 M	Week 8 P50	Week 12 M	Week 12 P50	p-value*
Pain	4.46	5	3.15	3	2.86	2	2.84	2	2.82	2	3.37	3	< 0.0001
Tiredness	4.96	5	5.46	6	5.24	6	4.98	5	4.90	5	4.83	5	0.0043
Nausea	1.50	0	1.64	0	1.44	0	1.28	0	1.52	0	1.19	0	0.65
Depression	2.49	2	2.40	1	2.55	2	2.38	1	2.24	1	2.56	1	0.36
Anxiety	3.24	3	2.46	2	2.44	2	2.33	1	2.25	1	2.38	1	< 0.0001
Drowsiness	3.57	3	3.76	4	3.28	3	2.89	2	2.85	2	2.72	2	0.0015
Appetite	4.12	5	4.23	5	4.06	4	3.94	4	3.44	3	3.09	2	0.0071
Well Being	4.33	3	3.74	2	3.54	2	3.23	1	3.49	1	3.63	1	< 0.0001
Shortness of Breath	2.24	1	1.82	0	2.00	0	1.97	0	2.17	1	1.78	0	0.07

*p-value of week was obtained by general linear mixed model and indicated significance of ESAS symptoms change over time in all patients.

Table 3. Percent change in all ESAS symptoms from baseline to last FU

ESAS Symptoms	Increase	Decrease	No Change
Pain	40.5	50.9	8.6
Tiredness	52.8	39.4	7.8
Nausea	27.2	40.3	32.5
Depression	38.9	41.2	19.9
Anxiety	32.6	49.3	18.2
Drowsiness	36.9	52.6	10.5
Appetite	46.7	41.4	11.9
Sense of Well-Being	47.7	40.9	11.4
Shortness of Breath	29.5	46.0	24.6

At week 8 both anxiety and drowsiness were significantly better in responders. The greatest number of symptoms with a significant difference between responders and non-responders occurred at week 12. Pain, nausea, anxiety, drowsiness and appetite were all significantly better in responders when compared with non-responders at week 12.

When comparing those patients who responded to radiation to those who did not from weeks 1 through 12, all symptoms showed a significant difference except for shortness of breath (see table 5). Pain, tiredness, nausea, depression, anxiety, drowsiness, appetite and overall sense of well being were all significantly better in responders when compared to the non-responders. The only symptom which showed no significant difference between the responder and non-responder populations was shortness of breath.

Table 4. Percentage change of ESAS symptoms in responders and non-responders at weeks 4, 8 and 12

ESAS symptom	Responder Increase (%)	Responder Decrease (%)	Responder No Change (%)	Non-responder Increase (%)	Non-responder Decrease (%)	Non-responder No Change (%)	p-value*
At week 4							
Pain	22.4	67.2	10.4	43.2	49.2	7.6	0.0015
Tiredness	44.4	45.9	9.8	49.2	38.6	12.1	0.47
Nausea	21.8	32.3	45.9	23.5	42.4	34.1	0.12
Depression	33.8	42.9	23.3	33.6	38.9	27.5	0.70
Anxiety	26.5	57.6	15.9	32.1	42.0	26.0	0.029
Drowsiness	32.6	54.5	12.9	35.6	50.0	14.4	0.76
Appetite	36.1	51.9	12.0	46.2	38.6	15.2	0.096
Sense of Well-Being	25.8	62.9	11.4	38.6	40.9	20.5	0.0015
Shortness of Breath	29.9	45.5	24.6	28.8	40.2	31.1	0.48
At week 8							
Pain	33.0	60.6	6.4	43.4	53.3	3.3	0.19
Tiredness	43.1	50.5	6.4	52.5	43.4	4.1	0.33
Nausea	24.8	34.9	40.4	27.9	45.9	26.2	0.066
Depression	28.4	49.5	22.0	40.8	38.3	20.8	0.12
Anxiety	20.4	63.9	15.7	39.2	46.7	14.2	0.0074
Drowsiness	25.9	57.4	16.7	41.8	51.6	6.6	0.0077
Appetite	30.3	57.8	11.9	43.4	49.2	7.4	0.094
Sense of Well-Being	33.9	58.7	7.3	41.0	49.2	9.8	0.34
Shortness of Breath	33.9	45.0	21.1	36.1	37.7	26.2	0.49
At week 12							
Pain	37.8	54.1	8.2	53.7	44.2	2.1	0.029
Tiredness	40.8	57.1	2.0	57.9	40.0	2.1	0.056
Nausea	22.4	35.7	41.8	31.6	49.5	18.9	0.0026
Depression	33.0	50.5	16.5	44.2	35.8	20.0	0.12
Anxiety	17.5	66.0	16.5	46.8	43.6	9.6	0.0001
Drowsiness	28.6	64.3	7.1	47.9	47.9	4.3	0.021
Appetite	22.4	62.2	15.3	50.5	44.2	5.3	0.0001
Sense of Well-Being	38.8	56.1	5.1	44.7	48.9	6.4	0.60
Shortness of Breath	34.7	41.8	23.5	24.2	53.7	22.1	0.20

* p-value was obtained by Chi-squared test to see the relationship between response effect and percentage change of ESAS symptom at week 4, 8, and 12.

Discussion

The symptoms included in ESAS are very appropriate for analyzing an advanced cancer patient's overall response after their course of radiation treatment. In a recent study by Walsh et al (10) involving 1,000 advanced cancer patients, many of the symptoms included in ESAS were among the most prevalent in the overall population. The most distressing symptoms according to this study were pain (84%), tiredness (69%), lack of appetite (66%), drowsiness (61%) and shortness of breath (50%). Walsh et al (10) also noted that many advanced cancer patients are polysymptomatic and although one symptom be the most dominant, all symptoms contribute to a patient's overall QOL. They also showed that advanced cancer symptoms are, for the most part, independent of age, gender, performance status and primary cancer site (10).

Table 5. Average of ESAS symptoms between responders (R) and non-responders (NR) from week 1 to 12

ESAS Symptom	Week 1 R	Week 1 NR	Week 2 R	Week 2 NR	Week 4 R	Week 4 NR	Week 8 R	Week 8 NR	Week 12 R	Week 12 NR	p-value Response effect[†]
Pain	2.33	3.92	2.08	3.64	1.81	3.89	2.29	3.28	2.52	4.22	< 0.0001
Tired	4.84	6.05	4.53	5.94	4.61	5.36	4.28	5.45	3.97	5.75	< 0.0001
Nausea	1.42	1.84	1.09	1.79	1.02	1.55	1.32	1.71	1.02	1.36	0.049
Depression	2.11	2.68	2.06	3.08	2.32	2.44	1.73	2.73	2.09	3.05	0.0004
Anxiety	2.21	2.69	1.99	2.94	2.20	2.47	1.48	2.99	1.83	2.96	< 0.0001
Drowsiness	3.06	4.42	2.52	4.08	2.78	2.99	2.13	3.54	1.94	3.55	< 0.0001
Appetite	3.87	4.57	3.26	4.86	3.44	4.44	2.91	3.92	2.35	3.87	0.015
Well Being	3.23	4.20	2.99	4.09	2.76	3.74	3.03	3.95	3.10	4.25	0.0007
Shortness of Breath	1.66	1.97	1.66	2.34	2.14	1.80	2.06	2.27	1.88	1.67	0.32

[†]*p-value of response effect* indicates significance of comparing symptoms change from week 1 to week 12 between responders and non-responders, when adjusting for week variable. General linear mixed model was performed in the analysis.

Radiotherapy for palliation of bone metastases has been proven to be an effective treatment for reducing pain and increasing patients' overall QOL (1,2,6). For patients with bone metastases, severe pain is often the most prevalent symptom for over 70% of these individuals, which is why palliation of pain using radiation is a primary concern (2,6,11-13). Limited mobility, fracture, hypercalcemia, reduced KPS, impaired daily functioning and diminished QOL are all noted consequences of bone metastases (2,14). In our study, most ESAS symptoms were shown to improve after radiation in all patients and the majority of those who responded to radiotherapy achieved a significant improvement within the first week after the start of radiation. In an overview of pain and QOL (15), they suggested that as a patient is cognitively aware that their radiation treatment is providing pain relief, their anxiety, depression and overall sense of well being also improved. This finding was also noticed in our overall study population when analyzing the change in their symptom scores from baseline to last follow-up. The only symptom that was negatively affected in all patients was tiredness.

Radiation induced tiredness is experienced by 80-90% of all cancer patients. On average 69% of advanced cancer patients experience tiredness on a regular basis irrespective of radiation treatment (6,10). Tiredness has a significant impact on the QOL of cancer patients and it is caused primarily by cancer pathology and other systemic treatments (7). Even though the responders did not show a significant increase or decrease in tiredness following radiation, it was the only symptom which had the highest consistent mean and median score before and after radiation treatment. Tiredness was also the only negatively effected ESAS symptom reported by all patients after radiation treatment.

In a study by Strauss et al (16) data from a sample of 239 cancer patients receiving radiotherapy showed a high negative correlation between tiredness and QoL. They found tiredness to be the most dominant factor in cancer patient suffering. Other studies have shown that exercise such as walking can significantly reduce the effects of radiotherapy induced tiredness in cancer patients but only a very limited number of studies have focused on tiredness in the palliative population (17-19). In one such study by Brown et al., a multidisciplinary program which included physical therapy, stretching, cognitive behavioral strategies, discussion and support was shown to be unsuccessful in reducing tiredness in palliative cancer patients (6). Overall, psychosocial and physical intervention in the treatment of tiredness among all palliative cancer patients has been shown to be inconclusive and more research is needed to combat the very negative effects of tiredness on QOL (6).

For those who responded to radiation treatment, all symptoms with the exception of shortness of breath had a significantly lower ESAS scores when compared with those who did not respond to radiation treatment. Furthermore, the greatest number of significant differences in symptoms between responders and non-responders were noted at week 12. As a possible explanation for these results, Niv and Shulamith reported that patients who are able to either reduce or stabilize their opiate consumption in turn decrease the side effects of these drugs which can include nausea, respiratory depression and confusion (15). This could partially explain why responders do appreciably better from weeks 1 through 12 in all but one ESAS symptom when compared with non-responders. In a study by Kovner et al (15) of 42 metastatic patients who received palliative radiotherapy for pain, those who responded with pain reduction also had a decrease in depression, anxiety and had increased vigor, curiosity, and overall QOL. The results from our respondent cohort were also consistent with this finding but when considering all 518 patients, depression scores did not change after radiation treatment. Depression is not an inevitable response to cancer or radiation treatment, which explains the consistency in depression scores for all patients before and after radiation in our study (8).

Kovner et al (15) also stated that those patients who were more active, had more anxiety and depression prior to treatment and had greater spirituality were shown to have a better response to radiation treatment and a greater QOL. Though we did not analyze predetermining factors to radiation response in this study, this could possibly be an area of further research and analysis. We also found in our study that patients who did not respond to radiation treatment not only had poor pain response but also worsened or showed no improvement in all other ESAS symptoms as well, with the exception of shortness of breath. This implies that radiation not only effectively relieves pain in respondents, but also improves many other problematic symptoms that are commonly experienced by patients with advanced cancer in conjunction with other systemic therapies.

Our study was limited to only English speaking patients. Also only 67% of the patients interviewed at baseline could be reached to complete at least one follow-up. Another limitation to this study was that only the change in ESAS symptoms were assessed and other advanced cancer symptoms such as constipation and dry mouth were not followed throughout a patient's course of radiation treatment. Lastly any changes in other systemic therapies were not considered in this study.

Conclusions

Our study has shown that overall pain, anxiety, drowsiness, appetite and sense of well being all improved following palliative radiation for bone metastases. Tiredness was the only symptom which worsened after radiation. All other ESAS symptoms (nausea, depression and shortness of breath) showed no significant difference post radiation. The greatest number of ESAS symptoms which showed a significant difference between responders and non-responders occurred at week 12. When comparing those who responded to radiation to those who did not, all but one symptom showed a significant difference in favour of responders. Shortness of breath was the only symptom which showed no significant difference between responders and non-responders. Non-responders not only achieved lack of adequate pain relief from radiation but did poorly in almost all ESAS symptoms as well when compared to those who responded to palliative radiation. We strongly recommend palliative radiation treatment be offered to patients with bone metastases.

Acknowledgments

The studentship was funded by the Michael and Karyn Goldstein Cancer Research Fund. We thank Ms Stacy Lue for her secretarial assistance. Conflict of interest: none.

References

[1] Jasmin C, Capanna R, Coia L, Coleman R, Saillant G. Textbook of bone metastases. Hoboken, NJ: Wiley, 2005.
[2] Falkmer U, Jarhult J, Wersall P, Cavallin-Stahl E. A systematic overview of radiation therapy effects in skeletal metastases. Acta Oncol 2003;42(5-6):620-33.
[3] Chow E, Harris K, Fan G, Tsao M, Sze W. Palliative radiotherapy trials for bone metastases: A systematic review. J Clin Oncol 2007; 25(11):1423-36.
[4] Riechelmann RP, Krzyzanowska MK, O'Carroll A, Zimmermann C. Symptom and medication profiles among cancer patients attending a palliative care clinic. Support Care Cancer 2007;15(12):1407-12.
[5] Bruera E, Kuehn N, Miller MJ, Selmser P, Macmillan K. The edmonton symptom assessment system (ESAS): A simple method for the assessment of palliative care patients. J Palliat Care 1991;7(2):6-9.
[6] Brown P, Clark MM, Atherton P, Huschka M, Sloan JA, Gamble G, Girardi J, Frost MH, Piderman K, Rummans TA. Will improvement in quality of life (QOL) impact fatigue in patients receiving radiation therapy for advanced cancer? Am J Clin Oncol 2006;29(1):52-8.
[7] Greenberg DB, Sawicka J, Eisenthal S, Ross D. Fatigue syndrome due to localized radiation. J Pain Symptom Manage 1992;7(1):38-45.
[8] Jenkins C, Carmody TJ, Rush AJ. Depression in radiation oncology patients: A preliminary evaluation. J Affect Disord 1998;50(1):17-21.
[9] Chow E, Wu JS, Hoskin P, Coia LR, Bentzen SM, Blitzer PH. International consensus on palliative radiotherapy endpoints for future clinical trials in bone metastases. Radiother Oncol 2002;64(3):275-80.

[10] Walsh D, Donnelly S, Rybicki L. The symptoms of advanced cancer: Relationship to age, gender, and performance status in 1,000 patients. Support Care Cancer 2000;8(3):175-9.
[11] Gaze MN, Kelly CG, Kerr GR, Cull A, Cowie VJ, Gregor A, Howard GC, Rodger A. Pain relief and quality of life following radiotherapy for bone metastases: A randomised trial of two fractionation schedules. Radiother Oncol 1997; 45(2):109-16.
[12] Hoegler D. Radiotherapy for palliation of symptoms in incurable cancer. Curr Probl Cancer 1997;21(3):129-83.
[13] Janjan NA, Payne R, Gillis T, Podoloff D, Libshitz HI, Lenzi R, Theriault R, Martin C, Yasko A. Presenting symptoms in patients referred to a multidisciplinary clinic for bone metastases. J Pain Symptom Manage 1998;16(3):171-8.
[14] Barton MB, Dawson R, Jacob S, Currow D, Stevens G, Morgan G. Palliative radiotherapy of bone metastases: An evaluation of outcome measures. J Eval Clin Pract 2001;7(1):47-64.
[15] Niv D, Shulamith K. Pain and quality of life. Pain Medicine 2001;1(2):150-61.
[16] Strauss B, Brix C, Fischer S, Leppert K, Fuller J, Roehrig B, Schleussner C, Wendt TG. The influence of resilience on fatigue in cancer patients undergoing radiation therapy (RT). J Cancer Res Clin Oncol 2007;133(8):511-8.
[17] Winsor P, Potter J, Nicol K. A randomized, controlled trial of aerobic exercise for treatment-related fatigue in men receiving radical external beam radiotherapy for localized prostate carcinoma. Cancer 2004; 101 (3) 550-7.
[18] Sarna L, Conde F. Physical activity and fatigue during radiation therapy: a pilot study using actigraph monitors. Oncology Nursing Forum 2001; 28 (6): 1043-6.
[19] Mock V, Dow K, Meares L, Grimm P, Dienemann J, Haisfield-Wolde M, Quitasol W, Mitchile S, Chakravarthy A, Gage I. Effect of exercise on fatigue, physical functioning and emotional distress during radiation therapy for breast cancer. Oncology Nursing Forum 1997; 24(6): 991-1000.

Chapter 40

IMPACT OF PAIN FLARE ON PATIENTS TREATED WITH PALLIATIVE RADIOTHERAPY FOR SYMPTOMATIC BONE METASTASES

Amanda Hird, BSc(C)[1], Rebecca Wong, MD[2], Candi Flynn, BSc[1], Stephanie Hadi, BSc(C)[1], Eric de Sa, BSc[1], Liying Zhang, PhD[1], Carlo DeAngelis, PharmD[3] and Edward Chow, MBBS[1]*

[1]Rapid Response Radiotherapy Program, Department of Radiation Oncology, Odette Cancer Centre, Sunnybrook Health Sciences Centre, University of Toronto, Toronto, Ontario
[2]Palliative Radiotherapy Oncology Program, Department of Radiation Oncology, Princess Margaret Hospital, University of Toronto, Toronto Ontario and
[3]Pharmacy Department, Odette Cancer Centre, Sunnybrook Health Sciences Centre, University of Toronto, Toronto, Ontario, Canada

Abstract

Purpose: Pain flare following palliative radiotherapy (RT) for painful bone metastases is well-recognized with incidence rates of 2-44% reported in the literature. Our Oobjective was to investigate the impact of pain flare on patients with bone metastases treated with external beam RT. Methods: A five-item 'Pain Flare Qualitative Questionnaire' was developed to assess the psychological and functional impacts of the pain flare phenomenon. Results: Thirteen patients with pain flare completed the interview. There were three males and 10 females. The median age was 59 years (range: 48-89). The majority of participants had primary breast (9/13) or prostate cancer (2/13). Pain flare severely impacted patients' functional activity and and carried resulted in negative mood and isolation from family and friends due to unbearable pain. Breakthrough pain medications were not adequate to control the pain increase in more than three quarters75% of the interviewed patients. Prophylactic medication was preferred as opposed to management with breakthrough analgesia. Although patients felt the RT

---

* Correspondence: Edward Chow, MBBS, PhD, FRCPC, Department of Radiation Oncology, Odette Cancer Centre, Sunnybrook Health Sciences Centre, 2075 Bayview Avenue, Toronto, ON M4N 3M5, Canada. Tel: 416-480-4998; Fax: 416-480-6002; E-mail: Edward.Chow@sunnybrook.ca

was worthwhile, there was hesitation to repeat the treatment if necessary due to the previously experienced flare effect. Conclusions: Pain flare is a common side effect following palliative RT for painful bone metastases. Based on our patient interviews, this event was debilitating and worrisome. Patients should be informed of this potential side effect and health care professionals should ensure patients are equipped with sufficient analgesia to manage this increase in metastatic bone pain. However, prevention of the pain flare as opposed to management with breakthrough pain medications was preferable in this study.

Keywords: Bone metastases, pain flare, impact, qualitative survey.

Introduction

Pain is the most prevalent symptom associated with bone metastases and is experienced by 60-75% of patients. Palliative radiotherapy (RT) is a well-established and effective treatment option for symptomatic bone metastases with overall pain response rates approaching 80% (1-3).

'Pain flare' is a temporary worsening of pain in the treated bony metastatic site immediately following RT. Pain flare has been a well-recognized side effect following treatment of painful bone metastases, particularly following radionucleotide therapy (4-12). However, reported rates of pain flare following external beam RT range from 2-44% and suggest a higher risk for patients treated with a single fraction (13-17). Hird and colleagues recently reported an overall pain flare incidence rate of 38% across three Canadian outpatient radiation clinics (18). Dexamethasone, a corticosteroid and anti-inflammatory medication, has been employed as an effective prophylactic agent for prevention of the pain flare phenomenon in the first two days following a single 8 Gy when prescribed at baseline. Specifically, the incidence of pain flare in the two days immediately following RT decreased from 60% to 3% in a recent pilot study (19).

Seemingly, pain flare occurs in a significant portion of patients treated for symptomatic bone metastases. However, the impact of pain flare on these patients has not been investigated. The purpose of this qualitative study was to examine the impact of pain flare on bone metastases patients treated with external beam RT, and to investigate patients' preference for pain flare prophylaxis versus management with breakthrough pain medications.

Methods

In February 2006, an observational study across three Canadian cancer centres: Odette Cancer Centre (OCC, Toronto, Ontario); Princess Margaret Hospital (PMH, Toronto, Ontario); Tom Baker Cancer Centre (TBCC, Calgary, Alberta), was initiated to determine the incidence of pain flare following palliative RT for bone metastases (18). An interim analysis was completed in October 2007. It was found that 35 out of 93 evaluable patients (38%) experienced a pain flare.

Anecdotally, the study investigators noted a significant burden to several of the patients experiencing a pain flare, as expressed by the patients during the telephone follow-up assessments. Therefore, the investigators developed a qualitative questionnaire to assess the impact of the flare experienced byon these patients.

Brainstorming with palliative radiation oncologists produced the 5-item Pain Flare Qualitative Questionnaire (see Table 1). Open-ended questions were employed in order to facilitate open and unbiased responses from patients. Patients were eligible if they had experienced a pain flare in the incidence study by Hird et al (18). Patients were interviewed (by telephone) by a trained research assistant. Patient responses were recorded verbatim and analyzed for common themes between responders. Ethics approval was obtained from the hospital research ethics board to conduct the retrospective interviews.

Table 1. Pain Flare Qualitative Questionnaire Interviewer Guideline

Introduction to the interview
In *(insert date here)*, you received radiation to *(site)*. In the 10 days following your treatment, you indicated that your pain got a little bit worse. Do you recall this event? Would you mind if we asked you a total of 5 easy questions about this experience? We want to find out how the pain flare affected each patient, so there are no right or wrong answers to any of these questions.
Interview Questions
1. What did the pain increase mean to you at the time of the flare? (For example, what went through your mind when you were experiencing the flare?)   *2. Did the increase in pain interfere with your daily functioning? (For example, general activity, mood, walking ability, normal work, relations with others, sleep, enjoyment of life?)*   *3. What did you do to manage the increase in pain? (For example: extra pain medications, sitting, lying down, etc.)*   *4. In retrospect, what does the pain flare mean to you now?*   *5. Overall, do you feel the radiation treatment was worthwhile?*

In the pain flare incidence trial (18), patients completed the Brief Pain Inventory (BPI) before RT. The patient also kept a daily diary during treatment (if receiving multiple fractions) and for 10 days after RT. The diary collected the patients worst pain score for the preceding 24 hour period on a scale of 0-10, where 0 was the absence of pain and 10 was the worst possible pain; the patient's total intake of analgesia for the previous 24 hours, which was converted into an oral morphine equivalent dose (OMED); and a description of the worst pain as "worse", "the same", or "better" when compared to the baseline level. It was made clear to the patient that each pain score was to be based solely on the site treated with the RT.

Pain flare was defined (a priori) as a two-point increase in the worst pain score when compared to baseline on an 11-point scale (0-10) with no decrease in analgesic intake; or a 25% increase in analgesic intake employing OMED with no decrease in worst pain score. If the baseline worst pain was 9/10, pain flare was identified if the follow up worst pain score was 10/10 accompanied with a description of the current worst pain as "worse" when compared to the baseline worst pain. If the baseline worst pain was 10/10, pain flare was identified if the follow-up worst pain score was 10/10 with a description of the current worst pain level as "worse" than baseline worst pain. To distinguish pain flare from progression of pain, the worst pain score and OMED value must have returned back to baseline after the increase/flare.

The Wilcoxon rank-sum test or Fisher exact test was applied to compare patients from Hird et al.'s study population who experienced pain flare versus patients who completed the qualitative interview. Results were considered significant at the 5% critical level ($p < 0.05$). All calculations were performed using SAS (version 8.2 for Windows; SAS Institute, Cary, NC).

Results

From February 2006 to October 2007, 111 patients were enrolled in the pain flare incidence study (see table 2) (18). There were 93 evaluable patients. From this cohort, 35 patients (38%) experienced pain flare. A total of 13/35 (37%) patients completed the qualitative interview. Ten out of 35 (29%) were deceased/hospitalized, 8/35 (23%) were unreachable, and 4/35 (11%) were from TBCC and not included in the analysis. The demographics of the cohort contacted for this analysis is compared to all patients experiencing a pain flare from Hird et al.'s study in Table 3. There were no statistically significant differences between Hird et al cohort of pain flare patients (18) and those included in the current study ($p > 0.05$).

Table 2. Patient demographics of the enrolled patients in the pain flare incidence study from the Odette Cancer Centre and Princess Margaret Hospital (N=111)

Sex	
Male	55 (50%)
Female	56 (50%)
Age (years) – Median (Range)	64 (40-89)
Oral Morphine Equivalent at Baseline (mg/day) – Median (Range)	12 (0-880)
Worst Pain Score at Baseline – Median (Range)	7 (0-10)
Radiation Dose	
8Gy	81 (73%)
20Gy/5 or 30Gy/10	30 (27%)
Primary Cancer Site	
Breast	43 (39%)
Prostate	27 (24%)
Lung	19 (17%)
Gastrointestinal	10 (9%)
Others	12 (11%)

*All patients enrolled in the ongoing pain flare incidence investigation by Hird et al across three Canadian cancer centres (18).

Table 3. Patient demographics of pain flare patients (n=35) versus those contacted for the interview (n=13)

	Contacted Pain Flare Patients (n=13)*	Patients Experiencing a Pain Flare (n=35) †	*p-value*
Sex			
Male	3 (23%)	12 (34%)	0.73
Female	10 (77%)	23 (66%)	
Age (years) – Median (Range)	59 (48-89)	60 (40-89)	0.99
Oral Morphine Equivalent at Baseline (mg-day) – Median (Range)	0 (0-190)	3 (0-590)	0.85
Worst Pain Score at Baseline – Median (Range)	4 (0-9)	6 (0-10)	0.33
Radiation Dose			
8Gy	8 (62%)	23 (66%)	0.79
20Gy/5 or 30Gy/10	5 (38%)	12 (34%)	
Primary Cancer Site			
Breast	9 (69%)	19 (54%)	0.78
Prostate	2 (15%)	5 (14%)	
Lung	0 (0%)	4 (11%)	
Gastrointestinal	0 (0%)	1 (3%)	
Others	2 (15%)	6 (17%)	

* Patients from Hird et al.'s cohort who were interviewed in the current study.
† All patients experiencing a pain flare from the Odette Cancer Centre or Princess Margaret Hospital from Hird et al.'s cohort (18).
p-values were obtained by Wilcoxon rank-sum test or Fisher exact test for comparing two groups. There were no significant differences between the pain flare cohort from Hird et al.'s study (18) and the patients interviewed in the current study.

The following sections outline the patient responses for each item from the Pain Flare Qualitative Questionnaire.

- *Question 1*: What did the pain increase mean to you at the time of the flare? (For example, what went through your mind when you were experiencing the flare?). Patients indicated their fear that the "cancer was getting worse" and that their "cancer pain was never going to end". Some believed the RT was not effective. One patient mentioned feeling confused – the RT was meant to improve bone pain rather than make it worse. Specifically, one patient described the flare as "a thousand times worse" when compared to the pain he had experienced at initial consultation in the clinic. Another described her pain flare experience as "excruciating". Generally, patients who were well informed of the possibility of a flare up of pain were not concerned by the experience. In fact, one patient mentioned feeling a sense of optimism – she believed that the flare meant that the RT was working. Nevertheless, some patients who were informed of the possibility of experiencing a pain flare reported feeling as though they were caught off guard, which in turn resulted in a great deal of worry and stress. Despite having the research study and the pain flare phenomenon explained to her prior to enrolment in the original pain flare incidence trial, one patient in particular was unaware this was a potential side effect of the RT. She was not pre-medicated in anticipation of this event, and a lack of understanding on pain flare prevented her from being psychologically prepared to deal with this pain increase.

- *Question 2:* Did the increase in pain interfere with your daily functioning? (For example, general activity, mood, walking ability, normal work, relations with others, sleep, enjoyment of life?). Overall, 10 patients indicated some level of functional interference while experiencing the pain flare, with the majority indicating that the pain flare completely interfered with daily activities. One patient specifically indicated that the pain interfered with his relationships and put him in a "down" mood. He described himself as a "hermit" in the sense that he did not interact with people because the pain was so severe. Additionally, his wife described him as lethargic and said she could hear him "moaning during the night because of his pain". Another indicated that she needed assistance from her family with basic daily tasks. A female patient indicated she had to lie completely still because the pain significantly increased with the slightest movement. In general, patients indicated that daily activities had to be modified considerably during the time of the flare so as not to aggravate the pain they were experiencing.

- *Question 3:* What did you do to manage the increase in pain? (For example: extra pain medications, sitting, lying down, etc). Over three quarters of patients indicated they increased their pain medications. However, nine patients failed to achieve adequate control of the RT-induced flare pain despite this increase in OMED. Furthermore, some patients stated that they were reluctant to take additional breakthrough pain medications to control the pain flare due to the unfavourable side effects that may result (i.e. constipation, dry mouth, and fatigue). Alternative methods of pain flare management included rest, limited movement, and/or use of a hot water bottle.

- *Question 4:* In retrospect, what does the pain flare mean to you now? Most patients had not thought about this aspect of their pain flare experience. One patient indicated that she now knows that any pain relief she will obtain from RT comes with a discomfort. Similarly, another explained that she is now aware of what to expect in terms of what a pain flare feels like and how long it will last. Beyond this, patients experiencing adequate management of the flare with breakthrough pain medications did not have a response to this item. A single patient who did not recall the flare stated, "I don't know what the pain flare means at all".

- *Question 5:* Overall, do you feel the radiation treatment was worthwhile? The majority of patients indicated that RT was worthwhile, despite experiencing that pain flare. One patient mentioned that although the pain flare was problematic, the RT improved her daily functioning. Yet another expressed that if she wanted to improve functioning, she would have no choice but to experience the pain flare since RT seemed to be the only effective method of sustained pain relief. One patient expressed that she would have delayed RT since she achieved adequate pain relief following hormone therapy. Another patient indicated that the pain flare caused a significant amount of stress and did not result in any subsequent pain relief. The remaining patients were unsure whether the pain relief was from RT or due to pain medications.

At the end of the interview patients were asked if they would prefer the prevention of the pain flare altogether as opposed to management with breakthrough pain medications. Eleven out of 13 patients explicitly stated that they would prefer the prevention of the pain flare.

Discussion

Pain flare is common following external beam RT for symptomatic bone metastases. Our qualitative interview with patients experiencing a pain flare revealed several important trends. Not only was the pain flare debilitating to this cohort of patients by interfering with daily activities and general functioning, but it also resulted in the need for many patients to remain bed-bound. Furthermore, patients expressed anxiety and stress over treatment success. Increases in analgesia were not adequate to control RT-induced pain in the majority of patients. Although our study was limited by a small sample size, there was an overwhelming consensus to prevent the flare as opposed to managing it with breakthrough pain medications (85%).

Pain flare prophylaxis is preferential for two additional reasons: in order for the pain flare to be managed with as-needed pain medications, the patient in question must first experience a pain increase. Moreover, increases in pain medications can lead to increased side effects; including constipation, dry mouth, and drowsiness. The aforementioned situations may cause a further impairment in patient quality of life. Studies to explore prophylactic strategies for the prevention of the pain flare phenomenon are needed. Only through pain flare prevention can we completely eliminate additional and unnecessary patient suffering. Until this goal is reached, we encourage physicians to adequately educate their patients of the potential flare effect, ensure their patients are equipped with adequate breakthrough analgesia, and be attentive to the potential adverse effects of high dose opioid therapy.

Acknowledgments

This study was generously supported by the Michael and Karyn Goldstein Cancer Research Fund.

References

[1] Nielsen OS. Palliative radiotherapy of bone metastases: there is now evidence for the use of single fractions. Radiother Oncol 1999;52:95.
[2] Berk L. Prospective trials for the radiotherapeutic treatment of bone metastases. Am J Hosp Palliat Care 1995;12:24.
[3] Arcangeli G, Giovinazzo G, Saracino B, et al. Radiation therapy in the management of symptomatic bone metastases: The effect of total dose and histology on pain relief and response duration. Int J Rat Onc Biol Phys 1998;42:1119.

[4] Silberstein EB. Teletherapy and radiopharmaceutical therapy of painful bone metastases. Semin Nucl Med 2005;35(2):152-8.

[5] Kraeber-Bodere F, Campion L, Rousseau C, et al. Treatment of bone metastases of prostate cancer with strontium-89 chloride: efficacy in relation to the degree of bone involvement. Eur J Nucl Med 2000;27(10):1487-93.

[6] Roka R, Sera T, Pajor L, et al. Clinical experience with rhenium-188 HEDP therapy for metastatic bone pain. Orv Hetil 2000;141(19):1019-23.

[7] Slovin SF, Scher HI, Divgi CR, et al. Interferon--gamma and monoclonal antibody 131I-labeled CC49: outcomes in patients with androgenindependent prostate cancer. Clin Cancer Res 1998;4(3):643-51.

[8] Schoeneich G, Palmedo H, Dierke-Dzierzon C, et al. Rhenium-186 HEDP: palliative radionuclide therapy of painful bone metastases. Preliminary results. Scand J Urol Nephrol 1997;31(5):445-8.

[9] Limouris GS, Shukla SK, Condi-Paphiti A, et al. Palliative therapy using rhenium-186-HEDP in painful breast osseous metastases. Anticancer Res 1997;17(3B):1767-72.

[10] de Klerk JM, van het Schip AD, Zonnenberg BA, et al. Phase 1 study of rhenium-186-HEDP in patients with bone metastases originating from breast cancer. J Nucl Med 1996;37(2):244-9.

[11] Dafermou A, Colamussi P, Giganti M, et al. A multicentre observational study of radionuclide therapy in patients with painful bone metastases of prostate cancer. Eur J Nucl Med 2001;28(7):788-98.

[12] Bubley GJ. Is the flare phenomenon clinically significant? Urology 2001;58(2Suppl1):5-9.

[13] Kirkbride P, Aslanidis J. Single fraction radiation therapy for bone metastases - a pilot study using a dose of 12 Gy. [Abstract 581]. Clin Invest Med1996;19(4):S87.

[14] Foro P, Algara M, Reig A, et al. Randomized prospective trial comparing three schedules of palliative radiotherapy. Preliminary results. [Spanish]. Oncologia 1998;21(11):55-60.

[15] Loblaw DA, Wu JSY, Warde P, et al. Pain flare in patients with bone metastases after palliative radiotherapy: a nested randomized controlled trial. Sup Care Canc 2007;15(4):451-5.

[16] Chow E, Ling A, Davis L, et al. Pain flare following external beam radiotherapy and meaningful change in pain scores in the treatment of bone metastases. Radiother Oncol 2005;75:64-9.

[17] Roos DE, Turner SL, O'Brien PC, et al. Randomized trial of 8 Gy in 1 versus 20 Gy in 5 fractions of radiotherapy for neuropathic pain due to bone metastases (Trans-Tasman Radiation Oncology Group, TROG 96.05). Radiother Oncol 2005;75:54-63.

[18] Hird A, Hadi S, Loblaw A, et al. Pain flare following radiotherapy for painful bone metastases: a joint effort of three cancer centres to determine the incidence. Int J Rad Onc Biol Phys 2007;69(3) S32-3.

[19] Chow E, Loblaw DA, Harris K, et al. Dexamethasone for the prophylaxis of radiation-induced pain flare after palliative radiotherapy for bone metastases - a pilot study. Supp Care Canc 2007;15:643-7.

In: Pain Management Yearbook 2009
Editor: Joav Merrick

ISBN: 978-1-61209-666-7
©2012 Nova Science Publishers, Inc.

Chapter 41

VALIDATION OF MEANINGFUL CHANGE IN PAIN SCORES IN THE TREATMENT OF BONE METASTASES

Edward Chow, MBBS[*1], *Amanda Hird, BSc(C)*[2],
Rebecca Wong, MD[2], *Liying Zhang, PhD*[1], *Jackson Wu, MD*[3],
Lisa Barbera, MD[1], *May Tsao, MD*[1], *Elizabeth Barnes, MD*[1]
and Cyril Danjoux, MD[1]

[1]Odette Cancer Centre, Sunnybrook Health Sciences Centre, University of Toronto, Toronto, Ontario, [2]Princess Margaret Hospital, University Health Network, University of Toronto, Toronto, Ontario and [3]Tom Baker Cancer Centre, University of Calgary, Calgary, Alberta, Canada

Abstract

The purpose wasPurpose: Our objective was to validate what constitutes athe meaningful change in pain scores following palliative radiotherapy (RT) forin the treatment of bone metastases. Methods: Patients with bone metastases treated with external beam radiotherapy RT were asked to score their 'worst' pain on a scale of 0-10 before treatment (baseline), daily during treatment and for 10 days after completion of external beam radiationRT. Patients were also asked to indicate if their pain at the time of follow up was "worse", "the same", or "better" when compared to the pre-treatment level. Thus, Tthe change in pain score was accompanied with patient perception. Results: One hundred and seventy-eight patients were evaluated in this study. There were 82 male and 96 female patients with the median age of 65.5 years. A total of 1431 pain scorings were obtained. Patients perceived an improvement in pain when their self-reported pain score decreased by at least two points. Conclusion: Our current study validates the previous finding of meaningful change in pain score as reduction of patient self reported pain score by at least two points. This finding of the meaningful change in pain scores supports the investigation-defined partial response in clinical trials and the international consensus endpoints.

---

[*] **Correspondence:** Edward Chow, MBBS, PhD, FRCPC, Department of Radiation Oncology, Odette Cancer Centre, Sunnybrook Health Sciences Centre, 2075 Bayview Avenue, Toronto, Ontario, Canada M4N 3M5. Tel: 416-480-4998; Fax: 416-480-6002; E-mail: Edward.Chow@sunnybrook.ca

Keywords: Bone metastases, palliative radiotherapy, meaningful change.

Introduction

The benefits of palliative radiotherapy (RT) for bone metastases are mainly assessed by the change in pain intensity often measured by pain scores. Previous studies have shown that clinicians and family members tend to overestimate the benefits of treatment interventions (1-8). Patient self-assessment should therefore be the preferred measure of the benefit or success of the treatment.

Patients are often not uninformed of what pain score they provided at baseline when they are asked to score their current pain at a follow-up assessment. However, we have noticed that patients may inform whether their pain score is increasing/worsening in numbers but at the same time state their pain is getting better or vice versa. It is therefore important to determine a meaningful improvement or decline in scores to assess the benefits of the treatment such as palliative RT. In our previous study of 797 pain scorings from 88 patients, patients were able to perceive their current pain to be less than the baseline pain when they reported a decline of their pain score of two or more from the baselinepoints (9). The current study was to validate the above finding in a separate population.

Methods

Patients with bone metastases treated with external beam RT were eligible. Patients were asked to score their 'worst' pain on a scale of 0 – 10 with the Brief Pain Inventory (zero means0 is the absence of pain and 10 is the worst possible pain) before treatment, daily during treatment and for 10 days after the completion of external beam RT. Patients either recorded the information in a diary or requested a telephone follow- up by the research assistant.

At each follow -up, they were asked to compare their current 'worst' pain with their pretreatment 'worst' pain using the following categories based on their own perception: worse, the same, or better. Changes in pain score with respect to the baseline pain score were compared with patient perception of changes in pain at baseline and each follow-up assessment. When theA negative change in pain score indicatesis a negative value, it means the patient's current 'worst' pain score was is lower than the baseline pretreatment 'worst' pain score. A positive change in pain score indicates the patient's current 'worst' pain score is higher than the baseline pretreatment 'worst' pain score.

The analgesic intake was recorded at baseline and at each follow up and converted into daily oral morphine equivalent dose (OMED). Patients with pathological fractures, spinal cord compression, or language barrier were excluded. Ethics approval was obtained for the study.

Statistical methods

Descriptive statistics were reported as percentages for proportions, and as medians and ranges for continuous variables. All statistical analyses were performed using version 9.1 of the Statistical Analysis System (SAS).

Results

From February 2006 to March 2008, one hundred and seventy-eight patients were enrolled from three cancer centres in Canada (Odette Cancer Centre, 90; Princess Margaret Hospital, 80; Tom Baker Cancer Centre, 8). There were 82 male and 96 female patients. Their median age was 65.5 years. The median 'worst' pain score before treatment for all patients was 7 (range 0 – 10).

The median analgesic intake in daily oral morphine equivalentOMED was 6 mg (range 0 – 880). Breast, prostate and lung were the most common primary sites. Other patient characteristics are listed in Ttable 1.

The radiation dose fractionations employed are listed in Ttable 2 and sites of irradiation in Ttable 3.

Table 1. Patient characteristics (n=178)

Gender	
Male	82 (46%)
Female	96 (54%)
Age	
Median	65.5 years
Range	40-90 years
Primary Cancer Site	
Breast	64 (36%)
Prostate	42 (24%)
Lung	39 (22%)
Bladder + Kidney	12 (7%)
Gastrointestinal	10 (6%)
Others	11 (6%)
Worst Pain	
Mean ± SD	6.3 ± 2.7
Median (range)	7 (0-10)
Daily Total Oral Morphine Equivalent (mg)	
Mean ± SD	54.6 ± 115.3
Median (range)	6 (0-880)

Table 2. Radiation dose fractions (n=178)

Radiation Regimens	Number of Patients
8 Gy in 1 fraction	99 (56%)
20 Gy in 5 daily fractions	55 (31%)
30 Gy in 10 daily fractions	8 (4%)
Other multiple fractions	16 (9%)

Table 3. Sites of irradiation (n=178)

Site of Radiation	Number of Patients
Spine	73 (41%)
Extremities	54 (30%)
Pelvis	38 (21%)
Others	13 (7%)

A total of 1,431 pain scorings were obtained in the study cohort. Table 4 lists the change in pain score and patient perception of pain. From our data, there was consistency of the change in pain score with the patient perception when the change in pain score was from -10 to -2. The majority of patients reported feeling better when compared with theo baseline;. Hhowever, when the change in pain score was only -1, 39% of patients reported the same and 41% of patients reported better when compared with the baseline. When there was no change in pain score, 66% of patients reported same when compared with the baseline. For change in pain score from +1 to +9, the majority of patients gave the response of 'worse' when compared with to the baseline.

Table 4. Pain perception in 1,431 scorings

Change in Pain Score	Patient Perception		
	Pain Level	Frequency	%
-10 (n=4)	W	0	0%
	S	0	0%
	B	4	100%
-9 (n=17)	W	0	0%
	S	1	6%
	B	16	94%
-8 (n=31)	W	0	0%
	S	10	32%
	B	21	68%
-7 (n=42)	W	0	0%
	S	5	12%
	B	37	88%
-6 (n=41)	W	1	2%
	S	6	15%
	B	34	83%
-5 (n=52)	W	1	2%
	S	14	27%
	B	37	71%
-4 (n=121)	W	6	5%
	S	44	36%
	B	71	59%

Table 4. (Continued)

Change in Pain Score	Patient Perception		
	Pain Level	Frequency	%
-3 (n=117)	W	9	8%
	S	18	15%
	B	90	77%
-2 (n=217)	W	18	8%
	S	68	31%
	B	131	60%
-1 (n=234)	W	46	20%
	S	92	39%
	B	96	41%
0 (n=289)	W	72	25%
	S	190	66%
	B	27	9%
+1 (n=117)	W	78	67%
	S	24	20%
	B	15	13%
+2 (n=63)	W	45	71%
	S	10	16%
	B	8	13%
+3 (n=44)	W	33	75%
	S	7	16%
	B	4	9%
+4 (n=19)	W	19	10%
	S	0	0%
	B	0	0%
+5 (n=9)	W	9	100%
	S	0	0%
	B	0	0%
+6 (n=8)	W	8	100%
	S	0	0%
	B	0	0%
+7 (n=4)	W	4	100%
	S	0	0%
	B	0	0%
+8 (n=1)	W	1	100%
	S	0	0%
	B	0	0%
+9 (n=1)	W	1	100%
	S	0	0%
	B	0	0%

Change in pain score = current pain score – baseline pain score.
Patient perception = current pain compared with baseline pain.
W, worse; S, same; B, better.

Contributions of pain scorings varied from one patient to another depending on the dose fractionations they received. We were able to capture 65% of the anticipated pain score data. Thus, we randomly selected the same contributions from all patients and reanalyzed the data, but found no change in outcome (data not shown). We also removed the baseline pain scores near the ceiling (i.e. 9 or 10) to account and correct for the ceiling effect, but again our findings remained unchanged (data not shown). The change in pain score reflects a combined effect of RT and concurrent systemic therapies including analgesics.

Discussion

In our previous study, except when the change in pain score was -7, there was consistency of the change in score with the patient perception for change of pain score from -10 to -2. When the change in pain score was -2, 78% of the pain scorings were accompanied with a response of 'better' (9). Our current study showed consistency of the change in score with the patient perception from of change in pain score from -10 to -2. When the change in pain score was -2, 60% of the pain scorings were accompanied with a response of 'better'.

For the previous study, when the change in pain score was -1, the responses for the 'same' and 'better' categories were similar in frequency (9). The current study had the same findings: 39% vs. 41%. In the previous study, for change in pain score from 0 to +5, there was no consistent pattern in patient perception. For the change in pain score of +6 or above, 67% of pain scorings were accompanied with a response of 'worse' (9). In our current study, when there was no change in pain score, 66% of pain scorings were accompanied with a response of 'same'. For change in pain score from +1 to +9, the majority of pain scorings were accompanied with a response of 'worse'.

In our study, we asked patients their pain score and pain perception over a period of 11 days (for patients who received a single treatment) to 22–24 days (for patients who received 10 daily treatments). It is unlikely that during this time frame, patients' internal frame of reference may would have changed.

With our two studies, we are confident that patients perceived the current pain to be less than the baseline pain when they reported a decline of their pain score of two or more from the baseline. Recent bone metastases randomized trials (10,11) and international consensus in palliative RT endpoints for future clinical trials in bone metastases (12) defined partial response as a reduction of pain score by two or more points on a pain scale of 0-10. This definition appears to be supported by our data. Our current study however only focused on the pain score. The international consensus takes both pain score and analgesic consumption into consideration when defining partial response.

Our study suggests if the change in pain score was zero, the pain seemed to be stable. However for a positive change even from +1 onwards, patients in our study cohort reported worse pain. This finding, which should draw the attention of the health care professionals and. This needs to be taken into account when trialists define pain progression.

Acknowledgments

We thank Ms. Stacy Lue for secretarial support. This study was generously supported by Michael and Karyn Goldstein Cancer Research Fund. We thank staff and research assistants at the three cancer centres for the accrual. Conflicts of interest notification: None.

References

[1] Brunelli C, Constantini M, Di Giulio P, et al. Quality-of-life evaluation: when do terminal cancer patients and health-care providers agree? J Pain Symptom Manage 1998;15:151–8.

[2] Grossman SA, Sheidler VR, Swedeen K, Mucenski J, Piantadosi S. Correlation of patient and caregiver ratings of cancer pain. J Pain Symptom Manage 1991;6:53–7.

[3] Higginson IJ, McCarthy M. Validity of the support team assessment schedule: do staffs' ratings reflect those made by patients or their families? Palliat Med 1993;7:219–28.

[4] Higginson IJ. Can professionals improve their assessment? [commentary] J Pain Symptom Manage 1998;15:149–50.

[5] Nekolaichuk CL, Bruera E, Spachynski K, MacEachern T, Hanson J, Maguire TO. A comparison of patient and proxy symptom assessments in advanced cancer patients. Palliat Med 1999;13:311–23.

[6] Slevin ML, Plant H, Lynch D, Drinkwater J, Gregory WM. Who should measure quality of life, the doctor or the patient? Br J Cancer 1988;57:109–12.

[7] Sneeuw KCA, Aaronson NK, Sprangers MAG, Delmar SB, Wever LDV, Schornagel JH. Value of caregiver ratings in evaluating the quality of life of patients with cancer. J Clin Oncol 1997;15:1206–17.

[8] Sprangers MAG, Aaronson NK. The role of health care providers and significant others in evaluating the quality of life of patients with chronic disease: a review. J Clin Epidemiol 1992;45:743–60.

[9] Chow E, Ling A, Davis L, Panzarella T, Danjoux C. Pain flare following external beam radiotherapy and meaningful change in pain scores in the treatment of bone metastases. Radiat Oncol 2005;75:64-9.

[10] Hartsell WF, Scott C, Brunner DW, et al. Phase III randomized trial of 8 Gy in fraction vs. 30 Gy in 10 fractions for palliation of painful bone metastases: preliminary results of RTOG 97-14. Int J Radiat Oncol Biol Phys 2003;57:S124.

[11] Steenland E, Leer JW, van Houwelingen H, et al. The effect of a single fraction compared to multiple fractions on painful bone metastases: a global analysis of the Dutch bone metastasis study. Radiother Oncol 1999;52:101–9.

[12] Chow E, Wu J, Hoskin P, Coia L, Bentzen S, Blitzer P on behalf of the International Bone Metastases Consensus Working Party. International consensus on palliative radiotherapy endpoints for future clinical trials in bone metastases. Radiother Oncol 2002;64:275–80.

[13] Steenland E, Leer JW, van Houwelingen H, et al. The effect of a single fraction compared to multiple fractions on painful bone metastases: a global analysis of the Dutch bone metastasis study. Radiother Oncol 1999;52:101–9.

[14] Chow E, Wu J, Hoskin P, Coia L, Bentzen S, Blitzer P on behalf of the International Bone Metastases Consensus Working Party. International consensus on palliative radiotherapy endpoints for future clinical trials in bone metastases. Radiother Oncol 2002;64:275–80.

Chapter 42

EXPLORING THE OPTIMAL DEFINITIONS OF PARTIAL RESPONSE AND PAIN PROGRESSION IN PATIENTS RECEIVING RADIATION TREATMENT FOR PAINFUL BONE METASTASES? A PRELIMINARY ANALYSIS

Roseanna Presutti, BSc(C), Liying Zhang, PhD, Amanda Hird, BSc(C), Melissa Deyell, BMSc and Edward Chow, MBBS[*]

Rapid Response Radiotherapy Program, Department of Radiation Oncology, Odette Cancer Centre, Sunnybrook Health Sciences Centre, University of Toronto, Toronto, Ontario, Canada

Abstract

Purpose was to explore optimal definitions for partial response and pain progression in patients receiving palliative radiotherapy (RT) for painful bone metastases. Methods: Patients referred to the Rapid Response Radiotherapy Program (RRRP) for palliative RT from May 2003 to November 2007 were evaluated. The Brief Pain Inventory (BPI) evaluates worst, current, and average pain, as well as seven items of functional interference on an 11-point (0-10) numeric scale. The BPI was administered at baseline, 1- and 2-months following RT for all patients. Analgesic intake was collected and converted into an oral morphine equivalent dose (OMED). The total sum score of the BPI items was calculated at baseline and at subsequent follow-ups. The follow-up sum score was subtracted from the baseline sum score to determine the difference in the BPI sum score. Various cut-points for difference in worst pain score and percent change in analgesic intake were determined using multivariate analysis of variance (MANOVA).

---

[*] **Correspondence:** Edward Chow, MBBS, PhD, FRCPC, Department of Radiation Oncology, Odette Cancer Centre, Sunnybrook Health Sciences Centre, 2075 Bayview Avenue, Toronto, ON M4N 3M5, Canada. Tel: 416-480-4998; Fax: 416-480-6002; E-mail: Edward.Chow@sunnybrook.ca

Results: A total of 400 patients were evaluated, 235 males and 165 females, with a median age of 68 years (range: 30-91). The median Karnofsky Performance Status (KPS) was 70 (range: 30-90). At baseline, the mean worst pain score and OMED were 7.4 and 102mg/day respectively. Worst pain scores significantly decreased at the 1- and 2-month follow-up. Thirteen statistically significant and clinically relevant cut-points were identified in patients with BPI improvement or deterioration at 1- and 2-month follow-up.

Conclusion: The present study was a preliminary analysis and further investigation is required to validate our initial findings.

Keywords: Bone metastases, palliative radiotherapy, partial response, pain progression.

Introduction

Bone metastases are a common manifestation in advanced cancer. Pain is the most frequent complication reported, and over two thirds of patients will experience severe pain as a result of their bone metastases (1). External beam radiotherapy (RT) is an effective modality for the palliation of such metastases. Various randomized control trials have attempted to determine the optimal dose fractionation for alleviating metastatic bone pain. Bone metastases trials conducted by the Radiation Therapy Oncology Group (RTOG7402) initially concluded that low-dose, short-course schedules were as effective as high-dose, protracted schedules (2). However, when the data was reanalyzed using both pain score and analgesic intake, with or without retreatment, it was suggested that protracted fractionation schedules led to an improved complete response rate (3).

Subsequently, the Canadian Bone Metastases Trial compared a single 8Gy to 20Gy in five daily fractions in the treatment of bone metastases and found that pain relief—defined as reduction in the pain score at the treated site with reduced analgesics, or a pain score of zero at the treated site without an increase in analgesics—was significantly higher in patients receiving multiple fractions. However, when analgesic consumption was not included in the definition, the response rate was the same for both the single and fractionated arms (4). As the RTOG and Canadian trials demonstrate, different conclusions can be reached depending on the endpoint definitions employed.

In light of this, an International Bone Metastases Consensus Working Party on endpoint measurements was established in April 2000. Two years later, the Working Party published an international consensus on RT endpoints for future bone metastases clinical trials. Pain score and analgesic consumption were both incorporated into the RT response definition. According to these endpoints, a complete response (CR) is defined as a pain score of zero at the treated site, with no concomitant increase in analgesic intake. Partial response (PR) is defined as either a pain reduction of two or more at the treated site on a scale of zero to ten, without an increase in analgesic intake; or an analgesic reduction of 25% or more from baseline, without a concurrent increase in pain score. Finally, pain progression (PP) is defined as an increase in pain score of two or more points above baseline at the treated site, with stable analgesic intake; or an increase of 25% or more in analgesics relative to baseline measures, with a stable pain score or pain score + one point above baseline (5).

The aforementioned endpoints were reached through consensus from previous bone metastases trials investigators and others with a recognized interest in bone metastases. Although the definition of complete response seems very reasonable, the definitions of partial response and disease progression may require more concrete parameters. The purpose of the current study was to explore the optimal definitions of partial response and pain progression following palliative RT for bone metastases.

Methods

This study is a secondary analysis of data collected from a prospective database that examined the effectiveness of palliative RT on alleviating the severity of both pain and functional interference. From May 2003 to November 2007, all patients referred to the Rapid Response Radiotherapy Program (RRRP) with painful metastatic bone lesions for palliative RT were evaluated. Patients were eligible if they could speak and understand English, were competent to complete the survey, had radiographic evidence of bone metastases and provided verbal consent. Ethics approval was obtained from Sunnybrook Health Sciences Centre Research Ethics Board.

Prior to RT, basic demographic information was collected for each patient, including primary cancer site and Karnofsky Performance Status (KPS). Using the Brief Pain Inventory (BPI), patients rated their worst, average and current pain intensity on an 11-point scale of 0 (no pain) to 10 (pain as bad as you can imagine). Patients were also asked to rate the level of pain interference for seven functional items—general activity, mood, walking ability, normal work, relations with other people, sleep and enjoyment of life—on a scale of 0 (no interference) to 10 (complete interference). In the present study, only worst pain scores were used when calculating response to RT. Previous investigations have found that worst pain scores correlate most strongly with the seven items of interference on the BPI and recommend that an 11-point scale evaluating worst pain scores be used when evaluating response rates to RT (6). Thus, only worst pain scores as assessed by the BPI are included in the present study. Additionally, analgesic consumption was recorded for each patient and converted into a daily oral morphine equivalent (OMED). Follow-up telephone interviews were conducted by a research assistant at 1- and 2-month intervals following RT, in order to collect analgesic intake and administer the BPI.

Statistical analysis

Descriptive statistics and distributions were generated for patient demographics and disease-related characteristics. To determine the optimal definitions of partial response and pain progression, the total sum score of the BPI (i.e. the sum of the seven functional interference items) was calculated at baseline and at the 1- and 2-month follow-ups. The change in BPI sum score was determined by subtracting the follow up sum score from the baseline sum score. In the present study, patients were considered to have BPI improvement if the difference in sum score was > 0. On the contrary, if the change was < 0, patients were considered to have deterioration in the BPI.

The difference in the worst pain score and the percent change in OMED were calculated from baseline to follow-up. All possible combinations for the difference of the worst pain score and the percentage change of OMED were created and related to the set of seven functional interference items from the BPI using multivariate analysis of variance (MANOVA). A multivariate Wilk's Lambda, Pillai's trace and Hotelling-Lawley Trace F statistics were calculated based on the effect of variance/covariance matrix. Two-sided p-values less than 0.05 were considered statistically significant. All analyses were performed using the Statistical Analysis Software (SAS Institute, version 9.1 for Windows) package.

Results

Between May 2003 and November 2007, a total of 400 patients receiving palliative RT for painful bone metastases were evaluated. The median age was 68 years (range: 30-91) with more males (59%) than females (41%). The median KPS score was 70 (range: 30-90). Breast, lung and prostate were the most common primary cancer sites, each representing approximately a quarter of the study population (Table 1). The most common irradiated painful bony sites were the extremities (34%), followed by the spine (32%), pelvis (22%), ribs (6%) and others (6%). The majority of patients (61%) received a single dose of 8Gy.

Table 1. Patient characteristics (n=400)

	Number of Patients (%)
Sex	
Male	235 (58.8%)
Female	165 (41.2%)
Age (years)	
Median (range)	68 (30 – 91)
Karnofsky Performance Status	
n	385
Mean ± SD	70.2 ± 13.4
Median (range)	70 (30 – 90)
Primary cancer sites	
Breast	102 (25.5%)
Lung	99 (24.8%)
Prostate	98 (24.5%)
Kidney and Bladder	37 (9.3%)
Gastrointestinal	31 (7.8%)
Unknown	19 (4.8%)
Others	14 (3.5%)
Site of radiation treatment	
Extremities	135 (33.8%)
Spine	129 (32.3%)
Pelvis	86 (21.5%)
Ribs	25 (6.3%)
Others	25 (6.3%)
Radiation Dose/fraction	
8Gy/1	243 (60.8%)
20Gy/5	133 (33.3%)
30Gy/10	11 (2.8%)
Others	13 (3.3%)

At baseline, the mean worst pain score with standard deviation (SD) was 7.4 ± 2.4, with a mean (±SD) analgesic intake of 102 (±218) mg/day (Table 2). The mean (±SD) and median values for the seven functional interference items at baseline are outlined in Table 2. Following palliative RT, the mean (±SD) worst pain score was reduced to 4.11±3.14 and 3.71 ± 3.15 at the 1- and 2-month follow-up, respectively. Table 3 outlines the corresponding values for functional interference and analgesic intake at the 1- and 2-month follow-up.

Tables 4a and 5a list the possible cut-points (CP) for the worst pain score and percent change in OMED at the 1- and 2-month follow-up, respectively, for patients with improvement in their BPI sum score.

Table 2. Worst pain scores, seven interference items and analgesic consumption at baseline

Symptom	Mean ± SD	Median
Worst pain	7.4 ± 2.4	8
General activity	6.6 ± 3.2	8
Mood	5.0 ± 3.4	5
Walking ability	5.8 ± 3.6	7
Normal work	6.8 ± 3.5	8
Relations with others	3.4 ± 3.5	2
Sleep	4.8 ± 3.5	5
Enjoyment of life	6.5 ± 3.3	7
Total Daily Oral Morphine Equivalent (mg/day)	102 ± 218	24

Table 3. Worst pain, seven interference items and analgesic consumption at 1-month or at 2-month follow-up

At 1-month

	Mean ± SD	Median
Worst pain	4.11 ± 3.143.14	4
General activity	4.24 ± 3.773.77	4
Mood	3.05 ± 3.553.55	2
Walking ability	3.64 ± 3.693.69	3
Normal work	4.65 ± 4.174.17	5
Relations with others	2.05 ± 3.163.16	0
Sleep	2.64 ± 3.283.28	1
Enjoyment of life	4.14 ± 3.663.66	4
Total Daily Oral Morphine Equivalent (mg/day)	96.45 ± 172.9	20

At 2-month

	Mean ± SD	Median
Worst pain	3.71 ± 3.15	3
General activity	3.65 ± 3.63	3
Mood	2.73 ± 3.21	1
Walking ability	3.22 ± 3.65	2
Normal work	3.80 ± 3.94	3
Relations with others	1.84 + 2.94	0
Sleep	1.91 ± 2.76	0
Enjoyment of life	3.38 ± 3.46	2
Total Daily Oral Morphine Equivalent (mg/day)	76.10 ± 126.1	16

Table 4a. All possible combinations between changes in worst pain score and oral morphine equivalent in patients with BPI improvement at month 1 (n=84)

	Cutpoint	No. of patients
1	CP4,-100	1
2	CP4,20	1
3	CP4,50	1
4	CP4,60	2
5	CP4,90	1
6	CP4,100	15
7	CP4,-50	1
8	CP4,-10	1
9	CP5,-100	3
10	CP5,0	1
11	CP5,50	1
12	CP5,90	1
13	CP5,100	5
14	CP5,-30	1
15	CP5,-10	2
16	CP6,-100	3
17	CP6,0	2
18	CP6,10	1
19	CP6,20	1
20	CP6,50	1
21	CP6,60	1
22	CP6,100	12
23	CP,30	1
24	CP7,-100	1
25	CP7,10	1
26	CP7,100	2
27	CP7,-10	1
28	CP8,-100	2
29	CP8,0	1
30	CP8,30	1
31	CP8,70	1
32	CP8,100	5
33	CP9,0	1
34	CP9,50	1
35	CP9,60	1
36	CP9,70	1
37	CP9,90	1
38	CP9,100	3
39	CP10,40	1
40	CP10,80	1
41	CP10,100	5

	Cutpoint	No. of patients
42	CP10,-20	2
43	CP,100	1
44	CP-3,-100	1
45	CP-2,-100	2
46	CP-2,-40	1
47	CP-1,-100	2
48	CP-1,70	1
49	CP-1,100	1
50	CP-1,-10	1
51	CP0,-100	7
52	CP0,0	1
53	CP0,30	1
54	CP0,50	1
55	CP0,100	2
56	CP0,-50	1
57	CP0,-40	1
58	CP0,-30	1
59	CP0,-20	1
60	CP0,-10	1
61	CP1,-100	3
62	CP1,10	1
63	CP1,80	1
64	CP1,100	6
65	CP1,-50	1
66	CP1,-40	2
67	CP2,-100	5
68	CP2,0	1
69	CP2,20	2
70	CP2,40	1
71	CP2,50	1
72	CP2,70	1
73	CP2,100	8
74	CP2,-50	1
75	CP2,-30	1
76	CP3,-100	4
77	CP3,0	2
78	CP3,50	1
79	CP3,60	2
80	CP3,-80	1
81	CP3,100	11
82	CP3,-30	1

Table 4b. Multivariate analysis of variance (MANOVA) on all possible 66 combinations of cutpoints and the improvement of 7 interference items at month 1

Cutpoint	Statistic	Value	F statistic*	p-value*
CP9,100	**Wilks' Lambda**	**0.8412**	4.02	0.0005
CP9,100	Pillai's Trace	0.1588		
CP9,100	Hotelling-Lawley Trace	0.1888		
CP10,100	**Wilks' Lambda**	**0.8650**	3.32	0.0026
CP10,100	Pillai's Trace	0.1350		
CP10,100	Hotelling-Lawley Trace	0.1561		
CP5,-30	**Wilks' Lambda**	**0.8795**	2.92	0.0069
CP5,-30	Pillai's Trace	0.1205		
CP5,-30	Hotelling-Lawley Trace	0.1370		
CP5,90	**Wilks' Lambda**	**0.8961**	2.47	0.0200
CP5,90	Pillai's Trace	0.1039		
CP5,90	Hotelling-Lawley Trace	0.1160		
CP-1,-100	**Wilks' Lambda**	**0.8994**	2.38	0.0245
CP-1,-100	Pillai's Trace	0.1006		
CP-1,-100	Hotelling-Lawley Trace	0.1119		
CP0,30	**Wilks' Lambda**	**0.9021**	2.31	0.0290
CP0,30	Pillai's Trace	0.0979		
CP0,30	Hotelling-Lawley Trace	0.1085		
CP0,-40	**Wilks' Lambda**	**0.9036**	2.27	0.0317
CP0,-40	Pillai's Trace	0.0964		
CP0,-40	Hotelling-Lawley Trace	0.1067		
CP-1,70	Wilks' Lambda	0.9126	2.04	0.0538
CP-1,70	Pillai's Trace	0.0874		
CP-1,70	Hotelling-Lawley Trace	0.0958		
CP2,-30	Wilks' Lambda	0.9162	1.95	0.0661
CP2,-30	Pillai's Trace	0.0838		
CP2,-30	Hotelling-Lawley Trace	0.0915		
CP10,-20	Wilks' Lambda	0.9184	1.89	0.0746
CP10,-20	Pillai's Trace	0.0816		
CP10,-20	Hotelling-Lawley Trace	0.0889		
CP2,20	Wilks' Lambda	0.9225	1.79	0.0936
CP2,20	Pillai's Trace	0.0775		
CP2,20	Hotelling-Lawley Trace	0.0840		
CP0,-20	Wilks' Lambda	0.9226	1.79	0.0942
CP0,-20	Pillai's Trace	0.0774		
CP0,-20	Hotelling-Lawley Trace	0.0839		
CP8,100	Wilks' Lambda	0.9268	1.68	0.1175
CP8,100	Pillai's Trace	0.0732		

Cutpoint	Statistic	Value	F statistic*	p-value*
CP8,100	Hotelling-Lawley Trace	0.0790		
CP5,100	Wilks' Lambda	0.9275	1.66	0.1219
CP5,100	Pillai's Trace	0.0725		
CP5,100	Hotelling-Lawley Trace	0.0782		
CP4,60	Wilks' Lambda	0.9305	1.59	0.1428
CP4,60	Pillai's Trace	0.0695		
CP4,60	Hotelling-Lawley Trace	0.0747		
CP2,50	Wilks' Lambda	0.9311	1.57	0.1471
CP2,50	Pillai's Trace	0.0689		
CP2,50	Hotelling-Lawley Trace	0.0740		
CP10,40	Wilks' Lambda	0.9315	1.57	0.1500
CP10,40	Pillai's Trace	0.0685		
CP10,40	Hotelling-Lawley Trace	0.0735		
CP9,70	Wilks' Lambda	0.9317	1.56	0.1518
CP9,70	Pillai's Trace	0.0683		
CP9,70	Hotelling-Lawley Trace	0.0733		
CP2,70	Wilks' Lambda	0.9329	1.53	0.1611
CP2,70	Pillai's Trace	0.0671		
CP2,70	Hotelling-Lawley Trace	0.0719		
CP1,80	Wilks' Lambda	0.9337	1.51	0.1671
CP1,80	Pillai's Trace	0.0663		
CP1,80	Hotelling-Lawley Trace	0.0711		
CP2,100	Wilks' Lambda	0.9349	1.48	0.1777
CP2,100	Pillai's Trace	0.0651		
CP2,100	Hotelling-Lawley Trace	0.0696		
CP4,-100	Wilks' Lambda	0.9351	1.48	0.1791
CP4,-100	Pillai's Trace	0.0649		
CP4,-100	Hotelling-Lawley Trace	0.0695		
CP7,100	Wilks' Lambda	0.9353	1.47	0.1817
CP7,100	Pillai's Trace	0.0647		
CP7,100	Hotelling-Lawley Trace	0.0691		
CP2,-100	Wilks' Lambda	0.9364	1.44	0.1915
CP2,-100	Pillai's Trace	0.0636		
CP2,-100	Hotelling-Lawley Trace	0.0679		
CP4,-10	Wilks' Lambda	0.9369	1.43	0.1962
CP4,-10	Pillai's Trace	0.0631		
CP4,-10	Hotelling-Lawley Trace	0.0673		
CP-3,-100	Wilks' Lambda	0.9385	1.40	0.2110
CP-3,-100	Pillai's Trace	0.0615		
CP-3,-100	Hotelling-Lawley Trace	0.0656		
CP5,0	Wilks' Lambda	0.9427	1.29	0.2571

Table 4b. (Continued)

Cutpoint	Statistic	Value	F statistic*	p-value*
CP5,0	Pillai's Trace	0.0573		
CP5,0	Hotelling-Lawley Trace	0.0608		
CP-2,-100	Wilks' Lambda	0.9452	1.23	0.2877
CP-2,-100	Pillai's Trace	0.0548		
CP-2,-100	Hotelling-Lawley Trace	0.0580		
CP3,0	Wilks' Lambda	0.9463	1.21	0.3017
CP3,0	Pillai's Trace	0.0537		
CP3,0	Hotelling-Lawley Trace	0.0568		
CP9,50	Wilks' Lambda	0.9484	1.16	0.3301
CP9,50	Pillai's Trace	0.0516		
CP9,50	Hotelling-Lawley Trace	0.0544		
CP3,60	Wilks' Lambda	0.9496	1.13	0.3475
CP3,60	Pillai's Trace	0.0504		
CP3,60	Hotelling-Lawley Trace	0.0531		
CP3,-80	Wilks' Lambda	0.9513	1.09	0.3731
CP3,-80	Pillai's Trace	0.0487		
CP3,-80	Hotelling-Lawley Trace	0.0512		
CP4,100	Wilks' Lambda	0.9525	1.06	0.3918
CP4,100	Pillai's Trace	0.0475		
CP4,100	Hotelling-Lawley Trace	0.0498		
CP8,30	Wilks' Lambda	0.9529	1.05	0.3977
CP8,30	Pillai's Trace	0.0471		
CP8,30	Hotelling-Lawley Trace	0.0494		
CP1,-40	Wilks' Lambda	0.9529	1.05	0.3980
CP1,-40	Pillai's Trace	0.0471		
CP1,-40	Hotelling-Lawley Trace	0.0494		
CP-1,100	Wilks' Lambda	0.9531	1.05	0.4008
CP-1,100	Pillai's Trace	0.0469		
CP-1,100	Hotelling-Lawley Trace	0.0492		
CP0,-10	Wilks' Lambda	0.9585	0.92	0.4924
CP0,-10	Pillai's Trace	0.0415		
CP0,-10	Hotelling-Lawley Trace	0.0432		
CP5,-10	Wilks' Lambda	0.9616	0.85	0.5473
CP5,-10	Pillai's Trace	0.0384		
CP5,-10	Hotelling-Lawley Trace	0.0400		
CP6,0	Wilks' Lambda	0.9637	0.80	0.5871
CP6,0	Pillai's Trace	0.0363		
CP6,0	Hotelling-Lawley Trace	0.0377		
CP2,-50	Wilks' Lambda	0.9638	0.80	0.5886

Cutpoint	Statistic	Value	F statistic*	p-value*
CP2,-50	Pillai's Trace	0.0362		
CP2,-50	Hotelling-Lawley Trace	0.0376		
CP7,10	Wilks' Lambda	0.9647	0.78	0.6055
CP7,10	Pillai's Trace	0.0353		
CP7,10	Hotelling-Lawley Trace	0.0366		
CP1,-50	Wilks' Lambda	0.9652	0.77	0.6163
CP1,-50	Pillai's Trace	0.0348		
CP1,-50	Hotelling-Lawley Trace	0.0360		
CP4,50	Wilks' Lambda	0.9672	0.72	0.6543
CP4,50	Pillai's Trace	0.0328		
CP4,50	Hotelling-Lawley Trace	0.0339		
CP6,60	Wilks' Lambda	0.9679	0.70	0.6679
CP6,60	Pillai's Trace	0.0321		
CP6,60	Hotelling-Lawley Trace	0.0331		
CP3,50	Wilks' Lambda	0.9710	0.64	0.7250
CP3,50	Pillai's Trace	0.0290		
CP3,50	Hotelling-Lawley Trace	0.0299		
CP6,-100	Wilks' Lambda	0.9711	0.63	0.7274
CP6,-100	Pillai's Trace	0.0289		
CP6,-100	Hotelling-Lawley Trace	0.0298		
CP1,10	Wilks' Lambda	0.9729	0.59	0.7616
CP1,10	Pillai's Trace	0.0271		
CP1,10	Hotelling-Lawley Trace	0.0278		
CP0,0	Wilks' Lambda	0.9732	0.59	0.7664
CP0,0	Pillai's Trace	0.0268		
CP0,0	Hotelling-Lawley Trace	0.0275		
CP6,100	Wilks' Lambda	0.9736	0.58	0.7735
CP6,100	Pillai's Trace	0.0264		
CP6,100	Hotelling-Lawley Trace	0.0271		
CP,30	Wilks' Lambda	0.9768	0.51	0.8292
CP7,-100	Pillai's Trace	0.0232		
CP7,-100	Hotelling-Lawley Trace	0.0238		
CP0,-30	Wilks' Lambda	0.9781	0.48	0.8498
CP0,-30	Pillai's Trace	0.0219		
CP0,-30	Hotelling-Lawley Trace	0.0224		
CP8,70	Wilks' Lambda	0.9786	0.47	0.8584
CP8,70	Pillai's Trace	0.0214		
CP8,70	Hotelling-Lawley Trace	0.0219		
CP1,100	Wilks' Lambda	0.9798	0.44	0.8763
CP1,100	Pillai's Trace	0.0202		
CP1,100	Hotelling-Lawley Trace	0.0206		

Table 4b. (Continued)

Cutpoint	Statistic	Value	F statistic*	p-value*
CP1,-100	Wilks' Lambda	0.9827	0.38	0.9156
CP1,-100	Pillai's Trace	0.0173		
CP1,-100	Hotelling-Lawley Trace	0.0176		
CP9,60	Wilks' Lambda	0.9829	0.37	0.9187
CP9,60	Pillai's Trace	0.0171		
CP9,60	Hotelling-Lawley Trace	0.0174		
CP0,-100	Wilks' Lambda	0.9848	0.33	0.9404
CP0,-100	Pillai's Trace	0.0152		
CP0,-100	Hotelling-Lawley Trace	0.0154		
CP5,50	Wilks' Lambda	0.9854	0.32	0.9458
CP5,50	Pillai's Trace	0.0146		
CP5,50	Hotelling-Lawley Trace	0.0148		
CP2,40	Wilks' Lambda	0.9854	0.31	0.9464
CP2,40	Pillai's Trace	0.0146		
CP2,40	Hotelling-Lawley Trace	0.0148		
CP5,-100	Wilks' Lambda	0.9874	0.27	0.9641
CP5,-100	Pillai's Trace	0.0126		
CP5,-100	Hotelling-Lawley Trace	0.0128		
CP8,-100	Wilks' Lambda	0.9893	0.23	0.9775
CP8,-100	Pillai's Trace	0.0107		
CP8,-100	Hotelling-Lawley Trace	0.0108		
CP-1,-10	Wilks' Lambda	0.9893	0.23	0.9775
CP-1,-10	Pillai's Trace	0.0107		
CP-1,-10	Hotelling-Lawley Trace	0.0108		
CP0,100	Wilks' Lambda	0.9893	0.23	0.9775
CP0,100	Pillai's Trace	0.0107		
CP0,100	Hotelling-Lawley Trace	0.0108		
CP7,-10	Wilks' Lambda	0.9906	0.20	0.9845
CP7,-10	Pillai's Trace	0.0094		
CP7,-10	Hotelling-Lawley Trace	0.0095		
CP3,100	Wilks' Lambda	0.9911	0.19	0.9867
CP3,100	Pillai's Trace	0.0089		
CP3,100	Hotelling-Lawley Trace	0.0090		
CP3,-100	Wilks' Lambda	0.9912	0.19	0.9872
CP3,-100	Pillai's Trace	0.0088		
CP3,-100	Hotelling-Lawley Trace	0.0089		
CP2,0	Wilks' Lambda	0.9917	0.18	0.9894

Cutpoint	Statistic	Value	F statistic*	p-value*
CP2,0	Pillai's Trace	0.0083		
CP2,0	Hotelling-Lawley Trace	0.0084		

*Wilk's lamba, Pillai's trace and Hotelling-Lawley trace have same values for F-statistic and exact p-value. P-value < 0.05 was considered as significant.

For instance, CP4, 20 identified in Table 4a indicates that at follow-up the worst pain score was reduced by four points on the 0 to 10 scale of the BPI and there was also a concurrent reduction of 20% in OMED. Tables 4b and 5b show the multivariate analysis of variance (MANOVA) and the possible cut-point combinations for patients with improvement on the BPI. Cut-points with statistically significant values imply a partial response.

Table 5a. All possible combinations between changes in worst pain score and oral morphine equivalent in patients with BPI improvement at month 2 (n=92)

	Cutpoint	No. of patients
1	CP4,-100	1
2	CP4,0	2
3	CP4,10	1
4	CP4,60	2
5	CP4,70	1
6	CP4,100	5
7	CP4,-40	1
8	CP4,-30	1
9	CP5,-100	4
10	CP5,0	1
11	CP5,20	1
12	CP5,80	1
13	CP5,100	6
14	CP5,-20	2
15	CP6,-100	4
16	CP6,10	1
17	CP6,20	1
18	CP6,40	1
19	CP6,70	1
20	CP6,100	8
21	CP6,-30	1
22	CP7,-100	1
23	CP7,50	1
24	CP7,80	1
25	CP7,90	1
26	CP7,100	10
27	CP8,-100	1
28	CP8,10	1
29	CP8,40	1
30	CP8,100	6

Table 5a. (Continued)

	Cutpoint	No. of patients
31	CP9,0	1
32	CP9,60	1
33	CP9,70	1
34	CP9,90	1
35	CP9,100	3
36	CP10,-100	1
37	CP10,70	1
38	CP10,100	6
39	CP,100	1
40	CP-3,-50	1
41	CP-2,-100	1
42	CP-2,20	1
43	CP-2,-70	1
44	CP-1,0	1
45	CP-1,100	1
46	CP0,-100	5
47	CP0,0	1
48	CP0,20	1
49	CP0,50	1
50	CP0,100	3
51	CP0,-50	1
52	CP1,-100	5
53	CP1,0	1
54	CP1,20	1
55	CP1,40	1
56	CP1,70	2
57	CP1,100	8
58	CP1,-50	1
59	CP2,-100	4
60	CP2,0	1
61	CP2,20	1
62	CP2,100	2
63	CP2,-70	1
64	CP3,-100	5
65	CP3,0	1
66	CP3,60	1
67	CP3,100	9

Table 5b. Multivariate analysis of variance (MANOVA) on all possible 53 combinations of cut points and the improvement of 7 interference items at month 2

Cutpoint	Statistic	Value	F statistic*	p-value*
CP10,100	**Wilks' Lambda**	**0.8004**	**4.45**	**0.0002**
CP10,100	Pillai's Trace	0.1996		
CP10,100	Hotelling-Lawley Trace	0.2493		
CP8,10	**Wilks' Lambda**	**0.8558**	**3.01**	**0.0059**
CP8,10	Pillai's Trace	0.1442		
CP8,10	Hotelling-Lawley Trace	0.1686		
CP7,90	**Wilks' Lambda**	**0.8803**	**2.43**	**0.0229**
CP7,90	Pillai's Trace	0.1197		
CP7,90	Hotelling-Lawley Trace	0.1360		
CP2,100	**Wilks' Lambda**	**0.8842**	**2.34**	**0.0282**
CP2,100	Pillai's Trace	0.1158		
CP2,100	Hotelling-Lawley Trace	0.1309		
CP8,-100	**Wilks' Lambda**	**0.8861**	**2.29**	**0.0311**
CP8,-100	Pillai's Trace	0.1139		
CP8,-100	Hotelling-Lawley Trace	0.1285		
CP9,100	Wilks' Lambda	0.8963	2.07	0.0519
CP9,100	Pillai's Trace	0.1037		
CP9,100	Hotelling-Lawley Trace	0.1157		
CP1,0	Wilks' Lambda	0.9021	1.94	0.0689
CP1,0	Pillai's Trace	0.0979		
CP1,0	Hotelling-Lawley Trace	0.1086		
CP-1,100	Wilks' Lambda	0.9030	1.92	0.0721
CP-1,100	Pillai's Trace	0.0970		
CP-1,100	Hotelling-Lawley Trace	0.1074		
CP-1,0	Wilks' Lambda	0.9137	1.69	0.1183
CP-1,0	Pillai's Trace	0.0863		
CP-1,0	Hotelling-Lawley Trace	0.0944		
CP5,20	Wilks' Lambda	0.9161	1.64	0.1314
CP5,20	Pillai's Trace	0.0839		
CP5,20	Hotelling-Lawley Trace	0.0916		
CP1,-100	Wilks' Lambda	0.9164	1.63	0.1331
CP1,-100	Pillai's Trace	0.0836		
CP1,-100	Hotelling-Lawley Trace	0.0912		
CP2,20	Wilks' Lambda	0.9178	1.60	0.1415
CP2,20	Pillai's Trace	0.0822		
CP2,20	Hotelling-Lawley Trace	0.0896		
CP3,100	Wilks' Lambda	0.9236	1.48	0.1813
CP3,100	Pillai's Trace	0.0764		
CP3,100	Hotelling-Lawley Trace	0.0827		
CP8,100	Wilks' Lambda	0.9258	1.43	0.1985
CP8,100	Pillai's Trace	0.0742		
CP8,100	Hotelling-Lawley Trace	0.0802		

Table 5b. (Continued)

Cutpoint	Statistic	Value	F statistic*	p-value*
CP2,-100	Wilks' Lambda	0.9275	1.39	0.2132
CP2,-100	Pillai's Trace	0.0725		
CP2,-100	Hotelling-Lawley Trace	0.0781		
CP4,-40	Wilks' Lambda	0.9352	1.24	0.2869
CP4,-40	Pillai's Trace	0.0648		
CP4,-40	Hotelling-Lawley Trace	0.0693		
CP9,70	Wilks' Lambda	0.9374	1.19	0.3120
CP9,70	Pillai's Trace	0.0626		
CP9,70	Hotelling-Lawley Trace	0.0668		
CP0,50	Wilks' Lambda	0.9417	1.11	0.3636
CP0,50	Pillai's Trace	0.0583		
CP0,50	Hotelling-Lawley Trace	0.0619		
CP4,0	Wilks' Lambda	0.9430	1.08	0.3803
CP4,0	Pillai's Trace	0.0570		
CP4,0	Hotelling-Lawley Trace	0.0605		
CP0,100	Wilks' Lambda	0.9434	1.07	0.3858
CP0,100	Pillai's Trace	0.0566		
CP0,100	Hotelling-Lawley Trace	0.0600		
CP6,100	Wilks' Lambda	0.9437	1.07	0.3899
CP6,100	Pillai's Trace	0.0563		
CP6,100	Hotelling-Lawley Trace	0.0597		
CP2,0	Wilks' Lambda	0.9438	1.06	0.3905
CP2,0	Pillai's Trace	0.0562		
CP2,0	Hotelling-Lawley Trace	0.0596		
CP6,20	Wilks' Lambda	0.9449	1.04	0.4052
CP6,20	Pillai's Trace	0.0551		
CP6,20	Hotelling-Lawley Trace	0.0584		
CP4,100	Wilks' Lambda	0.9459	1.02	0.4201
CP4,100	Pillai's Trace	0.0541		
CP4,100	Hotelling-Lawley Trace	0.0572		
CP0,-100	Wilks' Lambda	0.9473	0.99	0.4396
CP0,-100	Pillai's Trace	0.0527		
CP0,-100	Hotelling-Lawley Trace	0.0556		
CP-3,-50	Wilks' Lambda	0.9474	0.99	0.4407
CP-3,-50	Pillai's Trace	0.0526		
CP-3,-50	Hotelling-Lawley Trace	0.0555		
CP7,100	Wilks' Lambda	0.9475	0.99	0.4415
CP7,100	Pillai's Trace	0.0525		
CP7,100	Hotelling-Lawley Trace	0.0555		
CP5,-20	Wilks' Lambda	0.9481	0.98	0.4511
CP5,-20	Pillai's Trace	0.0519		
CP5,-20	Hotelling-Lawley Trace	0.0547		
CP-2,-70	Wilks' Lambda	0.9496	0.95	0.4730

Cutpoint	Statistic	Value	F statistic*	p-value*
CP-2,-70	Pillai's Trace	0.0504		
CP-2,-70	Hotelling-Lawley Trace	0.0530		
CP7,80	Wilks' Lambda	0.9501	0.94	0.4794
CP7,80	Pillai's Trace	0.0499		
CP7,80	Hotelling-Lawley Trace	0.0526		
CP4,60	Wilks' Lambda	0.9511	0.92	0.4943
CP4,60	Pillai's Trace	0.0489		
CP4,60	Hotelling-Lawley Trace	0.0515		
CP9,0	Wilks' Lambda	0.9511	0.92	0.4946
CP9,0	Pillai's Trace	0.0489		
CP9,0	Hotelling-Lawley Trace	0.0514		
CP3,-100	Wilks' Lambda	0.9514	0.91	0.5001
CP3,-100	Pillai's Trace	0.0486		
CP3,-100	Hotelling-Lawley Trace	0.0510		
CP6,40	Wilks' Lambda	0.9538	0.86	0.5363
CP6,40	Pillai's Trace	0.0462		
CP6,40	Hotelling-Lawley Trace	0.0484		
CP5,0	Wilks' Lambda	0.9539	0.86	0.5380
CP5,0	Pillai's Trace	0.0461		
CP5,0	Hotelling-Lawley Trace	0.0483		
CP9,60	Wilks' Lambda	0.9590	0.76	0.6192
CP9,60	Pillai's Trace	0.0410		
CP9,60	Hotelling-Lawley Trace	0.0427		
CP5,-100	Wilks' Lambda	0.9596	0.75	0.6290
CP5,-100	Pillai's Trace	0.0404		
CP5,-100	Hotelling-Lawley Trace	0.0421		
CP2,-70	Wilks' Lambda	0.9606	0.73	0.6440
CP2,-70	Pillai's Trace	0.0394		
CP2,-70	Hotelling-Lawley Trace	0.0411		
CP10,70	Wilks' Lambda	0.9609	0.73	0.6489
CP10,70	Pillai's Trace	0.0391		
CP10,70	Hotelling-Lawley Trace	0.0407		
CP0,-50	Wilks' Lambda	0.9636	0.68	0.6927
CP0,-50	Pillai's Trace	0.0364		
CP0,-50	Hotelling-Lawley Trace	0.0378		
CP1,100	Wilks' Lambda	0.9641	0.67	0.7006
CP1,100	Pillai's Trace	0.0359		
CP1,100	Hotelling-Lawley Trace	0.0373		
CP5,80	Wilks' Lambda	0.9652	0.64	0.7196
CP5,80	Pillai's Trace	0.0348		
CP5,80	Hotelling-Lawley Trace	0.0360		
CP0,0	Wilks' Lambda	0.9656	0.64	0.7256
CP0,0	Pillai's Trace	0.0344		
CP0,0	Hotelling-Lawley Trace	0.0356		
CP4,70	Wilks' Lambda	0.9667	0.62	0.7420

Table 5b. (Continued)

Cutpoint	Statistic	Value	F statistic*	p-value*
CP4,70	Pillai's Trace	0.0333		
CP4,70	Hotelling-Lawley Trace	0.0345		
CP1,20	Wilks' Lambda	0.9716	0.52	0.8166
CP1,20	Pillai's Trace	0.0284		
CP1,20	Hotelling-Lawley Trace	0.0292		
CP7,-100	Wilks' Lambda	0.9741	0.47	0.8514
CP7,-100	Pillai's Trace	0.0259		
CP7,-100	Hotelling-Lawley Trace	0.0266		
CP1,70	Wilks' Lambda	0.9766	0.43	0.8831
CP1,70	Pillai's Trace	0.0234		
CP1,70	Hotelling-Lawley Trace	0.0240		
CP6,70	Wilks' Lambda	0.9774	0.41	0.8931
CP6,70	Pillai's Trace	0.0226		
CP6,70	Hotelling-Lawley Trace	0.0231		
CP1,-50	Wilks' Lambda	0.9789	0.38	0.9099
CP1,-50	Pillai's Trace	0.0211		
CP1,-50	Hotelling-Lawley Trace	0.0215		
CP4,10	Wilks' Lambda	0.9797	0.37	0.9178
CP4,10	Pillai's Trace	0.0203		
CP4,10	Hotelling-Lawley Trace	0.0208		
CP6,-100	Wilks' Lambda	0.9803	0.36	0.9247
CP6,-100	Pillai's Trace	0.0197		
CP6,-100	Hotelling-Lawley Trace	0.0201		
CP1,40	Wilks' Lambda	0.9835	0.30	0.9525
CP1,40	Pillai's Trace	0.0165		
CP1,40	Hotelling-Lawley Trace	0.0168		
CP5,100	Wilks' Lambda	0.9841	0.29	0.9576
CP5,100	Pillai's Trace	0.0159		
CP5,100	Hotelling-Lawley Trace	0.0161		

*Wilk's lamba, Pillai's trace and Hotelling-Lawley trace have same values for F-statistic and exact p-value. P-value < 0.05 was considered as significant.

All possible cut-points in worst pain score and percent change in OMED at 1- and 2-month follow-up are outlined in Tables 6a and 7a, respectively, for patients with deterioration in BPI sum score.

From Table 6a, CP-2,-30 indicates that at follow-up, the worst pain score increased by 2 and the OMED percent increased by 30%. Tables 6b and 7b show the MANOVA of the possible cut off point combinations for patients showing deterioration on the BPI. Statistical significance demonstrated by MANOVA ($p<0.05$) implies pain progression.

Table 6a. Possible cut-off points in patients with BPI deterioration at month 1 (n=56

	Cutpoint	No. of patients
1	CP4,-100	1
2	CP4,40	1
3	CP4,90	1
4	CP4,100	1
5	CP,10	1
6	CP-5,0	1
7	CP5,100	1
8	CP6,-100	1
9	CP-5,100	1
10	CP6,100	1
11	CP6,-30	1
12	CP7,-100	2
13	CP7,-40	1
14	CP,100	1
15	CP-4,90	1
16	CP-4,100	1
17	CP-3,-100	1
18	CP-3,-10	1
19	CP-2,-100	2
20	CP-2,-30	1
21	CP-1,30	1
22	CP-1,-80	1
23	CP-1,100	3
24	CP-1,-10	1
25	CP0,-100	4
26	CP0,30	1
27	CP0,100	4
28	CP0,-10	2
29	CP1,-100	1
30	CP1,0	1
31	CP1,100	1
32	CP1,-30	1
33	CP2,-100	1
34	CP2,0	1
35	CP2,20	1
36	CP2,80	1
37	CP2,-60	1
38	CP2,-20	1
39	CP3,-100	3
40	CP3,20	1
41	CP3,-80	1
42	CP3,100	2

Table 6b. Multivariate analysis of variance (MANOVA) on all possible 32 combinations of cut points and the deterioration of 7 interference items at month 1

Cutpoint	Statistic	Value	F statistic*	p-value*
CP7,-100	**Wilks' Lambda**	**0.3236**	**11.05**	**<.0001**
CP7,-100	Pillai's Trace	0.6764		
CP7,-100	Hotelling-Lawley Trace	2.0901		
CP-4,100	**Wilks' Lambda**	**0.6067**	**3.43**	**0.0063**
CP-4,100	Pillai's Trace	0.3933		
CP-4,100	Hotelling-Lawley Trace	0.6484		
CP3,20	**Wilks' Lambda**	**0.6839**	**2.44**	**0.0365**
CP3,20	Pillai's Trace	0.3161		
CP3,20	Hotelling-Lawley Trace	0.4622		
CP0,100	**Wilks' Lambda**	**0.6945**	**2.32**	**0.0452**
CP0,100	Pillai's Trace	0.3055		
CP0,100	Hotelling-Lawley Trace	0.4399		
CP0,30	Wilks' Lambda	0.7248	2.01	0.0804
CP0,30	Pillai's Trace	0.2752		
CP0,30	Hotelling-Lawley Trace	0.3797		
CP4,-100	Wilks' Lambda	0.7377	1.88	0.1012
CP4,-100	Pillai's Trace	0.2623		
CP4,-100	Hotelling-Lawley Trace	0.3555		
CP-3,-10	Wilks' Lambda	0.7491	1.77	0.1230
CP-3,-10	Pillai's Trace	0.2509		
CP-3,-10	Hotelling-Lawley Trace	0.3349		
CP3,-80	Wilks' Lambda	0.7574	1.69	0.1409
CP3,-80	Pillai's Trace	0.2426		
Cutpoint	Statistic	Value	F statistic*	p-value*
CP3,-80	Hotelling-Lawley Trace	0.3204		
CP4,40	Wilks' Lambda	0.7709	1.57	0.1747
CP4,40	Pillai's Trace	0.2291		
CP4,40	Hotelling-Lawley Trace	0.2972		
CP1,100	Wilks' Lambda	0.7784	1.50	0.1961
CP1,100	Pillai's Trace	0.2216		
CP1,100	Hotelling-Lawley Trace	0.2847		
CP0,-10	Wilks' Lambda	0.7865	1.43	0.2212
CP0,-10	Pillai's Trace	0.2135		
CP0,-10	Hotelling-Lawley Trace	0.2714		
CP1,-100	Wilks' Lambda	0.8063	1.27	0.2919
CP1,-100	Pillai's Trace	0.1937		
CP1,-100	Hotelling-Lawley Trace	0.2402		
CP-1,-80	Wilks' Lambda	0.8311	1.07	0.3993
CP-1,-80	Pillai's Trace	0.1689		
CP-1,-80	Hotelling-Lawley Trace	0.2032		
CP-2,-30	Wilks' Lambda	0.8381	1.02	0.4329
CP-2,-30	Pillai's Trace	0.1619		
CP-2,-30	Hotelling-Lawley Trace	0.1932		
CP6,100	Wilks' Lambda	0.8438	0.98	0.4611
CP6,100	Pillai's Trace	0.1562		
CP6,100	Hotelling-Lawley Trace	0.1852		

Cutpoint	Statistic	Value	F statistic*	p-value*
CP-5,100	Wilks' Lambda	0.8577	0.88	0.5339
CP-5,100	Pillai's Trace	0.1423		
CP-5,100	Hotelling-Lawley Trace	0.1659		
CP-1,100	Wilks' Lambda	0.8636	0.84	0.5653
CP-1,100	Pillai's Trace	0.1364		
CP-1,100	Hotelling-Lawley Trace	0.1580		
CP2,-60	Wilks' Lambda	0.8672	0.81	0.5850
CP2,-60	Pillai's Trace	0.1328		
CP2,-60	Hotelling-Lawley Trace	0.1532		
CP0,-100	Wilks' Lambda	0.8730	0.77	0.6165
CP0,-100	Pillai's Trace	0.1270		
CP0,-100	Hotelling-Lawley Trace	0.1455		
CP2,-20	Wilks' Lambda	0.8799	0.72	0.6545
CP2,-20	Pillai's Trace	0.1201		
CP2,-20	Hotelling-Lawley Trace	0.1365		
CP2,-100	Wilks' Lambda	0.8807	0.72	0.6589
CP2,-100	Pillai's Trace	0.1193		
CP2,-100	Hotelling-Lawley Trace	0.1355		
CP2,80	Wilks' Lambda	0.8855	0.68	0.6849
CP2,80	Pillai's Trace	0.1145		
CP2,80	Hotelling-Lawley Trace	0.1293		
CP5,100	Wilks' Lambda	0.9089	0.53	0.8064
CP5,100	Pillai's Trace	0.0911		
CP5,100	Hotelling-Lawley Trace	0.1002		
CP1,-30	Wilks' Lambda	0.9166	0.48	0.8421
CP1,-30	Pillai's Trace	0.0834		
CP1,-30	Hotelling-Lawley Trace	0.0910		
CP-2,-100	Wilks' Lambda	0.9269	0.42	0.8857
CP-2,-100	Pillai's Trace	0.0731		
CP-2,-100	Hotelling-Lawley Trace	0.0788		
CP7,-40	Wilks' Lambda	0.9329	0.38	0.9079
CP7,-40	Pillai's Trace	0.0671		
CP7,-40	Hotelling-Lawley Trace	0.0720		
CP2,0	Wilks' Lambda	0.9335	0.38	0.9102
CP2,0	Pillai's Trace	0.0665		
CP2,0	Hotelling-Lawley Trace	0.0712		
CP3,-100	Wilks' Lambda	0.9394	0.34	0.9296
CP3,-100	Pillai's Trace	0.0606		
CP3,-100	Hotelling-Lawley Trace	0.0645		
CP4,100	Wilks' Lambda	0.9427	0.32	0.9396
CP4,100	Pillai's Trace	0.0573		
CP4,100	Hotelling-Lawley Trace	0.0608		
CP2,20	Wilks' Lambda	0.9438	0.31	0.9427
CP2,20	Pillai's Trace	0.0562		
CP2,20	Hotelling-Lawley Trace	0.0595		
CP6,-100	Wilks' Lambda	0.9589	0.23	0.9765
CP6,-100	Pillai's Trace	0.0411		
CP6,-100	Hotelling-Lawley Trace	0.0429		

Table 6b. (Continued)

Cutpoint	Statistic	Value	F statistic*	p-value*
CP6,-30	Wilks' Lambda	0.9759	0.13	0.9954
CP6,-30	Pillai's Trace	0.0241		
CP6,-30	Hotelling-Lawley Trace	0.0247		

*Wilk's lamba, Pillai's trace and Hotelling-Lawley trace have same values for F-statistic and exact p-value. P-value < 0.05 was considered as significance.

Table 7a. Possible cut-off points in patients with BPI deterioration at month 2 (n=35)

	Cutpoint	No. of patients
1	CP-6,-100	1
2	CP4,50	1
3	CP5,90	1
4	CP6,100	1
5	CP7,-100	1
6	CP7,80	1
7	CP-5,-50	1
8	CP9,60	1
9	CP-4,0	1
10	CP-4,100	1
11	CP-3,-100	2
12	CP-3,60	1
13	CP-2,100	1
14	CP-1,-100	2
15	CP-1,-90	1
16	CP0,-100	3
17	CP0,10	1
18	CP0,100	1
19	CP1,-100	2
20	CP1,-90	1
21	CP1,-40	1
22	CP2,40	1
23	CP2,100	2
24	CP3,-100	2
25	CP3,10	1
26	CP3,-80	1
27	CP3,100	2

All statistically significant cut-points are summarized in Table 8. One month following RT, CP9, 100 showed the most statistical significance (p=0.0005), followed by CP10, 100 (p=0.0026), CP5,-30 (p=0.0069), CP5, 90 (p=0.0200) and CP0, 30 (p=0.0290), respectively, in patients experiencing improvement in the BPI. For patients experiencing deterioration in the BPI at 1-month follow-up, two cut-points, CP7,-100 (p=<0.0001) and CP-4,100 (p=0.0063), were found to be statistically significant. Two months following RT, five statistically significant cut-points were identified in patients with BPI improvement, and one statistically significant cut-point, CP7, 80 (p=0.0157), was identified in patients with BPI deterioration.

Table 7b. Multivariate analysis of variance (MANOVA) on all possible 19 combinations of cut points and the deterioration of 7 interference items at month 2

Cutpoint	Statistic	Value	F statistic*	p-value*
CP7,80	**Wilks' Lambda**	**0.4758**	**3.30**	**0.0157**
CP7,80	Pillai's Trace	0.5242		
CP7,80	Hotelling-Lawley Trace	1.1016		
CP0,100	Wilks' Lambda	0.5796	2.18	0.0794
CP0,100	Pillai's Trace	0.4204		
CP0,100	Hotelling-Lawley Trace	0.7254		
CP2,100	Wilks' Lambda	0.6061	1.95	0.1117
CP2,100	Pillai's Trace	0.3939		
CP2,100	Hotelling-Lawley Trace	0.6500		
CP9,60	Wilks' Lambda	0.6219	1.82	0.1352
CP9,60	Pillai's Trace	0.3781		
CP9,60	Hotelling-Lawley Trace	0.6081		
CP4,50	Wilks' Lambda	0.6490	1.62	0.1837
CP4,50	Pillai's Trace	0.3510		
CP4,50	Hotelling-Lawley Trace	0.5409		
CP3,-100	Wilks' Lambda	0.6496	1.62	0.1850
CP3,-100	Pillai's Trace	0.3504		
CP3,-100	Hotelling-Lawley Trace	0.5394		
CP2,40	Wilks' Lambda	0.6569	1.57	0.2000
CP2,40	Pillai's Trace	0.3431		
CP2,40	Hotelling-Lawley Trace	0.5222		
CP3,100	Wilks' Lambda	0.6845	1.38	0.2638
CP3,100	Pillai's Trace	0.3155		
CP3,100	Hotelling-Lawley Trace	0.4609		
CP7,-100	Wilks' Lambda	0.6933	1.33	0.2866
CP7,-100	Pillai's Trace	0.3067		
CP7,-100	Hotelling-Lawley Trace	0.4423		
CP-3,-100	Wilks' Lambda	0.7134	1.21	0.3428
CP-3,-100	Pillai's Trace	0.2866		
CP-3,-100	Hotelling-Lawley Trace	0.4018		
CP0,-100	Wilks' Lambda	0.7404	1.05	0.4267
CP0,-100	Pillai's Trace	0.2596		
CP0,-100	Hotelling-Lawley Trace	0.3507		
CP6,100	Wilks' Lambda	0.7510	0.99	0.4619
CP6,100	Hotelling-Lawley Trace	0.3316		
CP6,100	Pillai's Trace	0.2490		
CP3,-80	Wilks' Lambda	0.8360	0.59	0.7577
CP3,-80	Pillai's Trace	0.1640		
CP3,-80	Hotelling-Lawley Trace	0.1962		
CP5,90	Wilks' Lambda	0.8370	0.58	0.7611
CP5,90	Pillai's Trace	0.1630		
CP5,90	Hotelling-Lawley Trace	0.1948		
CP-1,-100	Wilks' Lambda	0.8669	0.46	0.8517
CP-1,-100	Pillai's Trace	0.1331		
CP-1,-100	Hotelling-Lawley Trace	0.1536		
CP-2,100	Wilks' Lambda	0.9041	0.32	0.9374
CP-2,100	Pillai's Trace	0.0959		
CP-2,100	Hotelling-Lawley Trace	0.1060		
CP1,-40	Wilks' Lambda	0.9274	0.23	0.9718

Table 7b. (Continued)

Cutpoint	Statistic	Value	F statistic*	p-value*
CP1,-40	Pillai's Trace	0.0726		
CP1,-40	Hotelling-Lawley Trace	0.0783		
CP-4,100	Wilks' Lambda	0.9399	0.19	0.9839
CP-4,100	Pillai's Trace	0.0601		
CP-4,100	Hotelling-Lawley Trace	0.0640		
CP-4,0	Wilks' Lambda	0.9805	0.06	0.9996
CP-4,0	Pillai's Trace	0.0195		
CP-4,0	Hotelling-Lawley Trace	0.0199		

*Wilk's lamba, Pillai's trace and Hotelling-Lawley trace have same values for F-statistic and exact p-value. P-value < 0.05 was considered as significant.

Table 8. Summary of all possible cut-points

	Cut-points			
	Worst Pain	Analgesic intake	F statistic*	p-value*
Patients with BPI improvement at 1-Month follow-up (FU)				
CP9,100	Reduce 9 scores	100% reduction or 0 at FU	4.02	0.0005
CP10,100	Reduce 10 scores or 0 at FU	100% reduction or 0 at FU	3.32	0.0026
CP5,-30	Reduce 5 scores	30% increase	2.92	0.0069
CP5,90	Reduce 5 scores	90% reduction	2.47	0.0200
CP0,30	No change	30% reduction	2.31	0.0290
Patients with BPI improvement at 2-Month FU				
CP10,100	Reduce 10 scores or 0 at FU	100% reduction or 0 at FU	4.45	0.0002
CP8,10	Reduce 8 scores	10% reduction	3.01	0.0059
CP7,90	Reduce 7 scores	90% reduction	2.43	0.0229
CP2,100	Reduce 2 scores	100% reduction or 0 at FU	2.34	0.0282
CP8,-100	Reduce 8 scores	100% increase	2.29	0.0311
	Worst Pain	Analgesic intake	F statistic*	p-value*
Patients with BPI deterioration at 1-Month FU				
CP7,-100	Reduce 7 scores	100% increase	11.05	<0.0001
CP-4,100	Increase 4 scores	100% reduction or 0 at FU	3.43	0.0063
Patients with BPI deterioration at 2-Month FU				
CP7,80	Reduce 7 scores	80% reduction	3.30	0.0157

* F-statistic and exact p-value was found by MANOVA Wilk's lambda or Pillai's trace or Hotelling-Lawley trace. P-value < 0.05 was considered as significance.

Discussion

The purpose of the present study was to explore optimal definitions for partial response and pain progression in patients receiving palliative RT for bone metastases. Numerous palliative RT trials for bone metastases have been conducted, in which a wide range of end-points were employed, especially in terms of partial response and pain progression. For instance, Steenland et al. defined partial response as a decrease in pain by two or more points and pain progression as an increase in pain, returning to initial pain score or higher when evaluated on an 11-point numeric scale in their 1999 trial (7). In contrast, Nielsen et al. used a visual analog scale (VAS), which used the descriptors none, mild, moderate and excruciating to evaluate pain and factored analgesic intake into their definition of pain progression. According to their study, partial response was a reduction of >50% on the VAS (8). Several trials did not provide a definition for partial response (4, 9-11) and others had no description for pain progression (4, 12). With such varying response definitions, it was recognized that the direct comparison of trial outcomes was invalid, and the unified definitions were necessary (13).

In 2002, the International Bone Metastases Consensus Group established definitions for complete response, partial response and pain progression. These endpoints were reached via the clinical experience of bone metastases experts and were not based on quantitative data. Individuals experiencing both a reduced worst pain score and increase in analgesic intake were not included in the response definitions, leading to a discrepancy in how to classify these patients. As a result, it has been recommended that the consensus response definitions be reassessed (14).

Based on our preliminary results, five clinically relevant and statistically significant cut-points were observed for partial response at both one and two months following RT. Although CP9, 100 (p=0.0005) and CP10, 100 (p=0.0026) had the greatest statistical significance at 1-month follow-up, these cut-points are closely related to the consensus definition for complete response. Cut-point 5,-30 (p=0.0069) represents a reduction in worst pain score by five points and a 30% increase in analgesic intake. This cut-point may be more relevant to defining partial response and also addresses the issue of calculating response in patients with decreased pain and increased analgesia. Furthermore, at the one month follow-up, CP0, 30 indicating no change in worst pain score and an analgesic reduction of 30%, was found to be statistically significant (p=0.029). This cut-point is similar to the International Consensus definition for partial response—analgesic reduction of 25% or more from baseline without an increase in worst pain score—and provides some degree of objectivity to the consensus definition.

Regarding patients with improvement in the BPI two months following RT, CP2, 100 (p=0.0282) represents a reduced worst pain by 2 scores with 100% reduction in analgesic intake or no analgesic intake at follow-up. This is also similar to the consensus definition of partial response (worst pain reduction of 2 or more at the treated site, without analgesic increase) in terms of worst pain score; however, differs in terms of analgesic consumption.

In an attempt to define pain progression, three cut-points were identified after the one and two-month follow-ups. However, CP7,80 (p=0.0157), which indicates a reduction of seven points in worst pain score and an 80% reduction in analgesic intake, is clinically irrelevant, and should be disregarded when considering pain progression. Only CP7,-100 (p=<0.0001) and CP-4,100 (p=0.0063) demonstrate both statistical significance and clinical relevance in the definition of progressive pain.

Although the primary objective of the present study is to explore the definition of partial response and pain progression using objective statistical analyses, it is also important to consider patient perspectives when defining response to palliative RT. We previously evaluated the meaningful change in pain scores as perceived by patients with bone metastases receiving palliative RT. It was found that when there was a decline in pain score of two or more on an 11-point numeric scale, patients perceived their current pain to be less than their baseline pain (15). In a similar investigation, the expectations of patients being treated with palliative RT for painful bone metastases were assessed in order to obtain a patient-derived definition for partial response. It was suggested that a pain score reduction of two-thirds from baseline as measured on an 11-point numeric scale may be indicative of partial response (16). A reduction of two-thirds is similar to the CP5,-30 identified in the present series which indicates a pain score reduction of approximately half on the 0-10 scale of the BPI. This cut-point demonstrates consistency with both statistical analyses and patient expectations when attempting to reach a more optimal definition for partial response. However, it is noted that patients were asked to consider pain scores only and not analgesic consumption in their expectation of partial response.

The present study was limited to only English speaking patients. Improvement and deterioration in the BPI were evaluated at 1- and 2-months post-RT. However, the International Bone Metastases Consensus Group recommends that pain response be assessed at 1-, 2- and 3-months post-RT (5). In order to maintain consistency, BPI sum scores may require evaluation 3-months following RT since we are attempting to reach a more optimal definition based on the International Consensus end-point definitions. On the other hand, one of our previous studies concluded that evaluating pain response 2-months post-RT may be more appropriate due to attrition rates and also because patients may require more than four weeks to achieve maximum pain relief (14). Therefore, the time intervals used in this study to measure BPI improvement and deterioration are supported.

Furthermore, cut-points that were statistically significant, but were not clinically relevant were removed from the analysis. Specifically, in patients found to have BPI improvement at 1-month follow-up, CP-1,-100 and CP0,-40 were eliminated. Also at 1-month follow up, CP 3, 20 and CP0, 100 were removed from the analysis for patients with deterioration in the BPI. Another possible limitation of this study lies in the method used to determine patient improvement or deterioration. Functional interference items were summed in order for such determination, which may not necessarily result in a linear relationship. Functional items of the BPI can be grouped into subscales of pain interference coupled with physical functions (general activity, walking ability and normal work) and psychological functions (mood, relations with other people, and enjoyment of life, sleep) (17, 18).

Response rates to RT are a function of the endpoint definition. The present study did not attempt to calculate response rate, rather it aimed to relate worst pain scores and percent change in analgesic intake to deterioration or improvement in the BPI. This would allow us to quantitatively define partial response and pain progression in patients with bone metastases. However, due to a small sample size, the present study was a preliminary analysis and the use of a larger sample size may result in more representative findings. Until our initial findings can be validated, the International Consensus end-points should continue to be used in order to maintain consistency when reporting RT response rates in bone metastases trials.

Acknowledgments

This study was supported by Michael and Karyn Goldstein Cancer Research Fund. We thank Stacy Lue for secretarial assistance. Conflict of Interest: None.

References

[1] von Moos R, Strasser F, Gillessen S, Zaugg K. Metastatic bone pain: treatment options with an emphasis on bisphosphonates. Support.Care Cancer 2008;16(10):1105-15.

[2] Tong D, Gillick L, Hendrickson FR. The palliation of symptomatic osseous metastases: final results of the Study by the Radiation Therapy Oncology Group. Cancer 1982;50(5):893-9.

[3] Blitzer PH: Reanalysis of the RTOG study of the palliation of symptomatic osseous metastasis. Cancer 1985;55:1468-72.

[4] Kirkbride P, Warde P, Panzarella A, et al: A randomized trial comparing the efficacy of single fraction radiation therapy plus ondansetron with fractionated radiation therapy in the palliation of skeletal metastases. Int J Radiat Oncol Biol Phys 2000;48(Suppl 3):185.

[5] Chow E, Wu JS, Hoskin P, Coia LR, Bentzen SM, Blitzer PH. International consensus on palliative radiotherapy endpoints for future clinical trials in bone metastases. Radiother Oncol. 2002;64(3):275-80.

[6] Harris K, Li K, Flynn C, Chow E. Worst, Average or Current Pain in the Brief Pain Inventory: Which Should be Used to Calculate the Response to Palliative Radiotherapy in Patients with Bone Metastases? Clin Oncol 2007;19:523-7.

[7] Steenland E, Leer JW, van Houwelingen H, Post WJ, van den Hout WB, Kievit J, et al. The effect of a single fraction compared to multiple fractions on painful bone metastases: a global analysis of the Dutch Bone Metastasis Study. Radiother Oncol 1999;52(2):101-9.

[8] Nielsen OS, Bentzen SM, Sandberg E, Gadeberg CC, Timothy AR. Randomized trial of single dose versus fractionated palliative radiotherapy of bone metastases. Radiother Oncol 1998;47(3):233-40.

[9] Koswig S, Budach V: Recalcification and pain relief following radiotherapy for bone metastases: A randomized trial of 2 different fractionation schedules (10 X 3 Gy vs. 1 X 8 Gy). Strahlenther Onkol 1999;175:500-8. [German]

[10] Kaasa S, Brenne E, Lund J, et al: Prospective randomized multicentre trial on single fraction radiotherapy (8 Gy X 1) versus multiple fractions (3 Gy X10) in the treatment of painful bone metastases: Phase III randomized trial. Radiother Oncol 2006;79:278-84.

[11] Haddad P, Behrouzi H, Amouzegar-Hashemi F, et al: Single versus multiple fractions of palliative radiotherapy for bone metastases: A randomized clinical trial in Iranian patients. Radiother Oncol 2006; 80:S65.

[12] Niewald M, Tkocz HJ, Abel U, Scheib T, Walter K, Nieder C, et al. Rapid course radiation therapy vs. more standard treatment: a randomized trial for bone metastases. Int J Radiat Oncol Biol Phys 1996;36(5):1085-9.

[13] Wu JS, Bezjak A, Chow E, Kirkbride P. Primary treatment endpoint following palliative radiotherapy for painful bone metastases: need for a consensus definition? Clin.Oncol (R Coll Radiol) 2002;14(1):70-7.

[14] Li KK, Hadi S, Kirou-Mauro A, Chow E. When should we define the response rates in the treatment of bone metastases by palliative radiotherapy? Clin Oncol 2008;20:83-9.

[15] Chow E, Chiu H, Doyle M, Hruby G, Holden L, et al. Patient expectation of the partial response and response shift in pain score. Support Cancer Ther 2007;4(2):110-8.

[16] Chow E, Ling A, Davis L, Panzarella T, Danjoux C. Pain flare following external beam radiotherapy and meaningful change in pain scores in the treatment of bone metastases. Radiother Oncol 2005; 75:64-9.

[17] Klepstad P, Loge JH, Borchgrevink PC, Mendoza TR, Cleeland CS, Kaasa S. The Norwegian brief pain inventory questionnaire: translation and validation in cancer pain patients. J Pain Symptom Manage 2002;24(5):517-25.

[18] Holen JC, Lydersen S, Klepstad P, Loge JH, Kaasa S. The Brief Pain Inventory: pain's interference with functions is different in cancer pain compared with noncancer chronic pain. Clin J Pain 2008; 24(3):219-25.

In: Pain Management Yearbook 2009
Editor: Joav Merrick

ISBN: 978-1-61209-666-7
©2012 Nova Science Publishers, Inc.

Chapter 43

A MULTIDISCIPLINARY BONE METASTASES CLINIC AT SUNNYBROOK ODETTE CANCER CENTRE: A REVIEW OF THE EXPERIENCE FROM 2006-2008

Janet Nguyen, BSc(C), Emily Sinclair, MRT (T), Albert Yee, MD, Joel Finkelstein, MD, Michael Ford, MD, Anita Chakraborty, MD, Macey Farhadian, RN, Robyn Pugash, MD, Gunita Mitera, MRT (T), Cyril Danjoux, MD, Elizabeth Barnes, MD, May Tsao, MD, Arjun Sahgal, MD and Edward Chow, MBBS[*]

Bone Metastases Site Group, Sunnybrook Health Sciences Centre,
University of Toronto, Toronto, Canada

Abstract

The purpose of this study is to review the coordinated, multidisciplinary approach to the management and care of cancer patients with metastatic bone disease at the one-stop bone metastases clinic (BMC) at the Odette Cancer Centre. Patients with symptomatic bone metastases are referred to the BMC and assessed by a team consisting of specialists in various disciplines such as interventional radiology, orthopedic surgery, palliative medicine, and radiation oncology. At initial consultation, patient demographics, reasons for referral, and case disposition were recorded. From June 2006 to December 2008, a total of 254 patients with bone metastases were seen at the BMC. The median age was 64 years (range 29-94) and median KPS score was 70 (range 10-100). The majority of patients arrived from home (85%), while 5% of patients came from a hospital. Approximately 16% of patients had 2 or more reasons for referral, yielding a total of 295 reasons. Bone pain was the main reason for referral (69%),

---

[*] **Correspondence:** Edward Chow, MBBS, PhD, FRCPC, Department of Radiation Oncology, Odette Cancer Centre, Sunnybrook Health Sciences Centre, 2075 Bayview Avenue, Toronto, Ontario, Canada M4N 3M5. Tel: 416-480-4998; Fax: 416-480-6002; E-mail: Edward.Chow@sunnybrook.ca

followed by a pathological fracture (10%) and impending fracture (8%). Out of 254 patients, only 240 case dispositions were recorded, with 3 patients receiving 2 treatment recommendations. Almost a third of patients (28%) received palliative radiation, 20% needed further investigation and/or imaging, 17% were referred to other support /specialist services such as palliative care or physiotherapy, and 15% of patients were offered surgery. A co-ordinated multidisciplinary clinic is useful in managing symptomatic bone metastases in cancer patients.

Keywords: Cancer, pain, bone metastases, multidisciplinary approach.

Introduction

In 2008, it is estimated that there will be 166,400 new cases of cancer and 73,800 deaths will result from cancer in Canada (1). Skeletal metastases are a frequent complication of cancer, particularly in breast, lung, prostate, thyroid, and renal cancers (2,3). Due to advances in systemic treatments, survival in cancer patients is increasing, and as a result the prevalence of patients with bone metastases is also expected to increase (3,4). Patients with breast and prostate cancer with bone-only metastases can have a relatively long median survival, ranging from 2 to 5 years (2,5). It is important that appropriate management and prevention of skeletal complications are achieved in order to maintain quality of life in these patients (6,7). There is a need to reassess the management strategies in patients with bone metastases due to the following reasons (2,6,8-13):

- Pain from bone metastases is the most common cause of cancer-associated pain;
- Bone metastases typically cause severe symptoms and these develop earlier than symptoms due to liver or lung metastases;
- Complications resulting from bone metastases are common and can seriously impact patients' quality of life. Pain and impaired mobility occur in 65-75% of patients with bone metastases; pathological fractures occur in 10-30% ; hypercalcemia occurs in 10-15%; and spinal cord compression or nerve root compression is seen in 5% of patients;
- There has been a noticeable increase in the prevalence of bone metastases due to longer survival duration of patients and;
- Multidisciplinary care of this group is needed to address specific problems in the management of bone metastases.

Pain is the most common symptom resulting from bone metastases, however bone pain is often under-treated (6,7). Treatment for bone metastases involves a multidisciplinary approach, which includes surgery, radiotherapy, chemotherapy, and other treatments (13). There have been clinical trials and reviews in a variety of disciplines addressing the optimal management of bone metastases, some of which discuss the potential of newer generations of bisphosphonates (5,9,14), the efficacy of radiotherapy, as well as the expanding need for effective surgical treatment (13). When bone pain is mechanical in origin, it cannot be adequately treated with radiotherapy or systemic therapies, and therefore surgical stabilization is recommended (2, 15).

In Janjan and colleagues' review of their multidisciplinary bone metastases clinic, they note that lack of coordination of care among many specialties contributes to inadequately treating cancer-related pain (6). Their report describes an integrated clinic model for the management of bone metastases, with 108 patients (seen by physicians from diagnostic radiology, nuclear medicine, pain and symptom management, physical medicine and rehabilitation, orthopedic surgery, medical oncology, and radiation oncology), being retrospectively evaluated. Presenting symptoms, extent of disease, past therapies, and evaluation of current treatment options were reviewed, and they concluded that coordination of care could overcome many practical difficulties in the management of metastatic disease in symptomatic patients. Surgery and radiotherapy are often used in combination with other treatments, therefore a multidisciplinary approach is especially important in reaching the goals of treatment for patients, some of which are to relieve pain, restore and maintain function, and to prevent skeletal related events (SREs). SREs are classified as the need for radiotherapy or surgery for palliation of pain, hypercalcemia, pathological fracture, or spinal cord compression (SCC) (6,8).

The Division of Orthopedics at Sunnybrook Health Sciences Centre and the Rapid Response Radiotherapy Program at Sunnybrook Odette Cancer Centre initiated a first-of-its-kind clinic, the Bone Metastases Clinic, at Sunnybrook Odette Cancer Centre in January 1999. The clinic aims to provide a coordinated multidisciplinary approach to the management of symptomatic bone metastases patients. This multidisciplinary service will also save the time and effort that a patient would otherwise expend during separate, sequential visits to various specialists for consultation.

A review of the BMC from 1999 to 2005 has previously been reported with a total of 272 patients seen at the BMC during that period 4. From 1999 to 2005, at initial consultation patient demographics, cancer history, disease status, and symptom profiles were collected, as well as patient Edmonton Symptom Assessment Scale (ESAS) scores. The purpose of this paper was to update our experience at the BMC from 2006 to 2008.

Methods

The BMC is managed by a team in various specialties: interventional radiology, nursing, orthopedic surgery, pain and palliative medicine, radiation oncology, and radiation therapy. The clinic is held on every second and fourth Friday of every month.

A prospective database has been set up for patients referred for assessment at BMC since January 1999. Pathological diagnosis of cancer and documentation of bone metastases either by pathological confirmation, clinical examination, or imaging, are required for referral to the BMC. Patients were entered into the database if they were able to speak English, give verbal consent, and respond to questions that assessed their symptoms. Patients were excluded from the database if they were confused, refused, or were unable to complete the symptom assessment. At initial consultation, patient demographics, cancer history, disease status, and symptom profiles were collected. Patients were asked to complete the Brief Pain Inventory (BPI) from June 2006 to May 2008. Then from May 2008 to December 2008, patients completed the EORTC Bone Metastases Module (EORTC QLQ-BM22). The BPI evaluates current, average, and worst pain on a scale of 0-10, as well as 7 questions evaluating the interference of pain in their daily life. The EORTC QLQ-BM22 consists of 22 questions assessing pain site(s), pain characteristics, functional interference, and psychosocial aspects, and rates on a scale of 1-4. Analgesic consumption, total pain relief, site(s) of bone metastases, and the risk of fractures at the initial visit were assessed and also recorded along with either the BPI or the EORTC QLQ-BM22. The functional status of the patient was scored as follows: normal with pain-free use of the extremity and spine; normal use with pain; significant limited use (i.e. use of prosthesis, walker, cane, crutches, and sling); and nonfunctional extremity/spine (wheelchair-bound, bedridden).

Patients were assessed by an orthopedic surgeon, a radiation oncologist, and a pain specialist at initial consultation. The team then made a joint recommendation based on their assessments, along with nursing and radiation therapy support. An interventional radiologist was consulted if the patient was considered a candidate for percutaneous vertebroplasty or cementoplasty.

Results

From June 2006 to December 2008, a total of 254 patients with bone metastases were referred to the BMC. One hundred and thirty-two patients were male (52%) and 122 were female (48%). Their median age was 64 years (range 29-94). The three most common primary sites were breast (22%), lung (17%), and renal cell (17%). The median KPS score at initial consultation was 70 (range 10-100). The majority of patients arrived from home (85%) while only 5% came from a hospital. Patients identified the spine (43%), pelvis and hips (21%), and lower limbs (17%) to be the most painful bony sites (see table 1). There were a total of 295 reasons for referral, where nearly one-fifth of patients (21%) had two or more reasons for referral. The top three reasons for referral were bone pain (69%), pathological fracture (10%), and impending fracture (8%) (see table 2).

Brief pain inventory scores are summarized in table 3. The median worst, average, and current pain score were 7, 4, and 3 respectively. Pain interfering with normal work was the most severe problem expressed by patients, with a median score of 8. Pain interfering with general activity, walking ability, and enjoyment of life came next at a median score of 7. There were only 91 patients who had analgesic intake recorded, measured by total daily oral morphine equivalent (OME) in milligrams. Sixteen of those patients had zero OME; therefore they may have been taking non-opioids or no pain medication(s) at all, however the names of the pain medication(s) were not recorded. The mean OME was 109.12 ± 144.21 mg, with a median of 36 mg (range 0 – 640 mg). Out of 91 patients with analgesic intake recorded, pain relief data was collected from 77 patients – with 0 being no relief and 100 being complete relief. The mean score was 69.31 ± 67.26, and median pain relief experienced by patients was 70 (range 0 – 100).

Scores from the EORTC QLQ-BM22 are summarized in table 4. A number of patients noted that they experience pain in the back, constant pain, pain not relieved by pain medication, and pain when walking quite a bit (median score of 3).

Table 1. Patient characteristics (n=254)

Sex	
Male	132 (52%)
Female	122 (48%)
Age (Years)	
Median (Range)	64 (29-94)
Mean ± SD	63.11 ± 12.72
Source of Referral	
SPEC: Previous patients reviewed in BMC for new reason	179 (70%)
FU: Previous Patients Followed-Up	62 (24%)
NP: New Patients	13 (5%)
Locations where cases arrived from	
Home	216 (85%)
Hospital	12 (5%)
Unknown	14 (6%)
Primary cancer site	
Breast	55 (22%)
Lung	53 (21%)
Renal Cell	43 (17%)
Prostate	37 (15%)
Gastrointestinal	23 (9%)
Unknown	10 (4%)
Bladder	7 (3%)
Gynecological	6 (2%)
Others	19 (7 %)
Painful bony sites	
Spine	109 (43%)
Pelvis/Hips	53 (21%)
Lower limbs	42 (17%)
Upper limbs	21 (8%)
Trunk (Ribs, Clavicle, Scapula)	7 (3%)
Karnofsky performance status	
Median (range)	70 (10-100)

Table 2. Reason(s) for referral*

Bone Pain	175 (69%)
Pathological Fracture	25 (10%)
Impending Fracture	20 (8%)
Review Recent Imaging	18 (7%)
Assess need for more treatment	15 (6%)
Lesion Seen in Diagnostic Imaging	13 (5%)
Neuropathic Pain	8 (3%)
Assess Progression of disease	8 (3%)
Post Surgery	6 (2%)
Cord Compression	2 (1%)
Others	13 (5%)

Note: *295 reasons in total for n = 254. Eighteen patients' reason(s) for referral were not listed.

Table 3. Pain scores and Analgesic intake according to the Brief Pain Inventory

	N	Mean	Standard Deviation	Median	Range
Worst pain in past day	92	6.47	3.00	7	0 – 10
Average pain in past day	90	4.39	2.47	4	0 – 10
Current Pain	92	3.40	2.87	3	0 – 10
General activity‡	88	5.77	3.59	7	0 – 10
Mood ‡	87	4.25	3.56	4	0 – 10
Walking ability‡	85	5.81	3.66	7	0 – 10
Normal work‡	82	7.12	3.34	8	0 – 10
Relations with other people‡	85	2.81	3.50	0	0 – 10
Sleeping‡	86	4.34	3.89	4	0 – 10
Enjoyment of life‡	87	6.23	3.57	7	0 – 10
Total Morphine Equivalent (mg)	91*	109.12	144.21	36	0 – 640
Pain relief experienced**	77	69.31	67.26	70	0-100

Notes: 0, no pain; 10, worst pain.
‡How much pain interferes with this issue. 0, no interference; 10, completely interferes.
*Out of 91 responses, 16 patients had 0 morphine equivalent.
**0, no relief; 100, complete relief.

Table 4. Pain scores according to the Bone Metastases Module (EORTC QLQ-BM22)*

	N	Mean	Standard Deviation	Median	Range
Pain in back	42	3	1.17	3	1 – 4
Pain in leg(s) or hip(s)	41	3	1.16	2	1 – 4
Pain in arm(s) or shoulder(s)	42	2	1.15	1	1 – 4
Pain in chest or rib(s)	42	1	3.59	1	1 – 4
Pain in buttock(s)	40	2	0.74	1	1 – 4
Constant pain	41	2	1.15	3	1 – 4
Intermittent pain	40	3	1.14	2	1 – 4
Pain not relieved by pain medication	36	2	1.15	3	1 – 4
Pain when sitting	42	2	3.89	4	1 – 4
Pain when lying down	42	2	1.14	2	1 – 4
Pain when trying to stand up	39	3	1.21	2	1 – 4
Pain when walking	38	3	1.17	3	1 – 4
Pain when bending/climbing stairs	32	2	1.14	2	1 – 4
Pain with strenuous activity	27	3	1.25	3	1 – 4
Trouble sleeping	42	2	1.18	2	1 – 4
Need to modify daily activities	39	2	1.16	2	1 – 4
Feel isolated from family/friends	38	2	1.22	1	1 – 4
Worried about loss of mobility	38	2	1.16	2	
Worried about being dependent on others	39	2	1.15	2	1 – 4
Worried about health in the future	38	2	1.26	2	1 – 4
Felt hopeful the pain will get better	37	4	0.90	4	1 – 4
Felt positive about health	38	3	1.01	3	1 – 4

Notes: *Refers to issues in the past week.
1, not at all; 2, a little; 3, quite a bit; 4, very much.

Table 5. Functional status of extremity/spine (n=201 orthopedic assessments filled out)

Status	
Normal use with pain	75 (37%)
Significant limited use	51 (25%)
Normal, pain free use of extremity/spine	26 (13%)
Nonfunctional extremity/spine	14 (7%)
Unknown	35 (17%)

Orthopedic assessment

The orthopedic surgeon's assessment was recorded at initial consultation with the patient. The functional status of the affected extremity/spine, the presence or risk of fractures, and the severity of the risk was recorded. The report was completed 79% of the time (n=201). The majority of patients had normal use with pain (37%), followed by significant limited use (25%) and normal, pain-free use of extremity/spine (13%). Only 7% of patients were reported to have nonfunctional use of the extremity/spine (see table 5).

At the orthopedic surgeon's assessment for presence or risk of fractures, 17% of patients had a high risk of fractures, 7% had low risk, and 25% had a present fracture at initial consultation (see table 6). Out of the 34 patients presenting with a high risk, 22 (65%) had a high risk of fractures at the extremities, with 41% (9/22) involving a lytic lesions = 2.5 cm in size, and 45% (10/22) having = 50% of the cortex involved. Seventeen patients were reported to have a high risk of fracture at the spine, with 47% (8/17) due to mechanical instability, 29% (5/17) because of spinal cord compression, and 24% (4/17) for cauda equine syndrome or = 2 nerve root deficits.

Table 6. Presence of bone metastasis fractures/risk of fracture (n=201)

Presence of fracture	
Pathological fracture	44 (22%)
Wedge	7 (3%)
Fracture risk assessment	
High risk	34 (17%)
Low risk	14 (7%)
Medium risk	2 (1%)
Extremities risks	
Lytic lesion 2.5 to 5 cm in size	6 (3%)
50-74% cortex involved	5 (2%)
≥ 75% cortex involved	5 (2%)
Lytic lesions ≥ 5 cm in size	3 (1%)
Subtrochanteric region of femur	3 (1%)
Spinal risks	
Mechanical instability	8 (4%)
Spinal cord compression	5 (2%)
Cauda equine syndrome OR ≥ 2 nerve root deficits	4 (2%)

Table 7. Case disposition and treatment recommendation(s) (n=240*)

Palliative radiation	67 (28%)
Further investigation required	48 (20%)
Referred to other support services	41 (17%)
Offered surgery	37 (15%)
No action	34 (14%)
Inappropriate referral	3 (1%)
Others	10 (4%)

Notes: *20 patient's case dispositions are unknown out of 254 patients. 3 patients received 2 treatment recommendations.

Case dispositions and recommendations

Following thorough examination of a patient's symptoms, the BMC physicians consulted to decide the best course of action to take. Out of 254 patients who were examined, only 240 case dispositions were recorded. Sixty-seven patients (28%) received palliative radiation, 20% required further investigation, 17% were referred to other support services such as physiotherapy, and 15% were offered surgery (see table 7).

Discussion

As many as two-thirds of patients with bone metastases experience severe pain, thus this is usually the reason for the significantly decreased quality of life in patients (10,11). Over 80% of bone metastases are located in the axial skeleton, with the spine, ribs, and hips being the most frequently involved sites (9). This concurs with the top three painful bony sites recorded for the 254 patients seen at the BMC. Patients with bone metastases are at risk for SREs (12). Radiotherapy remains the standard choice of treatment for bone pain, and is also used where there is a risk for pathological fracture, or neurological complications arising from SCC or cauda equine syndrome (7, 9,16). Surgery tends to be indicated where there is intractable pain, high risk of fractures, acute spinal cord injury, or in cases where the pain is mechanical and cannot be treated by radiotherapy or systemic therapies (2,13,15,17). Prophylactic surgery can allow for stabilization of significantly destructive lytic lesions, whereas support frames or surgical fusion can be used to prevent SCC (7). However, due to the risks that come with surgery, particularly in elderly patients, a thorough assessment of all the available treatment options will allow the physicians and the patient to make the best choice (7,10). Oetiker and colleagues did a review of palliative surgery for bone metastases patients. They state that it is important to plan early and effective treatment to maximize the quality of life for these patients, and surgery can be very effective in relieving pain and for stabilization. However, they do note that an orthopedic surgeon must recognize that there is a need to manage this group of patients from a multidisciplinary perspective to ensure the best possible care for the bone metastases patient (16).

Bisphosphonates are known to give impressive results for treating hypercalcemia, as well as possibly reducing symptoms from bone metastases and the incidence and severity of SREs

(5,7,17,18). In Brown and Coleman's review (5) of using bisphosphonates to manage bone metastases in breast cancer patients, they note that radiotherapy is the first-choice treatment for treating local pain in many bone metastases patients, and excellent results are frequently achieved. However, since many patients also have widespread, poorly localised and non-mechanical pain, bisphosphonates may be a valuable alternative (5). They have found several studies showing that using intravenous clodronate, ibandronate, pamidronate, and zoledronic acid showed pain relief in bone metastases patients, with reductions in analgesic intake and an improvement in quality of life (5).

Pain from bone metastases typically develop slowly, and become progressively more severe (4). In the early stages, pain can be managed with analgesics or anti-inflammatory agents, however patients may still experience intermittent pain, such as a flare of pain upon movement (19) – a common complaint among patients with bone metastases (20). This type of pain then interferes with patients' ability to function, as well as restricting them from normal activities. This is seen in the BPI scores recorded at the BMC, where a median score of 8 was seen for pain interfering with normal work.

Once pain from bone metastases progress, other treatments must be considered. External beam radiotherapy achieves good results in most situations where patients have well-localized bone pain (5), and generally used in conjunction with either systemic treatment or supportive care (ie. analgesic therapy or bisphosphonates) (10). One-fifth of all radiotherapy treatments are given for pain due to bone metastases, and more than 40% of patients achieve at least 50% pain relief at 1 month. However, patients may also experience episodes of pain flare shortly after receiving radiotherapy. Approximately 14% of patients receiving a single dose of radiation have pain flare on day one as well as day two. Thus it is important to provide symptom control when alternative treatments are considered. Since pain relief from radiotherapy is also not permanent, pain progression generally happens at a median 5 to 6 months after treatment (21).

In Mercadante and colleagues' review of management of painful bone metastases, they state that 20-30% of patients treated with radiotherapy and analgesic may not have optimal pain relief, and therefore this may be where minimally invasive procedures, such as percutaneous vertebroplasty (PV), can play an important role (10). A prospective study was done by Cheung et al. investigating the efficacy of PV on pain relief and improvement of quality of life on patients with metastatic bone fractures (22). They used the ESAS for common cancer symptoms, the Townsend Functional Assessment Scale (TFAS) to assess mobility, site-specific pain score, as well as recording analgesic intake to assess changes in quality of life and pain before and after the intervention. A significant improvement was found in TFAS scores, all nine symptoms on the ESAS, site-specific pain, and there was a general trend of reduced analgesic intake post-PVP.

There is a real need for reducing complications due to bone metastases, as well as to improve the quality of life in these patients (5). Efficient management of bone metastases in patients requires a multidisciplinary approach due to the associated symptoms, clinical presentations, and complex underlying medical conditions (6,9). Closer collaboration between different disciplines would lead to quantifying clinical strategies and targeting them efficiently to those patients who have the most to gain (2). It is generally agreed that treatment should be individualized according to each patient's life expectancy, performance status, and quality of life (8,10).

From the inception of the BMC in 1999 until 2005, a total of 272 patients were seen (4). The median age was 65 years (range 28-95) and median KPS score at initial consultation was 60 (range 30-90), and this is fairly similar to the numbers seen in this review. Approximately a third (28%) of patients seen had two or more reasons for referral, which is nearly double the 16% of patients who had two or more reasons for referral to the BMC in 2006 – 2008. The most common reasons for referral in Li and colleague's review of the BMC were bone pain (42%), bone metastases (21%), high risk for pathological fracture (12%), and pathological fracture (10%). Bone pain continues to be the prevalent reason for referral to the BMC from 2006 – 2008 (69%). Out of the 272 patients, 40% of patients received palliative radiotherapy, 19% received interventional surgery, 7% were referred to other support services, and 7% needed further investigation or imaging. Although radiotherapy continues to be the most common case disposition seen (28%), there was an increase seen for patients who required further investigation or imaging (20%) and/or other support services (17%) in the past 3 years. During the initial six years at the BMC, the ESAS was used to record patient's symptoms; therefore there was no information on analgesic intake at that time.

When the total of 272 patients seen from 1999 – 2005 is compared with the 254 patients seen at the BMC from 2006 – 2008, it is evident that the BMC did approximately the same amount of work in 3 years as it did in its first six years. This is indicative of the increased awareness and need for multidisciplinary care in this group of patients. It is likely that the number of referrals to the BMC will continue to rise, which means there will be also be a need for increased funding as well as human resources. The ultimate goal of the BMC is to improve the overall quality of life for patients with bone metastases by maintaining and expanding this one-stop clinic approach for more patients who require this care. This is important given that as the population ages, the burden of cancer and bone metastases may also increase.

The Odette Cancer Centre Bone Metastases Clinic's integrated approach to the care of bone metastases patients allows for more streamlined care, in addition to eliminating the inconvenience of separate visits to a variety of specialists for consultation. Patients referred to the BMC receive a multidisciplinary assessment to decide the best course of action in order to maximize the benefits and palliate present symptoms. In order to further improve patient care at the BMC, there should be one quality of life instrument tool employed in order to keep results consistent, (ie. the EORTC QLQ-BM22). Analgesic information should be carefully recorded as well. Methods should also improve to collect orthopedic assessments and patient-rated quality of life questionnaires, as there were a number of patients and orthopedic surgeons who did not complete the assessments. Patient satisfaction of and cost-effectiveness of the clinic may need to be investigated in order to ensure the BMC continues to give efficient multidisciplinary care to patients with bone metastases.

Acknowledgments

This study was supported by the Michael and Karyn Goldstein Cancer Research Fund and Novartis Oncology. We thank Stacy Lue for secretarial assistance.

References

[1] [CCS/NCIC] Canadian Cancer Society/National Cancer Institute of Canada. 2008. Canada Cancer Statistics 2008. Toronto, Canada: Canadian Cancer Society/National Institute of Canada.
[2] Coleman RE. Skeletal complications of malignancy. Cancer 1997;80(8 Suppl):1588-94.
[3] Andersson L, Chow E, Finkelstein J, Connolly R, Danjoux C, Szumacher E, Wong R, Stephen D, Axelrod T. The ultimate one-stop for cancer patients with bone metastases: New combined bone metastases clinic. Can Oncol Nurs J 1999;9(2):103-4.
[4] Li KK, Sinclair E, Pope J, Farhadian M, Harris K, Napolskikh J, Yee A, Librach L, Wynnychuk L, Danjoux C, Chow E. A multidisciplinary bone metastases clinic at Toronto Sunnybrook Regional Cancer Centre – A review of the experience from 1999 to 2005. J Pain Res 2008:1;43-8.
[5] Brown JE, Coleman RE. The present and future role of bisphosphonates in the management of patients with breast cancer. Breast Cancer Res 2002;4(1):24-9.
[6] Janjan NA, Payne R, Gillis T, Podoloff D, Libshitz HI, Lenzi R, Theriault R, Martin C, Yasko A. Presenting symptoms in patients referred to a multidisciplinary clinic for bone metastases. J Pain Sympt Manage 1998;16(3):171-8.
[7] Mystakidou K, Katsouda E, Stathopoulou E, Vlahos L. Approaches to managing bone metastases from breast cancer: The role of bisphosphonates. Cancer Treat Rev 2005;31(4):303-11.
[8] Schachar NS. An update on the nonoperative treatment of patients with metastatic bone disease. Clin Orthop 2001;382:75-81.
[9] Selvaggi G, Scagliotti GV. Management of bone metastases in cancer: A review. Crit Rev Oncol Hematol 2005;56(3):365-78.
[10] Mercadante S, Fulfaro F. Management of painful bone metastases. Curr Opin Oncol 2007;19(4):308-14.
[11] Carlin BI, Andriole GL. The natural history, skeletal complications, and management of bone metastases in patients with prostate carcinoma. Cancer 2000;88(12 Suppl):2989-94.
[12] Lipton A. Future treatment of bone metastases. Clin Cancer Res 2006;12(20 Pt 2):6305s-8s.
[13] Manabe J, Kawaguchi N, Matsumoto S, Tanizawa T. Surgical treatment of bone metastasis: Indications and outcomes. Int J Clin Oncol 2005;10(2):103-11.
[14] Kohno N. Treatment of breast cancer with bone metastasis: Bisphosphonate treatment - current and future. Int J Clin Oncol 2008;13(1):18-23.
[15] Coleman RE. Clinical features of metastatic bone disease and risk of skeletal morbidity. Clin Cancer Res 2006;12(20 Pt 2):6243s-9s.
[16] Oetiker RF, Meier G, Hefti F, Bereiter H. [Palliative surgery for bone metastases]. Ther Umsch 2001;58(12):738-45.
[17] Talbot M, Turcotte RE, Isler M, Normandin D, Iannuzzi D, Downer P. Function and health status in surgically treated bone metastases. Clin Orthop 2005;438:215-20.
[18] Chow E, Ling A, Davis L, Panzarella T, Danjoux C. Pain flare following external beam radiotherapy and meaningful change in pain scores in the treatment of bone metastases. Radiother Oncol 2005;75(1):64-9.
[19] Coleman RE. Future directions in the treatment and prevention of bone metastases. Am J Clin Oncol 2002;25(6 Suppl 1):S32-8.
[20] Portenoy RK, Hagen NA. Breakthrough pain: Definition, prevalence and characteristics. Pain 1990;41(3):273-81.
[21] Steenland E, Leer JW, van Houwelingen H, Post WJ, van den Hout WB, Kievit J, et al. The effect of a single fraction compared to multiple fractions on painful bone metastases: A global analysis of the dutch bone metastasis study. Radiother Oncol 1999;52(2):101-9.
[22] Cheung G, Chow E, Holden L, Vidmar M, Danjoux C, Yee AJ, Connolly R, Finkelstein J. Percutaneous vertebroplasty in patients with intractable pain from osteoporotic or metastatic

fractures: A prospective study using quality-of-life assessment. Can Assoc Radiol J 2006;57(1):13-21.

Chapter 44

THE TEST-RETEST RELIABILITY OF THE EUROPEAN ORGANIZATION FOR RESEARCH AND TREATMENT OF CANCER QUALITY-OF-LIFE GROUP BONE METASTASES MODULE (EORTC QLQ-BM22) QUESTIONNAIRE

Candi J Flynn, MSc(C)[1], Mark Clemons, MD[2], Liying Zhang, PhD[1] and Edward Chow, MBBS[*1]*

[1]Rapid Response Radiotherapy Program, Radiation Oncology, Odette Cancer Centre, Toronto, Ontario and [2]Medical Oncology, Princess Margaret Hospital and Campbell Family Institute for Breast Cancer Research, Toronto, Ontario, Canada

Abstract

Clinical trials in palliative care settings require reliable and brief quality-of-life (QOL) assessment tools in order to obtain valid results to minimize burden on participants. Traditionally, patients with bone metastases in clinical trials have completed general QOL instruments, which did not cover the key issues pertinent for this specific population. The EORTC QLQ-BM22 was developed to supplement the EORTC QLQ-C30 core questionnaire as a bone metastases specific qualify-of-life instrument with cross-culture relevance. Methods: One hundred and fourteen patients at the Odette Cancer Centre and Princess Margaret Hospital were enrolled. Patients completed the EORTC QLQ-BM22 questionnaire in person at baseline during their clinic appointment, and completed the follow-up BM22 questionnaire one week later by telephone. A follow-up report was completed at the time of the one week follow-up to record any changes in clinical conditions and/or treatments. Results: Employing a 95% confidence interval, an intraclass correlation coefficient (ICC) was used to assess agreement between the baseline and follow-up responses for each BM22 item. The ICC values (median = 0.80; range of 0.55-0.89) for

---

* **Correspondence:** Edward Chow, MBBS, PhD, FRCPC, Department of Radiation Oncology, Odette Cancer Centre, Sunnybrook Health Sciences Centre, 2075 Bayview Avenue, Toronto, ON M4N 3M5, Canada. Tel: 416-480-4998; Fax: 416-480-6002; E-mail: Edward.Chow@sunnybrook.ca

the 22 items revealed 'moderate' (2 items), 'good' (10 items), and 'very good' (10 items) reliability. Conclusion: Based on the overall consistent agreement between the baseline and follow-up interview results, the EORTC QLQ-BM22 appears to be a reliable instrument for cancer patients with bone metastases.

Keywords: EORTC QLQ-BM22, bone metastases, test-retest, reliability, quality of life.

Introduction

Bone metastases are common in patients with advanced cancers (1). Breast and prostate carcinomas are the most common to spread to bone, with an incidence of 75% and 68%, respectively (1). In addition, lung, thyroid, and renal carcinomas metastasize to bone in approximately 40% of cases (1).

Advances in effective systemic treatment and supportive care have substantially improved survival of patients with bone metastases. In fact, the prevalence of bone metastases in cancer patients is estimated to be double the number of new cases (2). For certain subsets of patients with bone metastases (e.g. breast and prostate cancer with predominately bone or bone-only metastases) life expectancies have increased to a range of approximately 2-5 years (3). With this increased survival, effective management of bone metastases has become essential in order to reduce skeletal complications and maximize patient quality-of-life (QOL).

A number of indicators of the need for reassessment of management strategies in patients with bone metastases have been identified (4). Such indicators include: i) pain arising from bone metastases is the most common symptom requiring treatment in cancer patients; ii) the symptoms of bone metastases are often severe; 50 to 75% of patients with bone metastases suffer from severe pain (1); iii) complications of skeletal metastases are common and can seriously impair patient QOL and function. Pain and impaired mobility occur in 65-75% of patients with bone metastases. Fractures of weight-bearing long bones occur in 10-20%; hypercalcaemia occurs in 10-15%; and spinal cord or nerve root compression occurs in 5%; iv) increasing incidence of bone metastases and longer survival duration of patients with bone metastases and v) increasing emphasis to assess the efficacy and side effects of existing and new interventions, as well as QOL from the patient's perspective.

According to the World Health Organization, health is described as 'a state of complete physical, mental and social well-being, and not merely the absence of disease or infirmity' (5). In palliative trials, symptom control as well as QOL is a major endpoint. Quality-of-life measurement is subjective in nature and is a multidimensional construct which reflects functional status, psychosocial well-being, health perceptions, and disease- and treatment-related symptoms from the patient's perspective (6). Quality-of-life incorporates a patient's expectations, satisfaction, value system and the other important aspects of his or her life. Since palliative interventions are unlikely to lead to survival prolongation and significant tumour regression, QOL is a more meaningful endpoint when compared with the traditional endpoints, such as survival times and local control. Thus, any palliative interventions should primarily aim to improve the QOL of patients with advanced cancer.

Some trials have employed the European Organization for Research and Treatment of Cancer QOL Group core questionnaire (EORTC QLQ-C30), version 3. There are a number of advantages to using this instrument, including extensive validation, available reference data, standardized procedures for scoring and translation, and a large number of published studies that have utilized this tool (7). However, it was not specifically designed to address the QOL issues relevant for cancer patients with bone metastases. There was, therefore, a need to develop a disease-specific QOL questionnaire for bone metastases patients to supplement the validated EORTC QLQ-C30. Consequently, the Bone Metastases Module (EORTC QLQ-BM22; from now on referred to as BM22) was created to address this need. This module addresses QOL issues that are particularly important to patients with bone metastases and are not sufficiently covered by the EORTC QLQ-C30. The instrument contains a total of 22 questions with 19 items that form three scales: Painful Sites (questions 1-5), Pain Characteristics (questions 6-8), Functional Interference (questions 9-15), and Psychosocial Aspects (questions 16-22).

The BM22 is presently undergoing large scale international field testing (Phase IV) as part of its development and validation. This phase of development aims to determine the test-retest reliability, validity and cross-cultural applicability of the module by testing the questionnaire in a large, international group of patients. The primary objective of the present study was to examine the test-retest reliability of the BM22, and in doing so determine the degree to which the instrument is free from random measurement error. The secondary objective was to verify the relevance of the 22 items to patients diagnosed with bone metastases.

Methods

Patients attending palliative radiation and medical oncology clinics at the Odette Cancer Centre and Princess Margaret Hospital in Toronto, Ontario between January and March 2008 were considered for study eligibility. Patients exhibiting radiological evidence of osseous metastases who were able to comprehend the survey and provide informed consent were approached to participate. Those who were not fit to complete the questionnaire or were unavailable for follow-up were excluded. In total, 114 patients were able to complete the study.

Once a patient was deemed eligible for study participation by their treating oncologist, he or she was approached by the clinical research assistant to discuss the study during his or her regularly scheduled appointment. All agreeable patients provided written informed consent and completed the BM22 questionnaire (Figure 1) by rating their general pain and the degree of provocation of their symptoms and emotions by various activities. The clinical research assistant was available to assist the patients if necessary and was responsible for collecting patient demographics, disease information and treatment history as baseline measurements. Patients were contacted for follow-up via telephone one week after their initial interview. At this point they were asked to complete the BM22 questionnaire again, and a follow-up report was compiled to record any changes in clinical condition and/or treatments. A one week period was selected as the appropriate time interval due to the recommendation that within this time frame patients are unlikely to both recall their previous responses and to experience significant changes in their condition relating to their bone metastases (7).

During the past week, Have you experienced:	Not at all	A Little	Quite a Bit	Very Much
1. pain in your back?	1	2	3	4
2. pain in your leg(s) or hip(s)?	1	2	3	4
3. pain in your arm(s) or shoulder(s)?	1	2	3	4
4. pain in your chest or rib(s)?	1	2	3	4
5. pain in your buttock(s)?	1	2	3	4
6. constant pain?	1	2	3	4
7. intermittent pain?	1	2	3	4
8. pain not relieved by pain medications?	1	2	3	4
9. pain while sitting or lying down?	1	2	3	4
10. pain when trying to stand up?	1	2	3	4
11. pain while walking?	1	2	3	4
12. pain with activities such as bending or climbing stairs?	1	2	3	4
13. pain with strenuous activity (e.g. exercise, lifting)?	1	2	3	4
14. pain interfered with your sleeping at night?	1	2	3	4
15. modify your daily activities?	1	2	3	4
16. felt isolated from those close to you (e.g. family, friends)?	1	2	3	4
17. thinking about your illness?	1	2	3	4
18. worried about loss of mobility?	1	2	3	4
19. worried about becoming dependent on others?	1	2	3	4
20. worried about your health in the future?	1	2	3	4
21. felt hopeful your pain will get better?	1	2	3	4
22. felt positive about your health?	1	2	3	4

Figure 1. The EORTC QLQ-BM22 Module.

The statistical methodology involved within this study included the Wilcoxon rank-sum test, the Fisher exact test, and Intraclass Correlation Coefficients. The Wilcoxon rank-sum test (for continuous variables) and the Fisher exact test (for categorical variables) were conducted to determine which variables predicted good concordance between both administrations of the questionnaire. Intraclass correlation coefficients (ICCs) were determined to assess the agreement between each BM22 item on the test and retest questionnaires. Intraclass correlation coefficient values range from 0.00 to 1.00 and measure inter-rater reliability. Intraclass correlation coefficients are classified as belonging to one of five categories: Poor (range 0-0.20), fair (range 0.21-0.40), moderate (range 0.41-0.60), good (range 0.61-0.80), or very good (range 0.81-1.00). Statistical Analysis Systems (SAS, version 9.1) Macro was employed to calculate the ICCs with 95% confidence intervals. Results were considered significant at the 5% critical level (two sided p-value < 0.05). The study proposal and consent forms were reviewed and approved by the institutional Research Ethics Boards at both of the participating centres.

Results

Patient characteristics are summarized in table 1. In total, 71 patients were female (62%) and 43 (38%) were male. The median age was 61 years with a range of 32-87 years. Breast and prostate cancers were most prevalent at 61% and 30%, respectively. Lung (4%) and renal cell (2%) carcinomas, as well as multiple myeloma (2%) were less common primaries. In general, patients were most often interviewed within medical oncology clinics (75%). This was followed by radiation oncology (17%) and multidisciplinary clinics (7%). With regards to the extent of patient metastases, the majority of those surveyed had two separate organ systems with metastatic disease (48%), with three (44%) and four (8%) metastatic locations being less frequently witnessed.

Table 1. Patient Characteristics (n=114)

Characteristics	Number of Patients N (%)
Gender	
Male	43 (38)
Female	71 (62)
Age (years)	
Median	61
Range	32-87
Primary Cancer Site	
Breast	69 (61)
Prostate	34 (30)
Lung	4 (4)
Renal Cell	2 (2)
Multiple Myeloma	2 (2)
Colon	1 (1)
Liver	1 (1)
Unknown	1 (1)
Number of Metastatic Sites	
2	23 (48)
3	21 (44)
4	4 (8)
Treatment	
Radiotherapy	87 (76)
Hormone Therapy	84 (76)
Surgery	72 (64)
Bisphosphonate	64 (58)
Chemotherapy	61 (54)

Concordance between test and re-test responses

Good concordance is defined as having the absolute difference between the test and the re-test responses equal to zero. The number of patients who obtained good concordance between the initial and follow-up questionnaires is shown in table 2. Overall, concordance ranged from 56.6% and 75.5% with a median value of 65.1%. Items 16 (felt isolated from those close to you?), 5 (pain in your buttocks?) and 4 (pain in your chest/ribs?) demonstrated the best concordance with 75.5%, 74.5% and 71.7% of responding patients obtaining good concordance, respectively.

The worst concordance was demonstrated by items 7 (intermittent pain?), 17 (thinking about your illness?), and 22 (felt positive about your health?) with only 56.6%, 58.1% and 59.2% of responding patients obtaining good concordance, respectively. Percentages were based on the number of respondents as not all participants answered each item on the questionnaire.

Table 2. Number of Patients with Good Concordance per Item on the EORTC QLQ-BM22

Question Number	Number with Good Concordance *	Total Number of Responses	Percentage
1	69	106	65.1
2	72	106	67.9
3	69	106	65.1
4	76	106	71.7
5	79	106	74.5
6	71	106	67.0
7	60	106	56.6
8	59	89	66.3
9	63	106	59.4
10	63	105	60.0
11	68	104	65.4
12	64	96	66.7
13	40	60	66.7
14	66	105	62.8
15	64	104	61.5
16	80	106	75.5
17	61	105	58.1
18	64	103	62.1
19	68	104	65.4
20	67	105	63.8
21	52	84	61.9
22	61	103	59.2

*The absolute difference between Test response and Re-Test response was calculated for each item, and the number of patients with zero difference was considered as the number with good concordance.

Few demographic variables were successful at consistently predicting good concordance. Only eight items on the questionnaire had significant predictive variables, including items 5 (pain in your buttocks?), 8 (pain not relieved by pain medications?), 9 (pain while sitting or lying down?), 11 (pain while walking?), 14 (pain interfered with your sleeping at night?), 16 (felt isolated from those close to you?), 19 (worried about becoming dependent on others?), and 20 (worried about your health in the future?). Predictors of good concordance for each of the items were as follows: item 5 - the clinic in which the patient was received (p = 0.0001) and their primary cancer site (p = 0.0020); item 8 – clinic (p = 0.0269) and previous radiotherapy treatment (p = 0.0370); item 9 – previous chemotherapy treatment (p = 0.0120); item 11 – previous radiotherapy treatment (p = 0.0037); item 14 – clinic (p = 0.0120); item 16 – age (p = 0.0244); item 19 – previous radiotherapy treatment (p = 0.0494); and item 20 – previous chemotherapy treatment (p=0.0171). The remaining items failed to demonstrate any significant predictors of good concordance.

Agreement between test and re-test items

The ICC values and their respective 95% confidence intervals for each item of the BM22 questionnaire are available in Table 3. Of the 22 items, 10 (45%) demonstrated 'very good' agreement, 10 (45%) demonstrated 'good' agreement, and 2 (9%) demonstrated 'moderate' agreement between the test and retest questionnaires. The ICC values ranged from 0.55 to 0.89 with a median value of 0.80. In general, items related to future perspectives, patient concerns or the impact of osseous metastases on activity demonstrated 'very good' agreement. Items that dealt with the characteristics or location of the pain often demonstrated 'good' agreement. The only location of pain that demonstrated moderate agreement was the buttocks. One's degree of social isolation also only demonstrated moderate agreement.

Table 3. Intraclass Correlation Coefficients (ICC) for Each Item on the EORTC QLQ-BM22

Question Number	ICC	95% Confidence Interval	Interpretation*
1	0.80	0.71-0.86	Good
2	0.84	0.77-0.89	Very Good
3	0.74	0.62-0.82	Good
4	0.65	0.49-0.76	Good
5	0.58	0.38-0.71	Moderate
6	0.76	0.66-0.84	Good
7	0.79	0.69-0.85	Good
8	0.65	0.48-0.76	Good
9	0.77	0.66-0.84	Good
10	0.81	0.73-0.87	Very Good
11	0.83	0.76-0.89	Very Good
12	0.87	0.80-0.91	Very Good
13	0.89	0.84-0.93	Very Good
14	0.76	0.65-0.83	Good
15	0.78	0.68-0.85	Good
16	0.55	0.35-0.69	Moderate
17	0.83	0.76-0.88	Very Good
18	0.81	0.73-0.87	Very Good
19	0.81	0.71-0.86	Very Good
20	0.88	0.82-0.91	Very Good
21	0.86	0.79-0.90	Very Good
22	0.76	0.65-0.83	Good

*The interpretation of the ICC values can be considered as: poor ≤ 0.20, fair 0.21 – 0.40, moderate 0.41 – 0.60, good 0.61 – 0.80, and very good 0.81 – 1.00.

Discussion

The European Organization for Research and Treatment of Cancer (EORTC) QOL Group has endorsed a modular approach to the evaluation of QOL in cancer patients involved in clinical trials since 1986. The development and validation of the C30 core questionnaire initiated this improvement in QOL assessment, and the subsequent cancer- and site-specific modules have continued this advancement (9,10). Detailed guidelines, published to ensure scientific rigour of module development, were strictly followed during the creation of the BM22 (11). The module development process consists of four phases, including: (I) Generation of the relevant QOL issues; (II) Operationalization; (III) Pretesting; and (IV) Large scale international field testing. Phase I includes a literature search and semi-structured interviews with patients and health care professionals to generate a list of potential QOL issues. Phase II involves operationalizing the list of QOL issues into questions while using the format and time frame of the C30 core questionnaire. Phase III aims to identify and solve potential problems in the questionnaire's administration (e.g. the phrasing of questions, the sequence of questions), as well as to determine the need for additional questions or the elimination of others. Phase IV, as previously mentioned, involves testing the module questionnaire in a larger, international group of patients in order to determine its test-retest reliability, validity and cross-cultural applicability. Once a module has been developed, it is administered along with the C30 core questionnaire (or the C15-PAL for palliative patients with low performance status) to obtain a comprehensive QOL assessment in cancer patients.

The present study served to determine the reliability of the BM22 questionnaire. Concordance or percent agreement was calculated for each item of the module and determined the proportion of all patients whom provided identical responses to test and retest questions (12). Overall, good concordance was consistently demonstrated by a majority of patients for each item of the questionnaire. The best concordance was obtained by items dealing with pain locations and social isolation. This finding is intuitive, as pain is expected to be found in the location of osseous lesions, which are unlikely to change within a week's time. In addition, a patient's interpreted level of social interaction is also anticipated to remain constant within the initial and follow-up interviews. The worst concordance occurred in the items dealing with intermittent pain and psychosocial aspects. These findings are also not unexpected, as intermittent pain, by definition, is presumed to vary, and future concerns may be altered in tune with these bodily changes. Not all participants answered each item on the questionnaire, and so percentages were merely based on the number of respondents. This may have affected the results obtained within the study. However, as the questions were generally answered by a great majority of the participants, it is unlikely that the results have been altered to any significant degree.

Good concordance was successfully predicted by few demographic variables. The clinic in which the patient was interviewed and having previous radiotherapy treatment both significantly predicted good concordance in three items each. Previous chemotherapy treatment was a successful predictor in two items, and age and primary care site both only predicted good concordance in one item of the questionnaire. Despite these significant findings, it is unlikely that these demographic variables are relevant for maximizing concordance in future module development, as no single variable was a consistent predictor throughout the entirety of the BM22 questionnaire. In addition, a large proportion of the interviewed sample was breast cancer patients. Therefore, it is possible that this heavily weighted group of individuals may have induced statistical significance of variables relevant to their own condition (e.g. clinic and previous treatment). For this reason, it is suggested that these findings be interpreted with due caution until future research can confirm their significance.

An important potential limitation when employing concordance is that this measure fails to account for agreement that chance alone could predict (12). Therefore, ICC's, which correct for chance agreement, may be a more suitable measure for determining the test-retest reliability of the BM22. As the majority of items demonstrated either 'very good' or 'good' reliability, it appears as if the module is a reliable instrument. No specific ICC cut-offs for identifying module reliability are available within the EORTC guidelines (11). Therefore, the results and conclusions of previously published EORTC studies were employed as a measure of which to compare our results and draw conclusions in regards to our own module's reliability (10,13,14).

The two items that only expressed moderate reliability may have been influenced by the varying circumstances under which the initial and follow-up questionnaires were administered. The baseline measures were acquired following regularly scheduled appointments in comparison to the telephone interviews that were conducted for the follow-up portion of the study. For example, pain may have been exacerbated in a patient's buttocks after traveling to the hospital and waiting in the clinic for his or her appointment. This pain may have been less severe when they were interviewed in the comfort of their home one week later by telephone. In addition, patients are often accompanied by their family or friends to their clinic appointments. This may have enhanced their feelings of social support and reduced their feelings of isolation. Consequently, one week after their appointment they have been alone in their home when contacted for follow-up. This may have altered their perception of their own personal isolation from their opinions the previous week.

To ensure the most accurate reliability of the measure, perhaps patients should have been interviewed in the same atmosphere for each administration of the questionnaire. However, in order to obtain informed consent, the patients had to be approached in person, and it would not be appropriate to insist that patients travel back to the clinic one week later to simply fill out the questionnaire again. This limitation may have served to reduce the true reliability of the BM22, but seems worthwhile to minimize the burden on those participating in the study. Failure to accept this slight limitation may have resulted in a significant reduction of in the number of patients agreeable to participate, or may have increased the number of individuals lost to follow-up. Therefore, it would seem as if this was a worthwhile sacrifice to make. The BM22 has undergone slight modification since the completion of our accrual.

The development and validation of a QOL assessment tool specifically for patients with bone metastases is vital. Such an instrument will enable better patient management as an identifier of effective treatments for cancer patients in a clinical setting. Furthermore, the establishment of a standardized instrument will facilitate cross-study comparisons for the development of new treatments in patients with bone metastases. The successful determination of the module's test-retest reliability within the present study will assist in achieving EORTC validation. However, completion of Phase IV large scale international field testing of the module is required before the module can be finalized for use in future clinical trials.

Based on the overall consistent agreement that was witnessed between the baseline and follow-up interviews, the BM22 appears to be a reliable instrument and will be a brief and suitable tool in future clinical trials involving palliative patients with bone metastases.

Acknowledgments

This study was supported by Michael and Karyn Goldstein Cancer Research Fund and Novartis Oncology. We thank the research assistants in the accrual and Stacy Lue for her secretarial assistance.

References

[1] InSightec.com: InSightec Image Guided Treatment Ltd. Pain palliation of bone metastases – overview. Accessed 2009 Feb 23. URL: http://www.insightec.com/135-en-r10/BoneMetastases.aspx

[2] Harrington KD. The management of acetabular insufficiency secondary to metastatic malignant disease. J Bone Joint Surg Am 1981;63:653-4.

[3] Harrington KD. Prophylactic management of impending fractures. In: Harrington KD. Orthopedic management of metastatic bone disease. St Louis, MO: CV Mosby, 1988:283-307.

[4] Patrick DL, Ferketich SL, Frame PS, Harris JJ, Hendricks CB, Levin B, et al. National Institutes of Health state-of-the-science conference statemen t: Symptom management in cancer: Pain, depression, and fatigue, July 15-17, 2002. J Natl Cancer Inst 2003;95(15):1110-7.

[5] World Health Organization. Constitution of the World Health Organization. Geneva, Switzerland: WHO Basic Documents, 1948.

[6] Soni MK and Cella D. Quality of life and symptom measures in oncology: An overview. Am J Manag Care 2002;8(18):S560-73.

[7] Streiner DL, Norman GR. Health measurement scales: a practical guide to their development and use. New York: Oxford Univ Press, 2003:126-52.

[8] Nunnally JC, Bernstein IH. Psychometric theory. New York: McGraw-Hill, 1994:264-5.

[9] Aaronson NK, Ahmedzai S, Bergman B, Bullinger M, Cull A, Duez NJ, Filiberti A, Flechtner H, Fleishman SB, de Haes JC, et al. The European Organization for Research and Treatment of Cancer QLQ-C30: A quality-of-life instrument for use in international clinical trials in oncology. J Natl Cancer Inst 1993;85(5):365-76.

[10] Chie W-C, Chang K-J, Huang C-S, K W-H. Quality of life of breast cancer patients in Taiwan: Validation of the Taiwan Chinese version of the EORTC QLQ-C30 and EORTC QLQ-BR23. Psychooncology 2003;12:729-35.

[11] Blazeby J, Sprangers M, Cull A, Groenvold M, Bottomley A. EORTC quality of life group: guidelines for developing questionnaire modules. Third edition revised. Accessed 2009 Feb 23. URL: http://groups.eortc.be/qol/downloads/200208module_development _guidelines.pdf

[12] Koepsell TD, Weiss NS. Epidemiologic methods: studying the occurrence of illness. New York, New York: Oxford Univ Press, 2003.

[13] Sprangers MAG, te Velde A, Aaronson NK. On behalf of the European Organization for Research and Treatment of Cancer Study Group on Quality of Life. The construction and testing of the EORTC colorectal cancer-specific quality of life questionnaire module (QLQ-CR38). Eur J Cancer 1999;35(2):238-47.

[14] Bloechle C, Izbicki JR, Knoefel WT, Kuechler T, Broelsch CE. Quality of life in chronic pancreatitis – results after duodenum-preserving resection of the head of the pancreas. Pancreas 1995;11(1):77-85.

In: Pain Management Yearbook 2009
Editor: Joav Merrick

ISBN: 978-1-61209-666-7
©2012 Nova Science Publishers, Inc.

Chapter 45

DETERMINING RELIABILITY OF PATIENT PERCEPTIONS OF IMPORTANT BONE METASTASES QUALITY OF LIFE ISSUES

*Sarah Campos, BSc(C), Liying Zhang, PhD and Edward Chow, MBBS**

Rapid Response Radiotherapy Program, Department of Radiation Oncology, Odette Cancer Centre, Sunnybrook Health Sciences Centre, University of Toronto, Toronto, Ontario, Canada

Abstract

The purpose of this study was to test the reliability of patient perceptions in important bone metastases quality of life (QOL) items. A secondary objective was to determine whether changes in disease progression or changes in treatment affected the reliability of their responses. Methods: Twenty seven patients were asked to complete the EORTC – QLQ BM61 Bone Metastases Module upon visiting the Odette Cancer Centre on two occasions between 2005 and 2008. Patients were asked to complete 61 items assessing quality of life, ranking each item on a scale of 1 to 4 based on their own experience, then indicating whether they would recommend inclusion on the final questionnaire for each item. Basic demographic information was collected from each patient on first and re-approaches, as well as information regarding patients' condition and treatment regimens. New complications and changes in therapies were recorded. Results: Patient perception of the important bone metastases QOL issues was overall reliable over time, but was found to be related to changes in treatment and complications of disease.

Conclusion: The finding should be kept in mind when developing QOL measurement tools based on patient perceptions of generated QOL issues, and when assessing the reliability of QOL measurement tools over time.

Keywords: Bone metastases, quality of life, patient perceptions.

---

* **Correspondence:** Edward Chow, MBBS, PhD, FRCPC, Department of Radiation Oncology, Odette Cancer Centre, Sunnybrook Health Sciences Centre, 2075 Bayview Avenue, Toronto, ON M4N 3M5, Canada. Tel: 416-480-4998; Fax: 416-480-6002; E-mail: Edward.Chow@sunnybrook.ca

Introduction

Metastases of cancer to the bone are a complication that occurs frequently in a wide population of individuals diagnosed with advanced cancer. Bone metastases are also much more common than primary bone tumors (1). Approximately 75% of breast cancer patients will develop bone metastases (2-4), along with 68% of those affected by prostate cancer (2,3). The incidence in renal, thyroid and lung cancer is slightly lower, but still amounts to about 40% of cases (2,3). Some cancers have relatively low incidence rates, such as gastric cancer with only 5% (4), however bone metastases has been identified in 70-80% of cancer patients on autopsy (2,3).

Patients with predominantly bone only disease can survive from 2-5 years after diagnosis, which is a marked improvement in recent years due to the use of more effective systemic therapies (3). Survival has thus been discarded as a primary endpoint for clinical trials of bone metastases, in favor of improved quality of life (QOL) (3,5). The importance of QOL is in fact, underscored by the increased survival times of these patients, as end of life care is often not imminent.

One of the most common symptoms of bone metastases is pain (2,3, 6,7), affecting at least 50-75% of bone metastases patients (3), with 50% of all cancer pain due to bone metastases (4), and severe pain reported in 45% of patients assessed in one study (8). Pain is frequently under treated (8,9) and this poses a major public health concern (9), as pain can significantly hinder patients' QOL and ability to carry out daily activities. A recent study found that of those patients complaining of moderate or severe pain, 34% were either only prescribed weak opiates, non opiates or no analgesics at all (8). Other frequent complications include pathological fractures (4,10), occurring in 25% of patients on average (11). These fractures also affect many aspects of QOL causing unmanageable pain, motor impairment, neurological complications (12), and even negatively affecting survival (13). Other prevalent symptoms reflecting quality of life include fatigue, drowsiness and a poor sense of well being (2).

Following the World Health Organization's definition of health as the complete state of physical, mental and social well being, notwithstanding the absence of disease or infirmity (14), QOL is a well accepted outcome for patients in clinical settings, including trials (5). The EORTC- QLQ- 30 is a widely available QOL measurement tool used in the cancer population that focuses on common symptoms and concerns faced by all cancer patients, including those of physical, emotional, social, and cognitive concern. It is supplemented by different modules applying to sub populations of cancer patients, including those affected by lung, and breast cancer. The EORTC- QLQ – C-30 has been validated in various populations internationally, and has been demonstrated to be a reliable tool (15).

More recently, a bone metastases module to supplement the EORTC- QLQ C-30 has been developed, after extensive interviews with bone metastases patients and health care professionals to determine the most commonly faced issues impacting patient quality of life. Development of this module was done in several stages. Stage I involved the generation of a tentative 61 item questionnaire, later to be refined in Stage II, for a final product at Stage III of an internationally validated 22 item questionnaire. The 61 item questionnaire, or EORTC – QLQ BM61, was administered to patients in 2005 to obtain feedback on the most important items to be included in the final questionnaire. The purpose of this study was to use that data, and re-approach patients at a later date to test the reliability of patients' responses, as well as their perception of the most important items on the questionnaire. A secondary objective was to determine whether changes in disease progression of patients during the interval between both approaches, as well as changes in treatment, affected the reliability of their responses.

Methods

In 2005, 130 patients were asked to complete the newly compiled EORTC – QLQ BM61 Bone Metastases Module (see appendix I): a 61 item precursor to the EORTC – QLQ BM22 (BM22) questionnaire. The BM22 was designed to meet the need for a QOL measurement tool specifically for cancer patients with metastases to the bone. The BM22 has demonstrated reproducibility and validity, and has been validated on an international basis (16). This questionnaire, having been refined for a lower patient burden, and validated in clinical settings, is a useful tool for helping clinicians uncovers patient concerns and symptoms. The patients were approached upon visiting the Rapid Response Radiotherapy clinic, or other clinics at the Odette Cancer Centre in Toronto, Ontario. All patients were asked to complete the 61 items assessing quality of life, rating each on a scale of 1 to 4, based on their own experience for that item. Patients were also asked to indicate, for each item, whether they considered that particular item relevant enough to be included on a final, condensed version of the questionnaire.

Between 2007 and 2008, 27 of these patients were re-approached upon a visit to a clinic at the Odette Cancer Centre. The follow ups were conducted on the basis of patient attendance to clinics, and thus varied in their intervals from baseline. Patients were again asked to complete the EORTC- QLQ BM61, ranking each item on a scale of 1 to 4 based on their own experience, then indicating whether they would recommend inclusion on the final questionnaire for each item. Written consent was obtained from patients both at first approach and re-approach, and the purpose, benefits and risks of the study was clearly explained to them at both times.

Outcomes and statistical analysis

Results were expressed as mean, standard deviation (SD), median and range for continuous variables, as proportion (%) for categorical variables. Basic demographic information was collected from each patient on first and re-approaches, as well as information regarding patients' condition and treatment regimens. Performance status, date of primary cancer diagnosis, date of bone metastasis diagnosis, time between original cancer diagnosis and diagnosis of bone metastasis, as well as primary cancer site and sites of metastasis were recorded both at baseline and at re-approach. Skeletal related events include spinal cord compression, cauda equina syndrome, pathological fractures, hypercalcaemia, surgical intervention to bone, or radiotherapy (RT) to bone. Dates of all skeletal related events were recorded for each patient at baseline and on re-approach. Patients' systemic therapy regimens included their use of hormonal therapy, bisphosphonates and chemotherapy. The type of treatment and specific drug was recorded at both time points, as were the start and stop dates.

Any RT was recorded, including the sites of RT, the doses received and the dates of treatment. This information was then compared at analysis to determine which patients had developed new sites of metastases and/or new skeletal related events since baseline. Changes in all therapies between baseline and re-approach were also noted. Fisher exact test was used to compare the QOL change (or Final Questionnaire FQ change) on the new complications and treatments. QOL or FQ change was considered as zero change or non-zero change between baseline and re-approach. Two-sided p-value of less than 0.05 was considered as statistical significance. Statistical Analysis Software (SAS Institute, version 9.1 for windows) was used in the study.

Results

The demographics of the 27 patients re-approached, including their ages, gender, performance status (measured by KPS), duration of cancer diagnosis, duration of cancer diagnosis before diagnosis of bone metastases, and primary cancer sites are given in table 1. Information regarding the clinic in which the patients were re-approached can also be found in table 1. Patients' complications and treatment regimens are listed in table 2.

Using the Fischer exact test, patients' responses to the 61 quality of life items on the EORTC-QLQ BM61 at baseline in 2005 and at re-approach in 2007-2008 were compared. Any changes in these responses reflect patients' perception of change in their quality of life in that time period. Of 61 items, item #1 assessing the patient's chronic pain, item #18, their ability to perform self-care, and item #43, their emotional stress related to receiving a diagnosis of advanced, incurable cancer, showed significant change. In terms of the items patients wished to include on the final questionnaire, no significant change was observed for all of the items.

Changes in patients' response to QOL items were significantly correlated to new complications or changes in treatments in 9 of 61 items (see table 3). Changes in response to item #15, difficulty planning activities outside the home, and in item #23, difficulty in standing up, and changes in response to item #55, worry about running out of medical treatments were related to new sites of RT. Item #25, difficulty sitting, showed correlation to new sites of metastases; item #27, difficulty lying flat was related to changes in hormonal therapy; and item #29, the presence of drowsiness was related to the incidence of new skeletal related events and new sites of RT.

QOL responses to item #42, mood changes and item #44, increased focus on spiritual issues were related to changes in bisphosphonates and chemotherapy, respectively.

Patients' selection of items for the final questionnaire was related to new complication and treatment in 10 of 61 items (see table 4). Changes in all ten items either showed correlation ($p<0.05$) to new skeletal related events, new RT, changes in chemotherapy or new sites of metastasis. Changes in selection of item #20, difficulty in completing daily tasks, #30, dizziness, #34, strength of relationship to family and friends, #35, the presence of a clear, alert mind, were only shown to be related to new skeletal related events. Changes in selection of item #52, worry about the future were only related to new RT. Changes in selection of item #38, reluctance to use pain medicines were related to changes in chemotherapy. Changes in items #29, drowsiness, and item #30, confusion were related to both new skeletal events and new RT. Changes in selection of item #41, frustration, for the final questionnaire was shown to be related to new sites of metastasis.

Table 1. Patient Baseline Demographics

Sex	
Male	9 (33.3%)
Female	18 (66.7%)
Age (years)	
n	27
Mean ± SD	60.5 ± 10.5
Median (range)	61 (41 – 82)
KPS	
n	26
Mean ± SD	78.8 ± 14.2
Median (range)	80 (50 – 100)
Duration of primary cancer diagnosis (years)	
n	26
Mean ± SD	6.22 ± 6.31
Median (range)	4.31 (0.003 – 18.4)
Duration of bone metastasis diagnosis (year)	
n	19
Mean ± SD	1.44 ± 1.13
Median (range)	1.33 (0 – 3.44)
Duration from cancer diagnosis to BM (year)	
n	19
Mean ± SD	5.08 ± 5.99
Median (range)	3.77 (0 – 17.4)
Location of re-approach	
Inpatient ward	2 (7.4%)
Medical Oncology Clinic	18 (66.7%)
Palliative Pain Outpatient Clinic	3 (11.1%)
Palliative Radiation Outpatient Clinic	2 (7.4%)
Radiation Oncology Clinic	2 (7.4%)
Primary cancer site	
Breast	15 (55.6%)
Prostate	2 (7.4%)
Lung	1 (3.7%)
Renal cell	2 (7.4%)
Multiple myeloma	4 (14.8%)
Others	3 (11.1%)

Table 2. Changes in Patient Disease Complications and Treatment

New sites of metastases	
No	19 (70.4%)
Yes	8 (29.6%)
New skeletal related events	
No	14 (51.9%)
Yes	13 (48.2%)
New pathological fracture	
No	24 (88.9%)
Yes	3 (11.1%)
Surgery since baseline	
No	26 (96.3%)
Yes	1 (3.7%)
New Radiotherapy	
No	15 (55.6%)
Yes	12 (44.4%)
Changes in Bisphosphonate therapy	
No	22 (81.5%)
Yes	5 (18.5%)
Changes in Chemotherapy	
No	9 (33.3%)
Yes	18 (66.7%)
Changes in Hormone therapy	
No	20 (74.1%)
Yes	7 (25.9%)
New sites of Radiotherapy	
No	15 (55.6%)
Yes	12 (44.4%)

Table 3. Comparison of QOL changes with New Complications and Treatments*

Item #	New site of metastases	New Skeletal events	New pathological fracture	Surgery since baseline	New Radio-therapy	Changes in Bisphosphonates	Changes in Chemo	Changes in Hormone therapy	New sites of radiation
11	0.3981	0.1283	0.5692	0.4444	0.0071	0.9999	0.2172	0.1850	0.2576
15	0.9999	0.2087	0.9999	0.9999	0.0433	0.9999	0.3748	0.9999	0.0433
23	0.4048	0.9999	0.9999	0.4074	0.9999	0.3705	0.0969	0.6618	0.0473
25	0.0433	0.7036	0.5692	0.9999	0.7068	0.3419	0.1266	0.6618	0.4408
27	0.6776	0.7064	0.9999	0.4815	0.1283	0.1647	0.6946	0.0329	0.7036
29	0.0687	0.0138	0.5385	0.3846	0.6891	0.3402	0.0873	0.6680	0.0426
42	0.9999	0.9999	0.9999	0.9999	0.9999	0.0391	0.4110	0.9999	0.4283
44	0.9999	0.2519	0.9999	0.4074	0.4517	0.6185	0.0417	0.0840	0.1302
55	0.9999	0.6483	0.5453	0.9999	0.0200	0.9999	0.9999	0.9999	0.6618

*Fisher exact test was used to compare QOL change (zero change vs. non-zero change) on new complications and treatments. The Item was not listed in the table if there is no any statistical significance on all complications and treatments.

Table 4. Comparison of Patient Selection for Final Questionnaire (FQ) and New Complications and Treatments*

Item #	New site of metastases	New Skeletal events	New pathological fracture	Surgery since baseline	New Radiotherapy	Changes in Bisphosphonates	Changes in Chemotherapy	Changes in Hormone therapy	New sites of radiation
20	0.5165	0.0440	0.5165	0.2000	0.5253	0.9999	0.5055	0.9999	0.2418
29	0.9999	0.0319	0.9999	0.3846	0.0319	0.9999	0.0754	0.9999	0.9999
30	0.9999	0.0150	0.5055	0.9999	0.0150	0.9999	0.2208	0.9999	0.0949
31	0.9999	0.0030	0.9999	0.3571	0.0909	0.9999	0.0859	0.9999	0.2657
32	0.1084	0.5105	0.4231	0.9999	0.0350	0.2308	0.9999	0.2028	0.2028
34	0.5604	0.0256	0.4762	0.2667	0.2352	0.9999	0.2308	0.5165	0.9999
35	0.5604	0.0256	0.4762	0.2667	0.2352	0.9999	0.2308	0.9999	0.2352
38	0.5055	0.0909	0.9999	0.3571	0.0909	0.9999	0.0310	0.5804	0.2657
41	0.0410	0.2448	0.5055	0.2857	0.9999	0.9999	0.2208	0.2507	0.5804
52	0.1538	0.9999	0.5165	0.9999	0.0440	0.3714	0.9999	0.5253	0.9999

*Fisher exact test was used to compare FQ change (zero change vs. non-zero change) on new complications and treatments. The Item was not listed in the table if there is no any statistical significance on all complications and treatments.

Discussion

QOL depends largely on many factors, including health status, financial status, job satisfaction, and living conditions. QOL that depends solely on an individual's health is known as Health Related Quality of Life (HR-QOL). In cancer patients, the morbidities associated with the disease often have such a huge impact on their lives that as symptoms worsen, QOL can be considered equivalent to HR-QOL (17). This is especially true for patients with bone metastases, where symptom control is often the primary goal of treatment. In the current study, bone metastases patients were asked about their QOL perceptions over three years, and it is almost certain that they would suffer from new complications due to disease progression during that time. These may take the form of new sites of metastasis, skeletal related events or increased pain. Systemic treatments, such as hormone therapy or chemotherapy are initiated in certain patients, depending on other disease related factors, but these therapies can only slow disease progression (4). It is therefore important to consider QOL as an endpoint for these patients.

QOL fluctuates frequently in bone metastases patients over time, as complications and their treatments can easily diminish or improve it. Treatments such as RT and bisphosphonates are used for symptom palliation and prevention of skeletal related events, which are a main cause of diminished QOL in these patients. RT has been shown to significantly improve pain, and help local control at sites of metastases (9,18,19). One study compared symptom distress of patients before and after RT. Patients who responded to RT, generally had decreased symptoms, including pain and fatigue as soon as two weeks after baseline, while symptoms in patients who did not respond stayed constant (2). Pathological fractures are another serious complication of bone metastases, and can cause pain, motor impairment, and neurological complications (6,7,20). The use of bisphosphonates can delay and prevent pathological fractures in many bone metastases patients (11,21, 22), thereby preventing further impaired QOL.

Significant change in QOL was observed in two of the 61 items on the EORTC–QLQ BM61, over nearly three years between baseline and re-approach, which is expected given the nature of our bone metastases population. One of those items was the ability to perform self care (item #18), which is very reflective of a patient's performance status and QOL. We also found that of the 61 items, change in QOL responses for 9, were correlated to new complications or altered treatment regimens, which is not surprising since those factors greatly influence QOL. This relationship is not an indication of the reliability of patients' perceptions, as it likely reflects real changes in their QOL as a result of treatment.

There was no significant change in the items that patients selected for the final questionnaire between baseline and re-approach. This indicates that their perceptions of relevant QOL items did not change over time. This shows good reliability of patient perceptions of important QOL issues, which is very important since most QOL measurement tools are developed from patient perceptions. Accurate QOL measurement based on patient perception is therefore the most meaningful evaluation of patient QOL.

When assessing the relationship of the change in items patients selected for the final questionnaire and complications and treatment, we found that 10 of the 61 items showed a significant value. This indicates that increased complications of disease and changes in treatment, can affect patients perceptions of important QOL items.

Patient perceptions of any disease endpoint are not static, and change according to their own disease experiences. This means that the experience of new complications and treatments likely affect patient perceptions on QOL. For example, early in their disease, a patient may not assign importance to QOL items regarding mobility, but once immobilized by a fracture their importance becomes clear.

This weakens the reliability of patient perceptions, but uncovers important information regarding patients' ever-evolving perceptions of QOL.

A limitation of the current study is the relatively small sample size. It is likely that if all the patients who were originally sampled had been re-approached, the results would have varied significantly. However, due to the longitudinal nature of our study, and the short lifespan of our patient population, it is likely that the patients re-approached are representative of those patients who survived since baseline. Furthermore, the performance status of this sample was considerably high (median 70), for a population of palliative cancer patients. This is again, likely a survival bias, as most patients who survived during the study period would be expected to have a low burden of disease. Nevertheless, high performance status is reflective of high QOL, and therefore perceptions related to that endpoint may be skewed.

QOL is considered a meaningful endpoint partially because it accounts for patient perspective, as well as responsiveness and change over time (3). This study was able to provide insight into how QOL is perceived by patient and how it evolves over time. Furthermore, it indicated the reliability of the BM61 in assessing patient QOL. Although the BM61 is not used on a large scale for this purpose, it represents a precursor to a validated QOL questionnaire developed through patient perceptions.

Many QOL measurement tools are developed in this way, and assessing the reliability of the BM61 ultimately provides insight on how patients perceive QOL in their own lives, as well as those of patients with similar conditions.

Conclusions

Patient perception of the importance of particular QOL issues was overall reliable over time, but was found to be related to changes in treatment and complications of disease. This should be kept in mind when developing QOL measurement tools based on patient perceptions of generated QOL issues, and when assessing the reliability of QOL measurement tools over time.

Acknowledgments

This project was funded by Michael and Karyn Goldstein Cancer Research Fund and Novartis Oncology. We thank Stacy Lue of her secretarial assistance. Conflicts of interest notification: None.

Appendix I: The EORTC-QLQ BM61 Tool

QUALITY OF LIFE ISSUES		i) Please indicate for each experience separately, the extent to which you have had it during your illness, on a scale of (1) "not at all" to (4) "very much."				ii) Include this issue on the final questionnaire? (circle Yes or No for each item)	
		Not At All (1)	A Little (2)	Quite a Bit (3)	Very Much (4)		
SYMPTOMS							
1	Long-term (or chronic) pain	1	2	3	4	Yes	No
2	Short-term (or acute), severe pain	1	2	3	4	Yes	No
3	Pain at rest (i.e. when sitting)	1	2	3	4	Yes	No
4	Pain with activity (i.e. when walking)	1	2	3	4	Yes	No
5	Pain aggravation with movement or weight-bearing	1	2	3	4	Yes	No
6	Uncontrolled, unmanageable pain not relieved by pain killers	1	2	3	4	Yes	No
7	Pain at night preventing sleep	1	2	3	4	Yes	No
8	Aches and stiffness	1	2	3	4	Yes	No
9	Lack of energy	1	2	3	4	Yes	No
10	Numbness	1	2	3	4	Yes	No
11	Tingling	1	2	3	4	Yes	No
12	Burning Sensation	1	2	3	4	Yes	No
13	Postural problems	1	2	3	4	Yes	No
FUNCTION							
14	Limited movement due to pain	1	2	3	4	Yes	No
15	Difficulty planning activities outside the home	1	2	3	4	Yes	No
16	Difficulty traveling outside the home (i.e. using public transportation, driving, sitting in car)	1	2	3	4	Yes	No

QUALITY OF LIFE ISSUES		i) Please indicate for each experience separately, the extent to which you have had it during your illness, on a scale of (1) "not at all" to (4) "very much."				ii) Include this issue on the final questionnaire? (circle Yes or No for each item)	
		Not At All (1)	A Little (2)	Quite a Bit (3)	Very Much (4)		
FUNCTION (continued)							
17	Difficulty in carrying out meaningful activity (including employment)	1	2	3	4	Yes	No
18	Able to perform self-care	1	2	3	4	Yes	No
19	Able to return to work promptly	1	2	3	4	Yes	No
20	Difficulty carrying out usual daily tasks (i.e. grocery shopping, work outside the home, housework)	1	2	3	4	Yes	No
21	Difficulty bending	1	2	3	4	Yes	No
22	Difficulty lifting	1	2	3	4	Yes	No
23	Difficulty standing up	1	2	3	4	Yes	No
24	Difficulty climbing stairs	1	2	3	4	Yes	No
25	Difficulty sitting	1	2	3	4	Yes	No
26	Difficulty lying in bed	1	2	3	4	Yes	No
27	Difficulty lying flat	1	2	3	4	Yes	No
28	Ability to have sex	1	2	3	4	Yes	No
SIDE EFFECTS FROM TREATMENT OF BONE METASTASES							
29	Drowsiness	1	2	3	4	Yes	No
30	Confusion	1	2	3	4	Yes	No
31	Dizziness	1	2	3	4	Yes	No
PSYCHOSOCIAL							
32	Able to perform role functioning (including domestic and family roles)	1	2	3	4	Yes	No
33	Feeling socially isolated	1	2	3	4	Yes	No

Appendix I. (Continued)

	QUALITY OF LIFE ISSUES	\multicolumn{4}{c	}{i) Please indicate for each experience separately, the extent to which you have had it during your illness, on a scale of (1) "not at all" to (4) "very much."}	\multicolumn{2}{c	}{ii) Include this issue on the final questionnaire? (circle Yes or No for each item)}
		Not At All (1)	A Little (2)	Quite a Bit (3)	Very Much (4)		
\multicolumn{8}{	l	}{PSYCHOSOCIAL (continued)}
34	Strengthened relationships with family and friends	1	2	3	4	Yes	No
35	Have a clear, alert mind	1	2	3	4	Yes	No
36	Feel in control, positive, and confident	1	2	3	4	Yes	No
37	Hope to live as long as possible	1	2	3	4	Yes	No
38	Reluctance to use pain medication	1	2	3	4	Yes	No
39	Fear of addiction to pain medication	1	2	3	4	Yes	No
40	Anxiety	1	2	3	4	Yes	No
41	Frustration	1	2	3	4	Yes	No
42	Mood changes	1	2	3	4	Yes	No
43	Emotional stress of diagnosis of advanced, incurable cancer	1	2	3	4	Yes	No
44	Increased focus on spiritual issues	1	2	3	4	Yes	No
45	Loss of interest in activities you normally enjoy	1	2	3	4	Yes	No
46	Loss of interest in sex	1	2	3	4	Yes	No
47	Worry about pain	1	2	3	4	Yes	No
48	Worry about suffering	1	2	3	4	Yes	No
49	Worry about loss of mobility compromising independence	1	2	3	4	Yes	No
50	Worry about becoming dependent on others	1	2	3	4	Yes	No
51	Worry about current health status	1	2	3	4	Yes	No

QUALITY OF LIFE ISSUES		i) Please indicate for each experience separately, the extent to which you have had it during your illness, on a scale of (1) "not at all" to (4) "very much."				ii) Include this issue on the final questionnaire? (circle Yes or No for each item)	
		Not At All (1)	A Little (2)	Quite a Bit (3)	Very Much (4)		
PSYCHOSOCIAL (continued)							
52	Worry about the future	1	2	3	4	Yes	No
53	Worry about becoming bed-bound	1	2	3	4	Yes	No
54	Worry about disease progression, deterioration in condition, and future complications	1	2	3	4	Yes	No
55	Worry about running out of medical treatments	1	2	3	4	Yes	No
56	Worry about hospitalization	1	2	3	4	Yes	No
57	Worry about ending days in a hospital or nursing home	1	2	3	4	Yes	No
58	Worry about death	1	2	3	4	Yes	No
TREATMENT EXPECTATIONS							
59	Hope for sustained pain relief (reduce pain for as long as possible)	1	2	3	4	Yes	No
60	Hope treatment will reduce pain as much as possible	1	2	3	4	Yes	No
OTHER ISSUES							
61	Financial burden due to the illness	1	2	3	4	Yes	No

References

[1] American Cancer Society. Cancer facts and figures. Atlanta, GA: Am Cancer Society, 1997.
[2] Chow E, Fan G, Hadi S, Filipczak L. Symptom clusters in cancer patients with bone metastases. Support Care Cancer 2007; 15(9):1035-43.
[3] Chow E, Hoskin P, van der Linden Y, Bottomley A, Velikova G. Quality of life and symptom end points in palliative bone metastases trials. Clin Oncol 2006;18(1):67-9.
[4] Kanis JA. Bone and cancer: Pathophysiology and treatment of metastases. Bone 1995;17(2 Suppl):101S-5S.
[5] Soni MK, Cella D. Quality of life and symptom measures in oncology: An overview. Am J Manag Care 2002;8(18 Suppl):S560-73.
[6] Kanis JA, O'Rourke N, McCloskey EV. Consequences of neoplasia-induced bone resorption and the use of clodronate. Int J Oncol 1994;5:713-31.
[7] Paterson AH. Bone metastases in breast cancer, prostate cancer and myeloma. Bone 1987;8(Suppl 1):S17-22.
[8] Yau V, Chow E, Davis L, Holden L, Schueller T, Danjoux C. Pain management in cancer patients with bone metastases remains a challenge. J Pain Sympt Manage 2004;27(1):1-3.

[9] Patrick DL, Ferketich SL, Frame PS, Harris JJ, Hendricks CB, Levin B, et al. National institutes of health state-of-the-science conference statement: Symptom management in cancer: Pain, depression, and fatigue, july 15-17, 2002. J Natl Cancer Inst 2004;Monogr(32):9-16.

[10] Saad F. Impact of bone metastases on patient's quality of life and importance of treatment. Eur Urol Suppl 2006;5:547-50.

[11] Saad F, Gleason DM, Murray R, Tchekmedyian S, Venner P, Lacombe L, et al. Long-term efficacy of zoledronic acid for the prevention of skeletal complications in patients with metastatic hormone-refractory prostate cancer. J Natl Cancer Inst 2004;96(11):879-82.

[12] Harrington KD. Orthopedic surgical management of skeletal complications of malignancy. Cancer 1997;80(8 Suppl):1614-27.

[13] Oefelein MG, Ricchiuti V, Conrad W, Resnick MI. Skeletal fractures negatively correlate with overall survival in men with prostate cancer. J Urol 2002;168(3):1005-7.

[14] World Health Organization. Constitution of the world health organization. Geneva, Switzerland: WHO, 1948.

[15] Osoba D, Zee B, Pater J, Warr D, Kaizer L, Latreille J. Psychometric properties and responsiveness of the EORTC quality of life questionnaire (QLQ-C30) in patients with breast, ovarian and lung cancer. Qual Life Res 1994;3(5):353-64.

[16] Chow E, Hird A, Velikova G, Johnson C, Dewolf L, Bezjak A, et al. The european organisation for research and treatment of cancer quality of life questionnaire for patients with bone metastases: The EORTC QLQ-BM22. Eur J Cancer 2008 Dec 17 [Epub ahead of print].

[17] Guyatt GH, Feeny DH, Patrick DL. Measuring health-related quality of life. Ann Intern Med 1993;118(8):622-9.

[18] Hoskin PJ. Radiotherapy for bone pain. Pain 1995;63(2):137-9.

[19] Tong D, Gillick L, Hendrickson FR. The palliation of symptomatic osseous metastases: Final results of the study by the radiation therapy oncology group. Cancer 1982;50(5):893-9.

[20] Weinfurt KP, Li Y, Castel LD, Saad F, Timbie JW, Glendenning GA, et al. The significance of skeletal-related events for the health-related quality of life of patients with metastatic prostate cancer. Ann Oncol 2005;16(4):579-84.

[21] Coleman RE. Bisphosphonates: Clinical experience. Oncologist 2004;9(Suppl 4):14-27.

[22] van Holten-Verzantvoort AT, Kroon HM, Bijvoet OL, Cleton FJ, Beex LV, Blijham G, et al. Palliative pamidronate treatment in patients with bone metastases from breast cancer. J Clin Oncol 1993;11(3):491-8.

In: Pain Management Yearbook 2009
Editor: Joav Merrick

ISBN: 978-1-61209-666-7
©2012 Nova Science Publishers, Inc.

Chapter 46

SHORTENING THE BONE METASTASES QUALITY OF LIFE INSTRUMENT TOOL

Lying Zhang, PhD, Janet Nguyen, BSc (C), Amanda Hird, BSc (C) and Edward Chow, MBBS[*]

Rapid Response Radiotherapy Program, Department of Radiation Oncology, Odette Cancer Centre, Sunnybrook Health Sciences Centre, University of Toronto, Toronto, Ontario, Canada

Abstract

Purpose was to shorten the 22-item bone metastases (BM22) quality of life (QOL) instrument tool for bone metastases patients with a low performance status. Methods: The BM22 was developed in patients with bone metastases from eight countries. It was divided into four scales: painful sites, pain characteristics, functional interferences, and psychosocial aspects. Differential item functioning (DIF), item response theory (IRT), and item information functions (IIFs) analyses were used to shorten the tool. A Bonferroni adjusted p-value of < 0.002 was considered statistically significant. Results: The data from four hundred and ninety four patients were analyzed in this study. There were 283 females (57%) and 211 males (43%). The median age was 62 years. The majority of patients had primary breast (46%), prostate (22%), or lung (12%) cancer. No significant DIF was found between translations of the questionnaire (62 patients) and the original English version (432 patients). Based on the IRT model and IIFs, eight items were removed from the original version. Both the shortened 14-item and the original 22-item versions predicted four scales with excellent agreement. Demographic group comparisons yielded the same conclusions on both the shortened and original versions with little or no loss of measurement efficiency. Conclusion: The BM22 can be condensed to 14 items, which may ease patient burden in completing baseline and follow-up quality of life assessments in future clinical trials.

Keywords: bone metastases, quality of life, item response theory (IRT), differential item functioning (DIF), item information functions (IIFs).

---

[*] **Correspondence:** Edward Chow, MBBS, PhD, FRCPC, Department of Radiation Oncology, Odette Cancer Centre, Sunnybrook Health Sciences Centre, 2075 Bayview Avenue, Toronto, Ontario, Canada M4N 3M5. Tel: 416-480-4998; Fax: 416-480-6002; E-mail: Edward.Chow@sunnybrook.ca

Introduction

Proper and timely assessment of patients' subjective symptomatology in a palliative care setting is important to ensure good quality of care. Patient-based self-assessment is the gold standard to gather information about the symptoms, functional, and psychosocial problems patients are experiencing (1). However, because patients with advanced disease often present with low performance status and limited life expectancy, there is a strong need to reduce responder burden when completing quality of life (QOL) questionnaires (1,2).

In view of this, the European Organization for Research and Treatment of Cancer core questionnaire (EORTC QLQ-C30) has been shortened to a core palliative version (EORTC QLQ-C15-PAL) for cancer palliative patients using item response theory (IRT) (1, 3). IRT seeks to make scores from a shortened questionnaire compatible with the scores from the original questionnaire (2). Additionally, disease-specific modules have been developed to accompany either the EORTC QLQ-C30 or EORTC QLQ-C15-PAL. The 22-item Bone Metastases Module (BM22) has recently been developed to assess quality of life in patients with bone metastases (4). The BM22 was developed in accordance to the EORTC Module Development Guidelines, which consists of four stages of development (4, 5). The objective of this analysis was to determine if the BM22 can be shortened further to reduce patient burden and thus increase the duration by which patients are able to continue the quality of life follow-up assessment in a routine clinical or clinical trial setting, while retaining the ability to reliably capture the overall issues relevant to the patient.

In the present study, we used differential item functioning (DIF) analyses with regard to different translations. Several methods for analysis of DIF have been used (6-9), which include contingency tables, logistic regression and IRT. The major objective was to retain as few items as possible within each scale while still allowing for an accurate estimation (i.e. prediction) of the original score. For unidimensional scales consisting of two or more items with categorical response choices, IRT is a very efficient statistical technique for item selection and score estimation (10,11). This approach to shortening scales was first described in Bjorner et al (3) and was further developed, applied and evaluated from EORTC Quality of Life Group (1-2,12). In the current paper, IRT was used to shorten the BM22. The agreement between the original and the shortened scales was explored, and the potential loss of statistical power was illustrated in demographic group comparisons.

Methods

Patients with bone metastases treated with chemotherapy, surgery, bisphosphonates, radiotherapy, and symptom management were eligible to participate. Patients were accrued in Argentina, Australia, China (Hong Kong), Canada, Germany, Greece, Spain and the United Kingdom. Five translations were presented in the study (English, Greek, Spanish, Chinese, and German). All patients provided written informed consent. Demographic variables including gender, age, and primary cancer site were collected, and all patients completed the BM22 questionnaire at baseline. Each item has four response categories: 1 = "Not at all", 2 = "A little", 3 = "Quite a bit", and 4 = "Very much". Note that items 21 and 22 have inversed responses comparing to other psychosocial questions (i.e., items 17 – 20).

The BM22 was divided into four scales (0 – 100): painful sites (PS; items 1 – 5), pain characteristics (PC; items 6 – 8), functional interferences (FI; items 9 – 16), and psychosocial aspects (PA; items 17 – 22). The four scale scores were constructed by summation and linear transformation of the scores on the items. For instance, the average (XPS) of items 1 to 5 was calculated and the PS scale was then computed by a linear transformation to convert to a 0 – 100 scale, {(XPS - 1) / 3} × 100. Scales were considered missing if fewer than 3 of the PS or PA items, fewer than 2 of the PC items, or fewer than 4 of the FI items were answered by patients. Patients were considered to have worse symptoms if the PS or PC scales were higher, and patients were classified to have better functioning if the FI or PA scales were higher.

Statistical analysis

Results were expressed as mean, standard deviation (SD), and median (range) for continuous variables, and proportion (%) for categorical variables. To compare other translations (German, Greek, Spanish or Chinese) versus English, three methods of differential item functioning (DIF) analyses were applied for each item of BM22 (6-9). Differential item functioning analyses include the Fisher exact test between the item responses and translations, ordinal logistic regression, and methods based on item response theory (IRT). All IRT-models predict the probability of choosing a particular response to an item as governed by characteristics of the item and characteristics of the person (the person's IRT score). We used the Generalized Partial Credit Model (GPCM) in the IRT analysis (13), which deals with two types of item characteristics (item parameters): threshold parameters and slope parameters. For example, Figure 1 shows the GPCM model predictions (response probability functions) for each response choice for item Q9 (pain while sitting?). The model has three threshold parameters due to four item responses (not at all, a little, quite a bit, very much). The slope parameter describes the item's ability to discriminate; the items with higher slope parameters are better at discriminating between people with good and poor QOL than items with lower slope parameters. The average of threshold parameters in other translations was compared to the average of thresholds in English for each BM22 item. In order to avoid many spurious positives, the Bonferroni adjusted p-value < 0.002 (0.05/22 items) was used as the significance criteria for the multiple comparisons. We considered the difference between translations if three DIF analyses have significant p-values for each BM22 item.

Based on the IRT model, we estimated the score distribution using the expected a posteriori (EAP) method and we calculated the item information functions (IIFs) for all items (14-16). The IIF can be seen as a function of the standard error of the latent score estimate and is a measure of how much information the item provides about the person score for various levels of the BM22 scales. By choosing the items with the largest information in the area where most patients were expected to be, we obtained the most accurate estimation of the IRT scores. The items with lower information in the area (lower slope parameters) were removed from the BM22 items, and the shortened scales were calculated.

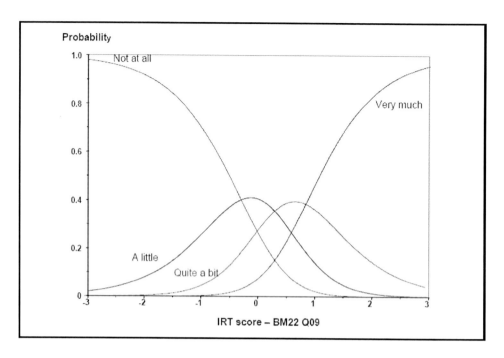

Note: The curved lines are the trace lines (response probability functions) for each response choice. The slope parameter describes the item's ability to discriminate; the items with higher slope parameters are better at discriminating between people with good and poor quality of life than items with lower slope parameters. The slope parameter for item 9 is 1.44.

Figure 1. Item trace lines – Generalized Partial Credit Model (GPCM) for item 9 (pain while sitting?).

To evaluate the shortened scales, Cronbach's alpha and Spearman coefficient were calculated between the original and shortened scales, and the group comparisons of demographics (age = 60 vs. < 60, males vs. females, and primary cancer site of breast, prostate or lung) were performed on the original and shortened scales using Wilcoxon rank-sum test or Kruskal-Wallis test.

IRT analyses were conducted using the PARSCALE (14, 17) computer program (version 4, Scientific Software International, Lincolnwood, IL). The item parameters were estimated using marginal maximum likelihood estimation. For all estimations, 75 quadrature points and a precision level for convergence of 0.01 were used. All observations with complete data on the four scales were used for estimation of the IRT model. Statistical Analysis Software (SAS, version 9.1 for Windows) was also used.

Results

Patient characteristics

Patient characteristics are summarized in table 1. Among 494 patients with bone metastases, the median age was 62 years (range: 53 – 72 years). There were 283 females (57%) and 211 males (43%). The most common primary cancer sites were breast (46%), prostate (22%) and lung (12%) patients. Participants were accrued from eight countries: Canada, Greece, Australia, UK, Hong Kong (China), Germany, Argentina and Spain. The majority of patients were accrued in Canada (83%). Four hundred and thirty-two patients (87%) completed the original English version, and 62 patients (13%) completed the translated non-English versions (29 in Greek, 14 in Spanish, 10 in Chinese, and 9 in German).

The BM22 consists of 22 items and forms four scales which were transformed to a 0-100 scale. The average (± SD) and median for the PS scale were 31.3 (± 24.1) and 26.7; for the PC scale they were 37.2 (± 28.5) and 33.3. Functioning scales have higher scores than symptoms scales. The average (± SD) and median for the FI scale was 56.9 (± 29.2) and 61.1; for the PA scale they were 58.8 (± 22.8) and 55.6.

Table 1. Demographics of the 494 patients

Age (years)		
n	486	
Mean ± SD	62.8 ±13.0	
Median (range)	62 (53 – 72)	
Gender		
Female	283	(57.3%)
Male	211	(42.7%)
Primary Cancer site		
Breast	225	(45.5%)
Prostate	107	(21.7%)
Lung	61	(12.3%)
Kidney	26	(5.3%)
Myeloma	22	(4.5%)
Bladder	12	(2.4%)
Colon	12	(2.4%)
Others	22	(4.5%)
Unknown	7	(1.4%)
Translations		
English	432	(87.5%)
Greek	29	(5.9%)
Spanish	14	(2.8%)
Chinese	10	(2.0%)
German	9	(1.8%)

DIF analyses

Table 2 summarizes the results of the DIF analyses, comparing the p-values between non-English versions and the English version. BM22 items with non-significant DIF are not shown. Using the Fisher exact test, significant DIF was found in 3 items [items 5, 6 and 7] involving two non-English versions (Greek or Spanish). Using ordinal logistic regression of item response on translation subgroups, only one item (item 6) was found to be significant between Greek and English versions. There were more significant DIF found using IRT method [items 9, 10, 18 – 20]. However, none of the findings had significant DIF from three methods at the same time.

Table 2. Test for differential item functioning (DIF) between translations and the original English using Fisher exact test, ordinal logistic regression, and IRT analysis

QOL item	p-value*		
	Fisher exact test	Ordinal logistic regression	IRT analysis
German vs. English			
9. pain while sitting or lying down?	0.804	0.424	0.001
Greek vs. English			
5. Pain in your buttock(s)?	0.0008	0.036	0.377
6. constant pain?	0.0004	0.0004	0.503
10. pain when trying to stand up?	0.070	0.195	0.001
Spanish vs. English			
7. intermittent pain?	0.0001	0.002	0.199
18. worried about loss of mobility?	0.055	0.564	0.001
19. worried about becoming dependent on others?	0.268	0.093	0.001
20. worried about your health in the future?	0.224	0.516	0.001
Chinese vs. English			
9. pain while sitting or lying down?	0.971	0.691	0.001
10. pain when trying to stand up?	0.945	0.795	0.001

*Bonferroni adjusted p-value < 0.002 was considered as significance for each test. We considered the difference between translations if three DIF analyses have significant p-values for each BM22 item. The non-significant BM22 items were not shown in the table.

IRT model and information functions

Table 3 shows the slope parameter (with standard error) in the IRT models for each BM22 item. This table illustrates the implications of the item parameters for the response probabilities for different levels of symptoms or functioning domain. Among 5 items from the painful site (PS) domain, item 3 (pain in the arm or shoulder) had a much smaller slope parameter than the four other items in the PS scale (0.331 for item 3; 0.406 for item 1; 0.523 for item 2; 0.460 for item 4 and 0.643 for item 5; respectively). This finding indicates that item 3 had a poorer ability to discriminate relative to the other items in the scale. Among 3 items from the PC domain, item 7 had a lower slope parameter than the other two items. Moreover, items 14 and 16 had lower slope parameters compared to the other items in the FI domain. Four items (17, 20, 21, and 22) had smaller slope parameters in the PA domain. The IIFs based on four different domains (PS, PC, FI, and PA) are shown in Figure 2a–d. Some BM22 items provided markedly less information than the other items, which had similar contributions to IRT model. For instance, Figure 2b shows that the item 7 provided less information on the Pain Characteristic (PC) score than other two items (Q6 and Q8).

Based on the IRT model and IIFs, eight items would be removed from the original version of the BM22, namely items 3, 7, 14, 16, 17, 20, 21, and 22. Table 4 shows the remaining items in the "shortened version" of BM22 for each symptom or functioning domain. Therefore, the shortened version includes 14 items.

Evaluation of shortened BM22

The PS, PC, FI and PA scales were calculated based on the shortened version of the BM22. The average (± SD) and median value for the shortened PS scale were 32.1 (± 25.7) and 25.0; for the shortened PC scale they were 33.0 (± 33.6) and 33.3. Shortened functioning scales have higher scores than symptoms scales. The average (± SD) and median for the shortened FI scale was 59.8 (± 30.1) and 66.7; for the shortened PA scale they were 47.6 (± 36.5) and 50.0.

Table 3. Slope parameter and corresponding standard error (SE) from the Item response theory (IRT) model for each bone metastases QOL tool

BM22	Slope parameter	SE
Painful Site (PS)		
1. Pain in your back?	0.406	0.053
2. Pain in your leg(s) or hip(s)?	0.523	0.064
3. Pain in your arm(s) or shoulder(s)?	0.331	0.047
4. Pain in your chest or rib(s)?	0.460	0.062
5. Pain in your buttock(s)?	0.643	0.077
Pain Characteristics (PC)		
6. constant pain?	1.163	0.198
7. intermittent pain?	0.239	0.041
8. pain not relieved by pain medications?	0.795	0.123
Functional Interference (FI)		
9. pain while sitting or lying down?	1.444	0.200
10. pain when trying to stand up?	1.347	0.175
11. pain while walking?	1.377	0.148
12. pain with activities such as bending or climbing stairs?	1.571	0.158
13. pain with strenuous activity (e.g. exercise, lifting)	1.532	0.188
14. pain interfered with your sleeping at night?	0.852	0.079
15. modify your daily activities?	1.073	0.105
16. isolated from those close to you (e.g. family, friends)?	0.886	0.101
Psychosocial Aspects (PA)		
17. thinking about your illness?	0.361	0.042
18. worried about loss of mobility?	1.309	0.172
19. worried about becoming dependent on others?	1.408	0.216
20. worried about your health in the future?	0.559	0.042
21. hopeful your pain will get better?	0.350	0.030
22. positive about your health?	0.122	0.033

Table 4. Summarization of shortened bone metastases QOL tool

			Shortened version	
QOL tool	Original version	Removed item	Remaining items	No. of items
Painful Site (PS)	Items 1 – 5	3	1, 2, 4, 5	4
Pain Characteristics (PC)	Items 6 – 8	7	6, 8	2
Functional Interference (FI)	Items 9 – 16	14, 16	9, 10, 11, 12, 13, 15	6
Psychosocial Aspects (PA)	Item 17 – 22	17, 20, 21, 22	18, 19	2

Table 5. Evaluation of shortened BM22 by group comparisons of demographics on painful site, painful characteristics, functional interference or psychosocial scales

		Original version		Shortened version	
Scale	Groups	Mean of scale	p-value*	Mean of scale	p-value*
Painful Site (PS)	Age ≥ 60	28.0	0.0144	34.3	0.0279
	Age < 60	33.5		28.9	
	Male	33.3	0.1511	33.7	0.1521
	Female	29.8		30.9	
	Breast cancer	25.5	0.0001	26.2	0.0001
	Prostate cancer	33.4		34.0	
	Lung cancer	38.6		40.2	
Painful Characteristics (PC)	Age ≥ 60	39.9	0.0064	35.2	0.0830
	Age < 60	32.8		29.3	
	Male	39.9	0.0643	35.4	0.1574
	Female	35.2		31.2	
	Breast cancer	30.2	0.0001	24.9	0.0001
	Prostate cancer	40.6		34.3	
	Lung cancer	48.3		48.6	
Functional Interference (FI)	Age ≥ 60	54.9	0.0504	57.8	0.0368
	Age < 60	59.9		63.1	
	Male	53.5	0.0235	56.6	0.0397
	Female	59.4		62.2	
	Breast cancer	64.7	0.0001	67.4	0.0001
	Prostate cancer	55.9		58.1	
	Lung cancer	45.2		49.3	
Psychosocial Aspects (PA)	Age ≥ 60	59.4	0.8176	48.1	0.8746
	Age < 60	58.5		47.3	
	Male	58.2	0.5395	45.5	0.2646
	Female	59.3		49.2	
	Breast cancer	62.0	0.0284	55.3	0.0138
	Prostate cancer	61.7		49.8	
	Lung cancer	53.2		40.2	

*Wilcoxon rank-sum statistic was used for comparing patients with age ≥ 60 vs. age < 60, or comparing males vs. females; Kruskal-Wallis statistic was used for comparing breast, prostate or lung primary cancer. Bonferroni adjusted p-value < 0.002 was considered as significance.

The Cronbach's alpha and Spearman correlation coefficient between the original version and the shortened version of the BM22 were 0.98 and 0.95 for the PS scale, 0.96 and 0.92 for the PC scale, 0.99 and 0.98 for the FI scale, and 0.92 and 0.87 for the PA scale, respectively. As the final step in the development of a shortened version, the group comparisons was performed on four original scales and on four shortened scales. The group comparisons included: age = 60 vs. age < 60; males vs. females; breast vs. prostate vs. lung primary cancer site (Table 5). The p-values were similar in original version and in shortened version. Primary cancer site had a significant difference on all scales. Age and gender had no difference on the scales for both versions. These findings indicate that the shortened version is able to detect a significant group difference with at least the same level of measurement efficiency as the original version of the BM22.

Discussion

The results of this study have shown that the BM22 can be shortened down to 14 items, while still maintaining the important QOL issues relevant to the patient and producing a QOL score comparable to that obtained using the original version. It is crucial that the items are correctly translated when comparing results from health status questionnaires across countries (18-20). Three methods were used to compare responses in translations: Fisher exact test of contingency tables, ordinal logistic regression of item responses, and IRT method. In each analysis, the translated item was compared against the English original. Due to the small sample size of item responses on translations (29 in Greek, 14 in Spanish, 10 in Chinese, and 9 in German, respectively), we considered a significant DIF when three tests have significant p-values for each item of the BM22. There was not any significant DIF between translations and the original English version; however, further validation of these findings in a larger sample of patients from different countries is necessary.

Several studies have used IRT methodology in recent years to shorten QOL questionnaires, such as the shortening of the EORTC QLQ-C30 core questionnaire to the EORTC QLQ-C15-PAL core questionnaire for palliative cancer patients (1-3,21-23). The results from the present study confirmed the analytical and theoretical advantages of IRT modeling for the development of a shortened BM22 questionnaire. This approach was successful in reducing the full 22–item questionnaire to 14 items. The shortened PS scale consists of items 1, 2, 4, and 5; the PC scale consists of items 6 and 8; the FI scale consists of items 9, 10, 11, 12, 13, and 15; and the PA scale consists of items 18 and 19. The differences between shortened scales and the original scales were small and their correlations (Cronbach's alpha and Spearman correlation) were also high. Separate group comparisons confirmed that our shortened symptom or functioning scales worked well as the original scales.

The BM22 was subsequently tested in an additional cohort of 170 patients from 9 different countries. This phase is critical to determine whether the module items compiled are comparable cross-culturally, as well as to make any amendments to the BM22 if necessary prior to undergoing large-scale field-testing. There was a consensus from participants to modify two items on the BM22. The first was item 9, "pain while sitting or lying down?", where 27 patients (16%) recommended this item be divided into two separate items. Many of the participants who suggested this modification only had pain during one of these activities. The second recommendation was to delete item 17, "thinking about your illness?", where five patients expressed that this was an obvious question, and two patients found this upsetting.

The BM22 was amended in response to these issues prior to beginning ongoing large scale field-testing.

Readers are cautioned that the BM22 used in this study was the original version prior to the recommendation from the additional 170 participants. We recognize that this exercise of shortening needs to be repeated after the final version from the large scale field testing in light of the fact that there may be additional changes made to the questionnaire based on patient recommendations. However, the current study will provide methodology to shorten the final quality of life instrument tool, which may help ease patient burden in clinical trials, and allow for the comparison of QOL scores for patients with a better performance status to those of patients with a poor performance status.

Acknowledgments

This study was supported by the Michael and Karyn Goldstein Cancer Research Fund and Novartis Oncology. We would also like to thank Stacy Lue for her secretarial assistance.

References

[1] Groenvold M, Petersen MA, Aaronson NK, Arraras JI, Blazeby JM, et al. EORTC Quality of Life,Group. The development of the EORTC QLQ-C15-PAL: A shortened questionnaire for cancer patients in palliative care. Eur J Cancer 2006;42(1):55-64.

[2] Petersen MA, Groenvold M, Aaronson N, Blazeby J, Brandberg Y, et al. European Organisation for Research and Treatment of Cancer Quality of Life Group. Item response theory was used to shorten EORTC QLQ-C30 scales for use in palliative care. J Clin Epidemiol 2006;59(1):36-44.

[3] Bjorner JB, Petersen MA, Groenvold M, Aaronson N, Ahlner-Elmqvist M, et al. European Organisation for Research and Treatment of Cancer Quality of Life Group. Use of item response theory to develop a shortened version of the EORTC QLQ-C30 emotional functioning scale. Qual Life Res 2004;13(10):1683-97.

[4] Chow E, Hird A, Velikova G, Johnson C, Dewolf L, et al. European Organisation for Research and Treatment of Cancer Quality of Life Group. The European Organisation for Research and Treatment of Cancer Quality of Life Questionnaire for patients with Bone Metastases: The EORTC QLQ-BM22. Eur J Cancer 2008 Dec 17 [Epub ahead of print]

[5] Blazeby J, Sprangers M, Cull A, et al. EORTC Quality of Life Group: guidelines for developing questionnaire modules. 3rd ed. revised. August 2002. <http://groups.eortc.be/qol/downloads/2008module_development_guidelines.pdf>.

[6] Holland PW, Wainer H. Differential Item Functioning. Hilsdale, NJ: Lawrence Erlbaum, 1993.

[7] French AW, Miller TR. Logistic regression and its use in detecting differential item functioning in polytomous items. J Educ Meas 1996; 33:315-32.

[8] Swaminathan H, Rogers HJ. Detecting differential item functioning using logistic-regrssion procedures. J Educ Meas 1990;27:361-70.

[9] Teresi JA, Kleinman M, Ocepek-Welikson K. Modern psychometric methods for detection of differential item functioning: Application to cognitive assessment measures. Stat Med 2000;19:1651-83.

[10] Hambleton RK. Principles and selected applications of item response theory. In: Linn RL, ed. Educational measurement. New York: Macmillan, 1989:143–200.

[11] Van der Linden WJ, Hambleton RK. Handbook of modern item response theory. Berlin: Springer, 1997.
[12] Petersen MA, Groenvold M, Aaronson N, Brenne E, Fayers P, et al. European Organisation for Research and Treatment of Cancer Quality of Life Group. Scoring based on item response theory did not alter the measurement ability of EORTC QLQ-C30 cales. J Clin Epidemiol 2005;58:902-8.
[13] Muraki E. A generalized partial credit model. In: van der Linden WJ, Hambleton RK, eds. Handbook of modern item response theory. Berlin: Springer; 1997:153-68.
[14] Muraki E, Bock RD. Parscale – IRT based test scoring and item analysis for graded open-ended exercises and performance tasks. Chicago: Sci Software, 1996.
[15] Bock RD, Mislevy RJ. Adaptive EAP estimation of ability in a microcomputer environment. Appl Psychol Meas 1982;6:431-44.
[16] Muraki E. Information functions of the generalized partial credit model. Appl Psychol Meas 1993;17:351-63.
[17] Du Toit M. IRT from SSI Manual. Lincolnwood: Sci Software, 2003.
[18] Petersen MA, Groenvold M, Bjorner JB, Aaronson N, Conroy T, et al. European Organisation for Research and Treatment of Cancer Quality of Life Group. Use of differential item functioning analysis to assess the equivalence of translations of a questionnaire. Qual Life Res 2003;12:373-85.
[19] Bjorner JB, Kreiner S, Ware JE, Damsgaard MT, Bech P. Differential item functioning in the Danish translation of the SF-36. J Clin Epidemiol 1998;51:1189-202.
[20] Crane K, Gibbons LE, Jolley L, Van Bell G. Differential item functioning analysis with ordinal logistic regression techniques. Med Care 2006;44(Suppl 3):S115-123.
[21] Orlando M, Sherbourne CD, Thissen D. Summed-score linking using item response theory: Application fo depression measurement. Psychol Assess 2000;12:354-59.
[22] Maydeu-Olivares A, Drasgow F, Mead AD. Distinguishing among parametric item response models for polychotomous ordered data. Appl Psychol Meas 1994;18:245-56.
[23] Badia X, Prieto L, Roset M, Diez-Perez A, Herdman M. Development of a short osteoporosis quality of life questionnaire by equating items from two existing instruments. J Clin Epidemiol 2002;55:32.40.

In: Pain Management Yearbook 2009
Editor: Joav Merrick

ISBN: 978-1-61209-666-7
©2012 Nova Science Publishers, Inc.

Chapter 47

SURGICAL STABILIZATION OF SEVERELY DESTRUCTIVE UPPER CERVICAL LYTIC BONE METASTASES

*Janet Nguyen, BSc(C)[1], Matthew Chung, BSc(C)[1], Michael Ford, MD[2], Philiz Goh, BSc[1], Joel Rubenstein, MD[3], Emily Sinclair, MRT(T)[1], Gunita Mitera, MRT(T)[1] and Edward Chow, MBBS, PhD, FRCPC[*1]*

[1]Department of Radiation Oncology
[2]Department of Orthopedics
[3]Department of Diagnostic Radiology, Sunnybrook Health Sciences Centre,
University of Toronto, Toronto, Ontario, Canada

Abstract

The spinal column is the most frequent site for skeletal metastases. Complications from spinal metastases include pain, neurological deficits, and mechanical instability – all of which may require treatment. Upper cervical metastases are rare when compared to its spinal counterparts, however when they do occur, because of anatomic characteristics of that region, instability or pathological fractures may be perceived as life-threatening. Although radiotherapy is considered the standard treatment for spinal metastases, it has a delayed effect on pain, and is not able to treat any mechanical instability a patient may have. We report a case where a breast cancer patient required surgical stabilization due to a severely destructive lesion in the upper cervical region.

Keywords: Breast cancer, orthopedic stabilization, upper cervical metastases.

---

* **Correspondence:** Edward Chow, MBBS, PhD, FRCPC, Department of Radiation Oncology, Odette Cancer Centre, Sunnybrook Health Sciences Centre, 2075 Bayview Avenue, Toronto, ON M4N 3M5, Canada. Tel: 416-480-4998; Fax: 416-480-6002; E-mail: Edward.Chow@sunnybrook.ca

Introduction

Skeletal metastases are very frequent in cancer patients. One out of every three patients becomes symptomatic, causing neurological deficits, biomechanical instability, and severe pain (1,2). Local pain is the prevalent symptom noted by patients. The spinal column is the most common site for skeletal metastases (3,4). Breast carcinoma has a 75% incidence of developing bone metastases (5). Primary breast cancer patients with metastases to the spine have a longer survival prognosis in comparison to other primary cancers (6), while the occurrence of metastases to the upper cervical area has a specifically shorter survival prognosis in comparison to its spinal counterparts (7). Cervical metastases may have a poorer prognosis due to a longer detection time. The cervical region is wider when compared to the thoracic, causing lesions to grow to a larger size before it can be detected (7). A late diagnosis would tend to indicate severe destruction of the vertebral body, consequently resulting in spinal instability and may be perceived as critical due to stabilizing characteristics of the upper cervical spine (8,9).

We present a case of a patient with primary breast cancer with extensive metastatic lesions to the upper cervical area of the C1 and C2 who presented with chronic neck pain.

Case study

A 66 year-old woman was treated with a right partial mastectomy with limited lymph node resection in February 2008 and prescribed Tamoxifen. She had presented with chronic neck pain, dizziness and decreased hearing in the left ear since the beginning of that year. Investigations suggested that her chronic pain was related to degenerative changes caused by spondylosis of the C5-7. The patient was given narcotic analgesics for her pain.

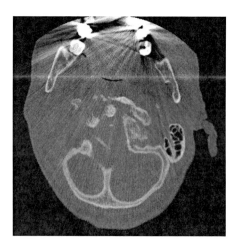

Figure 1. Axial CT image through the craniocervical junction showing extensive lytic destruction of the right lateral mass of C1 with rotation of the C1 vertebra to the left.

With the progressive neck pain, she became bedridden. Another CT scan was performed in July 2008 which confirmed bone metastases and showed that the neck was very unstable, due to a large lytic destructive lesion involving the right C1 with minimal involvement of the upper C2 body and lateral odontoid (see figures 1 and 2).

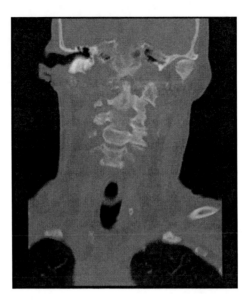

Figure 2. Coronal reformatted CT image showing lytic destruction of the right lateral mass of C1 with lateral subluxation of the left lateral mass of C1 at C1-2.

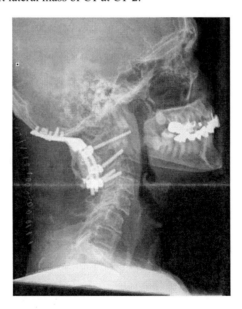

Figure 3. Postoperative lateral view of the cervical spine with posterior craniocervical instrumentation from the occiput to C3.

The patient was referred to an orthopedic surgeon who prompted an immediate need for fitting of a neck brace due to the severe instability of the neck, followed by a radical operation – an occipital cervical fusion from the occiput to the C3 (see figure 3). Since the C1 region had significant destructive lesion, polymethylmethacrylate (PMMA) was used as reinforcement and was placed onto the posterior portion of the spine, continuing up onto the skull. Degenerative changes were noted in the lower cervical spine, as well as first degree anterior spondylolisthesis at the levels of C5 on C6 and C6 on C7. Radiotherapy was delivered postoperatively to the neck, 2000 cGy in 5 fractions.

She recovered uneventfully and was able to move her head freely in a vertical motion and a 50-60% capability of horizontal rotation. She was able to ambulate, her pain was much improved and her pain medication was reduced.

Discussion

The spinal column is the most common site for skeletal metastases, however it is estimated that only 5% of those spinal metastases encountered actually cause symptoms (10). Once pain and local tenderness do occur, complications such as neurological deficits are expected to occur in up to 80% of those symptomatic patients within two months. Klekamp et al. reported on the surgical outcome for spinal metastases, and found that 86% of their 105 patients claimed local pain at the affected spinal level to be the first symptom (10). Heidecke et al (8) performed a retrospective study, with 100% of their 62 patients with cervical metastases presenting with local pain as a symptom. Nakamura et al (9) had a similar finding, with 100% of their thirteen patients complaining of neck pain as a symptom for their upper cervical metastases. Two of their patients had almost their entire atlas and axis infiltrated by tumor tissue, due to being left untreated for a long period of time.

Upper cervical metastases are also rare in its occurrence in comparison to thoracic, lumbar and sacral regions (7,11). It is estimated that thoracic spine metastases tend to occur in 50-60% of all vertebral metastases, with lumbar at 30-35%, followed by the cervical spine at 10-15% 8. A delay in the diagnosis of upper cervical metastases could be the reason why it has a poorer prognosis when compared to thoracic or lumbar regions (7-9). Sciubba et al (7) did a study regarding the prognosis variables in breast cancer patients undergoing spinal surgery, and suggested that one reason for such a delay is that the upper cervical canal is wider, able to tolerate a higher degree of tumor infiltration before cord compression occurs, thereby allowing the tumor time to grow before it is detected. After the initial presentation of pain, the manifestation of neurological symptoms is rapid, within a matter of days to weeks for the lumbar spine, however in the cervical and thoracic spine it may occur over a period of weeks to months (9,12).

Treatment options for skeletal metastases include surgery, radiation, hormonal manipulation, bisphosphonates and/or chemotherapy (13). Radiation is known to be effective in treating local bone pain, however the benefits are not usually immediate, and some patients may experience a temporary period of pain flare (2,14,15). Although evidence is inconclusive as to what type of surgery should be performed for spinal metastases (13), surgical intervention and various combination modality treatments have shown improvements in ambulation and patients' quality of life (9,16). Irradiation before or after surgical intervention have had conflicting support, however, these schools of thought have both agreed upon the factors in determining the most appropriate modality on a case by case basis, which include: spinal instability, vertebral collapse, radiation resistant tumors, and the risk of neurologic deficit (15,17). Aebi (12) did mention, however, that irradiation done prior to surgery has a significantly negative effect on the outcome of the surgery, therefore it should be administered postoperatively whenever possible. The aims of surgery include stabilization, ambulatory mobility, pain reduction, and improvement in the quantity and quality of life. However, Colak et al (18) and Shehadi et al (2) stated that surgical intervention for skeletal metastases to the spine should be an available option only for palliative patients with an estimated life expectancy of at least three months. Improving quality of life is especially important considering that metastases to the spine can quickly become a major burden on the patient, due to a reduced capacity for physical activity as well as ambulation (12).

Once surgery is performed, patients are known to experience significant pain relief and improved ambulatory function (9,19). Weigel et al. did a retrospective study concerning the use of surgical intervention to manage symptomatic metastases to the spine. They found that 83% of their 72 patients were ambulatory postoperatively (19). Out of 20 patients who were non-ambulatory prior to surgery, 14 (70%) were able to walk again after surgery (19). Nakamura et al (9) reported on the treatment of metastases of the upper cervical spine, and found that 10 out of 11 patients operated on had such remarkable pain relief, they were able to ambulate as soon as a week post-surgery with a simple neck brace. In a retrospective study done by Heidecke et al., they found that spinal fusion had few complications with a good rate of permanent stabilization for the cervical spine in question (8).

Recurrence in the form of spinal metastases from a primary in breast cancer is the most common in skeletal metastases, with an overall occurrence, in the cervical area, of 10% in all spine metastases patients (2,5,20,21). Chataigner et al (14) found that administering postoperative radiotherapy did not lower the risk of local recurrence in their patients. Radiotherapy is used for palliation of pain and is recommended for those patients who are in a poor condition or those without neurological deficits (5). Radiotherapy cannot correct spinal instability (14,15). Neoplasm to the upper cervical spine are rare in comparison to cases that have been reviewed, where C3-7 is the common ground (4). There is increased mechanical risk of rotatory instability or craniocervical dislocation in cases of metastases to the atlas or axis in the spine (3). In a study by Lee (21), a relapse in the form of metastases occurred in 24% in patients with less than three positively confirmed nodules after undergoing a masectomy. Kasai et al (6) found that metastatic spine carcinoma with a primary in breast or thyroid cancer have better prognosis in an increased life expectancy as opposed to other metastatic spine cases where the primary arises elsewhere. However, Sciubba (7) determined that cervical metastases had a negative prognostic value and a shorter median survival as opposed to metastases to other areas of the spine. It is generally agreed, however, that the type of primary tumor, the degree of metastatic spread, along with the general well being of the patient is what dictates the overall survival time and long term prognosis (8).

Surgery for bone metastases in general is often reserved for palliation, and is generally only considered for those patients with neurological deficits, intractable pain, mechanical instability, or radiation resistant tumors (2,7). Surgery as a palliative treatment modality can make improvements in the quality of life, reduce pain, and improve ambulatory movement (9,16) as illustrated in our case.

Acknowledgments

This study was supported by the Michael and Karyn Goldstein Cancer Research Fund. We thank Stacy Lue for secretarial assistance.

References

[1] Raycroft JF, Hockman RP, Southwick SO. Metastatic tumors involving the cervical vertebrae: Surgical palliation. J Bone Joint Surg 1978;60(6):763-8.
[2] Shehadi JA, Sciubba DM, Suk I, Suki D, Maldaun MV, et al. Surgical treatment strategies and outcome in patients with breast cancer metastatic to the spine: A review of 87 patients. Eur Spine J 2007;16(8):1179-92.
[3] Atanasiu JP, Badatcheff F, Pidhorz L. Metastatic lesions of the cervical spine. A retrospective analysis of 20 cases. Spine 1993;18(10):1279-84.
[4] Colak A, Kutlay M, Kibici K, Demircan MN, Akin ON. Two-staged operation on C2 neoplastic lesions: Anterior excision and posterior stabilization. Neurosurg Rev 2004l;27(3):189-93.
[5] Coleman RE, Rubens RD. The clinical course of bone metastases from breast cancer. Br J Cancer 1987;55(1):61-6.
[6] Kasai Y, Kawakita E, Uchida A. Clinical profile of long-term survivors of breast or thyroid cancer with metastatic spinal tumours. Int Orthop 2007;31(2):171-5.
[7] Sciubba DM, Gokaslan ZL, Suk I, Suki D, Maldaun MV, McCutcheon IE, Nader R, Theriault R, Rhines LD, Shehadi JA. Positive and negative prognostic variables for patients undergoing spine surgery for metastatic breast disease. Eur Spine J 2007;16(10):1659-67.
[8] Heidecke V, Rainov NG, Burkert W. Results and outcome of neurosurgical treatment for extradural metastases in the cervical spine. Acta Neurochir 2003;145(10):873-81.
[9] Nakamura M, Toyama Y, Suzuki N, Fujimura Y. Metastases to the upper cervical spine. J Spinal Disord 1996;9(3):195-201.
[10] Klekamp J, Samii H. Surgical results for spinal metastases. Acta Neurochir (Wien) 1998;140(9):957-67.
[11] Laus M, Pignatti G. Malaguti MC (1996) Anterior extraoral surgery to the cervical spine. Spine 1996;21(14):1687-93.
[12] Aebi M. Spinal metastasis in the elderly. Eur Spine J 2003;12(Suppl 2):S202-13.
[13] Tomita K, Kawahara N, Kobayashi T, Yoshida A, Murakami H, Akamaru T. Surgical Strategy for Spinal Metastases. Spine 2001;26(3):298-306.
[14] Chataigner H, Onimus M. Surgery in spinal metastasis without spinal cord compression: Indications and strategy related to the risk of recurrence. Eur Spine J 2000;9(6):523-7.
[15] Hirabayashi H, Ebara S, Kinoshita T, Yuzawa Y, Nakamura I, et al. Clinical outcome and survival after palliative surgery for spinal metastases: Palliative surgery in spinal metastases. Cancer 2003;97(2):476-84.
[16] Thongtrangan I, Balabhadra RS, Le H, Park J, Kim DH.Vertebral body replacement with an expandable cage for reconstruction after spinal tumor resection. Neurosurg Focus 2003;15(5):E8.
[17] Sundaresan N, Rothman A, Manhart K, Kelliher K. Surgery for solitary metastases of the spine: Rationale and results of treatment. Spine 2002;27(16):1802-6.
[18] Colak A, Kutlay M, Kibici K, Demircan MN, Akin ON. Two-staged operation on C2 neoplastic lesions: Anterior excision and posterior stabilization. Neurosurg Rev 2004;27(3):189-93.
[19] Weigel B, Maghsudi M, Neumann C, Kretschmer R, Muller FJ, Nerlich M. Surgical management of symptomatic spinal metastases. Postoperative outcome and quality of life. Spine 1999;24(21):2240-6.
[20] Esteva FJ, Valero V, Pusztai L, Boehnke-Michaud L, Buzdar AU, Hortobagyi GN. Chemotherapy of metastatic breast cancer: What to expect in 2001 and beyond. Oncologist 2001;6(2):133-46.
[21] Lee YT. Breast carcinoma: Pattern of recurrence and metastasis after mastectomy. Am J Clin Oncol 1984;7(5):443-9.

In: Pain Management Yearbook 2009
Editor: Joav Merrick

ISBN: 978-1-61209-666-7
©2012 Nova Science Publishers, Inc.

Chapter 48

WHEN ALL ELSE FAILS: SIMPLE BRACING FOR THE RELIEF OF INTRACTABLE PAIN

Roseanna Presutti, BSc(C)[1], Sarah Campos, BSc(C)[1], Joel Finkelstein, MD[2], Joel Rubenstein, MD[3], Emily Sinclair, MRTT[1], Gunita Mitera, MRTT[1] and Edward Chow, MBBS[*1]*

[1]Department of Radiation Oncology
[2]Department of Orthopedics
[3]Department of Diagnostic Radiology, Sunnybrook Health Sciences Centre,
University of Toronto, Toronto, Ontario, Canada

Abstract

Approximately 33% of patients with renal cell cancer develop bone metastases, most of which tend to be osteolytic in nature. Renal cell cancer is known to have a limited response to chemotherapy and radiation. In the present study, we describe a patient with renal cell cancer suffering from painful bone metastases in the left humerus. Despite surgical fixation and repeated palliative radiotherapy, the disease progressed leading to intractable pain. With no further palliative systemic, orthopedic or radiation treatments to offer as a means of pain relief, a simple brace was given to the patient. Fortunately, such bracing provided satisfactory symptom relief.

Keywords: Bone metastases, bracing, palliative radiotherapy, renal cell cancer.

---

[*] **Correspondence:** Edward Chow, MBBS, PhD, FRCPC, Department of Radiation Oncology, Odette Cancer Centre, Sunnybrook Health Sciences Centre, 2075 Bayview Avenue, Toronto, ON M4N 3M5, Canada. Tel: 416-480-4998; Fax: 416-480-6002; E-mail: Edward.Chow@sunnybrook.ca

Introduction

Bone metastases are a common occurrence in patients with advanced cancer, with a prevalence of 70-85% post-mortem (1). Approximately 40% of lung, thyroid and renal cell carcinomas metastasize to the bone (2). The site of bone metastasis varies, but approximately one third occur in the appendicular skeleton (3). Only 20% develop in the upper extremities with the humerus being the most common metastatic site (4). The life expectancy of patients with bone metastases has greatly improved with recent advances in systemic therapies (5,6). As a result, skeletal complications including pain and pathological fracture (6,8) are becoming more prevalent with pathological fracture of a long bone arising in 10% (9). Such events are debilitating, and can severely reduce quality of life (QOL) in patients with metastatic cancer. In the current study, we present the case of a patient with renal cell carcinoma (RCC) suffering from intractable pain due to bony metastasis in the left humerus.

Case study

A 62-year old gentleman, with clear cell RCC, initially treated with right nephrectomy in 2000, was referred to the Rapid Response Radiotherapy Program (RRRP) in December 2006 complaining of pain in the left humerus. Plain x-ray and MRI revealed a large lytic lesion with erosion of the medial cortex into the surgical neck (see figure 1).

After an orthopedic consultation, the patient was considered to be at high risk for pathological fracture and was scheduled for prophylactic surgical fixation. Prior to the planned surgery, the patient suffered a pathological fracture of the left proximal humerus and received pre-operative embolization followed by an intramedullary (IM) nailing in late January 2007. A Zimmer humerus nail secured by one distal and three proximal screws was used to stabilize the extremity.

Post-operatively, the patient was started on sunitinib. The patient was treated with palliative radiotherapy (RT), 20 Gy in five fractions, to the left humerus and shoulder in March 2007. He experienced significant pain relief post-RT. He developed cardiomyopathy with depressed cardiac function as a result of the sunitinib, and systemic therapy was therefore withheld.

In January 2008 the patient returned to the RRRP with recurring left shoulder pain. Both computed tomography (CT) and plain x-ray images showed progressive destruction of the surgical neck of the left humerus. Plain x-ray revealed stable configuration of the IM nail and therefore, further surgical intervention was not necessary. He was treated with a second course of 20Gy of RT in five fractions to the left humerus and shoulder. Post-RT, the patient continued to experience pain along the entire length of the left arm and difficulty elevating the left shoulder.

As a result of increased and unmanageable pain, the patient returned in October 2008 for consideration of further RT. Plain x-ray revealed progression of the metastatic disease with extensive lytic destruction along the entire length of the left humerus and in the left shoulder (Figure 2). A final course of palliative RT, 20Gy in ten fractions, was delivered; however, pain relief was not experienced. Following the completion of RT, he was referred to an orthopedic surgeon for a final opinion, where it was determined that further surgery was not possible, leaving the patient with limited options for pain relief.

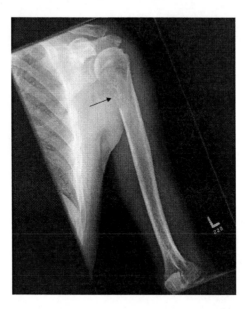

Figure 1. AP view shows a large lytic lesion in the proximal humerus with destruction of the medial cortex.

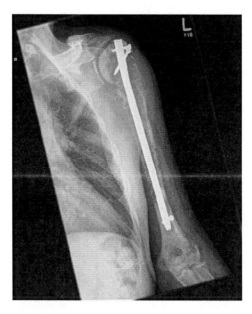

Figure 2. AP view shows fixation of the humerus with a static locking intramedullary nail and extension of the lytic destruction to involve the proximal 2/3 of the humerus.

Thus, with the failure of palliative systemic therapy, RT and surgical intervention to relieve the patient's pain, a Sarmiento shoulder and humeral brace was prescribed (see figure 3). The brace, traditionally used by orthopedic surgeons for individuals with humeral shaft fractures, successfully provided the patient with pain relief from late October 2008 to January 2009.

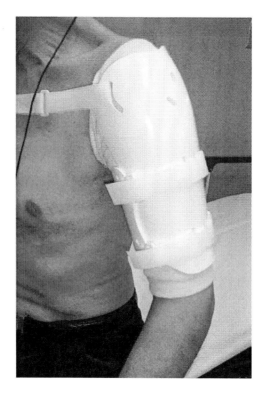

Figure 3. A Sarmiento shoulder and humeral brace was fitted and provided the patient with satisfactory pain relief where surgery, systemic therapy and palliative RT failed.

Discussion

Bone lesions arising from RCC develop in around approximately one third of patients and tend to be highly aggressive, hypervascular and osteolytic in nature (7,10-12). Osteolytic lesions involving erosion of the medial cortex are at high risk for pathological fracture, and often require surgical fixation. Due to the hypervascularity of metastatic RCC, preoperative embolization is a standard measure in order to decrease blood loss and morbidity (12,13). Furthermore, it is routine to deliver fractionated courses of palliative RT after surgical fixation of a pathological fracture (14).

The use of an interlocking IM nail for the fixation of humeral fractures is an intervention for pain relief. In a study by Sarahrudi et al (9), 11 of 27 patients with a pathological fracture of the humerus received surgical fixation by means of an IM nailing. Post operatively, all patients experienced good local pain relief (9). Tomé et al (4) found that of 12 patients with established humeral fractures treated with IM nailing, good to excellent pain relief was achieved post-operatively. Finally, in a retrospective study by Redmond et al (15), 12 out of 13 patients with humeral shaft fractures stabilized by interlocking IM nailing had good to excellent pain relief. Similar to the present study, after two-months of good function and pain relief our one patient had return of pain despite receiving the conventional 20 Gy postoperative RT.

Furthermore, it is well known that metastatic RCC shows limited response to RT and chemotherapy (8,10,16,17). Despite reported radioresistance, RT can be a beneficial modality to relieve bony pain in RCC patients (11,18,19). In a study by Halperin et al (20), bone pain responded to RT at 77% of the irradiated sites in patients with RCC. Response was defined as a decrease in analgesic intake due to decreased pain at the treated site or patient/family reported decrease in pain at the irradiated site. In addition, Durr et al (18) reported that RT provided bony pain relief in almost all RCC patients, with up to 55% of patients experiencing complete relief. In a prospective Phase II trial by Lee et al (19), palliative RT was delivered to 31 RCC patients, 81% of whom had bone metastases. A dose of 30Gy in 10 fractions delivered to all patients was found to provide significant local pain relief for patients with bony metastases from RCC. Another study by Reichel et al (10) evaluated response to RT for 36 bony metastatic sites in RCC patients. Re-irradiation was necessary at 26% of the painful sites. However, pain returned to pre-RT levels in a median time of 2 months for all evaluable patients. Although the relief provided by palliative RT may be short lived in RCC patients, it is nevertheless a useful modality for treating bone metastases in this the palliative population.

Metastatic RCC responds very poorly to many traditional cancer therapies including chemotherapy, and cytokine therapies, such as interferon-alfa (IFN-α) and interleukin-2 (IL-2), with chemotherapy and cytokines having response rates of 6% and 10-15% respectively (21,22). Sunitinib is a tyrosine kinase inhibitor that specifically targets vascular endothelial growth factor receptor 1-3 and platelet-derived growth factor α and β, and is a feasible treatment option when chemotherapy and cytokine therapies are unsuccessful (16,21-23). In patients with advanced RCC, sunitinib has an objective response of approximately 40% compared to 2-5% for cytokine therapy (22). Motzer et al (16) reported a similar objective response rate of 44% in patients with cytokine refractory metastatic clear cell RCC, with the duration of response lasting for a median of 10 months.

Despite its anti-tumor and anti-antigenic effects, sunitinib has been associated with cardiotoxicity. In a study by Telli et al (23), 15% of their patients suffered from grade 3/4 left ventricular dysfunction and symptomatic heart failure while receiving sunitinib. Similarly, Izzedine et al (22) reported incidence rates of left ventricular dysfunction and hypertension at 15% and 28% respectively in their review of sunitinib side effects in advanced metastatic RCC patients. Similar to these findings, in the present case, the use of sunitinib resulted in the development of cardiomyopathy resulting in the discontinuation of systemic therapy.

When no further palliative or surgical interventions were possible, a Sarmiento brace, traditionally employed for treatment of humeral shaft fractures, was prescribed to our patient. This simple, functional bracing technique was developed by Sarmiento in 1967. Muscular compression by the device forms an "inner splint" and external stabilization ensures fracture alignment and maintains limb length, allowing for mobilization of both the elbow and shoulder joint (24). In a review of 87 patients suffering from humeral shaft fractures treated with this functional bracing technique, 86% had no limitation in range of motion in the adjacent joints, with 65% of patients having no pain at follow-up assessment (24). Similarly, in a study by Rangger et al (25), all patients achieved full restoration and function in the shoulder and elbow after bracing. To our knowledge, implementation of this form of bracing has not been documented in cancer patients following surgical stabilization and post-operative RT.

The current study presented the case of a patient suffering from intractable pain due to osteolysis of the left proximal humerus. Despite surgical fixation, repeated post-operative RT and palliative systemic therapy, the patient's pain persisted. A simple brace was therefore employed in an attempt to provide symptom relief. Prior to bracing, the patient rated his worst pain as 10/10 using the Brief Pain Inventory (BPI). Immediately following implementation of the brace, the patient's worst pain was reduced to 4/10. The patient self-reported that when the brace was used, his pain was significantly reduced. Thus, when standard practice fails, and no further treatment is possible, a simple brace should be considered for the relief of intractable metastatic bony pain.

Acknowledgment

This study was supported by the Michael and Karyn Goldstein Cancer Research Fund. We would also like to thank Stacy Lue for her secretarial assistance.

References

[1] Tubiana-Hulin M. Incidence, prevalence and distribution of bone metastases. Bone 1991;12:S9-10.
[2] Pain palliation of bone metastases. Overview. InSightec.com.[homepage on the Internet]. InSightec Image Guided Treatment Ltd. 2005 1 April 2005. Available from: http://www.insightec.com/135-en-r10/BoneMetastases.aspx.
[3] Hage WD, Aboulafia AJ, Aboulafia DM. Incidence, location, and diagnostic evaluation of metastatic bone disease. Orthop Clin North Am 2000;31(4):515-28.
[4] Tome J, Carsi B, Garcia-Fernandez C, Marco F, Lopez-Duran Stern L. Treatment of pathologic fractures of the humerus with seidel nailing. Clin Orthop 1998(350):51-5.
[5] Falkmer U, Jarhult J, Wersall P, Cavallin-Stahl E. A systematic overview of radiation therapy effects in skeletal metastases. Acta Oncol 2003;42(5-6):620-33.
[6] Pavlakis N, Stockler M. Bisphosphonates for breast cancer.update in cochrane database syst rev. Cochrane Database Syst Rev 2002(1):003474 and 2005;(3):CD003474.
[7] Lipton A, Theriault RL, Hortobagyi GN, et al. Pamidronate prevents skeletal complications and is effective palliative treatment in women with breast carcinoma and osteolytic bone metastases: Long term follow-up of two randomized, placebo-controlled trials. Cancer 2000;88(5):1082-90.
[8] Kollender Y, Bickels J, Price WM, et al. Metastatic renal cell carcinoma of bone: Indications and technique of surgical intervention. J Urol 2000;164(5):1505-8.
[9] Sarahrudi K, Hora K, Heinz T, Millington S, Vecsei V. Treatment results of pathological fractures of the long bones: A retrospective analysis of 88 patients. Int Orthop 2006;30(6):519-24.
[10] Reichel LM, Pohar S, Heiner J, Buzaianu EM, Damron TA. Radiotherapy to bone has utility in multifocal metastatic renal carcinoma. Clin Orthop 2007;459:133-8.
[11] Adiga GU, Dutcher JP, Larkin M, Garl S, Koo J. Characterization of bone metastases in patients with renal cell cancer. BJU Int. 2004;93(9):1237-40.
[12] Sun S, Lang EV. Bone metastases from renal cell carcinoma: Preoperative embolization. J Vasc Interv Radiol 1998;9(2):263-9.
[13] Chatziioannou AN, Johnson ME, Pneumaticos SG, Lawrence DD, Carrasco CH. Preoperative embolization of bone metastases from renal cell carcinoma. Eur Radiol 2000;10(4):593-6.
[14] Hoegler D. Radiotherapy for palliation of symptoms in incurable cancer. Curr Problems Cancer 1997;21(3):131-83.
[15] Redmond BJ, Biermann JS, Blasier RB. Interlocking intramedullary nailing of pathological fractures of the shaft of the humerus. J Bone Joint Surg Am 1996;78(6):891-6.

[16] Motzer RJ, Rini BI, Bukowski RM, et al. Sunitinib in patients with metastatic renal cell carcinoma. JAMA 2006;295(21):2516-24.
[17] Jung ST, Ghert MA, Harrelson JM, Scully SP. Treatment of osseous metastases in patients with renal cell carcinoma. Clin Orthop 2003(409):223-31.
[18] Durr HR, Maier M, Pfahler M, Baur A, Refior HJ. Surgical treatment of osseous metastases in patients with renal cell carcinoma. Clin Orthop 1999(367):283-90.
[19] Lee J, Hodgson D, Chow E, et al. A phase II trial of palliative radiotherapy for metastatic renal cell carcinoma. Cancer 2005;104(9):1894-1900.
[20] Halperin EC, Harisiadia L. The Role of Radiation Therapy in the Management of Metastatic Renal Cell Carcinoma.Cancer 1983; 51(4):614-7.
[21] Chouhan JD, Zamarripa DE, Lai PH, Oramasionwu CU, Grabinski JL. Sunitinib (sutent): A novel agent for the treatment of metastatic renal cell carcinoma. J Oncol Pharm Pract 2007;13(1):5-15.
[22] Izzedine H, Buhaescu I, Rixe O, Deray G. Sunitinib malate. Cancer Chemother Pharmacol 2007;60(3):357-64.
[23] Telli ML, Witteles RM, Fisher GA, Srinivas S. Cardiotoxicity associated with the cancer therapeutic agent sunitinib malate. Ann Oncol 2008;19(9):1613-1618.
[24] Wallny T, Westermann K, Sagebiel C, Reimer M, Wagner UA. Functional treatment of humeral shaft fractures: Indications and results. J Orthop Trauma 1997;11(4):283-7.
[25] Rangger C, Kathrein A, Klestil T. Immediate application of fracture braces in humeral shaft fractures. J Trauma 1999;46(4):732-5.

In: Pain Management Yearbook 2009
Editor: Joav Merrick

ISBN: 978-1-61209-666-7
©2012 Nova Science Publishers, Inc.

Chapter 49

CEMENTED HEMIARTHROPLASTY, PERCUTANEOUS ACETABULAR CEMENTOPLASTY AND POST OPERATIVE RADIATION FOR A HIGH RISK LESION OF THE HIP

Jocelyn Pang, BSc(C)[1], Richard Jenkinson, MD[2], Gunita Mitera, MRTT[1], Andrea Donovan, MD[3], Robyn Pugash, MD[3], Maureen Trudeau, MD[4], Cindy Quinton, MD[4], Emily Sinclair, MRTT[1], Janet Nguyen, BSc(C)[1], Roseanna Presutti, BSc(C)[1] and Edward Chow, MBBS[1]*

[1]Department of Radiation Oncology
[2]Orthopaedic Surgery
[3]Medical Imaging
[4]Medical Oncology, Sunnybrook Health Sciences Centre,
University of Toronto, Ontario, Canada

Abstract

We present a case of a 45 year-old premenopausal patient with breast cancer who developed multiple sites of bone metastases. She presented with severe pain in her right femur and hip with inability to weight-bear. Imaging demonstrated extensive lytic destruction of the femoral neck and acetabulum. A combined approach with right hip hemiarthroplasty to treat the high risk proximal femoral lesion, cementoplasty to stabilize the acetabular lesion and palliative radiation was used. The patient suffered minimal procedural morbidity and was discharged after a 2 day inpatient stay. She had significant pain relief and rapidly regained functional independence with full weight bearing.

---

* **Correspondence:** Edward Chow, MBBS, PhD, FRCPC, Department of Radiation Oncology, Odette Cancer Centre, Sunnybrook Health Sciences Centre, 2075 Bayview Avenue, Toronto, ON M4N 3M5, Canada. Tel: 416-480-4998; Fax: 416-480-6002; E-mail: Edward.Chow@sunnybrook.ca

Keywords: Cemented hemiarthroplasty, bone metastases, femoral lesion, cementoplasty, radiation treatment.

Introduction

Bone metastases are a common development in breast cancer and patients (1). Nearly two thirds of patients with bone metastases will develop complications, which can include pathological fractures, severe pain, hypercalcemia, spinal cord compression, need for surgery and radiation treatment (2). Fractures are most common in long weight bearing bones, with the femur being the most frequent site. When patients present with pain related to bone metastases before a fracture has occurred, surgical intervention can decrease morbidity related to completed pathological fracture (3). Surgical reconstruction of the pelvis and acetabulum in patients with metastatic disease can be technically challenging and exposes the patient to surgical morbidity and potential complications (4). To address this problem, percutaneous cementoplasty techniques have been developed in recent years (5). We present a case of a 45 year-old woman to illustrate the potential utility of a combined treatment with arthroplasty and cementoplasty for treatment of osseous metastasis around the hip.

Case story

A 45 year-old premenopausal female was referred in February 2007 for a second opinion regarding treatment of her breast cancer. She had undergone a left lumpectomy in December 2006 for a 1.7 cm, grade III, infiltrating ductal carcinoma. The tumor was estrogen and progesterone positive, and HER2/neu positive. Subsequent axillary lymph node dissection revealed two out of six lymph nodes positive for metastatic adenocarcinoma. The metastatic work up was negative. She was recommended Fluorouracil, Epirubicin, Cyclophosphamide, Docetaxel (FEC-D) chemotherapy followed by Tamoxifen and Herceptin as adjuvant treatment for her breast cancer. Unfortunately, her first dose of chemotherapy brought upon severe palpitations and functional decline. Her second cycle of FEC-D chemotherapy was accompanied by Neulasta because she had developed neutropenia during her treatment. The drug induced more side effects leaving her bed-ridden due to bone pain. Rather than continuing the chemotherapy treatment, the patient decided to pursue naturopathic medications. Thus, she did not receive any Tamoxifen, Herceptin, hormonal therapy or adjuvant radiation.

In March 2008, patient reported bone pain and a bone scan was performed. The scan revealed increased activity in axial and appendicular skeleton compatible with bone metastases. She received multiple treatments of palliative radiation over several months to a variety of sites. She was also prescribed various analgesics to manage her pain. Additionally, she was started on Pamidronate alongside with Zoladex and Tamoxifen; however the Zoladex caused nausea and lack of appetite. Nevertheless her illness progressed despite the hormone therapy. Therefore, in October 2008, the patient was started on Taxol chemotherapy.

Very soon after that, she began to report severe pain in her right thigh when bearing weight, and became wheel-chair bound. Physical examination revealed pain on internal rotation of the right hip and tenderness in the upper thigh on deep palpation. Radiographs revealed changes in the pelvis and proximal femora, and sclerotic lesions in the right distal femur (see figure 1).

Destructive osteolysis in the right proximal femur was at high risk for a pathologic fracture. She was referred for an orthopedic consultation. One option was a complete pelvic reconstruction with a total hip arthroplasty. However, the relatively small, contained lesion in her right acetabulum made her a good candidate for cementoplasty. It was therefore possible to avoid the surgical morbidity associated with a pelvic reconstruction by instead performing a replacement of the proximal femur, followed by a minimally invasive cementoplasty.

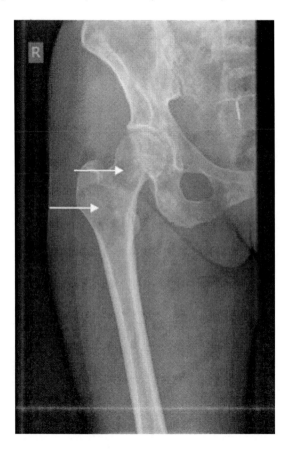

Figure 1. Right hip radiograph shows mixed lytic and sclerotic lesions in the right hemipelvis and the proximal right femur. The lytic lesion in the right femoral neck extending into the subtrochanteric femur is at high risk for a pathologic fracture (arrows).

She underwent a long stemmed cemented bipolar hemiarthroplasty in November 2008. The procedure was tolerated well by the patient with minimal blood loss and no immediate complication. The patient was discharged two days post-operatively when mobilizing independently with minimal discomfort. The preoperative pain was decreased substantially after her proximal femoral reconstruction. She was treated with appropriate DVT prophylaxis.

Three weeks after the operation her incision had healed and her staples were removed. Her function was reported at a much higher level in comparison to pre-operation, however, she had not recovered normal endurance. After approximately 100 meters of walking she would require rest due to hip/groin pain. The patient received postoperative cementoplasty to her right acetabulum in December 2008 (Figure 2). Further, she also received postoperative radiation therapy to her right hip in January 2009 with 2000 cGy in 5 fractions. These treatments improved her mobility to the point that it was no longer limited by hip pain.

At 8- week follow up post surgery, she did not have any leg length discrepancy and her right leg was neurovascularly intact. She had also regained a wide range of motion in her right hip. Radiographs showed hemiarthroplasty in good position and cement at the acetabulum demonstrated good filling of the lesion. There were no fractures or hardware complications (see figure 3).

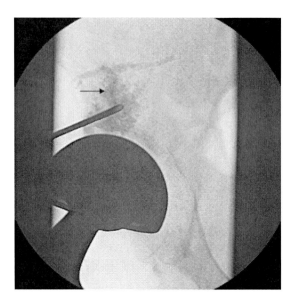

Figure 2. Fluoroscopic image of the right hip shows administration of cement via a percutaneous approach (arrow). Note right bipolar hemiarthroplasty in place.

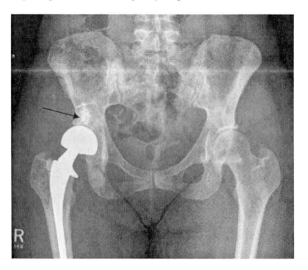

Figure 3. Radiograph of the pelvis following right bipolar hemiarthroplasty and cementoplasty of the right acetabulum. There are widespread mixed sclerotic and lytic lesions in the pelvis and proximal femora.

Discussion

The incidence of bone metastases is highest in breast and prostate cancer patients, with breast cancer accounting for the highest frequency of pathological fracture (6). As with this patient's experience, one of the most significant symptoms of bone metastases is pain (1,2,6); if the sensation is persistent in weight bearing bones, pain can also raise suspicion of an impending pathological fracture (7). In this situation, surgical intervention should be strongly considered (6). In the hip region, impending fractures are typically stabilized through metal implants, bone cement and joint replacement; however, there are currently no evidence-based guidelines for surgical management for these lesions (4). As a result, these patients require an individualized approach to their treatment.

When considering surgical treatment for an impending fracture, both the lesion and patient are taken into consideration. This patient's lesion was lytic rather than blastic, involved a large area of the proximal femur and caused pain that precluded weight bearing. This called for immediate intervention (6). Her principal lesion involved the femoral neck which could be addressed with proximal femoral reconstruction using a hemiarthroplasty. This restored immediate independent weight bearing function to this patient with minimal surgical morbidity. Her acetabular lesion was significant but amenable to urgent outpatient treatment with percutaneous cementoplasty after her femoral surgery. This spared the patient the added surgical morbidity of a pelvic reconstruction and total hip arthroplasty.

Implant selection is affected by several factors. In general, cemented prosthesis are preferred as they provide immediate stability and allow full weight bearing. Uncemented components rely on a biological response from the surrounding bone tissue. This is often compromised by ongoing chemotherapy and radiation. A Cochrane review of the general hip fracture population revealed that pain is reported more often and with increased severity in patients who underwent arthroplasty at the proximal femur without cement. This review also reported that patients who had received bone cement regained better mobility post operation (8). These findings would likely be even more pronounced in a pathologic fracture group where failure rates of uncemented fixation would be predictably higher.

After the hemiarthroplasty, a peri-acetabular lesion underwent cementoplasty. Basile et al (5) report that cementoplasty is a safe and efficient method of managing pain associated with small lesions from bone metastases. Their entire patient group (100% of patients) reported pain relief. With respect to mobility, 80% of the treated showed improvement (5). We used radiation therapy post-surgery to minimize possible disease progression (6). As Townsend et al. showed in their study, surgery alongside radiation provides for the best possibility of reaching and maintaining a level of normal functioning (9).

While this patient has shown improvement in pain and mobility after surgery, further follow up is recommended. The short term outcome of pain and mobility from a bipolar hemiarthroplasty is more or less equal to outcomes associated with a total hip replacement. Longer term outcomes in hemiarthroplasty patients of ten years or longer reveal more complications including increased pain and occasionally a need for revision to total hip arthroplasty (10). The goal of this surgery is palliative to immediately improve mobility, decrease pain and improve quality of life (11). Currently, patients with bone metastases have a life span of approximately 2-5 years (12), the immediate advantages of the less invasive hemiarthroplasty should outweigh the future implications.

We report a successful early outcome of a multidisciplinary treatment strategy in a patient with metastatic breast carcinoma to the hip. Hemiarthroplasty was chosen as a less invasive surgical option over total hip arthroplasty with pelvic reconstruction. Post-operative cementoplasty and radiotherapy treatment were able to further improve mobility, decrease pain, and potentially limit spread of disease in this patient.

Acknowledgments

This study was supported by the Michael and Karyn Goldstein Cancer Research Fund. We would also like to thank Stacy Lue for her secretarial assistance. Conflict of interest: none.

References

[1] Solomayer E, Diel IJ, Meyberg GC, Gollan C, Bastert G. Metastatic breast cancer: Clinical course, prognosis and therapy related to the first site of metastasis. Breast Cancer Res Treat 2000;59(3):271-8.
[2] Coleman RE, Rubens RD. The clinical course of bone metastases from breast-cancer. Br J Cancer 1987;55(1):61-6.
[3] Johnson SK, Knobf MT. Surgical interventions for cancer patients with impending or actual pathologic fractures. Orthop Nurs 2008;27(3):160-71.
[4] Kreder HJ. Factors affecting outcome after surgical treatment of acetabular and femoral metastatic lesions. Tech Orthop 2004;19(1):38-44.
[5] Basile A, Giuliano G, Scuderi V, Motta S, Crisafi R, Coppolino F, et al. Cementoplasty in the management of painful extraspinal bone metastases: Our experience. Radiol Med 2008;113(7):1018-28.
[6] Swanson KC, Pritchard DJ, Sim FH. Surgical treatment of metastatic disease of the femur. J Am Acad Orthop Surg 2000;8(1):56-65.
[7] Riccio AI, Wodajo FM, Malawer M. Metastatic carcinoma of the long bones. Am Fam Physician 2007;76(10):1489-94.
[8] Parker MJ, Gurusamy KS. Arthroplasties (with and without bone cement) for proximal femoral fractures in adults (review). Cochrane DB Syst Rev. 2006;3:1.
[9] Townsend PW, Smalley SR, Cozad SC, Rosenthal HG, Hassanein RES. Role of postoperative radiation therapy after stabilization of fractures caused by metastatic disease. Int J Radiat Oncol 1995;31(1):43-9.
[10] Muraki M, Sudo A, Hasegawa M, Fukuda A, Uchida A. Long-term results of bipolar hemiarthroplasty for osteoarthritis of the hip and idiopathic osteonecrosis of the femoral head. J Orthop Sci 2008;13(4):313-7.
[11] Stephen D. Management of metastatic osseous lesions of the lower extremity. Tech Orthop. 2004;19(1):15-24.
[12] Chow E, Hoskin P, van der Linden, Y., Bottomley A, Velikova G. Quality of life and symptom end points in palliative bone metastases trials. Clin Oncol 2006(18):67-9.

In: Pain Management Yearbook 2009
Editor: Joav Merrick
ISBN: 978-1-61209-666-7
©2012 Nova Science Publishers, Inc.

Chapter 50

REMINERALIZATION OF AN IMPENDING FRACTURE FROM AN OSTEOLYTIC METASTASIS IN A BREAST CANCER PATIENT FROM PALLIATIVE RADIOTHERAPY AND BISPHOSPHONATE. A CASE REPORT

Gunita Mitera, BSc, MRT(T)[*1], *Joel Rubenstein, MD*[2],
Joel Finkelstein, MD[3], *Melanie TM Davidson, PhD*[4]
and Edward Chow, MBBS[1]

[1]Rapid Response Radiotherapy Program, Department of Radiation Oncology
[2]Department of Radiology
[3]Department of Orthopedic Surgery
[4]Department of Physics, Sunnybrook Health Sciences Centre,
University of Toronto, Toronto, Ontario, Canada

Abstract

Metastatic disease to the bone is a common manifestation of breast cancer. A skeletally related event (SRE) may occur in up to two-thirds of patients with bone metastases. An SRE may include pathological fractures, severe pain, hypercalcemia, spinal cord compression, need for surgery and radiation treatment. This case report highlights the management for an impending pathological fracture that most frequently presents in the femur, a weight-bearing area. This case study presents a patient with an osteolytic lesion within the intertrochantic region of the right femur. She was offered prophylactic fixation of the right hip and femur and post-operative radiotherapy, but she refused surgical intervention. Given the heightened concern for an impending pathological fracture, we

---

[*] **Correspondence:** Gunita Mitera BSc, MRT(T), Department of Radiation Therapy, Odette Cancer Centre, Sunnybrook Health Sciences Centre, 2075 Bayview Avenue, Toronto, ON, Canada M4N 3M5. Tel: 416-480-6100 ext 7543; Fax: 416-480-6002; E-mail: Gunita.Mitera@sunnybrook.ca

managed her using radiotherapy with Clodronate, a bisphosphonate to stabilize and promote bone growth in the metastatic area. Based on our case study, we confirm radiotherapy in addition to bisphophonates may help to stabilize an osteolytic impending fracture from breast histology if patient is not a surgical candidate or refuses surgery if offered.

Keywords: Cancer, radiotherapy, breast cancer, pain.

Introduction

Metastatic disease to the bone is a common manifestation of breast cancer (1). A skeletally related event (SRE) may occur in up to two-thirds of patients with bone metastases. An SRE may include pathological fractures, severe pain, hypercalcemia, spinal cord compression, need for surgery and radiation treatment (2). This case report highlights the management for an impending pathological fracture that most frequently presents in the femur, a weight-bearing area (3). This case study presents a patient with an osteolytic lesion within the intertrochantic region of the right femur. She was offered prophylactic fixation of the right hip and femur and post-operative radiotherapy; however, she refused surgical intervention. Given the heightened concern for an impending pathological fracture, we managed her using radiotherapy with Clodronate, a bisphosphonate to stabilize and promote bone growth in the metastatic area.

Case study

A 55-year old female was diagnosed with a stage I, Estrogen-receptor equivocal and Progesterone-receptor positive left-sided breast cancer in 1997. Her treatment included breast conserving surgery with axillary node dissection and radiotherapy. Subsequently, her oncologist followed her on an annual basis for her breast cancer. In 2003 she suffered from local recurrence and was treated with a mastectomy, four cycles of doxorubicin and cyclophosphamide (AC) chemotherapy and Tamoxifen.

In January of 2008, she complained of right hip pain. Bone scan revealed an intense uptake in the right intertrochanteric region. Plain x-rays of the right pelvis and femur revealed an extensive mixed osteolytic and osteosclerotic focus within the right femoral neck and intertrochanteric area, along with cortical permeation. Furthermore, a computed tomography (CT) volumetric scan showed an extensive irregular lytic, permeative lesion in the proximal femoral diaphysis, extending to the lesser tuberosity and femoral neck, consistent with metastasis. It also confirmed extensive cortical permeation at the posterolateral femoral head, encompassing approximately 25% of the circumference. There was an additional focal cortical permeation at the anterior aspect of the mid-femoral neck. Radiographically, this was concerning for a significantly high risk of fracture (see figure 1).

Based on the imaging studies, the patient was immediately referred to the orthopedic surgeon for consideration of prophylactic fixation of the right hip and femur prior to radiotherapy. Prophylactic surgery was offered to the patient; however, she refused surgery. Hence, it was recommended that the patient walk with a cane to avoid the possibility of a fracture. Due to the high risk of fracture, as an alternative option the patient was offered palliative radiotherapy to the right hip and femur with 3000 cGy in 10 fractions.

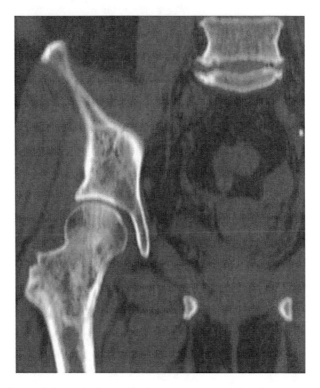

Figure 1. CT of right hip and femur before radiotherapy treatment showing permeative lytic destruction of bone in the proximal femur.

During a response assessment at three weeks, the patient reported reduced pain level and no longer walked with a limp, and discontinued the use of a cane. At two and four weeks post-radiotherapy, plain x-rays of the right hip and femur revealed no significant changes. Two months post-radiotherapy, the patient reported the pain to have resolved and was able to walk comfortably.

On her four-month follow-up, the patient still had complete relief of her pain and her activity level had increased such that she was able to dance again. X-rays reveal evidence of bone filing and no pathological fracture. Consequently, the surgeon declared the risk of fracture of the right femur to be minimal. The patient had also been prescribed Femara 2.5mg daily and Clodronate. Almost one-year post-radiotherapy treatment, the patient reported excellent range of motion of her right hip. X-rays continued to report no pathological fracture, with minimal changes. However, at this time there were two new noted sclerotic foci in the supraacetabular ilium. Since they were clinically asymptomatic, they were not treated with radiotherapy. Finally, 14-months post-radiotherapy, follow-up CT scan revealed sclerotic lesions in the radiated right hip and femur, compatible with treatment related response with significant improvement (figures 2 and 3).

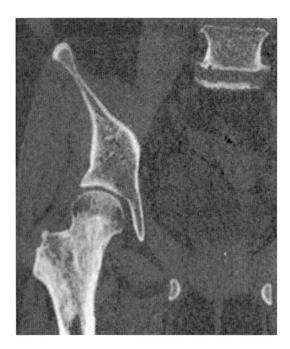

Figure 2. CT of right hip and femur 14-months after radiotherapy treatment showing sclerotic new bone formation in the region of previous lytic destruction

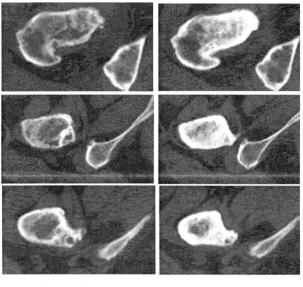

Pre-radiation   Post-radiation

Figure 3. An enhanced view of the pre-radiation lytic destruction and post-radiation sclerosis within the right hip and femur.

Discussion

Approximately 75% of breast cancer patients with recurrent disease will develop bone metastases during the course of their disease, and for one third of patients this is the first sign of recurrence (4). Breast cancer patients with bone metastases alone have a life expectancy of several years. This is longer when compared with patients who have visceral metastases from the same primary histology (5-8). Hence, it is important to evaluate the long-term efficacy of any offered treatment regimen in order to promote an improved quality of life for our patients (9).

Osteolytic bony metastases from breast histology may result in intractable pain and a high risk of pathologic fracture. Once bone has lost its structural integrity and is not yet fractured, they may be unable to support weight-bearing function for months. Under these circumstances, quality of life may be directly related to intact limb function that is necessary for ambulatory ability and activities of daily living (10).

When either patient dysfunction or pain is rated as severe, a treatment option that provides quick resolve of pain as well as quality of life should be considered. Treatment options in the management of metastatic bone disease are not mutually exclusive. Hence, an upfront multi-disciplinary approach is imperative for appropriate and timely decision-making. For example, surgical stabilization may revive functionality, while post-operative radiotherapy or chemotherapy may be required for pain relief and tumor control (10).

For impending pathological fractures routine follow-up with imaging and physical examination is recommended in order to prevent a fracture. The morbidity associated with a pathological fracture is not only devastating for the patient; moreover, it also narrows the range of treatment options, mitigates against full functional restoration, and demands a rehabilitation hiatus (10).

For clinicians to determine the risk of pathological fracture, Mirels (11) developed an objective scoring system that is governed by both clinical and radiographic evidence for each patient. It was developed with the intent to be used as an objective measure to help determine the risk of pathological fracture, and hopefully to prevent it from happening at all.

This system allots one, two, or three points to each risk factor based on both clinical and radiographic evidence for each patient. The maximum obtainable score is 12 points and the summation of these factors equips a clinician with an individualized accuracy for a given risk of fracture, as compared to evaluating any individual factor alone. A score of 9 suggests a 33% chance of fracture and is considered to the most accurate in Mirels' study (11) due to the 0% false positive rate. However, scores of 7 and 8 were associated with a smaller risk of fracture, but were confounded with a higher false positive rate within the study. Mirels (11) recommended that lesions with scores of 8 or higher require prophylactic internal fixation prior to radiotherapy, and lesions that obtain scores of 7 or lower can be safely irradiated without a risk of fracture. Table 1 demonstrates this scoring system.

Using Mirel's criteria (11), our patient would be assigned a score of 10, and this would equate to a high risk for pathological fracture. Surgical stabilization is recommended to be the first line of treatment for such clinical scenarios, however, beyond the scoring criteria, other considerations should include the location of the metastasis, primary tumor, ability to withstand general anesthesia, life expectancy and expected clinical response to non-operative therapy (10,12).

Radiotherapy is an established treatment for metastatic bone pain (10,14); however, its role in remineralization of osteolytic lesions as an upfront therapy for high-risk bony metastases remains unclear. While the literature recommends post-operative radiotherapy (11,12,14), there is a paucity of evidence to determine the optimal radiotherapy dose fractionation schedule to promote bone healing and prevent fracture (12-14). We previously reviewed 25 breast cancer patients with osteolytic metastases who had CT scans before and three months after palliative radiotherapy. The median percent density change following a single 8 Gy, 20 Gy in 5 treatments, and 30 Gy in 10 treatments were demonstrated to be 128 (range 98–255), 141 (range 79–342), and 145 (range 65–235), respectively. It was feasible to evaluate remineralization of osteolytic lesions with palliative radiotherapy using CT imaging (13). However, beyond its feasibility the appropriate dose fractionation scheme is still controversial.

A study by the Radiation Therapy Oncology Group (RTOG) observed an increased risk of pathological fracture after 40.5 Gy as compared with after 25 Gy (12). In contrast, there has been a randomized study that has evaluated the effects of pain relief and remineralization for patients with histologically proven breast, lung, prostate or kidney cancer and radiologically confirmed bone metastases. These patients were randomized to either a single 8 Gy or 30 Gy in 10 fractions. Pain relief was determined using pain score, analgesic usage and subjective perception of pain.

Remineralization was measured using CT imaging. Results were captured prior to radiotherapy, the day after, 6 weeks, 3 and 6 months post-treatment. Of 107 patients, there was no significant difference in overall (81% versus 78%) and complete (33% versus 31%) pain response for the use of 8 Gy versus 30 Gy respectively. However, the remineralization rate proved to be significantly different between patients in the fractionated group (173%) and the single dose group (120%, $p < 0.0001$). Specifically, this trend was highly significant for patients with a primary breast histology ($p < 0.001$) (15).

Table 1. Scoring system for risk of pathological fracture

VARIABLE	SCORE		
	1	2	3
Site	Upper limb	Lower limb	Peritrochanter
Pain	Mild	Moderate	Functional (Severe)
Lesion	Blastic	Mixed	Lytic
Size	<1/3	1/3 – 2/3	>2/3

Another treatment modality, bisphosphonates, has demonstrated promise within in vivo studies to prevent or delay SREs. More interestingly, Krempien demonstrate that the use of early bisphosphonates administration in conjunction with radiotherapy improves remineralization and restabilization of osteolytic bone metastases in animal tumor models (16). For example, in a mouse model of tumor-induced osteolysis, concurrent administration of zoledronic acid with radiation therapy was found to improve bone density, biomechanical strength and microarchitecture (17). Particularly, there is in vitro evidence for synergistic effects between zoledronic acid and radiation when demonstrated on breast cancer cells (18). Furthermore, a pilot study conducted by Vassiliou et al (19), delivered 30-40 Gy of radiotherapy delivered over 3 - 4.5 weeks combined with 10 cycles of monthly intravenous ibandronate. This was demonstrated to provide substantial bone pain relief and increased bone density for patients. The majority of these patients had primary breast (29%), lung (29%), or prostate (13%) cancers. Therefore, these studies support the idea that under circumstances where surgical intervention is either technically not feasible or the patient does not wish to have surgery for an impending fracture, perhaps these combined treatment interventions may be less invasive alternative options to help stabilize an osteolytic impending fracture from a breast histology.

Comprehensive management of patients with metastatic bone disease requires the participation of an orthopedic surgeon early in the clinical course. Early consultation and mutual follow-up will benefit the patient in maintaining independent function and avoid a possible fracture that may be devastating to the patient (10). When a pathological fracture has occurred, the primary goal is to provide pain relief. Secondary intentions are to achieve stability and to restore function. Unless medical contraindications exist, or unless life expectancy is extremely short, surgery is usually recommended. Based on our case study, we confirm radiotherapy in addition to bisphophonates may help to stabilize an osteolytic impending fracture from breast histology if patient is not a surgical candidate or refuses surgery if offered.

Acknowledgment

Conflict of interest: None.

References

[1] Solomayer E, Diel IJ, Meyberg GC, et al. Metastatic breast cancer: Clinical course, prognosis and therapy related to the first site of metastasis. Breast Cancer Res Treat 2000;59(3):271-8.
[2] Coleman RE, Rubens RD. The clinical course of bone metastases from breast-cancer. Br J Cancer 1987;55(1): 61-6.
[3] Johnson SK, Knobf MT. Surgical interventions for cancer patients with impending or actual pathologic fractures. Orthop Nurs 2008;27(3):160-71.
[4] Stoll B. Natural history, prognosis and staging of bone metastasis. In: Stroll BA, Parbhoo S, eds. Bone metastasis: Monitoring and treatment. New York: Raven Press, 1983:1-20.
[5] Perez JE, Machiavelli M, Leone BA, et al. Bone-only versus visceral-only metastatic pattern in breast cancer: analysis of 150 patients. A GOCS study. Am J Clin Oncol 1990;13(4):294-8.
[6] Toma S, Venturino A, Sogno G, et al. Metastatic bone tumors. Nonsurgical treatment. Outcome and survival. Clin Orthop 1993;295:246-51.
[7] Brown JE, Coleman RE. The present and future role of bisphosphonates in the management of patients with breast cancer. Breast Cancer Res 2002;4(1):24-9.
[8] Coleman RE. Skeletal complications of malignancy. Cancer 1997;80(8 Suppl):1588-94.
[9] Rasmussen B, Vejborg I, Jensend AB, et al. Irradiation of bone metastases in breast cancer patients: a randomized study with 1 year follow-up Radiother Oncol 1995;34:179-84.
[10] Colyer RA. Surgical stabilization of pathological neoplastic fractures Curr Probl Cancer 1986;10(3):117-68.
[11] Mirels H. Metastatic disease in long bones A proposed scoring system for diagnosing impending pathologic fractures Clin Orthop Relat Res 2003;415S: S4-13.
[12] Andreson PR, Coia LR. Fractionation and outcomes with palliative radiation therapy Semin Radiat Oncol 2000;10(3):191-9.
[13] Chow E, Holden L, Rubenstein J, et al. Computed tomography (CT) evaluation of breast cancer patients with osteolytic bone metastases undergoing palliative radiotherapy—a feasibility study. Radiother Oncol 2004;70:291-4.

[14] Chow E, Harris K, Fan G, et al. Palliative radiotherapy trials for bone metastases: a systematic review. J Clin Oncol 2007;25(11):1423-36.
[15] Koswig S, Budach V. Recalcification and pain relief following radiotherapy for bone metastases: A randomized trial of 2 different fractionation schedules (10 X 3 Gy vs. 1 X 8 Gy). Strahlenther Onkol 1999;175:500-8. [German].
[16] Krempien R, Huber P, Hrms W, et al. Combination of early bisphosphonate administration and irradiation leads to improved remineralization and restabilization of osteolytic bone metastases in an animal tumor model. Cancer 2003;98(6):1318-24.
[17] Arrington SA, Damron TA, Mann KA, et al. Concurrent administration of zoledronic acid and irradiation leads to improved bone density, biomechanical strendgth and microarchitecture in a mouse model of tumor-induced osteolysis. J Surg Oncol 2008;97(3):284-90.
[18] Ural AU, Avcu F, Candir M, et al. In vitro synergistic cyroreductive effects of zoledronic acid and radiation on breast cancer cells, Breast Cancer Res 2006;8(4): R52.
[19] Vassiliou V, Kalogeropoulou C, Christopoulos C, et al. Combination ibandronate and radiotherapy for the treatment of bone metastases: clinical evaluation and radiologic assessment. Int J Radiat Oncol Biol Phys 2007;67(1):264-72.

Chapter 51

NEED FOR POST PROCEDURE RADIATION THERAPY AFTER KYPHOPLASTY OR VERTEBROPLASTY/CEMENTOPLASTY FOR BONY METASTATIC DISEASE

Edward Chow[*], MBBS, May Tsao, MD, Arjun Sahgal, MD, Elizabeth Barnes, MD, Cyril Danjoux, MD, Gunita Mitera, MRT(T) and Emily Sinclair, MRT(T)

Rapid Response Radiotherapy Program, Department of Radiation Oncology, Sunnybrook Health Sciences Centre, Odette Cancer Centre, University of Toronto, Toronto, Ontario, Canada

Postoperative radiation therapy has been routinely administered following the orthopedic stabilization of impending and pathological fractures due to metastatic bone disease. There have been no randomized studies conducted to date to verify the benefits of this practice. Townsend et al (1,2) retrospectively reviewed the benefits of postoperative radiation therapy in 60 patients with pathological or impending pathologic fracture after 64 orthopedic stabilization procedures. They compared the outcomes of 35 patients treated with adjuvant postoperative radiation therapy versus 29 patients treated with surgery alone. The delivery of post-op radiation therapy resulted in more patients regaining normal use of their extremity (with or without pain) and fewer reoperations to the same site (1,2). This supports the benefits of postoperative radiation therapy in this setting. Unless patients have very limited survival, we recommend the referral of patients after the orthopedic stabilization for a radiation oncology consult.

---

[*] **Correspondence:** Edward Chow, MBBS, PhD, FRCPC, Department of Radiation Oncology, Odette Cancer Centre, Sunnybrook Health Sciences Centre, 2075 Bayview Avenue, Toronto, ON M4N 3M5, Canada. Tel: 416-480-4998; Fax: 416-480-6002; E-mail: Edward.Chow@sunnybrook.ca

Kyphoplasty, vertebroplasty and cementoplasty have gained popularity as minimally invasive surgical procedures in patients with bone metastases. Some patients have been treated with these procedures alone. There have been few comparative studies addressing the benefits of adjuvant post procedure radiation therapy. Gerszten et al (3) did report using a combined kyphoplasty and spinal radiosurgery treatment in 26 patients with histologically confirmed pathological fractures, and an improvement in pain was seen in 24 patients. We encourage more prospective or retrospective research in this expanding area. Until then, extrapolating the evidence of benefits of adjuvant postoperative radiation therapy from the one retrospective study following the open orthopedic stabilization, we recommend patients likewise be treated with post procedure radiation therapy after kyphoplasty, vertebroplasty, or cementoplasty, unless they have received prior radiation to that site.

References

[1] Townsend P, Rosenthal H, Smalley S, et al. Impact of postoperative radiation therapy and other perioperative factors on outcome after orthopedic stabilization of impending or pathologic fractures due to metastatic disease. J Clin Oncol. 1994;12(11):2345-50.
[2] Townsend P, Smalley S, Cozad S, et al. Role of postoperative radiation therapy after stabilization of fractures caused by metastatic disease. Int J Radiat Oncol Biol Phys 1995;31(1):43-9.
[3] Gerszten P, Germanwala A, Burton S et al. Combination kyphoplasty and spinal radiosurgery: a new treatment paradigm for pathological fractures. Neurosurg Focus 2005;18(3):E8.

Section Five – Acknowledgments

ABOUT THE EDITOR

Joav Merrick, MD, MMedSci, DMSc, is professor of pediatrics, child health and human development affiliated with Kentucky Children's Hospital, University of Kentucky, Lexington, United States and the Zusman Child Development Center, Division of Pediatrics, Soroka University Medical Center, Ben Gurion University, Beer-Sheva, Israel, the medical director of the Division for Mental Retardation, Ministry of Social Affairs, Jerusalem, the founder and director of the National Institute of Child Health and Human Development. Numerous publications in the field of pediatrics, child health and human development, rehabilitation, intellectual disability, disability, health, welfare, abuse, advocacy, quality of life and prevention. Received the Peter Sabroe Child Award for outstanding work on behalf of Danish Children in 1985 and the International LEGO-Prize ("The Children's Nobel Prize") for an extraordinary contribution towards improvement in child welfare and well-being in 1987.

Contact:
Office of the Medical Director, Division for Mental Retardation, Ministry of Social Affairs, POBox 1260, IL-91012 Jerusalem, Israel.
E-mail: jmerrick@zahav.net.il
Website: www.nichd-israel.com
Home-page: http://jmerrick50.googlepages.com/home

ABOUT THE NATIONAL INSTITUTE OF CHILD HEALTH AND HUMAN DEVELOPMENT IN ISRAEL

The National Institute of Child Health and Human Development (NICHD) in Israel was established in 1998 as a virtual institute under the auspicies of the Medical Director, Ministry of Social Affairs and Social Services in order to function as the research arm for the Office of the Medical Director. In 1998 the National Council for Child Health and Pediatrics, Ministry of Health and in 1999 the Director General and Deputy Director General of the Ministry of Health endorsed the establishment of the NICHD.

Mission

The mission of a National Institute for Child Health and Human Development in Israel is to provide an academic focal point for the scholarly interdisciplinary study of child life, health, public health, welfare, disability, rehabilitation, intellectual disability and related aspects of human development. This mission includes research, teaching, clinical work, information and public service activities in the field of child health and human development.

Service and academic activities

Over the years many activities became focused in the south of Israel due to collaboration with various professionals at the Faculty of Health Sciences (FOHS) at the Ben Gurion University of the Negev (BGU). Since 2000 an affiliation with the Zusman Child Development Center at the Pediatric Division of Soroka University Medical Center has resulted in collaboration around the establishment of the Down Syndrome Clinic at that center. In 2002 a full course on "Disability" was established at the Recanati School for Allied Professions in the Community, FOHS, BGU and twice a year seminars for specialists in family medicine. In 2005 collaboration was started with the Primary Care Unit of the faculty and disability became part of the master of public health course on "Children and society". In the academic year 2005-2006 a one semester course on "Aging with disability" was started as part of the master of science program in gerontology in our collaboration with the Center for Multidisciplinary Research in Aging.

Research activities

The affiliated staff has over the years published work from projects and research activities in this national and international collaboration. In the year 2000 the International Journal of Adolescent Medicine and Health and in 2005 the International Journal on Disability and Human development of Freund Publishing House (London and Tel Aviv), in the year 2003 the TSW-Child Health and Human Development and in 2006 the TSW-Holistic Health and Medicine of the Scientific World Journal (New York and Kirkkonummi, Finland), all peer-reviewed international journals were affiliated with the National Institute of Child Health and Human Development. From 2008 also the International Journal of Child Health and Human Development (Nova Science, New York), the International Journal of Child and Adolescent Health (Nova Science) and the Journal of Pain Management (Nova Science) affiliated.

National collaboration

Nationally the NICHD works in collaboration with the Faculty of Health Sciences, Ben Gurion University of the Negev; Department of Physical Therapy, Sackler School of Medicine, Tel Aviv University; Autism Center, Assaf HaRofeh Medical Center; National Rett and PKU Centers at Chaim Sheba Medical Center, Tel HaShomer; Department of Physiotherapy, Haifa University; Department of Education, Bar Ilan University, Ramat Gan, Faculty of Social Sciences and Health Sciences; College of Judea and Samaria in Ariel and recently also collaborations has been established with the Division of Pediatrics at Hadassah, Center for Pediatric Chronic Illness, Har HaZofim in Jerusalem.

International collaboration

Internationally with the Department of Disability and Human Development, College of Applied Health Sciences, University of Illinois at Chicago; Strong Center for Developmental Disabilities, Golisano Children's Hospital at Strong, University of Rochester School of Medicine and Dentistry, New York; Centre on Intellectual Disabilities, University of Albany, New York; Centre for Chronic Disease Prevention and Control, Health Canada, Ottawa; Chandler Medical Center and Children's Hospital, Kentucky Children's Hospital, Section of Adolescent Medicine, University of Kentucky, Lexington; Chronic Disease Prevention and Control Research Center, Baylor College of Medicine, Houston, Texas; Division of Neuroscience, Department of Psychiatry, Columbia University, New York; Institute for the Study of Disadvantage and Disability, Atlanta; Center for Autism and Related Disorders, Department Psychiatry, Children's Hospital Boston, Boston; Department of Paediatrics, Child Health and Adolescent Medicine, Children's Hospital at Westmead, Westmead, Australia; International Centre for the Study of Occupational and Mental Health, Düsseldorf, Germany; Centre for Advanced Studies in Nursing, Department of General Practice and Primary Care, University of Aberdeen, Aberdeen, United Kingdom; Quality of Life Research Center, Copenhagen, Denmark; Nordic School of Public Health, Gottenburg, Sweden; Scandinavian Institute of Quality of Working Life, Oslo, Norway; Centre for Quality of Life of the Hong Kong Institute of Asia-Pacific Studies and School of Social Work, Chinese University, Hong Kong.

Targets

Our focus is on research, international collaborations, clinical work, teaching and policy in health, disability and human development and to establish the NICHD as a permanent institute at one of the residential care centers for persons with intellectual disability in Israel in order to conduct model research and together with the four university schools of public health/medicine in Israel establish a national master and doctoral program in disability and human development at the institute to secure the next generation of professionals working in this often non-prestigious/low-status field of work. For this project we need your support. We are looking for all kinds of support and eventually an endowment.

Contact

Professor Joav Merrick, MD, MMedSci, DMSc
Medical Director, Division for Mental Retardation
Ministry of Social Affairs, POBox 1260
IL-91012 Jerusalem, Israel
E-mail: jmerrick@internet-zahav.net
Website: www.nichd-israel.com;

SECTION SIX - INDEX

#

20th century, 88, 90, 91

A

abuse, 139, 140, 146, 150, 396, 407, 587
access device, 66
acetabulum, 569, 570, 571, 572
acetic acid, 311
acetylcholine, 294, 337, 419, 422
acid, 256, 305, 321, 432, 433, 434, 440, 442, 443, 444, 515, 542, 580, 582
ACLS (Advanced Cardiology Life Support), 187
action potential, 268, 274, 291, 331, 354, 401, 407, 408
activity level, 577
adaptive functioning, 23, 35
adenocarcinoma, 570
adenosine, 294, 320
adolescents, 7, 16, 24, 28, 34, 62, 76, 77, 79, 84, 172, 181, 182, 183, 193, 202
adulthood, 4, 5, 13, 21, 172, 181
adults, xi, 10, 11, 13, 14, 15, 18, 19, 20, 21, 30, 34, 35, 45, 46, 47, 48, 56, 57, 58, 62, 63, 70, 73, 84, 126, 166, 171, 172, 248, 311, 342, 398, 408, 574
advanced cancer symptoms, 446, 454, 458, 460
adverse effects, 31, 140, 141, 143, 312, 326, 333, 389, 469
adverse event, 150, 151, 292, 414, 432
aerobic exercise, 297, 462
aetiology, 351
affective dimension, 308, 397, 398, 407
affective disorder, 347, 348, 349, 355, 357

aging process, 248
aging society, 140
agonist, 258, 277, 290
alcohol dependence, 333
algorithm, 145, 146, 147, 149, 150
alpha activity, 304
alternative treatments, 515
alters, 28, 206, 260
altruism, 43
ambivalence, 118, 121
American Heart Association, 190
American Psychiatric Association, 143
amino acids, 311, 321
amplitude, 128, 264, 266, 269, 274, 275, 289, 330, 338, 353, 354, 356, 388, 401, 413
amputation, 211, 254, 256, 259, 260, 347, 349, 351, 357, 358, 396
amygdala, 257, 313, 397
amyotrophic lateral sclerosis, 339
anaesthesiologist, 194, 373
analgesic, 8, 17, 31, 61, 66, 74, 128, 143, 187, 306, 307, 324, 342, 343, 346, 349, 357, 359, 399, 401, 412, 418, 419, 423, 424, 425, 426, 432, 434, 437, 438, 439, 440, 441, 444, 446, 447, 455, 465, 472, 473, 476, 479, 480, 481, 482, 483, 503, 504, 510, 515, 516, 565, 580
anatomy, 39, 92, 269, 356, 379, 402
androgen, 435
anesthesiologist, 403
anesthetics, 344
ANOVA, 50, 52, 129, 139, 140, 141, 142, 216, 304, 307, 415, 416, 445, 447, 449, 450
ANS, 382, 383
anterior cingulate cortex, 40, 42, 255, 261, 397
antibiotic, 96
anticonvulsant, 145, 146, 147, 292

antidepressant medication, 302
antidepressant(s), 146, 297, 299, 300, 302, 303, 311, 314, 393, 421
anti-inflammatory agents, 300, 515
anus, 93
anxiety, 4, 6, 15, 23, 47, 141, 142, 154, 156, 171, 172, 174, 175, 179, 180, 181, 182, 183, 186, 196, 219, 221, 236, 239, 255, 258, 261, 303, 307, 310, 313, 322, 397, 399, 401, 414, 416, 418, 419, 445, 446, 447, 450, 451, 453, 454, 456, 457, 459, 460, 461, 469
aphasia, 305, 339, 389
apnea, 4, 342
apoptosis, 432, 433, 435, 441
appendicular skeleton, 562, 570
appetite, 336, 409, 421, 445, 446, 447, 453, 454, 455, 456, 457, 458, 461, 570
appointments, 527
apraxia, 4
arousal, 28, 32, 40, 92, 94, 95, 172, 179, 180, 346
arrest, 3, 9, 315, 389, 441
arterial hypertension, 186
arthritis, 46, 48, 51, 158, 159, 176, 193, 201, 202, 238, 240, 311
arthroplasty, 570, 573
Asociación Chilena de Seguridad (ACHS), 205, 206, 208, 211
aspartate, 261, 279, 321
asphyxia, 66
assessment tools, xii, 13, 16, 46, 47, 62, 357, 519
asymptomatic, 577
ataxia, 4, 353
ATLS (Advanced Trauma Life Support), 187
ATP, 320
atrophy, 322, 368, 370, 383, 386
auditory cortex, 315
autism, 10, 17, 24, 62, 74, 76
autobiographical memory, 77, 78, 79, 80, 81, 82
autogenic training, 130
automatic processes, 257
autonomic nervous system, 299
autopsy, 530
avoidance, 103, 140, 142, 155, 182, 192, 201
avoidance behavior, 182
awareness, 15, 21, 89, 92, 516
axial skeleton, 514
axon terminals, 256
axonal degeneration, 327
axons, 7, 268, 274, 275, 288, 305, 315, 321, 354, 356, 362, 401

B

back pain, 101, 102, 104, 105, 107, 108, 111, 112, 113, 114, 115, 116, 117, 118, 119, 120, 121, 124, 125, 126, 140, 141, 143, 193, 201, 202, 203, 205, 214, 215, 220, 221, 240, 249, 255, 260, 261, 270, 271, 300, 311
background information, 196
barriers, 27, 29, 30, 126, 142, 190
basal ganglia, 255
Beck Depression Inventory, 302, 303, 414, 416
behavioral assessment, 33
behavioral change, 29, 270
behavioral problems, xi
behavioral science, 88
behaviors, xi, xii, 5, 6, 9, 16, 18, 25, 28, 32, 206, 258
behavioural scales, 13
benchmarking, 131, 132, 138
bending, 315, 512, 522, 549
beneficial effect, 302
benefits, 108, 113, 115, 117, 118, 143, 206, 216, 326, 353, 406, 412, 419, 431, 440, 441, 442, 472, 516, 531, 558, 583, 584
benign, 182, 202
benzodiazepine, 141
bias, 104, 224, 403, 536
biological processes, 31
biomarkers, 32, 33, 268
biopsychosocial domain, 123
bisphosphonate treatment, 444
Bisphosphonates, viii, 431, 432, 443, 444, 451, 514, 542, 566
bleeding, 353, 370, 375, 384
blood, 30, 259, 298, 299, 302, 313, 320, 355, 362, 363, 397, 404, 564, 571
blood flow, 259, 302, 313, 320, 355, 362
blood pressure, 299, 363, 397
BMI, 416, 418
body mass index, 416, 418
bone form, 578
bone growth, 576
Bone Metastases Clinic, 509, 516
bone resorption, 541
bone scan, 570
bone tumors, 530, 581
borderline personality disorder, 306
bowel, 176, 299
brachial plexus, 357, 358, 367, 375, 381, 382, 383
bracing, x, 561, 565
bradykinin, 320
brain activity, 9, 260, 291, 306, 316, 335, 348, 355, 356, 358
brain chemistry, 261

brain damage, 386
brain functioning, 305
brain polarization, 293, 339, 395, 408, 412, 421
brain stem, 390
brain structure, 257, 265, 274, 300, 306, 330, 349, 354, 355
brainstem, 8, 11, 12, 306, 322, 359, 373, 390, 396
branching, 8, 9, 322
breast cancer, x, 432, 433, 436, 437, 442, 443, 444, 462, 470, 515, 517, 526, 528, 530, 541, 542, 550, 555, 556, 558, 559, 560, 566, 569, 570, 573, 574, 575, 576, 578, 580, 581, 582
bruxism, 4

C

calcitonin, 298
calcium, 146, 256, 290, 292, 294, 303, 362, 432
calcium channel blocker, 290, 303
calvarium, 350
CAM, 87, 182, 190
candidates, 146, 147, 363, 386
cannabinoids, 258, 261
capsule, 348, 349, 359
carbamazepine, 373
carcinoma, 556, 559, 560, 562, 566, 570, 574
cardiac surgery, 84, 167
cardiomyopathy, 562, 565
caregivers, 14, 18, 19, 20, 22, 27, 28, 30, 47, 63, 64, 83, 249
cartoon, 224, 229, 231, 232
case study, 328, 362, 575, 576, 581
catastrophes, 23
catecholamines, 130
category a, 247
catheter, 165, 168
cation, 292
cauda equina, 531
cauda equina syndrome, 531
causal inference, 161
causalgia, 424
causality, 28, 180, 338
causation, 116
CCA, 259, 427
cell body, 302, 354
cell cycle, 441
cell death, 256, 292
cell differentiation, 432
cell line, 433, 435, 443, 444
cell lines, 443
cell size, 176
Cemented hemiarthroplasty, x, 569, 570

cementoplasty, x, 510, 569, 570, 571, 572, 573, 574, 583, 584
central nervous system, 7, 128, 129, 258, 297, 298, 301, 321, 361, 367, 396, 412, 413
central neuropathic pain, 145, 146, 149, 150, 365, 366, 374, 378, 381, 386, 391
cerebellum, 42, 300, 302
cerebral blood flow, 300, 302, 311, 312, 313, 355, 373, 393
cerebral cortex, 287, 293, 294, 377, 398
cerebral hemorrhage, 389
cerebral palsy, 17, 20, 24, 25, 46, 51, 59
cerebrospinal fluid, 8, 11, 272, 326
cerebrum, 7, 8
challenges, 27, 28, 30, 33, 46, 349
channel blocker, 290, 303
charge density, 292
chemical, 7, 9, 268, 321, 331, 344, 396, 432
chemotherapy, 149, 508, 525, 526, 531, 532, 535, 544, 558, 561, 564, 565, 570, 573, 576, 579
Choice reaction time (CRT), 127, 128, 129
cholinesterase, 291
chronic fatigue syndrome, 310
chronic illness, 154, 214
circulation, 51, 63, 265
classification, 153, 154, 155, 162, 163, 169, 265, 266, 336, 376, 377, 378, 392
classroom, 174, 232
cluster headache, 349, 355, 356, 360, 362
clusters, 106, 121, 541
CNS, 260, 261, 315, 321
CO2, 435
coagulopathy, 351
cocaine, 143
coefficient of variation, 129
cognition, 28, 39, 42, 84, 179, 202, 237, 261, 268, 311, 408
coherence, 337
collaboration, xi, 30, 515, 589, 590
colorectal cancer, 528
combination therapy, 431, 432, 433, 440
combined effect, 476
commercial, 269
common symptoms, 453, 530
communication, xii, 20, 25, 28, 37, 41, 46, 49, 50, 58, 92, 123, 268, 270, 305, 311, 316, 356, 362
community support, 238
comorbidity, 181, 258, 407
compensation, 206, 207
complex interactions, 274
Complex Regional Pain Syndrome I (CRPS/RSD), viii, 325, 327, 334, 339, 423, 424, 426

complications, 141, 269, 353, 369, 370, 373, 389, 446, 508, 514, 515, 517, 520, 529, 530, 532, 534, 535, 536, 537, 542, 558, 559, 562, 566, 570, 572, 573, 581
comprehension, 23, 160, 166
compression, 93, 432, 446, 472, 508, 509, 513, 520, 531, 558, 560, 565, 570, 575, 576
computed tomography, 300, 302, 311, 313, 351, 355, 369, 434, 562, 576
computer, 358, 413, 546
computing, 19, 50, 157
conceptualization, 246
concordance, 522, 524, 526, 527
conditioned response, 257
conditioning, 257, 261, 276, 277, 278
conductor, 264, 315
configuration, 268, 275, 354, 356, 562
conflict, 87, 90, 330, 443
conflict of interest, 443
Congress, 34, 162, 328, 427
connective tissue, 93, 298
connectivity, 256, 276, 281, 315, 352, 358
conscious perception, 7
consciousness, 87, 90, 344
consensus, 95, 102, 104, 142, 146, 186, 226, 451, 461, 469, 471, 476, 477, 480, 503, 505, 551
consent, 48, 95, 174, 216, 226, 369, 481, 509, 522, 531
consolidation, 280, 284, 294, 337, 419
constipation, 48, 51, 150, 342, 460, 468, 469
construct validity, 46, 52, 231
construction, 106, 235, 248, 528
consulting, 102, 174
consumption, 187, 355, 440, 442, 460, 476, 480, 481, 483, 503, 504, 510
contingency, 544, 551
contralateral hemisphere, 400
contrast sensitivity, 289
control group, 41, 74, 79, 80, 81, 82, 127, 128, 129, 193, 200, 300
controlled studies, 292, 325, 334, 424, 426
controlled trials, 126, 326, 341, 345, 376, 442, 566
controversial, 5, 353, 382, 580
convergence, 546
convulsion, 388
coordination, 335, 508
coping strategies, 153, 156, 163, 191, 192, 201, 236, 237, 246, 247, 248, 249
coronary heart disease, 126
correlation, 32, 50, 52, 55, 56, 64, 67, 68, 69, 143, 157, 158, 159, 242, 243, 246, 304, 311, 314, 326, 377, 382, 384, 388, 391, 418, 425, 450, 456, 460, 519, 522, 532, 550, 551

cortical neurons, 8, 273, 274, 279, 400
Cortical plasticity, 253
corticotropin, 299
cortisol, 25, 299
cranial nerve, 367
craniotomy, 369, 375, 383, 385, 389
cranium, 265
craving, 336, 338
cross cultural pain drawings, 223
cross-validation, 249
CSF, 8, 9
CST, 275, 280
CT scan, 556, 577, 580
cultural differences, 29, 232
cultural influence, 37
cultural norms, 20
culture, 20, 96, 107, 111, 114, 223, 228, 232, 305, 519
cure(s), 89, 91, 95, 97, 107, 108, 112, 113, 114, 115, 116, 154, 186, 214, 216, 219, 220, 239, 241
curriculum, 232
cutaneous innervation, 327
cycles, 92, 438, 439, 576, 580
cycling, 372
cyclophosphamide, 576
cytoarchitecture, 392
cytochrome, 31
cytokines, 297, 298, 300, 310, 320, 326, 565

D

daily living, 49, 50, 140, 155, 326, 579
data analysis, 76, 205, 232, 236
data collection, 50, 226, 246, 248
data set, 131, 369, 371
database, 235, 236, 443, 481, 509, 566
declarative memory, 257, 314, 337, 409
decoding, 43
deep brain stimulation, 271, 272, 347, 358, 359, 360, 361, 362, 363, 367, 389
deficiencies, 420
deficiency, 311, 338
deficit, 78, 368, 371, 558
deinstitutionalization, 58
delta wave, 314
dementia, 14, 74
demographic characteristics, 70, 175, 176, 248
demographic data, 207
dendrites, 303, 354, 401
dental care, 10
Department of Education, 27, 590
dependent variable, 216, 244, 245, 307, 415
depolarization, 275, 291, 321, 356, 400

depressive symptoms, 182, 300, 306, 312
deprivation, 314
depth, xii, 4, 104, 352
desensitization, 326
despair, 40, 124
destruction, 367, 368, 432, 556, 557, 562, 563, 569, 577, 578
detachment, 384
detectable, 371
detection, 14, 128, 143, 175, 176, 289, 316, 345, 372, 412, 552, 556
developing brain, 11, 12
developing countries, 143
developmental disorder, 3, 32
developmental process, 30
developmental psychology, 43
developmental psychopathology, 84
deviation, 245
diabetes, 389
diabetic neuropathy, 312
Diagnostic and Statistical Manual of Mental Disorders, 302
diagnostic criteria, 298
diaphoresis, 186
diaphysis, 576
diarrhea, 299
differential item functioning (DIF), 543, 544, 545, 547, 548, 551, 552, 553
diffusion, 286, 352, 369, 390
diodes, 128
Direct current stimulation, 285, 294, 335
disability, xi, 4, 11, 13, 16, 27, 28, 30, 31, 32, 33, 34, 46, 48, 51, 59, 102, 108, 112, 140, 143, 155, 162, 180, 183, 195, 205, 206, 207, 211, 214, 235, 236, 237, 238, 241, 242, 243, 246, 247, 248, 249, 300, 312, 396, 424, 587, 589, 591
discomfort, 59, 92, 160, 219, 220, 231, 286, 343, 399, 400, 468, 571
discrimination, 257, 259, 327, 398
discrimination training, 257
disease progression, 481, 529, 531, 535, 573
diseases, 161, 206, 211, 285, 330, 366, 390
dislocation, 353, 370, 559
disorder, 4, 9, 11, 12, 28, 46, 160, 166, 174, 176, 180, 181, 258, 297, 300, 301, 347, 349, 360, 367, 396, 411, 413, 420
dispersion, 81
displacement, 51, 254
disposition, 507, 514, 516
dissatisfaction, 103, 122, 214
distress, 4, 6, 15, 28, 30, 39, 40, 47, 83, 95, 108, 112, 153, 156, 159, 160, 161, 163, 165, 169, 186, 235, 236, 237, 238, 246, 247, 248, 249, 258, 535

distribution, 108, 194, 293, 337, 375, 408, 420, 545, 566
diversity, 106, 108, 186, 215
dizziness, 532, 556
doctors, 93, 105, 133, 137, 142, 219, 239
dominance, 104, 122, 123
dopamine, 130, 300, 306, 311, 316, 336
dopaminergic, 291, 302
dorsal horn, 7, 8, 298, 300, 321
dorsolateral prefrontal cortex, 261, 303, 317, 333, 337, 397, 398, 412, 413, 417, 421
dosage, 271, 372, 447
dosing, 267, 269
double blind study, 382
double-blind trial, 374, 375, 378, 382, 392
Down syndrome, 4, 84
drawing, 103, 224, 226, 229, 230, 231, 232, 233
drug abuse, 142, 368
drug action, 344
drug addiction, 143
drug metabolism, 31, 141
drugs, 96, 129, 143, 186, 206, 221, 256, 294, 303, 324, 344, 400, 460
DSM-IV, 139, 143
duodenum, 528
dura mater, 383, 385, 386, 399
dynamism, 125
dysarthria, 374
dysmenorrhea, 51
dyspareunia, 87, 93, 94, 96, 97, 99
dysphoria, 342
dystonia, 339, 348, 353, 390, 393

E

edema, 93, 319, 320
education, 89, 97, 156, 157, 175, 176, 193, 194, 195, 220
educational background, 122
EEG patterns, 286
ejaculation, 88, 96, 99
elaboration, 24
elderly population, 141, 142
electric current, 39, 265, 383, 396, 399, 401, 406
electric field, 268, 272, 274, 281, 305, 315
electrical properties, 268, 320, 354
electricity, 264, 267, 268
electroconvulsive therapy, 297, 301, 313
electrodes, 264, 265, 266, 267, 269, 270, 273, 275, 286, 293, 303, 325, 330, 331, 333, 334, 336, 344, 348, 352, 355, 356, 358, 359, 369, 383, 385, 387, 396, 399, 401, 405, 413, 414, 425, 426
electroencephalogram, 254, 271

electroencephalography, 412
electromagnetic, 274, 305, 400
Electrotherapy, 263, 264, 265, 269, 270
elongation, 7, 8
elucidation, 407
emboli, 562, 564, 566
embolization, 562, 564, 566
emergency, 185, 186, 187, 188, 189, 190
EMG, 273, 275
emission, 300, 302, 311, 313, 355, 373, 378
emotion, 37, 38, 39, 40, 42, 43, 107, 108, 111, 112, 117, 118, 231, 242, 243, 247, 248, 397, 407, 421
emotional distress, 153, 154, 156, 157, 159, 160, 161, 462
emotional experience, 166, 206
emotional problems, 88, 90, 94, 96, 97, 202
emotional reactions, 22
emotional responses, 309, 397
emotional state, 322
emotional stimuli, 412
emotionality, 261
empathy, 38, 40, 41, 42, 43, 231, 261
employment, 117, 156, 157, 237, 240
employment status, 156, 157, 240
encoding, 10
endocrine, 397
endorphins, 8, 9
endorsements, 237
endothelial cells, 272
endurance, 336, 421, 571
energy, 63, 88, 91, 107, 111, 114, 305, 437
environment, 22, 38, 56, 342, 553
environmental factors, 180
enzymatic activity, 31
EORTC, ix, 509, 510, 512, 516, 519, 520, 522, 524, 525, 526, 527, 528, 529, 530, 531, 532, 536, 538, 542, 544, 551, 552, 553
epidemiology, 33, 35, 181
epidural hematoma, 384
epilepsy, 294, 396, 408
episodic memory, 257
epithelium, 5
equipment, 131, 132, 134, 137, 307, 344, 403
erectile impotency, 96, 97
erosion, 562, 564
ERPs, 309
estrogen, 570
ethical implications, 95, 349
ethical issues, 29
ethical standards, 413
ethics, 95, 216, 413, 455, 465
ethnicity, 175, 176, 179
etiology, 31, 48, 96, 154, 182, 183, 269, 299, 397

event-related potential, 309
everyday life, 14, 107, 111, 118, 120, 130
evoked potential, 5, 11, 254, 260, 267, 271, 273, 281, 286, 289, 293, 294, 309, 311, 314, 317, 335, 337, 338, 369, 378, 379, 385, 399, 400, 420
examinations, 94, 373
excision, 560
excitability, 254, 255, 256, 258, 260, 272, 276, 277, 278, 279, 280, 282, 283, 285, 286, 287, 288, 289, 290, 291, 292, 293, 294, 298, 303, 314, 315, 319, 320, 321, 323, 326, 330, 331, 335, 336, 337, 344, 354, 398, 400, 401, 408, 413, 418, 420, 421, 422, 424
excitation, 274, 290, 305, 315, 354, 362
excitatory synapses, 256
excitotoxicity, 292
exclusion, 106, 116, 117, 193, 238
execution, 167, 168, 188, 357, 377
executive function, 396
executive functioning, 396
exercise, 89, 92, 98, 115, 460, 462, 522, 549, 552
experimental design, 213, 312
explicit memory, 257
exposure, 31, 39, 258, 299, 443
external locus of control, 192
extinction, 257, 258, 259, 261, 419
extraction, 74, 109
eye movement, 70

F

Facial Action Coding, 62, 75
facial expression, 16, 17, 20, 38, 39, 40, 43, 76, 225, 336
facial muscles, 38
facial pain, 271, 357, 358, 366, 367, 368, 374, 375, 377, 378, 379, 392
facial palsy, 374
facilitators, 196, 200, 214
factor analysis, 56, 76, 109, 126, 236
false positive, 372, 579
families, 28, 32, 101, 141, 174, 206, 477
family history, 41
family members, 472
FDA, 270, 348, 349
FDI, 279
fear(s), 6, 18, 92, 95, 126, 140, 171, 172, 175, 179, 180, 182, 183, 196, 198, 202, 215, 261, 397, 467
feelings, 37, 38, 41, 92, 94, 161, 192, 196, 200, 397, 527
FEM, 271
female partner, 88, 96, 97
femoral lesion, 569, 570

femur, 436, 513, 569, 570, 571, 573, 574, 575, 576, 577, 578
fetus, 169
fever, 300
fiber, 8, 261, 272, 315, 327, 393
fibers, 279, 298, 309, 321, 322, 390, 398
fibrositis, 298, 311
financial, 215, 297, 535
fitness, 237
fixation, 561, 562, 563, 564, 565, 573, 575, 576
fixed costs, 403
flashbulb memory, 81
flexibility, 263, 269, 434
flexor, 279
flexor carpi radialis, 279
fluctuations, 260
fluid, 8, 12, 311
fluoxetine, 317
focal seizure, 370, 373
food, 54, 333
force, 114, 336, 339, 421
forebrain, 8
fractures, 6, 46, 59, 186, 205, 208, 210, 432, 441, 446, 472, 508, 510, 513, 514, 515, 517, 528, 530, 531, 535, 542, 555, 563, 564, 565, 566, 567, 570, 572, 573, 574, 575, 576, 579, 581, 583, 584
free radicals, 320
freezing, 6
friction, 89
frontal cortex, 255, 293, 315, 316, 337, 345, 355, 408
frontal lobe, 362
full capacity, 7
functional activation, 256
functional changes, 255, 260
functional electrical stimulation, 263
functional imaging, 260, 377, 379, 391
functional MRI, 313, 315, 362, 373
funding, 516
fusion, 10, 11, 74, 75, 141, 371, 514, 557

G

GABA, 256, 268, 290, 323, 362
gait, 4, 353
ganglion, 8
gender differences, 220
gene expression, 321
general anesthesia, 342, 344, 345, 353, 383, 579
General Health Questionnaire, 238, 239, 249
general practitioner, 102, 104, 126, 135
generalizability, 56
generalized anxiety disorder, 172

genetic factors, 180
genetics, 29, 32
genitals, 91, 97
gerontology, 589
gestational age, 165, 167
glia, 300
glial cells, 298, 327, 354
globus, 361, 362
glucose, 355, 393
glutamate, 298, 303, 305, 321, 362
grants, 98
gratings, 289
gray matter, 11, 260, 306, 359, 361
group intervention, vii, 191, 193, 200, 201, 202
group size, 413
grouping, 123, 141, 299
growth, 4, 22, 29, 92, 256, 314, 320, 451, 565
growth factor, 314, 320, 565
guidance, 21, 33, 131, 137, 188, 267, 370, 377, 379
guidelines, 103, 104, 125, 138, 139, 140, 142, 147, 258, 269, 272, 355, 373, 376, 379, 526, 527, 528, 552, 573
guiding principles, 122
gynecologist, 94

H

habituation, 257, 420
hair, 229, 231
hardness, 87, 96
harmful effects, 130
head injuries, 205, 206, 208
headache, 126, 182, 193, 201, 202, 203, 205, 208, 211, 333, 338, 355, 373, 377, 389
healing, 98, 194, 437, 579
heart failure, 565
heart murmur, 182
heart rate, 299, 311
heat transfer, 272
hegemony, 123
height, 309
helplessness, 14, 192, 236
hematoma, 389, 403
hemiparesis, 374
hemisphere, 276, 278, 282, 323, 338, 384, 408, 414
hemorrhage, 389
herniated, 141, 207, 211
herniated nucleus pulposus, 141
heterogeneity, 35, 150, 269
hip arthroplasty, 571, 573, 574
hip fractures, 10
hip replacement, 573
hippocampus, 306, 315

histogram, 275, 443
histology, 469, 576, 579, 580, 581
history, 20, 22, 23, 37, 41, 102, 154, 200, 249, 322, 348, 351, 383, 413, 424, 509, 517, 521, 581
HIV, 181
holistic health, 88, 100
holistic medicine, 98, 99
homeostasis, 33
homovanillic acid, 313
hormone(s), 215, 305, 310, 315, 468, 535, 570
hospitalization, xi, 4, 142, 166, 206, 403, 404
host, 108, 216, 297
hostility, 156
House, 138, 143, 374, 590
HPA axis, 300
HTLV, 319
hyperactivity, 7, 331, 389, 398, 432
hypercalcemia, 432, 446, 459, 508, 509, 514, 570, 575, 576
hyperesthesia, 371
hyperplasia, 321
hyperpnea, 4
hypersensitivity, 5, 297, 327
hypertension, 565
hypertrophy, 321
hyperventilation, 11
hypnosis, 77, 78, 79, 82, 83, 255, 309
hypnotherapy, 84
hypochondriasis, 196, 202
hypotension, 186, 299, 311
hypothalamus, 322, 348, 349, 360, 397
hypothesis, 12, 43, 71, 99, 178, 246, 299, 306, 389, 451
hypothesis test, 451
hypoxia, 186

I

IASP, 12, 147, 166, 206, 211, 328, 366, 427
iatrogenic, 366
ICC, 45, 50, 55, 519, 525, 527
idiopathic, 260, 300, 311, 574
IFN, 565
IL-8, 300
ilium, 577
imagery, 78, 84, 310, 337, 377
imaging modalities, 369
immune system, 397
immunization, 16, 20, 73, 75
immunoglobulins, 321
impairments, 10, 20, 23, 30, 33, 35, 62, 66, 70, 73, 74, 75, 78, 126
implants, 353, 573

implicit memory, 253
improvements, 280, 291, 338, 349, 400, 408, 412, 418, 419, 558, 559
impulses, 321, 390
impulsiveness, 336
in vitro, 272, 362, 580
in vivo, 261, 313, 580
incidence, 23, 30, 31, 33, 46, 183, 205, 211, 300, 312, 359, 363, 440, 463, 464, 465, 466, 468, 470, 514, 520, 530, 532, 556, 565, 573
independent variable, 245
indirect measure, 355
induction, 31, 274, 290, 302, 372, 399, 400, 433
industrialized societies, 143
industry, 88, 98
infancy, 90, 309
infants, 14, 17, 24, 34, 167, 169, 170
infarction, 368, 374, 392
infection, 96, 353, 389
inferences, 274, 276, 281
inflammation, 7, 29, 326, 366
inflation, 84, 175
information processing, 419
informed consent, 48, 63, 155, 173, 174, 216, 413, 521, 527, 544
infrared spectroscopy, 355
inhibition, 31, 74, 254, 256, 258, 260, 276, 277, 278, 279, 280, 282, 283, 288, 291, 293, 294, 299, 303, 305, 316, 322, 323, 330, 335, 343, 356, 361, 362, 390, 398, 400, 402, 432
inhibitor, 290, 291, 299, 565
initial state, 106
injections, 6, 62, 213, 215, 217, 218, 219
insertion, 17, 62, 66, 165, 168, 370, 373, 384
insomnia, 142, 239, 292, 314
institutions, 46, 79
insulin, 314
integration, 122, 197, 379
Integrative medicine, 88
integrity, 93, 323, 432, 579
intellectual and developmental disabilities (IDD), 4, 6, 13, 27, 28, 29, 30, 31, 32, 33
intellectual disability(ies) (ID), xi, xii, 4, 13, 14, 15, 16, 17, 18, 19, 20, 21, 22, 23, 25, 27, 45, 46, 47, 48, 51, 56, 57, 58, 59, 61, 62, 63, 73, 74, 76, 77, 78, 79, 80, 81, 82, 83, 261, 415, 587, 589, 591
intensity values, 64
intensive care unit, 64, 165
interaction effect, 175, 178, 179, 249
interaction effects, 175, 178, 179, 249
intercourse, 90, 91, 94, 97
interest groups, 146
interface, 264, 330, 331

interference, 258, 420, 468, 479, 481, 482, 483, 486, 493, 498, 501, 504, 505, 509, 512, 550
interferon, 565
internal consistency, 50, 52, 56, 156, 175, 194, 196, 241
internal environment, 22
internal fixation, 579
International Association for Study of Pain, 166
International Classification of Diseases, 183, 312
International Narcotics Control, 142
interneurons, 275, 277, 303, 305
interpretative bias, 182
interpretive problem, 30
interstitial cystitis, 99
intervention, 25, 90, 119, 121, 123, 161, 165, 191, 192, 193, 199, 200, 201, 202, 215, 218, 220, 258, 259, 291, 347, 396, 404, 460, 515, 558, 564, 573
intracortical circuits, 282
intramuscular injection, 25, 165
intravenously, 342
Invasive pain management, vii, 213
ion channels, 287, 290, 354
ipsilateral, 254, 255, 276, 283, 300, 325, 333, 338, 373
IRC, 249
irradiation, 433, 443, 444, 473, 474, 558, 565, 582
irritable bowel syndrome, 299, 310
ischemia, 187
isolation, 14, 168, 193, 231, 433, 463, 525, 526, 527
issues, 14, 21, 27, 28, 29, 30, 31, 59, 97, 103, 119, 123, 156, 192, 197, 233, 270, 331, 360, 392, 444, 512, 519, 521, 526, 529, 530, 532, 536, 537, 544, 551, 552
item information functions (IIFs), 543, 545, 548, 549
item parameters, 545, 546, 548
item response theory, 543, 544, 545, 552, 553

J

joint pain, 138, 140
joints, 7, 565
Journal of Pain Management, xii, 590
jumping, 52, 56

K

kidney, 580
Kings Regional Rehabilitation Centre (KRRC), 45, 48, 49, 58

L

laminectomy, 211
language barrier, 472
languages, 20, 224
laparotomy, 344
latency, 275, 281, 289, 304
laterality, 313, 352
laws and regulations, 142
learning, 84, 181, 193, 202, 253, 257, 258, 273, 274, 278, 280, 281, 283, 315, 335, 336, 337, 409
learning process, 257
legal issues, 206
lesions, 292, 321, 353, 366, 368, 397, 432, 440, 442, 446, 481, 513, 514, 526, 556, 560, 564, 571, 572, 573, 574, 577, 579
life expectancy, 4, 515, 544, 559, 562, 579, 581
life quality, 56
lifetime, 102, 154, 298, 301
light, 3, 37, 40, 41, 92, 95, 97, 143, 158, 168, 181, 291, 292, 480, 552
limbic system, 130, 397, 398
linear model, 272
liver, 508
living conditions, 535
local anesthesia, 351, 384
local anesthetic, 214
local field potentials, 347
localization, 10, 306, 353, 377, 385, 392, 399, 401, 407
locus, 191, 192, 193, 194, 200, 201, 397
logistics, 49
longitudinal study, 181, 182, 259, 312
long-term memory, 420
loss of consciousness, 344
love, 96, 99
Low back pain, 101, 102, 107, 111, 114, 116, 117, 118, 120, 125
low risk, 513
LTD, 279, 290, 315
lumbar radiculopathy, 319
lumbar spine, 558
lung cancer, 442, 454, 530, 542
lung metastases, 508
lying, 465, 468, 512, 522, 525, 532, 548, 549, 551
lymph, 556, 570
lymph node, 556, 570

M

machinery, 403

magnetic field, 264, 266, 274, 305, 344, 355, 396, 400
magnetic resonance imaging (MRI), 12, 32, 255, 260, 267, 272, 286, 292, 293, 300, 311, 316, 317, 336, 337, 351, 352, 353, 355, 361, 362, 368, 369, 371, 377, 389, 390, 391, 392, 401, 408, 420, 562
magnetic resonance spectroscopy, 256, 261
magnetoencephalography, 347, 356, 362
magnetotherapy, 263
major depression, 271, 299, 305, 312, 314, 315, 330, 333, 338, 360, 368, 421
major depressive disorder, 298, 301, 310, 312
malignancy, 357, 517, 542, 581
mammals, 260
mania, 353
manipulation, 558
MANOVA, 479, 482, 486, 491, 493, 496, 498, 501, 502
manual sexological therapy, 95
mapping, 40, 91, 93, 328, 361, 367, 377, 391, 399, 408
mastectomy, 560, 576
matrix, 41, 110, 157, 482
mechanical testing, 436, 441
median, 64, 65, 128, 207, 216, 324, 349, 359, 369, 384, 447, 449, 450, 455, 459, 463, 471, 473, 480, 482, 507, 508, 510, 515, 516, 519, 523, 524, 525, 531, 536, 543, 545, 546, 547, 549, 559, 565, 580
mediation, 182, 237, 240, 244, 246, 247, 249
medical assistance, 160
medical care, 10, 201, 206
Medical Disability Evaluation Committee, 205, 206, 207
medical history, 389
medical science, 88
medication, 10, 74, 119, 121, 141, 192, 193, 239, 242, 243, 287, 291, 302, 317, 342, 351, 369, 371, 372, 374, 400, 413, 421, 425, 461, 463, 464, 510, 512, 558
medicine, 88, 91, 97, 99, 120, 122, 123, 126, 150, 188, 341, 343, 344, 507, 509, 589, 591
MEG, 356, 357, 362
membranes, 287, 291
memory, 77, 79, 81, 82, 128, 253, 257, 258, 259, 261, 271, 305, 315, 338, 396, 399, 402, 414, 420
memory formation, 259
memory performance, 261, 414
memory processes, 257
mental age, 23, 77, 78, 79
mental disorder, 143, 258, 302
mental health, 88, 91, 153, 154, 155, 156, 157, 158, 159, 160, 161
mental health component score (MHC), 154, 159

mental image, 77, 78, 79, 82, 83, 84
mental imagery, 77, 78, 79, 83
mental impairment, 206
mental retardation, 10, 46, 58, 59, 84
messages, 115, 121, 122, 124
meta-analysis, 126, 316, 346, 368, 377, 391, 396, 401, 407, 420
metabolic disorder, 32
metabolic disorders, 32
metabolism, 31, 215, 393
metabolites, 30, 311
metaphor, 123
metastasis, 433, 477, 505, 513, 517, 531, 532, 533, 535, 560, 562, 570, 574, 575, 576, 579, 581
metastatic cancer, 443, 562
metastatic disease, 440, 509, 523, 562, 570, 574, 583, 584
methodology, 30, 32, 101, 105, 108, 113, 121, 124, 126, 343, 382, 388, 522, 551, 552
MHC, 154, 159
microcephaly, 4
midbrain, 344, 356, 363
migraines, 176
migration, 321
milligrams, 510
mineralization, 434, 437, 441
Ministry of Education, 376
misconceptions, 141
mission, 589
misuse, 143, 146
mitogen, 327
model system, 288
modelling, 272, 354, 355
models, 7, 76, 161, 183, 249, 256, 298, 327, 349, 415, 416, 431, 433, 434, 441, 443, 545, 548, 553, 580
modifications, 146, 288, 290, 291, 319
modules, 526, 528, 530, 544, 552
mole, 66
molecular biology, 29, 32
molecules, 432
monoclonal antibody, 470
mood change, 302, 418, 532
mood disorder, 301, 313
morbidity, 94, 297, 301, 432, 441, 443, 517, 564, 569, 570, 571, 573, 579
morning stiffness, 154
morphine, 107, 112, 115, 117, 142, 144, 147, 150, 343, 346, 369, 382, 465, 472, 473, 479, 481, 484, 491, 510, 512
morphology, 261
mortality, 59
Moses, 11

motivation, 102
motor behavior, 274, 275, 278
motor control, 273, 281, 282
Motor cortex stimulation, 271, 363, 365, 377, 378, 379, 381, 391, 392, 393, 400, 407, 408, 420
motor evoked potential, 267, 273, 281, 294, 314, 335, 400
motor neurons, 293
motor skills, 4, 28, 49, 50
motor system, 254, 277, 306, 328
motor task, 280
movement disorders, 320, 348, 355, 357, 359, 361, 367, 377, 391
multidimensional, 15, 22, 37, 97, 104, 114, 154, 258, 520
multi-dimensional pain assessment tools, xii
multiple factors, 33
multiple myeloma, 523
multiple regression, 153, 157, 159, 160, 245
multiple regression analyses, 153, 160
multiple regression analysis, 245
multiple sclerosis, 271, 357, 363, 396
multivariate analysis, 479, 482, 491
multivariate statistics, 59, 76
muscle strain, 32
muscles, 7, 38, 39, 89, 90, 98, 254, 275, 278
music, 5, 78, 84, 168, 169, 170
mutations, 10
mutilation, 6
myalgia, 414
myocardium, 187
myringotomy, 66

N

Na$^+$, 290, 419
NaCl, 286, 293, 336, 425
narcotic, 143, 556
narcotic analgesics, 556
National Health Service, 108
National Institute of Child Health and Human Development, 2, xi, 587, 589, 590
National Institute of Mental Health, 181
National Institutes of Health, 528
National Survey, 131
nausea, 150, 292, 342, 445, 446, 447, 449, 450, 453, 454, 457, 460, 461, 570
navigation system, 385
near infrared spectroscopy, 362
necrosis, 292
negative affectivity, 163, 236, 237
negative effects, 108, 112, 114, 460
negative emotions, 226

negative mood, 299, 463
negativity, 192
neglect, 139, 140
neocortex, 320
Neonatal Facial Coding System (NFCS), 62
neonatal nursing, 166
neonates, 6, 75, 165, 167, 168, 169
neoplasm, 433
nephrectomy, 562
nervous system, 5, 7, 8, 9, 33, 34, 169, 253, 259, 268, 299, 320, 397
neural development, 9
neural network, 24, 305, 397, 398, 401, 402
neural networks, 401, 402
neural systems, 6
neuralgia, 148, 149, 366, 375, 392, 403
neurobiology, 336
neurodegeneration, 321
neuroimaging, 40, 300, 347, 355, 412
neurological disability, 25
neurologist, 135, 403, 404
neuroma, 211, 376
neuronal circuits, 288, 290, 402
neuropathy, 327, 396
neuropeptides, 321
neurophysiology, 326
neuropsychiatry, 314, 315
neuropsychopharmacology, 281
neuroscience, 32, 43, 84, 281
neurosurgery, 347, 351, 406
neurotransmission, 302
neurotransmitter, 9, 30, 256, 268, 299, 321
neurotransmitters, 9, 256, 268, 319, 321
neutral, 109, 118, 225
neutropenia, 570
next generation, 591
nitric oxide, 321
N-methyl-D-aspartic acid, 150
Nobel Prize, 587
nodes, 570
nodules, 559
Non-communicating Children's Pain Checklist, 13, 17, 19, 47, 62
non-pharmacological treatments, 300
non-steroidal anti-inflammatory drugs, 140
norepinephrine, 299, 300, 327
normal development, 4
normal distribution, 106, 197
NPT, 165, 167, 168, 169
NSAIDs, 140, 142
nuclei, 348, 359, 389, 398, 400
nucleus, 300, 306, 312, 316, 349, 359, 361, 362, 377, 397

nurses, 10, 101, 105, 122, 132, 133, 134, 186, 190
nursing, 122, 126, 142, 143, 165, 166, 167, 169, 185, 186, 190, 193, 509, 510
nursing home, 142, 143
nutrition, 170

O

obsessive compulsive disorder, 347, 349
obsessive-compulsive disorder, 360
obstruction, xii, 386
occipital cortex, 289, 333, 398, 401
occlusion, 99
occupational therapy, 122
oedema, 292
oil, 265
one dimension, 13
operant conditioning, 257, 261
operations, 367, 378
opiates, 8, 300, 530
Opioid dependence, vi, 139
opioids, 66, 73, 139, 140, 141, 142, 143, 144, 145, 146, 147, 151, 268, 343, 367, 510
optimism, 467
optimization, 270
oral antibiotic, 370
organ(s), 5, 89, 93, 268, 396, 523
organize, 34, 268
orgasm, 87, 90, 91, 95, 96, 97, 98, 99
orthopedic stabilization, 555, 583, 584
orthopedic surgeon, 206, 510, 513, 514, 516, 557, 563, 576, 581
oscillatory activity, 357, 401
osteoarthritis, 140, 163, 310, 314, 574
osteoporosis, 51, 140, 553
outcome relationship, 246
outpatients, 202, 312
overlap, 122, 236, 254, 301
ownership, 345
oxygen, 187, 355

P

pacing, 197, 354
pain beliefs, vi, vii, 101, 125, 126, 235, 236, 238, 242, 243, 245, 247, 248
Pain faces, 223
pain management, xi, xii, 12, 13, 14, 22, 23, 30, 32, 46, 47, 77, 78, 79, 82, 83, 101, 102, 105, 108, 115, 119, 121, 122, 123, 124, 125, 126, 131, 132, 133, 135, 136, 137, 140, 146, 150, 165, 166, 167, 169, 185, 187, 188, 190, 197, 202, 213, 218, 300, 308, 342, 343
pain service, 131, 132, 136, 137
pallor, 54
palpation, 91, 93, 94, 570
palpitations, 570
pancreas, 528
pancreatitis, 407, 528
panic attack, 172
panic disorder, 181
panic symptoms, 182
paralysis, 368, 371, 374
parietal cortex, 315, 389
parietal lobe, 367
paroxetine, 302
partial credit model, 553
partial mastectomy, 556
pathogenesis, 320
pathology, 9, 92, 267, 298, 459
pathophysiological, 161, 382
pathophysiology, 155, 298, 299, 300, 311
pathways, 7, 8, 9, 12, 40, 256, 269, 282, 283, 299, 302, 303, 321, 322, 323, 346, 354, 367, 376, 441
patient care, 104, 516
patient perceptions, ix, 529, 536, 537
Pavlovian conditioning, 257, 261
PCA, 61, 65, 69, 70, 74, 343
Pearson correlations, 156
pediatric pain, 13, 25, 62, 83, 179, 233
Pediatric Pain and Coping Inventory (PPCI), 78
pelvic floor, 88, 89, 91, 93, 97, 99
pelvic floor physical therapy, 99
pelvic physiotherapy, 93
pelvis, 93, 449, 455, 482, 510, 570, 571, 572, 576
penis, 89
peptides, 298
perceived control, 249
perceived outcome, 219
perfusion, 356, 362
perinatal, 66
perineum, 93, 94
periodicity, 275
periosteum, 399
peripheral nervous system, 214, 267, 268, 281, 366
peripheral neuropathy, 149, 366
permeation, 576
personality, 155, 237, 310, 396
personality traits, 155, 310
pessimism, 192
PET, 260, 286, 306, 316, 317, 355, 356, 373, 378, 389, 390, 393, 420
phantom limb pain, 254, 256, 259, 261, 327, 351, 356, 360, 366, 375, 377, 379, 383, 391, 392

pharmaceutical, 88, 98, 345
pharmacological treatment, 146, 185, 187, 188, 189, 215, 325, 351
pharmacology, 29, 32, 129, 187, 305
pharmacotherapy, 119, 327
phenomenology, 31, 33
phenotype, 319, 322
phobic anxiety, 156
phosphate, 432
photographs, 41, 75, 225
physical activity, 196, 559
physical exercise, 116
physical health component score (PHC), 154, 159
physical therapist, 194
physical therapy, 4, 93, 94, 95, 99, 460
physical well-being, 160, 446
physicians, 71, 88, 102, 103, 125, 141, 142, 143, 155, 186, 206, 214, 215, 342, 469, 509, 514
physiological mechanisms, 280
physiology, 29, 32, 89, 92, 269, 273, 277, 344
physiopathology, 187, 359
Picasso, 39
pilot study, 46, 47, 48, 191, 193, 200, 202, 289, 311, 313, 326, 342, 408, 420, 462, 464, 470, 580
placebo, 25, 96, 128, 150, 219, 233, 291, 304, 307, 308, 312, 317, 326, 359, 371, 372, 376, 382, 421, 431, 434, 437, 566
plasticity, 253, 256, 258, 259, 261, 273, 274, 278, 280, 281, 283, 285, 290, 291, 302, 320, 326, 327, 336, 337, 338, 339
plexus, 374, 375, 386
PLP, 366
PMMA, 557
polarity, 264, 266, 287, 288, 290, 330, 383, 401
polarization, 290, 291, 292, 293, 294, 335, 339, 395, 401, 408, 412, 420, 421
polymethylmethacrylate, 557
polymorphism, 299, 310
polymorphisms, 31
pons, 367, 371
poor performance, 56, 322, 552
positive relationship, 287
positron, 255, 260, 286, 300, 311, 313, 317, 355, 362, 373, 393
positron emission tomography, 255, 260, 286, 300, 311, 313, 317, 355, 362, 373, 393
postoperative outcome, 399
postoperative pain, viii, 10, 19, 35, 61, 62, 63, 169, 233, 306, 341, 342, 343, 345
postural control, 255, 260
potential benefits, 441, 443
pre- and post-quasi-experimental design, 213
preadolescents, 181, 182

prefrontal cortex, 8, 297, 306, 308, 315, 316, 322, 336, 338, 345, 346, 396, 398, 409, 421
premature infant, 170
preparation, 127, 220, 221, 379
pre-planning, 350
preschool, 24, 28, 75, 76, 230
preterm infants, 170
prevention, 14, 98, 126, 166, 170, 186, 202, 206, 220, 258, 432, 464, 469, 508, 517, 535, 542, 587
primacy, 115, 123
primary caregivers, 19
primary motor cortex, viii, 273, 275, 282, 283, 286, 297, 303, 307, 325, 334, 337, 346, 377, 379, 381, 383, 384, 386, 389, 390, 391, 392, 393, 398, 407, 409, 412, 413, 417
primary school, 226
primary tumor, 559, 579
primary visual cortex, 289, 294, 335, 337, 408
primate, 260
principles, 22, 117, 122, 187, 190, 257, 274, 348, 350, 353, 358, 396
private practice, 200
probability, 82, 158, 176, 275, 545, 546
proband(s), 298, 299
problem behavior, 202
problem behaviors, 202
procedural knowledge, 283, 284
processing pathways, 412
professional management, 123
professionalism, 95
professionals, xii, 10, 14, 15, 18, 21, 41, 75, 83, 95, 101, 102, 103, 104, 105, 106, 107, 111, 112, 117, 119, 121, 124, 125, 126, 141, 166, 186, 238, 403, 477, 589, 591
progesterone, 570
prognosis, 407, 556, 558, 559, 574, 581
programming, 269, 361
pro-inflammatory, 326
prolapse, 93
proliferation, 103
promoter, 310
prophylactic, 370, 464, 469, 562, 575, 576, 579
prophylaxis, 464, 469, 470, 571
proportionality, 108
prostaglandins, 298, 321
prostate cancer, 432, 443, 444, 463, 470, 508, 520, 523, 530, 541, 542, 573
prostate carcinoma, 444, 462, 517, 520
prosthesis, 257, 510, 573
protection, 95, 126, 373, 432
protein synthesis, 290, 294
proteins, 432
protons, 320

pruritus, 342
psychiatric disorders, 181, 299, 301, 351, 368
psychiatrist, 135, 180, 206
psychiatry, 301
psychoanalysis, 99
psychological distress, 235, 236, 237, 243, 248, 416, 417
psychological functions, 504
psychological processes, 215
psychological resources, 237
psychologist, 106, 107, 112, 116, 118, 135, 136, 180, 194, 196
psychology, 29, 32, 34, 122, 126, 203
psychometric properties, 13, 15, 21, 46, 50, 56, 57, 58, 126, 182, 233
psychopathology, 84, 182, 194
psychophysics, 127, 128, 130
psychoses, 351
psychosis, 368
psychosocial factors, 161, 162, 299, 310
psychosocial stress, 299
psychosomatic, 129
psychosurgery, 349
psychotherapy, 90, 91, 97, 99, 261, 297
psychoticism, 156
PTSD, 401
public health, 143, 530, 589, 591
public service, 589
puckering, 53
punishment, 38, 107, 111, 116, 167
P-value, 447, 491, 496, 500, 502
PVP, 515

Q

QLQ-BM22, ix, 509, 510, 512, 516, 519, 520, 521, 522, 524, 525, 542, 552
Q-methodology, 101, 105, 108, 113, 121, 124, 126
qualitative research, 126
quality improvement, 190

R

radiation therapy, 443, 444, 451, 461, 462, 470, 505, 509, 510, 542, 566, 572, 573, 574, 580, 581, 583, 584
radiculopathy, 327
radioresistance, 564
rating scale, 18, 78, 147, 224, 233, 325
reaction time, 128, 129, 278, 280, 286, 337, 339
reactions, 22, 39, 42, 92, 154, 300
reactivity, 30, 33, 42, 181, 328

recall, 77, 79, 82, 84, 465, 468, 521
Receiver Operating Characteristic (ROC), 50, 56
receptors, 7, 8, 166, 256, 285, 291, 303, 319, 321, 322
recognition, 27, 28, 32, 121, 123, 214, 219, 338
reconstruction, 369, 371, 560, 570, 571, 573, 574
recovery, 64, 66, 70, 71, 73, 74, 140, 214, 259, 281, 303, 314, 328, 389, 427
rectocele, 93
rectum, 93
recurrence, 307, 559, 560, 576, 579
redistribution, 315
redundancy, 236
reflex sympathetic dystrophy, 327, 423, 424
reflexes, 275, 322, 390, 397
regression, 4, 90, 160, 240, 244, 249, 388, 455, 520, 544, 545, 547, 548, 551, 552, 553
rehabilitation, 20, 123, 135, 206, 211, 220, 367, 509, 579, 587, 589
reinforcement, 257, 557
reinforcers, 257
relatives, 40, 43, 249, 298
relaxation, 92, 127, 128, 129, 130, 197
relevance, 113, 122, 123, 150, 257, 503, 519, 521
reliability, 16, 17, 19, 20, 21, 24, 25, 45, 47, 48, 50, 52, 56, 58, 64, 103, 156, 225, 360, 520, 521, 522, 526, 527, 529, 531, 536, 537
REM, 304
remission, 186, 306, 314
renal cell cancer, 440, 561, 566
renal cell carcinoma, 444, 562, 566, 567
replication, 307, 343, 346
RES, 574
research funding, 345
researchers, xi, xii, 8, 28, 39, 47, 68, 69, 91, 93, 94, 95, 97, 215, 219, 220, 238, 270, 298
resection, 528, 556, 560
resilience, 155, 160, 163, 462
resistance, 89, 90
resolution, 117, 291, 306, 356, 397
resources, 132, 236, 237, 246, 404
respiration, 63
respiratory failure, 141
responsiveness, 258, 344, 354, 536, 542
restoration, 98, 441, 565, 579
restrictions, 186
restructuring, 123
rhenium, 470
rheumatic diseases, 154, 201
rheumatoid arthritis, 149, 153, 154, 162, 163, 201, 202, 247, 249, 298, 310, 311
rheumatologist, 135, 413

risk, 4, 13, 14, 118, 140, 143, 172, 180, 182, 186, 201, 206, 211, 270, 312, 336, 342, 346, 353, 355, 356, 361, 384, 386, 388, 389, 396, 406, 407, 409, 413, 421, 432, 434, 464, 510, 513, 514, 516, 517, 531, 558, 559, 560, 562, 564, 569, 571, 576, 577, 579, 580
rodents, 348, 434
ROI, 313
root(s), 90, 161, 240, 327, 367, 368, 374, 508, 513, 520
rubber, 286, 401
rules, 95, 96, 201

S

sadness, 397
safety, 96, 265, 269, 270, 272, 286, 294, 301, 329, 330, 331, 333, 334, 335, 348, 353, 354, 355, 359, 395, 396, 408, 414
saliva, 25
sample variance, 109
samplings, 96
scaling, 47, 65, 233
scar tissue, 93
scarcity, 165, 167
schema, 122, 229, 232
schizophrenia, 91, 98, 99, 390
sciatica, 220, 327
science, 30, 32, 88, 91, 126, 248, 270, 528, 542, 589
sclerosis, 578
scoliosis, 51
scope, 30, 103, 124, 329
search terms, 433
secondary education, 195
sedatives, 62
seizure, 270, 301, 302, 305, 373, 388, 406
selective attention, 196
selectivity, 266, 277, 384
self-assessment, 233, 472, 544
self-confidence, 88
self-efficacy, 182, 193
self-perceptions, 174
self-portrait, 38
seminars, 589
semi-structured interviews, 102, 526
senescence, 142
sensation, 3, 4, 6, 7, 9, 10, 24, 89, 92, 160, 171, 172, 175, 179, 181, 196, 239, 246, 247, 255, 260, 287, 292, 303, 307, 308, 334, 352, 390, 397, 414, 425, 573
sensitivity, 5, 6, 7, 9, 46, 47, 50, 52, 56, 62, 63, 92, 98, 99, 141, 156, 171, 172, 181, 182, 183, 261, 289, 298, 299, 310, 356, 362, 382, 393

sensitization, 257, 261, 298, 300, 321, 389, 397
sensors, 5, 7, 9, 264, 356
sensory impairments, 32
sensory processing, 3, 4, 297, 300, 302
sensory systems, 260
serotonin, 130, 151, 221, 298, 299, 300, 310
serum, 286, 292, 298, 299, 311, 400
services, 48, 58, 123, 124, 131, 132, 136, 137, 138, 206, 312, 508, 516
severe intellectual disabilities, 63
sex, 87, 88, 89, 90, 91, 92, 93, 94, 95, 96, 97, 98, 99, 102, 171, 172, 174, 175, 176, 177, 178, 179, 180, 181, 182, 194, 211, 215, 216, 221, 224, 240, 299
shape, 90, 223, 226, 228, 230, 231, 264, 266, 267
shortness of breath, 445, 447, 453, 454, 455, 456, 457, 458, 460, 461
short-term memory, 43
showing, 5, 28, 31, 52, 141, 160, 276, 302, 305, 352, 390, 401, 406, 416, 496, 515, 556, 557, 577, 578
siblings, 298, 299
side chain, 432
side effects, 94, 95, 118, 141, 151, 186, 300, 302, 331, 333, 334, 353, 369, 396, 426, 432, 440, 460, 468, 469, 520, 565, 570
signals, xi, 7, 33, 265, 268, 321, 398
signs, 57, 102, 160, 186, 320, 326
SII, 255
skill acquisition, 280, 284
skin, 7, 38, 66, 264, 265, 291, 303, 304, 319, 320, 322, 327, 328, 331, 333, 384, 397, 400, 415
skin diseases, 38
sleep deprivation, 305
sleep disturbance, 299, 301, 303, 304, 416, 417
sleep stage, 314
smoking, 336
socialization, 49, 50
societal cost, 102, 403
society, 22, 123, 206, 377, 444, 589
socioeconomic status, 237
sodium, 256, 290, 321
software, 80, 81, 139, 140, 415, 455
soleus, 279
solid tumors, 437, 438, 439, 442
solution, 69, 71, 74, 87, 90, 97, 98, 117, 121, 293, 336
somatization, 156, 162
spastic, 16, 51, 54, 374
spasticity, 32, 33, 51
special education, 5
specialists, 107, 109, 112, 114, 121, 122, 124, 126, 133, 134, 136, 137, 320, 507, 509, 516, 589
specialization, 274
speculation, 342

speech, 10, 305, 315, 389
sphincter, 91
spirituality, 460
splint, 565
spondylolisthesis, 558
sponge, 264, 293, 325, 331, 333, 334, 336, 401, 413, 425, 426
spontaneous recovery, 103
sprouting, 256
SSI, 553
stability, 170, 573, 581
stabilization, 434, 508, 514, 555, 559, 560, 565, 574, 579, 581, 583, 584
staff members, 48, 49
staffing, 131, 133
standard deviation, 158, 176, 177, 198, 207, 245, 415, 447, 482, 531, 545
standard error, 417, 545, 548, 549
Statistical Analysis System (SAS), 207, 447, 455, 466, 473, 482, 522, 532, 546
statistics, 157, 211, 217, 240, 241, 473, 481, 482
stenosis, 149
sterile, 97
steroids, 150
stimulus, 6, 9, 10, 128, 170, 186, 275, 276, 277, 278, 279, 282, 309, 313, 331, 354, 361, 371, 372, 397, 399, 400, 407
stomach, 51
strabismus, 66
stress, 28, 32, 33, 78, 82, 83, 89, 128, 129, 130, 155, 161, 163, 176, 180, 181, 197, 235, 236, 237, 238, 239, 243, 245, 246, 247, 248, 258, 299, 300, 310, 311, 312, 451, 467, 468, 469, 532
stretching, 20, 93, 460
striatum, 257, 306
stroke, 281, 285, 292, 295, 303, 314, 330, 333, 334, 338, 339, 349, 357, 358, 360, 363, 365, 367, 378, 381, 382, 389, 390, 391, 392, 393, 396, 403, 418, 421
strontium, 470
structural changes, 253, 258
structure, 5, 21, 33, 65, 69, 73, 98, 126, 172, 182, 183, 249, 266, 289, 389
structuring, 79
subacute, 221
subarachnoid hemorrhage, 386
subcortical nuclei, 272
subdural hematoma, 389
subgroups, 32, 96, 547
subjectivity, 113, 121, 124, 126, 442
subluxation, 557
substance abuse, 142, 413
substrate, 27, 29, 32

substrates, 30, 40, 284, 301
success rate, 373, 376, 381
sucrose, 169
suicide, 239
support services, 514, 516
suppression, 277, 279, 315, 323, 338, 359, 400, 432, 433, 441
suprapubic, 92
surgical intervention, 99, 201, 531, 558, 559, 562, 563, 565, 566, 570, 573, 575, 576, 580
surgical technique, 347, 384
survival, 435, 437, 438, 442, 508, 520, 530, 536, 542, 556, 559, 560, 581, 583
survivors, 560
susceptibility, 83, 180
sustainability, 320
suture, 351
sweat, 223, 228, 229, 232
sympathetic nervous system, 311, 327
sympathy, 108, 113, 114, 119, 120
symptomology, 451
synapse, 7, 9, 275
synaptic strength, 419
synaptic transmission, 8
synchronization, 347
syndrome, 3, 4, 8, 9, 10, 11, 12, 31, 66, 96, 99, 100, 148, 149, 154, 160, 162, 174, 176, 221, 254, 259, 261, 299, 310, 311, 314, 319, 320, 321, 322, 326, 327, 328, 330, 339, 345, 349, 360, 363, 368, 392, 393, 396, 403, 407, 412, 420, 423, 427, 461, 513, 514
synergistic effect, 141, 431, 433, 441, 443, 580
synthesis, 211, 271, 299, 300
systemic lupus erythematosus, 154, 160, 162

T

tachycardia, 186
tachypnea, 186
tactics, 108, 112, 118
tactile stimuli, 323
tantra, 88, 91
target, 79, 161, 193, 240, 258, 264, 265, 266, 268, 269, 274, 281, 308, 315, 342, 351, 353, 356, 360, 361, 362, 385, 396, 398, 402, 412
target population, 402
teams, 105, 126, 136, 211, 349, 386
technician, 400, 403, 404, 406
techniques, 10, 37, 42, 65, 77, 78, 79, 93, 94, 121, 123, 134, 161, 187, 193, 197, 233, 274, 277, 285, 291, 297, 301, 302, 305, 309, 320, 342, 346, 348, 353, 373, 385, 399, 402, 405, 411, 414, 422, 444, 553, 570

technology(ies), 30, 32, 33, 99, 263, 264, 269, 270, 341, 342, 344, 345, 354, 391
telephone, 174, 203, 213, 216, 219, 447, 455, 464, 465, 472, 481, 519, 521, 527
temperature, 63, 128, 272
tendon, 66
tension, 38, 39, 40, 91, 92, 93, 105, 176, 371
tensions, 129
terminals, 7, 279
territory, 220, 424
test items, 525
test scores, 63
testing, 10, 19, 103, 129, 158, 224, 248, 311, 323, 368, 369, 372, 376, 388, 434, 436, 437, 521, 526, 527, 528, 551, 552
test-retest reliability, 175, 196, 519, 521, 526, 527
thalamus, 42, 300, 302, 306, 312, 321, 344, 347, 348, 349, 351, 352, 356, 357, 361, 362, 367, 373, 390, 393, 397, 398, 407
therapeutic agents, 33
therapeutic approaches, 29, 32, 396, 412, 440
therapeutic benefits, 347
therapeutic effects, 84, 292, 293
therapeutic interventions, 125, 154
therapeutic use, 271, 400, 409
therapist, 92, 93, 94, 95, 106, 135, 206
think critically, 104
thoracotomy, 149
threshold level, 298, 312
thyroid, 315, 508, 520, 530, 559, 560, 562
tibia, 436
tibialis anterior, 279
time commitment, 132
time frame, 22, 30, 403, 476, 521, 526
tin, 292, 303, 334, 415, 425
tinnitus, 292, 338, 367, 377
tissue, 11, 14, 29, 93, 166, 186, 194, 206, 264, 267, 268, 269, 270, 274, 291, 292, 293, 300, 315, 320, 330, 331, 333, 334, 353, 354, 356, 361, 401, 437, 558, 573
titanium, 350
TNF, 321, 326
TNF-alpha, 321, 326
toddlers, 62
tonic, 261, 291, 353
total costs, 404
toxic effect, 141
toxicity, 396, 441, 442
traditions, 29, 123
training, 21, 78, 92, 104, 122, 127, 128, 129, 130, 170, 186, 193, 202, 257, 258, 259, 280
trait anxiety, 175, 182, 414, 418
trajectory, 22, 101, 351

transection, 398
transference, 7, 90, 99
transformation, 156, 240, 403, 450, 545
trauma, 10, 41, 89, 190, 211, 299, 310, 320, 366, 396
traumatic brain injury, 66, 207
traumatic incident, 6
treatment evaluation, 191
tremor, 348, 354, 363, 377
tricyclic antidepressant, 145, 146, 147, 396
trigeminal nerve, 368, 375, 390
trigeminal neuralgia, 255, 260, 351, 357, 363, 368, 379
trigeminal neuropathic pain, 260, 365, 367, 374, 377, 378, 381, 382, 383, 386, 391, 392
triggers, 7, 25, 40, 299
tryptophan, 311
tumor(s), 368, 396, 413, 431, 432, 433, 434, 436, 441, 442, 443, 444, 558, 559, 560, 565, 570, 579, 580, 582
tumor cells, 434, 441, 444
twins, 179
Type I error, 175
tyrosine, 565

U

underlying mechanisms, 283, 347, 355
UNESCO, 24
unmasking, 256, 328
unstructured interviews, 106
upper cervical metastases, 555, 558
urethra, 99
urinary retention, 342
urinary tract, 165
uterus, 93
uti, 386

V

vaccinations, 20
vagina, 89, 90, 92, 93, 94, 96, 99
vagus, 265, 271
vagus nerve, 265, 271
variations, 181, 223, 228, 230, 232, 299, 355
varimax rotation, 109
vasculature, 327
vasoconstriction, 299, 322
vein, 386
venipuncture, 24, 78, 83, 165
ventricle, 352
venue, 34
vertebrae, 560

vessels, 386
Viagra, 87, 88, 90, 91, 96, 97
videotape, 17, 61, 63, 74, 75
viscera, 7
vision, 40, 305
Visual Analogue Scale (VAS), 17, 45, 49, 50, 51, 55, 63, 64, 65, 66, 67, 68, 69, 70, 71, 72, 73, 74, 78, 194, 198, 199, 216, 217, 302, 304, 305, 309, 324, 343, 349, 351, 357, 371, 375, 388, 390, 402, 404, 405, 406, 412, 413, 414, 415, 416, 417, 418, 503
visual area, 335
visual stimulus, 129
visualization, 271
vocabulary, 231
voiding, 99
vulnerability, 171, 172, 180, 255
vulva, 93
vulval pain, 99
vulvodynia, 409

weight loss, 342, 343
welfare, 108, 113, 115, 587, 589
well-being, 128, 161, 215, 520, 587
white matter, 322, 327, 353
WHO, 139, 140, 143, 150, 528, 542
withdrawal, 6, 139, 140, 155, 310
working memory, 333, 336, 337, 338, 398, 408, 409, 414, 419, 421
World Health Organization, 143, 144, 520, 528, 530, 542
worldview, 87
worry, 156, 160, 467, 532
wound infection, 373, 389

X

X chromosome, 3
XPS, 545
x-rays, 576, 577

W

walking, 460, 465, 468, 481, 504, 510, 512, 522, 525, 549, 571
waste, 107, 112, 119, 120
water, 265, 389, 468
weakness, 87, 89, 371, 374, 386

Y

yes/no, 19, 176, 240
yield, 32, 122, 154, 291
youth transition, 21